Clinical Guidelines In Primary Care:

A Reference and Review Book

Amelie Hollier
Rhonda Hensley

Advanced
Practice
Education
Associates

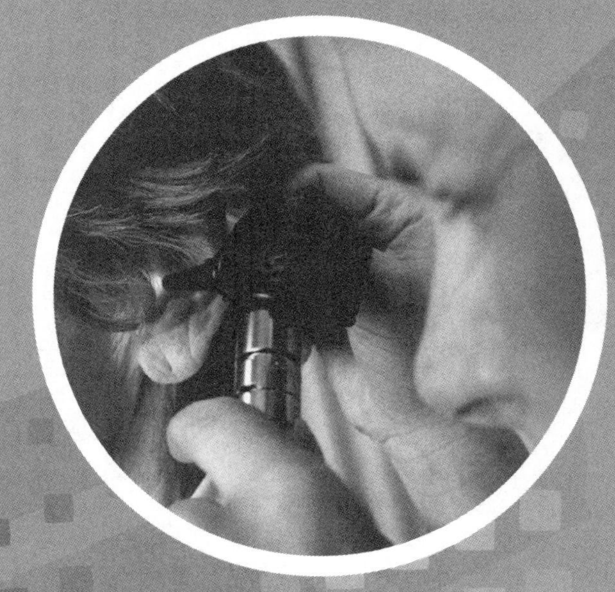

Clinical Guidelines in Primary Care: A Reference and Review Book

Amelie Hollier, DNP, FNP-BC, FAANP
Rhonda Hensley, EdD, APRN, BC

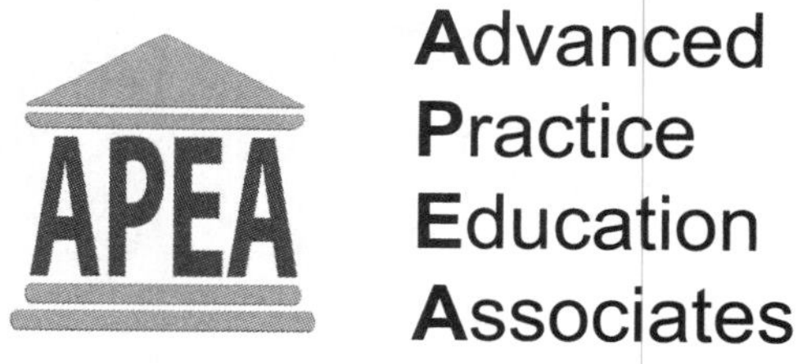

Clinical Guidelines in Primary Care: A Reference and Review Book

Amelie Hollier, DNP, FNP-BC, FAANP
Rhonda Hensley, EdD, APRN, BC

Published by: Advanced Practice Education Associates, Inc.
103 Darwin Circle
Lafayette, LA 70508 U.S.A.

ISBN 978-1-892418-16-6

Printed in the United States of America.

Acknowledgments

This book would not have been possible without many people who helped it become a reality. The contributions of some people were so great they deserve specific mention.

Dr. Rod Hicks provided guidance to the authors in writing, pharmacology expertise, and extensive proofreading. His efforts moved this project from start to finish and were critical to its completion.

Dr. Mary Neiheisel coordinated the work of reviewers and provided proofreading work. Her efforts improved the quality of every chapter.

Jeanie Doucet provided technical expertise, support at every venue, and coordinated the completion of the manuscript and distribution of the finished work.

Lisa Puckett worked tirelessly and diligently to create this work electronically. Her patience and computer expertise were invaluable.

REVIEWERS

The authors gratefully acknowledge the work of the following people who selflessly gave of their time to help review chapters in this first edition.

Christell O. Bray, PhD, RN, FNP, FAANP
Texas A&M University
Corpus Christi, Texas

Brenda S. Broussard, MSN, APRN-CNM, WHNP-BC
University of Louisiana at Lafayette
Lafayette, Louisiana

Elizabeth F. Ellis, DNP, APRN, FNP-BC, FAANP
Clinical Assistant Professor in Adult Health
University of South Alabama College of Nursing
Clinical Staff St. Joseph Physician Associates
Bryan, Texas

Angela Golden, DNP, FNP-BC, FAANP
Assistant Professor
Northern Arizona University
Flagstaff, Arizona

Elizabeth Goodwin, MSN, FNP-BC
Department of Gastroenterology
Veteran Administration
Jackson, MS

Janis Guilbeau, DNP, RN, FNP-BC
Assistant Professor of Nursing and SLEMCO Endowed Professor
University of Louisiana at Lafayette
Lafayette, Louisiana

Rodney W. Hicks, PhD, RN, FNP-BC, FAANP, FAAN
Chief Executive Officer: eLOGS
Lubbock, TX

Helen Hurst, DNP, RNC, APRN-CNM
Assistant Professor and LGMC/BORSF Endowed Professor
University of Louisiana at Lafayette
Lafayette, Louisiana

REVIEWERS

Michaelene Jansen, PhD, RN-C, GNP-BC, FNP-C, FAANP
Professor, College of Nursing and Health Sciences
University of Wisconsin – Eau Claire
Eau Claire, Wisconsin

Irma O. Jordan, DNP, APRN, FNP/PMHNP-BC
Assistant Professor, Primary Care and Public Health Department
University of Tennessee Health Science Center, College of Nursing
Memphis, TN
Family & Psychiatric Nurse Practitioner
Comprehensive Primary Care
Atoka, TN

Teresa Margaglio, APRN, EdD, FNP-BC, IBCLC, RLC
Certified Pediatric Nurse Practitioner
Nurse Practitioner & Lactation Consultant - Private Practice
Lafayette, Louisiana

Sheila Melander DSN, ACNP-BC, FAANP, FCCM
Professor, University of Tennessee at Memphis
Memphis, Tennessee
ACNP, Interventional Cardiology Practice
Santa Monica, California

Mary B. Neiheisel, RN, EdD, FNP-BC, CNS-BC, FAANP
Professor of Nursing/Pfizer/Ardoin Endowed Professor
University of Louisiana at Lafayette
Nurse Practitioner, Faith House
Lafayette, Louisiana

David G. O'Dell, DNP, FNP-BC
Associate Professor, College of Nursing
South University
West Palm Beach Campus

R. Mimi Clarke Secor, MS, MEd, APRN, FNP-BC, FAANP
Nurse Practitioner at Newton Wellesley ObGyn, Newton, Massachusetts
National NP Radio Host for Reach MD, "Partners in Practice"
National consultant and speaker

Laura B. Willsher, EdD APRN, FNP, PNP
Assistant Professor, Grambling State University
Grambling, Louisiana

Ken Wysocki, MS, RN, FNP-BC, FAANP
PhD Candidate, University of Arizona

Disclaimer

NOTICE:

Every effort has been made to ensure that the information provided in this book is accurate, up to date and complete, but no guarantee is made to that effect. Drug and treatment information may be time sensitive. Readers are advised to check the most current product information provided by the manufacturer of each drug to verify the recommended dose, the method and duration of administration, and contraindications. The ultimate responsibility of treatment with medication lies with the licensed prescriber. The absence of a warning for a given drug or combination is in no way intended to mean that it is safe, effective, or may be given to any patient. APEA does not assume any responsibility for any aspect of healthcare administered with the aid of the information in this book of clinical guidelines. The information included within is not intended to cover all possible patients, precautions, treatments, warnings, drug interactions, allergic reactions, or adverse effects. If you have questions about the patient you are treating, seek information from additional sources. The information contained in this book is intended for use in the United States. The publisher does not warrant that uses outside the United States are appropriate. **If you cannot agree to this disclaimer, please notify the publisher, APEA, prior to using any of the information in this book.**

Updates to this edition will be posted at www.apea.com/cgupdates.php.

TABLE OF CONTENTS

1. Cardiovascular Disorders 1

2. Dermatologic Disorders 83

3. Ear, Nose & Throat Disorders 171

4. Endocrine Disorders 225

5. Gastrointestinal Disorders 255

6. Health Promotion: Adult 307

7. Health Promotion: Pediatric 323

8. Hematologic Disorders 353

9. Lactation 383

10. Men's Health Disorders 395

11. Neurologic Disorders 421

12. Ophthalmic Disorders 461

13. Orthopedic Disorders 487

14. Pregnancy 535

15. Pulmonary Disorders 569

16. Sexually Transmitted Diseases 621

17. Social and Psychiatric Disorders 645

18. Urologic Disorders 683

19. Women's Health Disorders.. 715

Index.. 759

1

CARDIOVASCULAR DISORDERS

Cardiovascular Disorders

Hypertension 5

Chronic Heart Failure 22

Hyperlipidemia....29

Stable Angina 39

Acute Coronary Syndrome 52

Varicose Veins 65

Deep Vein Thrombosis 66

Peripheral Vascular Disease 68

* Congenital Heart Disease 70

Heart Murmurs....73

Rheumatic Fever 76

* Kawasaki Syndrome 78

References *80*

**Denotes pediatric diagnosis*

HYPERTENSION

(High Blood Pressure, Pregnancy-Induced Hypertension)

DESCRIPTION

Systolic and/or diastolic blood pressure that is higher than expected for age or pregnancy status. A presumptive diagnosis can be made if the average of 2 measurements ≥ 140 mm Hg systolic or ≥ 90 mm Hg diastolic on 2 separate visits. Hypertension is classified as either primary (essential) or secondary. Isolated systolic hypertension is common in older patients.

Target BP:
General population: < 140/90 mm Hg
Diabetics: < 130/80 mm Hg
Renal disease/proteinuria: 125/75 mm Hg

ETIOLOGY: ADULT

Causes of Primary Hypertension	
No known cause in 90% of cases	
Causes of Secondary Hypertension	
Renal	Acute glomerulonephritis Chronic renal failure Polycystic kidney disease Pyelonephritis
Vascular	Coarctation of the aorta Renal artery stenosis
Endocrine	Primary hyperaldosteronism Pheochromocytoma Cushing's syndrome Neuroblastoma Hyperthyroidism
Neurologic	Increased intracranial pressure Sleep apnea
Pharmacological	Oral contraceptives Corticosteroids Cocaine NSAIDS Decongestants Sympathomimetics
Stress	"White coat hypertension" Alcohol abuse

ETIOLOGY: PEDIATRIC

Causes of Primary Hypertension	
In children > 10 years, usually is primary, but secondary causes must be ruled out.	
Causes of Secondary Hypertension	
Renal	Most common cause (80%)
Vascular	Coarctation of the aorta (5-10% due to this)
Endocrine	Adrenal dysfunction Hyperaldosteronism Hyperthyroidism
Neurologic	Increased intracranial pressure Sleep apnea
Pharmacological	Oral contraceptives Corticosteroids Cocaine NSAIDS Decongestants Sympathomimetics

INCIDENCE

- Nearly 25% of U.S. population is hypertensive
- Reported rates of hypertensive children vary from 2-13% (highest in African- and Asian-American children)
- African-American adults have higher incidence than general population
- Males > Females
- Typically appears between 30-55 years
- Increased prevalence in the elderly
- 5-10% of all pregnancies

RISK FACTORS

- Family history
- Excessive alcohol intake
- Cigarette smoking
- Physical inactivity
- Dyslipidemia
- Age (> 55 yrs. males; > 65 yrs. females)
- Obesity is single most important factor in children; important in adults as well
- Stress

- Excessive dietary intake of sodium
- Pregnancy

ASSESSMENT FINDINGS

- Asymptomatic
- Occipital headaches
- Headache on awakening
- Blurry vision
- Exam of optic fundi: look for AV nicking, arteriolar narrowing, hemorrhages, exudates, and papilledema
- Left ventricular hypertrophy (after long standing hypertension)
- Pregnancy with hypertension and proteinuria, edema, and excessive weight gain
- Perform exam of symmetrical pulses, auscultate for carotid and abdominal bruits; auscultate over kidneys for bruits

Adult Classification of Hypertension	
Normal	SBP < 120 mm Hg AND DBP < 80 mm Hg
Pre-hypertension	120-139 mm Hg SBP OR 80-89 mm Hg DBP
Stage 1	SBP 140-159 mm Hg OR DBP 90-99 mm Hg
Stage 2	SBP ≥ 160 mm Hg OR DBP ≥ 100 mm Hg

Source: From "JNC VII" National Institutes of Health, 2003.

Pediatric Classification of Hypertension	
High Normal	90th - 94th percentile for age
Significant	95th - 99th percentile for age
Severe	> 99th percentile for age

Classified according to age and height.

DIFFERENTIAL DIAGNOSIS

- Secondary hypertension
- Hypertension worsened by pregnancy
- Pregnancy-induced hypertension (PIH)

DIAGNOSTIC STUDIES

- Hematocrit
- Urinalysis: may reveal proteinuria
- Electrolytes, creatinine, calcium
- Fasting lipid profile
- Fasting blood glucose
- Electrocardiogram (ECG)
- Other studies depending on history and physical exam
- Measure BP twice; 5 minutes apart; patient should be seated with proper cuff size and application (always assess contralateral arm to confirm elevated reading)

Goal of diagnostic studies is to identify target organ damage, an underlying cause, and/or additional risk factors.

PREVENTION

- Maintenance of healthy weight and BMI
- Smoking cessation
- Regular aerobic exercise
- Alcohol in moderation (< 1 oz/day)
- Stress management
- Compliance with medication regimen

NONPHARMACOLOGIC MANAGEMENT

- Initiate lifestyle modifications (see below) with abnormal BP readings
- DASH (Dietary Approaches to Stopping Hypertension) eating plan
- Compliance with medication regimen, diet, reduction or abstinence from alcohol intake, aerobic exercise (30 min/d), weight loss, and sodium restriction
- Identification and management of stressors
- Counseling about elimination of other cardiovascular risks (e.g., smoking cessation)
- Treatment of underlying disease, if applicable
- Twice weekly blood pressure checks during pregnancy if elevated
- Do not restrict salt intake during pregnancy
- Patient education regarding disease, treatment, prevention of complications, long term implications, diet changes, and lifestyle modifications

Effect of Lifestyle Modifications on SBP	
Modification	**Approximate Decrease in SBP (ranges)**
Weight loss	5-20 mm Hg/10kg loss
Adopt DASH diet	8-14 mm Hg
Reduce sodium	2-8 mm Hg
Physical activity	4-9 mm Hg
Moderate alcohol consumption	2-4 mm Hg

PHARMACOLOGIC MANAGEMENT

- A variety of agents may be used in adult, pediatric, and nonpregnant patients:
  - ◊ Diuretics: may decrease renal function if renal insufficiency present; or in patients with chronic renal failure
  - ◊ Angiotensin-converting enzyme inhibitors (ACE inhibitors)
  - ◊ Angiotensin II receptor blockers (ARB)
  - ◊ β-blockers
  - ◊ Calcium channel blockers
  - ◊ Vasodilators
  - ◊ Combination of the above
- In pregnant patients:
  - ◊ Vasodilators
  - ◊ β-blockers
  - ◊ Methyldopa (Aldomet®)
  - ◊ Avoid ARB & ACE inhibitors

PRESCRIBING STRATEGIES

- Thiazide diuretics are recommended first line for most patients
- Initial selection of agent depends on underlying patient diseases
- Consider ACE inhibitors or ARBs in patients with diabetes, proteinuria, heart failure; avoid during pregnancy
- β-blockers no longer recommended first line for uncomplicated hypertension, but consider in patients with heart failure, ischemic heart disease, migraines
- Calcium channel blockers (DHP) encouraged in isolated systolic hypertension, asthma, migraines, ischemic disease; consider for stroke prevention
- If patient has Stage 2 hypertension, consider initiating therapy with 2 drugs
- Selection of antihypertensives in children is similar to adults

HYPERTENSION PHARMACOLOGIC MANAGEMENT

Class	Drug Generic name (Trade name®)	Dosage How supplied	Comments
Thiazide Diuretics *Increase excretion of sodium and chloride and thus water; decrease circulating plasma volume* **General comments** Monitor for hypokalemia (check potassium level about 2 weeks after initiation & with increase in dose) Maintain potassium 4-5 mmol/L May worsen gout and elevate blood glucose and lipids	**hydrochlorothiazide (HCTZ)**	**Adult:** *Initial*: 25 mg/day *Usual*: 12.5-50 mg/day *Max*: 50 mg/day **Children:** *Initial*: 1-2 mg/kg/day in 1-2 divided doses < 6 mo: max 3 mg/kg/day 6 mo-2 yrs: max 37.5 mg/day 2-12 yrs: max 100 mg/day	• Considered first line for most patients • Pregnancy Category B (general) • Pregnancy Category D (if pregnancy induced HTN) • Relatively inexpensive • Contraindicated in sulfonamide allergy • Contraindicated in anuric patients
	Various generics (esidrix, HCTZ, HydroDiuril, Microzide, Oretic, thiazide)	*Caps: 12.5 mg* *Tabs: 25 mg, 50 mg, 100 mg*	
	chlorthalidone	**Adult:** *Initial*: 12.5-25 mg/day *Usual*: 12.5-50 mg/day *Max*: 50 mg/day **Children**: not recommended	• Pregnancy Category B • Chlorthalidone provides more consistent 24 hour blood pressure control than HCTZ
	Hygroton	*Tabs: 25 mg, 50 mg*	

HYPERTENSION PHARMACOLOGIC MANAGEMENT

Class	Drug Generic name (Trade name®)	Dosage How supplied	Comments
	chlorthalidone	**Adult**: *Initial*: 15 mg/day *Usual*: 30-45 mg/day *Max*: 50 mg/day **Children**: not recommended	
	Thalitone	*Tabs: 15 mg (Trade)* *Tabs: 30 mg, 50 mg (generic)*	• Do not interchange between trade and generic due to bioavailability differences • Higher doses predispose patients to hypokalemia
Loop Diuretics *Inhibit absorption of sodium and chloride in proximal/ distal tubules and loop of Henle* __General comments__ More potent diuretic action than thiazides Monitor for dehydration, electrolyte imbalances and hypotension May be used for patients who develop fluid overload Increases calcium excretion	**furosemide**	**Adult**: *Initial*: 20-40 mg twice daily *Usual*: Individualized for effect *Max*: 320 mg (split in 2-3 doses) do not exceed maximum adult dose **Children:** *Initial*: 2 mg/kg *Max*: 6 mg/kg	• Pregnancy Category C • Second line therapy after thiazides • Use lower doses in elderly • Diuretic of choice in reduced Cr Cl patients • Risk of ototoxicity
	Lasix	*Tabs: 20 mg, 40 mg, 80 mg* *Solution: 10 mg/mL, 40 mg/mL*	
	torsemide	**Adult**: *Initial*: 5 mg daily *Usual*: 5-10 mg/day *Max*: 10 mg (either daily or split between doses) **Children**: not recommended	• Pregnancy Category B • Second line therapy after thiazides • Contraindicated in patients with sulfonylurea allergy • May take without regard to meals • Risk of ototoxicity
	Demadex	*Tabs: 5 mg, 10 mg*	
Potassium-Sparing Diuretics *Enhance the action of thiazide & loop diuretics and counteract potassium loss by these agents*	**spironolactone**	**Adult**: *Initial*: 12.5 mg/day (either single or split dose) *Usual*: 25-50 mg daily *Max*: 200 mg/day (either single or split dose) **Children**: not recommended	• Pregnancy Category C • Usually not first line agent • Requires at least 2 weeks of therapy to determine effectiveness • Contraindicated in patients with anuria, acute renal insufficiency, hyperkalemia

continued

HYPERTENSION PHARMACOLOGIC MANAGEMENT

Class	Drug Generic name (Trade name®)	Dosage How supplied	Comments
	Aldactone	*Tabs: 25 mg, 50 mg, 100 mg*	
	triamterene	**Adult**: *Initial*: 100 mg twice daily after meal *Usual*: 100 mg twice daily *Max*: 300 mg/day **Children**: not recommended	• Pregnancy Category C • If on other diuretic or anti-HTN agent, must lower starting dose • Patients should not be receiving potassium supplementation
	Dyrenium	*Caps: 50 mg, 100 mg*	
Angiotensin Converting Enzyme Inhibitors (ACEI) *Inhibit the action of angiotensin converting enzyme (ACE) which is responsible for conversion of angiotensin I to angiotensin II; Angiotensin II causes vasoconstriction & sodium retention. Prevents breakdown of bradykinin* **General comments** First line agent End in "pril" Dry cough is common side effect; monitor for first dose hypotension, hyperkalemia, acute renal failure Angioedema is rare but more common in African-Americans Monitor for renal failure and worsening chronic heart failure Preferred in patients with diabetes and CHF Avoid use in patients with bilateral renal artery stenosis	**benazepril**	**For Patients NOT on Diuretics** **Adult**: *Initial*: 10 mg/day *Usual*: 20-40 mg/day *Max*: 80 mg/day **Children**: over 6 yrs: *Initial*: 0.2 mg/kg/day *Max*: 0.6 mg/kg/day (or 40 mg) **For Patients On Diuretics** **Adult**: *Initial*: 5 mg/day *Usual*: 20-40 mg/day *Max*: 80 mg/day **For Patients with Renal Impairment (Glomerular Filtration < 30mL)** *Initial*: 5 mg/day *Usual*: 20-40 mg/day *Max*: 40 mg/day	• Pregnancy Category D • Little additional effect noted at doses > 40 mg • Considered MONOTHERAPY in children • Avoid in children with glomerular filtration rates < 30 mL

continued

HYPERTENSION PHARMACOLOGIC MANAGEMENT

Class	Drug Generic name (Trade name®)	Dosage How supplied	Comments
	Lotensin	*Tabs: 5 mg, 10 mg, 20 mg, 40 mg*	
	catopril	**For Patients NOT on Diuretics** **Adult**: *Initial*: 25 mg two or three times/day *Usual*: 25-50 mg/day *Max*: 450 mg/day **Children**: not recommended **For Patients On Diuretics** **Adult**: *Initial*: 6.25-12.5 mg two or three times/day *Usual*: 25-150 mg two or three times/day *Max*: 450 mg/day **For Patients with Renal Impairment (Glomerular Filtration < 30mL)** *Initial*: 6.25-12.5 two or three times/day *Usual*: 12.5-75 mg/day	
	Capoten	*Tabs: 12.5 mg, 25 mg, 50 mg, 100 mg*	
	Enalapril maleate	**For Patients NOT on Diuretics** **Adult**: *Initial*: 5 mg/day *Usual*: 10-40 mg/day (either as single or two doses) *Max*: 40 mg/day **For Patients ON Diuretics** **Adult**: *Initial*: 2.5 mg/day *Usual*: 10-40 mg/day (either as single or two doses) *Max*: 40 mg/day	• Pregnancy Category D • Avoid potassium supplements • Use with caution in patients on lithium • Recommend holding diuretics 3 days prior to starting, if appropriate for patient • If patient on diuretic, must monitor for up to two hours after initial dose • If patient on dialysis, give only 2.5 mg on days of dialysis

continued

HYPERTENSION PHARMACOLOGIC MANAGEMENT

Class	Drug Generic name (Trade name®)	Dosage How supplied	Comments
		<u>For Patients with Renal Impairment (Glomerular Filtration < 30mL)</u> *Initial*: 2.5 mg/day *Usual*: 10-40 mg/day (either as single or two doses) *Max*: 40 mg/day **Children**: not recommended	
	Vasotec	*Tabs: 2.5 mg, 5 mg, 10 mg, 20 mg*	
	lisinopril	**<u>For Patients NOT on Diuretics</u>** **Adult**: *Initial*: 10 mg/day *Usual*: 20-40 mg/day *Max*: 80 mg/day **Children ≥ 6 yrs:** *Initial* 0.07 mg/kg *Usual*: Individualize *Max*: 0.61 mg/kg - do not exceed maximum adult dose **<u>For Patients on Diuretics</u>** **<u>OR</u>** **<u>For Patients with Renal Impairment (Glomerular Filtration < 30mL)</u>** **Adult:** *Initial*: 2.5 mg/day *Usual*: 2.5-5 mg/day *Max*: 5 mg/day **Children**: not recommended	• Pregnancy Category D • Recommend holding diuretics 3 days prior to starting, if appropriate for patient • Doses at 80 mg may not produce significantly greater effect compared to 40 mg
	Prinivil Zestril	*Tabs: 2.5 mg, 5 mg, 10 mg, 20 mg, 40 mg*	

continued

HYPERTENSION PHARMACOLOGIC MANAGEMENT

Class	Drug Generic name (Trade name®)	Dosage How supplied	Comments
	ramipril	**<u>For Patients NOT on Diuretics</u>** **Adult**: *Initial*: 2.5 mg/day for 7 days; 5 mg/day for 21 days; then 10 mg/day *Usual*: 2.5-20 mg/day (either as single or two doses) *Max*: 20 mg/day **Children**: Not recommended **<u>For Patients on Diuretics</u>** **<u>OR</u>** **<u>For Patients with Renal Impairment (Cr Cl < 40 mL/min)</u>** *Initial*: 1.25 mg/day for 7 days; 2.5 mg/day for 21 days; then 5 mg/day *Usual*: 2.5-5 mg/day (either as single or two doses) *Max*: 5 mg/day	• Pregnancy Category D • Requires initial titration of dosage schedule • May increase lithium levels
	Altace	*Caps 1.25 mg, 2.5 mg, 5 mg, 10 mg* *Tabs 1.25 mg, 2.5 mg, 5 mg, 10 mg*	
Angiotensin II Receptor Blockers (ARB) *Block vasoconstriction and sodium retention effects of AT II (angiotensin II) found in many tissues* **<u>General comments</u>** End in "sartan" Does not effect bradykinin; therefore, no cough as seen in ACE inhibitors. Good venoprotective action; therefore, good alternative in diabetics who cannot tolerate ACE inhibitors Monitor for hypotension and possible renal failure	**candesartan cilexetil**	**<u>For Patients NOT on Diuretics, Not Volume depleted</u>** **Adult:** *Initial*: 16 mg/day *Usual*: 8-32 mg/day (either as single or two doses) *Max*: 32 mg/day **Children < 1 yr:** not recommended **1- <6 yrs:** *Initial*: 0.2 mg/kg/day *Usual*: 0.05-0.4 mg/kg/day *Max*: do not exceed max adult dose	• Pregnancy Category D • Dose is individualized for effect • Initial response seen in ~ 2 weeks, full response in 4-6 weeks • **If patient has volume depletion or impaired renal function, must consider a lower dose and should be under close medical supervision**

continued

HYPERTENSION PHARMACOLOGIC MANAGEMENT

Class	Drug Generic name (Trade name®)	Dosage How supplied	Comments
		6-17 yrs: and Weight < 50 kg; *Initial*: 4-8 mg/day *Usual*: 2-16 mg/day *Max*: 16 mg/day **Weight > 50 kg**; *Initial*: 4-8 mg/day *Usual*: 2-16 mg/day *Max*: 4-32 mg/day	
	Atacand	*Tabs: 4 mg, 8 mg, 16 mg, 32 mg*	
	losartan	**For Patients NOT on Diuretics, Not Volume depleted** **Adult**: *Initial*: 50 mg/day *Usual*: 25-100 mg/day (either as single dose or split between 2 doses) *Max*: 100 mg/day **Children < 6 yrs:** not recommended **> 6 yrs:** *Initial*: 0.7 mg/kg/day *Usual*: 0.7-1.4 mg/kg/day *Max*: 1.4 mg/kg/day - do not exceed maximum adult dose **For Patients NOT on Diuretics, Not Volume depleted** **Adult**: *Initial*: 25 mg/day *Usual*: 25-100 mg/day (either as single dose or split between 2 doses) *Max*: 100 mg/day **Children**: not recommended	• Pregnancy Category D • Initial effect seen within 1 week, may take up to 3-6 weeks for maximum effect
	Cozaar	*Tabs: 25 mg, 50 mg, 100 mg*	

continued

HYPERTENSION PHARMACOLOGIC MANAGEMENT

Class	Drug Generic name (Trade name®)	Dosage How supplied	Comments
	eprosartan mesylate	**For Patients NOT on Diuretics, Not Volume depleted** **Adult**: *Initial*: 600 mg/day *Usual*: 400-800 mg/day (either as single dose or split between 2 doses) *Max*: 800 mg/day **Children**: not recommended	• Pregnancy Category D • **If patient has severe renal impairment, do not exceed 600 mg/day** • **Volume or salt-depleted patients must be closely monitored when starting treatment**
	Teveten	*Tabs: 400 mg, 600 mg*	
	olmesartan medoxomil	**For Patients NOT on Diuretics, Not Volume depleted** **Adult**: *Initial*: 20 mg/day *Usual*: 20-40 mg/day *Max*: 40 mg/day **Children**: **Weight: > 20 and < 35 kg** *Initial*: 10 mg/day *Usual: Individualize* *Max*: 20 mg/day **Weight: > 35 kg** *Initial*: 20 mg/day *Usual: Individualize* *Max*: 40 mg/day	• Pregnancy Category D • May be taken without regard to food • Doses must be individualized • Clinical effect seen within 2 weeks • Caution when initiating in patients with hepatic or severe renal impairment • At doses > 40 mg, recommend adding diuretic
	Benicar	*Tabs: 5 mg, 20 mg, 40 mg*	
	valsartan	**For Patients NOT on Diuretics, Not Volume depleted** **Adult**: *Initial*: 80 mg/day *Usual*: 80-320 mg/day *Max*: 320 mg/day **Children < 6 yrs**: not recommended **6-16 yrs:** *Initial*: 1.3 mg/kg/day *Usual*: Individualize *Max*: 160 mg/day	• Pregnancy Category D • May be taken without regard to food • Clinical effect seen within 2 weeks with maximum effect in 4 weeks • Caution when initiating in patients with hepatic or severe renal impairment • At doses > 80 mg, recommend adding diuretic
	Diovan	*Caps: 80 mg, 160 mg* *Tabs: 40 mg, 80 mg, 160 mg, 320 mg*	

continued

HYPERTENSION PHARMACOLOGIC MANAGEMENT

Class	Drug Generic name (Trade name®)	Dosage How supplied	Comments
Cardio-selective β-Blockers *Decrease sympathetic stimulation by β-blockade in the heart* **General comments** Consider post-MI, in CHF, ischemic heart disease Should be avoided (or used cautiously) in patients with airway disease, heart block Should be used with caution in diabetics (may mask the symptoms of hypoglycemia) and in those with peripheral vascular disease May cause exercise intolerance	**acebutolol** Sectral	**Adult**: *Initial*: 400 mg/day (either as single dose or split between 2 doses) *Usual*: 200-800 mg/day *Max*: 1200 mg/day **Children**: not recommended *Caps: 200 mg, 400 mg*	• Pregnancy Category B • **DO NOT ABRUPTLY STOP DRUG** • Twice daily dosing preferred as more effective than single dose • Has intrinsic sympathomimetic activity
	atenolol Tenormin	**Adult**: *Initial* 50 mg/day *Usual*: 50-100 mg/day *Max*: 100 mg/day **Children**: not recommended **Elderly or Patients with Renal Impairment** **Cr Cl 15-35 mL/min** *Initial*: 25 mg/day *Max*: 50 mg/day **Cr Cl < 15 mL/min** *Initial*: 25 mg/day *Max*: 25 mg/day *Tabs: 25 mg, 50 mg, 100 mg*	• Pregnancy Category D • **DO NOT ABRUPTLY STOP DRUG** • May titrate dose upwards after 1 week • Patients on dialysis should be monitored under hospital supervision for dosages given post treatment
	bisoprolol fumarate Zebeta	**Adult**: *Initial:* 5 mg/day *Usual:* Individualize *Max:* 20 mg/day **Patients with Renal or Hepatic Dysfunction** *Initial*: 2.5 mg/day *Usual*: Individualize *Max* 20 mg/day **Children**: not recommended *Tabs: 5 mg, 10 mg*	• Pregnancy Category C • **DO NOT ABRUPTLY STOP DRUG** • Individualize for patient effect • Advance from 5 mg to 10 mg to 20 mg as needed

continued

HYPERTENSION PHARMACOLOGIC MANAGEMENT

Class	Drug Generic name (Trade name®)	Dosage How supplied	Comments
	metoprolol succinate, extended release	**Adult**: *Initial:* 25-100 mg/day *Usual:* 100-400 mg/day *Max*: 400 mg/day **Children**: not recommended	• Pregnancy Category C • **DO NOT ABRUPTLY STOP DRUG; must be tapered over 2 weeks** • **NOTE different dosage forms; extended release form preferred for HTN control** • Individualize for patient effect • Advance dosage at weekly intervals
	Lopressor	*Ext. Rel. Tabs: 25 mg, 50 mg, 100 mg, 200 mg*	
	Toprol-XL	*Ext. Rel. Tabs: 25 mg, 50 mg, 100 mg, 200 mg*	
	metoprolol tartrate	**Adult**: *Initial:* 100 mg/day (single or divided dose) *Usual:* 100-400 mg/day (single or divided dose) *Max*: 450 mg/day (single or divided dose) **Children**: not recommended	• Pregnancy Category C • **DO NOT ABRUPTLY STOP DRUG; must be tapered over 2 weeks** • **NOTE different dosage forms; extended release form preferred for HTN control; single immediate doses may not offer 24 hour coverage** • Individualize for patient effect • Advance dosage at weekly intervals • **Should be given with meals**
	Lopressor	*Tabs: 25 mg, 50 mg, 100 mg, 200 mg*	
	Toprol-XL	*Tabs: 25 mg, 50 mg, 100 mg, 200 mg*	
Non-Cardioselective β-blockers *Block stimulation of both β1 (heart) and β2 (lungs) receptors causing decreased heart rate, blood pressure, and cardiac output (β1) as well as decreased central motor activity, inhibition of renin release from the kidneys, reduction of norepinephrine from neurons, and mild bronchoconstriction (β2)* **General comments**	**nadolol**	**Adult**: *Initial*: 20-40 mg/day *Usual*: 40-80 mg/day *Max*: 320 mg/day **Children**: not recommended **Special Dosing Schedule in Renal Impairment** *Initial*: 20 mg **Cr Cl > 50**: 24 hours **Cr Cl 31-50**: 24-36 hours **Cr Cl 10-30**: 24-48 hours **Cr Cl < 10**: 40-60 hours	• Pregnancy Category C • **DO NOT ABRUPTLY STOP DRUG; may take 2 weeks to withdraw drug while patient undergoes close monitoring** • Individualize therapy • May be taken without regard to meals • Note dosing schedule for renal dysfunction
End in "lol"	Corgard	*Tabs: 20 mg, 40 mg, 80 mg, 120 mg, 160 mg*	

continued

HYPERTENSION PHARMACOLOGIC MANAGEMENT

Class	Drug Generic name (Trade name®)	Dosage How supplied	Comments
Contraindicated in patients with bronchoconstrictive disease (i.e. asthma, COPD, etc.) Cautious use in diabetics because of masking signs and symptoms of hypoglycemia (tachycardia, blood pressure changes) Nonspecific β-blockade helpful in patients with tremors, anxiety and migraine headaches	**penbutolol**	**Adult**: *Initial:* 20 mg/day *Usual*: 20-40 mg/day *Max*: 80 mg/day **Children**: not recommended	• Pregnancy Category C • **DO NOT ABRUPTLY STOP DRUG; may take 2 weeks to withdraw drug while patient undergoes close monitoring** • Full effect seen within 2 weeks
	Levatol	*Tabs: 20 mg*	
	pindolol	**Adult**: *Initial*: 5 mg twice a day *Usual*: 10-30 mg/day *Max*: 60 mg/day **Children**: not recommended	• Pregnancy Category B • **DO NOT ABRUPTLY STOP DRUG** • Individualize therapy; adjust dose every 1-2 weeks • Has intrinsic sympathomimetic activity • Contraindicated with thioridazine
	Visken	*Tabs: 5 mg, 10 mg*	
	propranolol	**IMMEDIATE RELEASE** **Adult**: *Initial*: 40 mg twice daily *Usual*: 120-240 mg/day *Max*: 640 mg/day **Children**: *Initial*: 1 mg/kg/day (in two divided doses) *Usual*: 2-4 mg/kg/day (in two divided doses) *Max*: 16 mg/day (in two divided doses) or 640 mg/day **EXTENDED RELEASE** **Adult**: *Initial*: 80 mg/day *Usual*: 120-160 mg/day *Max*: 640 mg/day	• Pregnancy Category C • **DO NOT ABRUPTLY STOP DRUG** • **Ext. Release form has different kinetics, CANNOT switch between dosage forms on a 1:1 mg basis** • Titrate for effective BP; titration may vary from a few days to several weeks • Do not crush or chew tablets • Contraindicated with thioridazine
	Inderal	*Tabs: 10 mg, 20 mg, 40 mg, 60 mg, 80 mg*	
	Inderal LA	*Ext Rel Cap: 60 mg, 80 mg, 120 mg, 160 mg*	

continued

HYPERTENSION PHARMACOLOGIC MANAGEMENT

Class	Drug Generic name (Trade name®)	Dosage How supplied	Comments
Calcium Channel Blockers Dihydropyridine (DHP) *Inhibit movement of calcium ions across the cell membrane and vascular smooth muscle which depress myocardial contractility and increase cardiac blood flow* <u>General comments</u> End in suffix "pine" Does not cause bradycardia	**amlodipine besylate**	**Adult**: *Initial*: 5 mg/day *Usual*: 5-10 mg/day *Max*: 10 mg/day **Elderly, renal or hepatic patients:** *Initial*: 2.5 mg/day **Children > 6 years of age** *Initial*: 2.5 mg/day *Usual*: 2.5-5 mg/day *Max*: 5 mg/day	• Pregnancy Category C • Titrate for effect; increase doses at 7-14 day intervals; must reassess patient after each titration
	Norvasc	*Tabs: 2.5 mg, 5 mg, 10 mg*	
Monitor for hypotension and worsening of CHF, ankle edema Good choice in diabetics with proteinuria, patients with ISH (isolated systolic hypertension) for migraine prophylaxis and in patients with stable angina	**felodipine**	**Adult**: *Initial*: 2.5-5 mg/day *Usual*: 2.5-10 mg/day *Max*: 10 mg/day **Elderly or hepatic patients:** *Initial*: 2.5 mg/day **Children**: not recommended	• Pregnancy Category C • Titrate for effect; increase dose after minimum of 2 week interval • Do not crush or chew tablets • Bioavailability affected by meals; should take on empty stomach
Serious drug interactions with grapefruit juice	Plendil	*Ext. Rel. Tabs: 2.5 mg, 5 mg, 10 mg*	
Long acting DHP calcium channel blockers preferred for isolated systolic hypertension	**nicardipine HCL**	**<u>Immediate Release Formulation</u>** **Adult**: *Initial*: 20 mg three times/day *Usual*: 20-40 mg three times/day *Max*: 120 mg/day **Children**: not recommended **<u>Sustained Release Formulation</u>** **Adult**: *Initial*: 30 mg two times/day *Usual*: 30-60 mg two times/day *Max*: 60 mg two times/day **Children**: not recommended	• Pregnancy Category C • Individualize treatment • Lower doses required if impaired hepatic function • Effective response requires peak and trough BP measurements • Titrate dose after 3 days • Additional monitoring required if changing between dose formulations

continued

HYPERTENSION PHARMACOLOGIC MANAGEMENT

Class	Drug Generic name (Trade name®)	Dosage How supplied	Comments
	Cardene	*Caps: 20 mg, 30 mg*	
	Cardene SR	*Sust. Rel. Cap:* *30 mg, 45 mg, 60 mg*	
	nifedipine	**Adult***:* *Initial:* 30-60 mg/day *Usual:* 30-60 mg/day *Max:* 120 mg/day **Children**: not recommended	• Pregnancy Category C • Individualize treatment; advance doses at 1-2 week intervals • Use extended release formulations for HTN control • Take on empty stomach • Do not crush or chew extended release formulations • Must be withdrawn slowly if discontinued
	Procardia XL	*Ext. Rel. Tabs: 30 mg, 60 mg, 90 mg*	
	Adalat CC	*Ext. Rel. Tabs: 30 mg, 60 mg, 90 mg*	
	nisoldipine	**Adult**: *Initial*: 17 mg/day *Usual*: 8.5-34 mg/day *Max*: 34 mg/day **Elderly or those with Hepatic Dysfunction** *Initial*: 8.5 mg/day **Children**: not recommended	• Pregnancy Category C • Individualize treatment; advance doses at 1-2 week intervals • Take on empty stomach • Do not crush or chew
	Sular	*Ext. Rel. Tabs: 8.5 mg, 17 mg, 25.5 mg, 34 mg*	
Calcium Channel Blockers: Non-Dihydropyridine (Non-DHP) *Inhibit movement of calcium ions across the cell membrane and vascular smooth muscle which depress myocardial contractility and increase cardiac blood flow* **General comments** Watch for conduction defects	**diltiazem**	**Adult***:* *Initial:* 120-240 mg/day *Usual:* 240-360 mg/day *Max:* 480-540 mg/day* **> 60 years:** *Initial:* 120 mg/day **Children**: not recommended **See specific drug manufacturer for maximum dose limits*	• Pregnancy Category C • Use extended release formulations for HTN control • Available in multiple formulations (tablets and capsules) and strengths • Individualize therapy; titrate at bi-weekly intervals • Start with lowest dose possible, especially in elderly • Do not crush or chew • Incidence of side effects increases as dose increases
	Cardizem LA	*Ext. Rel. Tabs: 120 mg, 180 mg, 240 mg, 300 mg, 360 mg, 420 mg*	

continued

HYPERTENSION PHARMACOLOGIC MANAGEMENT

Class	Drug Generic name (Trade name®)	Dosage How supplied	Comments
Decreases heart rate Use cautiously or avoid with use of β-blockers Monitor for worsening of CHF, hypotension, bradycardia, constipation Consider in patients with atrial fibrillation with rapid ventricular response, in patients with angina, and in diabetics with proteinuria Serious drug interactions with grapefruit juice	Cardizem CD	*Ext. Rel. Caps: 120 mg, 180 mg, 240 mg, 300 mg, 360 mg*	
	Dilacor XR	*Ext. Rel. Caps: 120 mg 180 mg, 240 mg*	
	Tiazac	*Ext. Rel. Caps: 120 mg, 180 mg, 240 mg, 300 mg, 360 mg, 420 mg*	
	verapamil	**Adult**: *Initial*: 180 mg/day *Usual*: 180-240 mg/day *Max*: 360 mg/day (must be in divided doses)* **Children**: not recommended *Refer to specific product for additional guidelines	• Pregnancy Category C • Use extended release formulations for HTN control • Available in multiple formulations (tablets and capsules) and strengths. Refer to specific product for additional guidelines • Individualize therapy; titrate at bi-weekly intervals • **Elderly or small stature people may require lower starting dose**
	Calan SR	*Caplet: 120 mg, 180 mg, 240 mg*	
	Covera HS (Give at bedtime)	*Ext. Rel. Tabs: 120 mg, 240 mg*	
	Isoptin SR	*Sust. Rel. Tabs: 120 mg, 180 mg, 240 mg*	
	Verelan PM (Give at bedtime)	*Ext. Rel. Caps: 100 mg, 200 mg, 300 mg*	
Direct Renin Inhibitor *decreases plasma renin activity (PRA) and inhibits the conversion of angiotensinogen to Angiotensin I* General comments Monitor K+ levels in diabetics Caution with maximum doses of ACE inhibitors May be potentiated by statins and ketoconazole	**aliskiren hemifumarate**	**Adult***:* *Initial:* 150 mg/day *Usual:* 150-300 mg/day *Max:* 300 mg/day **Children***:* not recommended	• Pregnancy Category D • Individualize therapy; adjust dose after 2 weeks • Take on empty stomach • Use with caution in patients with renal impairment • Use in caution in patients with volume and/or salt depletion
	Tekturna	*Tabs: 150 mg, 300 mg*	

COMBINATION DRUGS FOR HYPERTENSION

Combination Type*	Fixed-Dose Combination, mg†	Trade Name
ACEIs and CCBs	Amlodipine-benazepril hydrochloride (2.5/10, 5/10, 5/20, 10/20) Enalapril-felodipine (5/5) Trandolapril-verapamil (2/180, 1/240, 2/240, 4/240)	Lotrel Lexxel Tarka
ACEIs and diuretics	Benazepril-hydrochlorothiazide (5/6.25, 10/12.5, 20/12.5, 20/25) Captopril-hydrochlorothiazide (25/15, 25/25, 50/15, 50/25) Enalapril-hydrochlorothiazide (5/12.5, 10/25) Fosinopril-hydrochlorothiazide (10/12.5, 20/12.5) Lisinopril-hydrochlorothiazide (10/12.5, 20/12.5, 20/25) Moexipril-hydrochlorothiazide (7.5/12.5, 15/25) Quinapril-hydrochlorothiazide (10/12.5, 20/12.5, 20/25)	Lotensin HCT Capozide Vaseretic Monopril/HCT Prinzide, Zestoretic Uniretic Accuretic
ARBs and diuretics	Candesartan-hydrochlorothiazide (16/12.5, 32/12.5) Eprosartan-hydrochlorothiazide (600/12.5, 600/25) Irbesartan-hydrochlorothiazide (150/12.5, 300/12.5) Losartan-hydrochlorothiazide (50/12.5, 100/25) Olmesartan medoxomil-hydrochlorothiazide (20/12.5,40/12.5,40/25) Telmisartan-hydrochlorothiazide (40/12.5, 80/12.5) Valsartan-hydrochlorothiazide (80/12.5, 160/12.5, 160/25)	Atacand HCT Teveten-HCT Avalide Hyzaar Benicar HCT Micardis-HCT Diovan-HCT
BBs and diuretics	Atenolol-chlorthalidone (50/25, 100/25) Bisoprolol-hydrochlorothiazide (2.5/6.25, 5/6.25, 10/6.25) Metoprolol-hydrochlorothiazide (50/25, 100/25) Nadolol-bendroflumethiazide (40/5, 80/5) Propranolol LA-hydrochlorothiazide (40/25, 80/25) Timolol-hydrochlorothiazide (10/25)	Tenoretic Ziac Lopressor HCT Corzide Inderide LA Timolide
Centrally acting drug and diuretic	Methyldopa-hydrochlorothiazide (250/15, 250/25, 500/30, 500/50) Reserpine-chlothalidone (0.125/25, 0.25/50) Reserpine-chlorothiazide (0.125/250, 0.25/500) Reserpine-hydrochlorothiazide (0.125/25, 0.125/50)	Aldoril Demi-Regroton, Regroton Diupres Hydropres
Diuretic and diuretic	Amiloride-hydrochlorothiazide (5/50) Spironolactone-hydrochlorothiazide (25/25, 50/50) Triamterene-hydrochlorothiazide (37.5/25, 75/50)	Moduretic Aldactazide Dyazide, Maxzide

* Drug abbreviations: BB, beta-blocker; ACEI, angiotensin converting enzyme inhibitor; ARB, angiotensin receptor blocker; CCB, calcium channel blocker.

† Some drug combinations are available in multiple fixed doses. Each drug dose is reported in milligrams.

Source: JNC 7 Express, The Seventh Report of the Joint National Committee on Prevention, Detection, Evaluation and Treatment of High Blood Pressure, U.S. Department of Health and Human Services, December 2003.

CONSULTATION/REFERRAL

- Referral to cardiologist for children with significant or severe hypertension
- Refer as needed for secondary causes of hypertension

FOLLOW-UP

- Inquire about compliance, side effects
- Monthly, until patient reaches goal; then every 3-6 months as appropriate

EXPECTED COURSE

- Only 25% of patients who are treated for hypertension are actually at goal; expect complications if inadequately managed
- Most patients require more than one medication to reach goal

POSSIBLE COMPLICATIONS

- Stroke
- Coronary artery disease
- Myocardial infarction
- Renal failure
- Heart failure
- Eclampsia (seizures)
- Pulmonary edema
- Hypertensive crisis

CHRONIC HEART FAILURE

DESCRIPTION

The heart is unable to meet the metabolic demands of the tissues. The left heart, right heart or both may be involved. Patients are classified using the New York Heart Association's (NYHA) classification system.

New York Heart Association Functional Classification	
Class I (none)	physical activity does not cause limitations
Class II (slight)	physical activity brings about "slight limitation" (fatigue, palpitations, dyspnea, anginal pain)
Class III (moderate)	physical activity brings about "marked limitations"; symptoms brought about by "less than ordinary activity"
Class IV (severe)	unable to participate in any physical activity without discomfort; symptoms at rest

Source: New York Heart Association Classification for CHF

ETIOLOGY

- Systolic and/or diastolic failure due to:
    - ◊ Left ventricular dysfunction
    - ◊ Volume overload
    - ◊ Myocardial infarction
    - ◊ Cardiomyopathy
    - ◊ Coronary artery disease
    - ◊ Cardiac drugs
    - ◊ Arrhythmias (especially atrial fibrillation)
    - ◊ Valvular abnormalities
    - ◊ Hyperthyroidism/hypothyroidism

INCIDENCE

- Depends on etiology
- Males > Females until age 75 years, then Males = Females
- More common in the elderly
- Most frequent cause of hospitalization in the U.S.

RISK FACTORS

- Underlying heart disease
- Noncompliance with medication and/or dietary modifications
- Pregnancy or postpartum cardiomyopathy
- Fluid or sodium excess
- Hyperthyroidism
- Long-standing hypertension
- Use of negative inotropic medications

ASSESSMENT FINDINGS

Mild failure symptoms	Crackles in lung bases S3 gallop Jugular vein distention Dyspnea on exertion Nocturia Tachycardia Diminished exercise capacity Fatigue and/or weakness Peripheral edema Weight gain
Moderate failure symptoms	Cough, especially nocturnal Crackles in lung bases Paroxysmal nocturnal dyspnea Tachypnea/shortness of breath (especially at rest) Tachycardia Hepatomegaly/ascites Edema (extremities, presacral, and scrotal)
Severe failure symptoms	Ascites Cyanosis Decreased level of consciousness Frothy sputum and/or pink sputum Hypotension

DIFFERENTIAL DIAGNOSIS

- Chronic obstructive pulmonary disease
- Asthma
- Cirrhosis
- Peripheral vascular disease with edema
- Dependent edema
- Pulmonary embolism

DIAGNOSTIC STUDIES

- Diagnosis can be made on clinical presentation but diagnostic studies may indicate complications
- BNP (B type natriuretic peptide): > 100 pg/mL (other conditions can elevate BNP levels e.g., renal failure, acute coronary syndromes, pulmonary embolism)
- Transthoracic echo and 2-D Doppler flow studies: mechanically evaluate heart and establish ejection fraction; if < 35-40%, then HF (best test for initial workup of HF)
- 12 lead EKG: assesses for arrhythmias, left ventricular hypertrophy, atrial arrhythmias, recent myocardial infarction
- Chest x-ray: establishes heart size, presence of pulmonary edema, pulmonary disease
- CBC: assesses anemia, infection
- Electrolytes: potassium, calcium, sodium, magnesium
- BUN/Creatinine: elevated Cr indicates renal failure and volume overload
- Urinalysis: proteinuria (less than one gram present)

PREVENTION

- Appropriate management of underlying conditions that can lead to CHF
- Compliance with medications and dietary modifications

NONPHARMACOLOGIC MANAGEMENT

- Surgery for underlying valve problems or other correctable etiologies
- Avoid smoking, alcohol
- Sodium restriction
- Fluid restriction when appropriate
- Daily weights for early identification of fluid overload
- Patient education regarding self-care, medication, diet, exercise, disease process
- Encourage exercise except in severe disease
- Consider evaluation for sleep apnea (if present, high pulmonary artery pressures evolve into pulmonary hypertension)

SPECIAL PHARMACOLOGICAL CONSIDERATIONS

- Most patients are managed on a combination of 3-4 drugs
- Mainstay of therapy is β-blockers and ACE inhibitors or ARBs
- Symptom relief may take several weeks once drug therapy begins
- Diuretics will provide quickest relief from HF symptoms but should be used in combination with other drugs
- Monitor potassium levels in patients taking diuretics and ACE inhibitors
- Monitor renal function and potassium 1-2 weeks after initiating ACE inhibitor, after dose increases; then periodically
- Initiate β-blockers at very low doses in a stable patient without evidence of fluid overload
- Do not initiate β-blockers or ACE inhibitors if systolic BP < 80 mm Hg; consider referral

CHRONIC HEART FAILURE PHARMACOLOGIC MANAGEMENT

Class	Drug Generic name (Trade name®)	Dosage How supplied	Comments
Angiotensin Converting Enzyme Inhibitors (ACEI) *Inhibit the action of angiotensin converting enzyme (ACE) which is responsible for conversion of angiotensin I to angiotensin II; Angiotensin II causes vasoconstriction & sodium retention. Prevents breakdown of bradykinin* **General comments** First line agent Commonly used post-MI for systolic dysfunction or in patients with clinical symptoms of CHF (SOB, fatigue, exercise intolerance) Monitor potassium levels: goal is 4-5 mmol/L Assess renal function and serum potassium within 1-2 weeks of drug initiation and after each dose change Start at low dose and titrate in 2-4 week increments Improvement of clinical symptoms is desired effect Preferred in patients with diabetes and CHF	**catopril**	**Adult**: *Initial*: 25 mg three times/day *Usual*: 50-100 mg three times/ day *Max*: 450 mg/day **Children**: not recommended **For Patients with salt/volume depletion or low blood pressure** *Initial*: 6.25-12.5 three times/ day *Usual*: Titrate for response	• Pregnancy Category D • Take 1 hour before meals and with diuretics • Adjust dose after 2 weeks to 50 mg three times/day if tolerated
	Capoten	*Tabs: 12.5 mg, 25 mg, 50 mg, 100 mg*	
	enalapril maleate	**Adult**: *Initial*: 2.5 mg twice/day *Usual*: 10-20 mg twice/day *Max*: 40 mg/day **Children**: not recommended	• Pregnancy Category D • Avoid potassium supplements • Use with caution in patients on lithium
	Vasotec	*Tabs: 2.5 mg, 5 mg, 10 mg, 20 mg*	
	fosinopril	**Adult**: *Initial*: 5-10 mg/day *Usual*: 20-40 mg/day *Max*: 40 mg/day **Children**: not recommended **Moderate to Severe Renal Failure or Salt/Volume Depletion** *Initial*: 5 mg/day *Usual*: Individualize *Max*: 40 mg/day	• Pregnancy Category D • Individualize therapy; increase over several weeks as needed • Use with caution in patients on lithium • Has been used in patients NOT currently taking digitalis
	Monopril	*Tabs: 10 mg, 20 mg, 40 mg*	

continued

CHRONIC HEART FAILURE PHARMACOLOGIC MANAGEMENT

Class	Drug Generic name (Trade name®)	Dosage How supplied	Comments
	lisinopril	**Adult**: *Initial*: 5 mg/day *Usual*: 5-40 mg/day *Max*: 40 mg/day **Children**: not recommended **For Patients with Renal Impairment (Glomerular Filtration < 30mL)** *Initial*: 2.5 mg/day *Usual*: 2.5-5 mg/day *Max*: 5 mg/day	• Pregnancy Category D • Individualize therapy; increase dose at 2 week intervals • Patients with significant renal impairment may require closer supervision
	Prinivil Zestril	*Tabs: 2.5 mg, 5 mg, 10 mg, 20 mg, 40 mg*	
	ramipril	**Adult**: *Initial*: 2.5 mg twice/day *Usual*: 5 mg twice/day *Max*: 10 mg/day **Children**: not recommended **For Patients with Renal Impairment (Cr Cl < 40 mL/min)** *Initial*: 1.25 mg twice/day *Usual*: 2.5-5 mg twice/day *Max*: 5 mg/day	• Pregnancy Category D • Requires initial titration of dosage schedule • May increase lithium levels
	Altace	*Caps: 1.25 mg, 2.5 mg, 5 mg, 10 mg* *Tabs: 1.25 mg, 2.5 mg, 5 mg, 10 mg*	
Loop Diuretics *Inhibit absorption of sodium and chloride in proximal/distal tubules and loop of Henle* **General comments** More potent diuretic action than thiazides	**bumetanide**	**Adult**: *Initial*: 0.25-2 mg/day *Usual*: 0.5-2 mg/day *Max*: 0.5-10 mg daily (split between 2-3 doses) **Children**: not recommended	• Pregnancy Category C • May use intermittent dosing • Contraindicated in anuric patients • Carries risk for ototoxicity • Caution in patients with allergies to sulfonamides • Contraindicated with lithium patients

continued

CHRONIC HEART FAILURE PHARMACOLOGIC MANAGEMENT

Class	Drug Generic name (Trade name®)	Dosage How supplied	Comments
Class of agents preferred in patients with reduced renal function	Bumex	*Tabs: 0.5 mg, 1 mg, 2 mg*	
Monitor for dehydration, electrolyte imbalances and hypotension May be used for patients who develop fluid overload Increases calcium excretion	**furosemide**	**Adult**: *Initial*: 20-80 mg/day *Usual*: Individualize for effect *Max*: 600 mg (split in 2-3 doses) **Children:** *Initial*: 2 mg/kg as single dose *Usual*: Individualize for effect *Max*: 6 mg/kg - do not exceed adult max	• Pregnancy Category C • Contraindicated in anuric patients • Allow 6-8 hours between doses • Patients with doses > 80 mg/day warrant close observation • Carries risk for ototoxicity
	Lasix	*Tabs: 20 mg, 40 mg, 80 mg* *Solutions: 10 mg/mL, 40 mg/mL*	
	torsemide	**Adult**: *Initial*: 10-20 mg/day *Usual*: Individualized for effect *Max*: 200 mg (either daily or split between doses) **Children**: not recommended	• Pregnancy Category B • May be given without regard to meals • Contraindicated in anuric patients • Contraindicated in patients with sulfonylurea allergy • Carries risk for ototoxicity • Titrate upwards by doubling dose to achieve desired effect
	Demadex	*Tabs: 5 mg, 10 mg, 20 mg, 100 mg*	
Digoxin *Increases intracellular concentration of calcium which increases force of myocardial contraction; decreases activation of the sympathetic nervous system* **General comments** Improved quality of life but no decrease in mortality	**digoxin**	**Rapid Digitalization** **Adult:** *Initial*: 1-1.5 mg split over 4 doses spanning 36 hours *Usual*: 0.125-0.5 mg/day **Gradual Digitalization in Adults < 70 yr with intact renal function** **Adult:** *Initial*: 0.25 mg/day *Usual*: 0.125-0.5 mg/day	• Pregnancy Category C • Individualize therapy based on lean body weight, renal function, age, and concomitant disease states, heart rate. All dosage selections must be based on clinical assessment of the patient. Half-life of drug is between 24-36 hours • If not on previous digitalization therapy, initiating oral therapy may take up to 3 weeks to achieve steady serum state (dependent upon renal function)

continued

CHRONIC HEART FAILURE PHARMACOLOGIC MANAGEMENT

Class	Drug Generic name (Trade name®)	Dosage How supplied	Comments
Use in patients with CHF secondary to poor myocardial contractility Correct hypokalemia before prescribing Do not use with heart block Cautious use with agent which decreases heart rate (β-blocker) Monitor for toxicity, anorexia, nausea, muscle weakness Consider in patients with atrial fibrillation with rapid ventricular response	Lanoxin	<u>**Gradual Digitalization in Adults > 70 yr or patients with impaired renal function**</u> **Adult**: *Initial*: 0.125 mg/day <u>**Marked renal impairment**</u> **Adult:** *Initial*: 0.0625 mg/day **Children < 2 yrs:** Consult references **> 2 yrs of age** *Initial*: 0.01 mcg/kg in divided doses *Max*: do not exceed maximum adult dose *Caps: 0.1 mg, 0.2 mg* *Elixir: 0.05 mg/mL* *Tabs: 0.125 mg; 0.25 mg*	• Requires regular laboratory monitoring of drug level and best obtained just prior to next dose or at least 6 hours after last dose. Consider more frequent lab monitoring in patients with marked renal impairment • There is different bioavailability when moving patients from digoxin injection to oral dosages • Patient must be able to monitor heart rate
<u>**β-Blockers**</u> *Decrease sympathetic stimulation by β-blockade in the heart* <u>**General comments**</u> Decreases morbidity and mortality associated with CHF Do not prescribe in an unstable patient or in patients with fluid overload; cautious use or avoid use in respiratory patients Used in conjunction with ACEIs, diuretics with/without digoxin; titrate dose to improve clinical symptoms	**carvedilol** Coreg (Immediate release) Coreg CR (Extended release)	<u>**Immediate Release**</u> **Adult: < 85 kg** *Initial:* 3.125 mg twice/day *Usual:* 25 mg twice/day *Max:* 25 mg twice/day **Adult: > 85 kg** *Initial:* 3.125 mg twice/day *Usual:* 50 mg twice/day *Max:* 50 mg twice/day <u>**Extended Release**</u> **Adult**: *Initial*: 10 mg/day *Usual*: Titrated *Max*: 80 mg/day *Tabs: 3.125 mg, 6.25 mg, 12.5 mg, 25 mg* *Ext. Rel. Caps: 10 mg, 20 mg, 40 mg, 80 mg*	• Pregnancy Category C but trimester specific risks exist • Do not abruptly withdraw medication; allow 1-2 weeks • Commonly used with diuretics, ACE inhibitors, and digitalis • Individualized therapy; requires close monitoring during phases of titration (minimum intervals of 2 weeks) • Reduce dose if pulse < 55/min • Take daily in AM with food • Do not crush or chew • Avoid in patients with severe hepatic impairment • Monitor glucose levels • Immediate release to extended release, consult references for bioequivalence and dosing schedules

continued

CHRONIC HEART FAILURE PHARMACOLOGIC MANAGEMENT

Class	Drug Generic name (Trade name®)	Dosage How supplied	Comments
	metoprolol succinate, extended release	<u>NYHA CLASS II</u> **Adult**: *Initial*: 25 mg/day *Usual*: Individualize *Max*: 200 mg/day <u>NYHA > CLASS II</u> **Adult**: *Initial*: 25 mg/day *Usual*: Individualize *Max*: 200 mg/day **Children**: not recommended	• Pregnancy Category C • **DO NOT ABRUPTLY STOP DRUG; must be tapered over 2 weeks** • Individualize for patient effect and advance dose at 2 week intervals • Avoid in patients with peripheral vascular disease
	Toprol-XL	*Ext. Rel. Tabs: 25 mg, 50 mg, 100 mg, 200 mg*	
Angiotensin II Receptor Blockers (ARB) *Block vasoconstriction and sodium retention effects of AT II (angiotensin II) found in many tissues* <u>**General comments**</u> End in "sartan" Does not effect bradykinin; therefore, no cough as seen in ACE inhibitors. Good renoprotective action; therefore, good alternative in diabetics who cannot tolerate ACE inhibitors Monitor for hypotension and possible renal failure	**candesartan cilexetil**	**Adult:** *Initial*: 4 mg/day *Usual*: 32 mg/day *Max*: 32 mg/day **Children:** not recommended	• Pregnancy Category D • NYHA Classes II-IV • Dose is individualized for effect; double dose at 2 week intervals
	Atacand	*Tabs: 4 mg, 8 mg, 16 mg, 32 mg*	
	valsartan	**Adult**: *Initial*: 40 mg twice/day *Usual*: 160 mg twice/day *Max*: 160 mg twice/day	• Pregnancy Category D • May be taken without regard to food • Clinical effect seen within 2 weeks with maximum effect in 4 weeks • Caution when initiating in patients with hepatic or severe renal impairment
	Diovan	*Caps: 80 mg, 160 mg* *Tabs: 40 mg, 80 mg, 160 mg*	

PREGNANCY/LACTATION CONSIDERATIONS

- Do not restrict sodium in diet
- Requires cardiology referral

CONSULTATION/REFERRAL

- Consult according to severity and patient objectives

FOLLOW-UP

- Variable depending on patient circumstances, but, generally daily, until exacerbation resolves, then 1-2 weeks until patient is symptom free; then, every 3-6 months

EXPECTED COURSE

- Chronic disease with frequent exacerbations
- Common diagnosis associated with frequent hospital admission
- 15% die within first year of diagnosis

HYPERLIPIDEMIA

DESCRIPTION

An elevated level of blood lipids: cholesterol, cholesterol esters, phospholipids, and/or triglycerides.

ETIOLOGY

- Inherited disorder of lipid metabolism
- High intake of dietary lipids
- Obesity, sedentary lifestyle
- Diabetes mellitus
- Hypothyroidism
- Anabolic steroid use
- Hepatic disorders: hepatitis, cirrhosis
- Renal disorders: uremia, nephrotic syndrome
- Stress
- Drug induced: thiazide diuretics, β-blockers, cyclosporine
- Alcohol and caffeine
- Metabolic Syndrome: characterized by hypertension, glucose intolerance, obesity, dyslipidemia, and/or coagulation abnormalities

INCIDENCE

- Hypercholesterolemia > 200 mg/dL; 100 million people in U.S.
- Hypercholesterolemia > 240 mg/dL; 35 million people in U. S.
- Males = Females; female onset delayed by 10-15 years compared to males
- Incidence increases as age increases

RISK FACTORS

- Family history of CHD [type 2 familial hypercholesterolemia (FH)]
- Physical inactivity
- Smoking
- Age: men > 45 years, women > 55 years or premature menopause without estrogen replacement
- Obesity
- Diet high in saturated fat
- Diabetes mellitus

ASSESSMENT FINDINGS

- Few physical findings
- Xanthomata
- Xanthelasma
- Corneal arcus prior to age 50 years
- Bruits
- Angina pectoris
- Myocardial infarction
- Stroke

DIFFERENTIAL DIAGNOSIS

- Consider secondary causes: hypothyroidism, pregnancy, diabetes, non-fasting state

DIAGNOSTIC STUDIES

- Fasting lipid profile (9-12 hours of fasting)
- Non-fasting sample: Total cholesterol, LDL and HDL values affected little by eating; triglycerides elevated by eating
- Glucose
- Urinalysis, creatinine (for detection of nephrotic syndrome which can induce dyslipidemia)
- TSH (for detection of hypothyroidism which may secondarily cause hypercholesterolemia)

PREVENTION

- 1% decrease in cholesterol decreases risk of CHD by 2%
- Adults and children > 2 years of age: reduce dietary intake of fats to < 30% of total calories; < 7% should be from saturated fat (estimated 10% reduction in LDL with this low fat diet)
- Total cholesterol intake < 200 mg/day
- Minimize use of trans fatty acids
- Increase intake of fiber, vegetables, fruits, and other whole grains
- Decreased intake of fat is *not* recommended for children < 1 year of age
- Identify and eliminate risk factors in children and adults
- Encourage an active lifestyle in children (decreases likelihood of obesity); adults should exercise at least 2.5 hours per week (sustained aerobic activity increases HDL, decreases total cholesterol)
- Weight control and avoidance of tobacco products
- Appropriate management of systemic diseases (e.g., diabetes mellitus, hypothyroidism, hypertension)

NONPHARMACOLOGIC MANAGEMENT

- Therapeutic lifestyle changes (TLC): Nutrition, weight reduction, increased physical activity (See Prevention)
- Patient education regarding risk factors, lifestyle modifications, diet, exercise, etc.

INDICATIONS FOR PHARMACOLOGICAL MANAGEMENT

- 3 risk categories delineate treatment options based on "CHD 10 year risk" calculation from Framingham and presence of major risk factors
- Primary lipid target is LDL

ATP III Classification of LDL, Total, and HDL\Cholesterol (mg/dL)	
LDL Cholesterol	
< 100	Optimal
100-129	Near or above optimal
130-159	Borderline high
160-189	High
> 190	Very high
Total Cholesterol	
< 200	Desirable
200-239	Bordeline high
> 240	High
HDL Cholesterol	
< 40	Low
> 60	High (negative risk factor)

Source: Adult Treatment Panel III, 2004

Pediatric patients	
Total Cholesterol	
< 170 mg/dL	Desirable
LDL Cholesterol	
< 110 mg/dL	Desirable

Lipid Screening Recommendation
• Screen women only if risk factors present for CHD otherwise, screen at age 45 years (A recommendation) • Screen women ages 20-45 if risk factors present (B recommendation) • Screen beginning at age 35 (men) and at age 20 if CHD risk factors are present • Optimal screening interval and age to stop screening is unknown

Source: U.S. Preventive Services Task Force Guide to Clinical Preventive Services, 2008.

Major Risk Factors
• Age (men ≥ 45 years or females ≥ 55 years) • Family history of premature CHD (first degree relatives, CHD in males < 55 yrs or females < 65 years) • Cigarette smoking • Hypertension (BP ≥ 140/90 mm Hg or on antihypertensive therapy) • HDL < 40 mg/dL, triglycerides > 200 mg/dL • Metabolic syndrome • Established CHD (history of MI, stable/unstable angina, previous CAD interventions • CHD risk equivalents (Peripheral artery disease, abdominal aortic aneurysm, carotid disease, diabetes mellitus)

Source: Third Report of the Expert Panel on Detection, Evaluation, and Treatment of High Blood Cholesterol in Adults (Adult Treatment Panel III) by the National Cholesterol Education Program (NCEP), 2004.

Summary of 2004 ATP III Updated Guidelines

Risk	Demographics	Lipid Goals/Pharmacologic Intervention
Low	0-1 risk factors and 10 year risk of CHD < 10%	Goal LDL < 160 mg/dL: if > 160, then trial of TLC; if goal not reached after trial, consider medication
Moderate	2+ risk factors; and 10 year CHD risk 10-20% or 10 year CHD risk < 10%	Goal LDL < 130 mg/dL; if > 130, then trial of TLC, if unable to achieve, then medication
High	2+ risk factors and 10 year CHD risk > 20%, established CHD or CHD equivalents	Goal LDL < 100 mg/dL (optional goal 70 mg/dL); if not at goal, initiate TLC and medication

Source: Third Report of the Expert Panel on Detection, Evaluation, and Treatment of High Blood Cholesterol in Adults (Adult Treatment Panel III) by the National Cholesterol Education Program (NCEP), 2004.

PHARMACOLOGIC MANAGEMENT

SUMMARY OF LIPID LOWERING AGENTS

DRUG CLASS	↓ LDL	↑ HDL	↓ TRIGS
Statins	19-54%	5-15%	7-30%
Bile Acid Sequestrants	15-30%	3-5%	Insignificant
Nicotinic Acid	5-25%	15-35%	20-50%
Fibric Acids	5-7%	10-20%	20-50%
Cholesterol Absorption Inhibitor	15-18%	3-3.5%	Insignificant

Framingham Scales

Table A - Age

Age (yr)	Male	Female
20-34	-9	-7
35-39	-4	-3
40-44	0	0
45-49	3	3
50-54	6	6
55-59	8	8
60-64	10	10
65-69	11	12
70-74	12	14
75-79	13	16

Table B - Systolic BP (mmHg)

Systolic BP mmHg	Male Treated	Male Untreated	Female Treated	Female Untreated
< 120	0	0	0	0
120-129	1	0	3	1
130-139	2	1	4	2
140-159	2	1	5	3
> 160	3	2	6	4

Table C - HDL-Cholesterol

HDL mg/dL	Male	Female
≥ 60	0	-1
50-59	0	0
40-49	1	1
< 40	2	2

Calculate 10-Year CHD Risk

Table A Points = _______ (+)
Table B Points = _______ (+)
Table C Points = _______ (+)
Table D Points = _______ (+)
Table E Points = _______ (+)

Table F Point Total = _______

Source: Framingham Heart Study Risk Chart and Adult Treatment Panel III by National Heart, Lung & Blood Institute.

Table D - Total Cholesterol

TC (mg/dL)	20-39 M	20-39 F	40-49 M	40-49 F	50-59 M	50-59 F	60-69 M	60-69 F	70-79 M	70-79 F
<160	0	0	0	0	0	0	0	0	0	0
160-199	4	4	3	3	2	2	1	1	0	1
200-239	7	8	5	6	3	4	1	2	0	1
240-279	9	11	6	8	4	5	2	3	1	2
≥ 280	11	13	8	10	5	7	3	4	1	2

M = Male F = Female

Table E - Smoking Status

Age	Non-smoker	Male Smoker	Female Smoker
20-39	0	8	9
40-49	0	5	7
50-59	0	3	4
60-69	0	1	2
70-79	0	1	1

Table F - POINT TOTAL

10-Year CHD Risk Assessment

Male Point Total	Male 10-Year Risk%	Female Point Total	Female 10-Year Risk%
<0	<1	< 9	< 1
1	1	9	1
2	1	10	1
3	1	11	1
4	1	12	1
5	2	13	2
6	2	14	2
7	3	15	3
8	4	16	4
9	5	17	5
10	6	18	6
11	8	19	8
12	10	20	11
13	12	21	14
14	16	22	17
15	20	23	22
16	25	24	27
≥17	≥30	≥25	≥30

10-Year Risk _______% 10-Year Risk _______%

Cardiovascular Disorders

LIPID LOWERING AGENTS

Class	Drug Generic name (Trade name®)	Dosage How supplied	Comments
HMG-CoA Reductase Inhibitors ("Statins") *Inhibit HMG-CoA, the enzyme which is partly responsible for cholesterol synthesis; decrease total cholesterol, LDL, minimal increase in HDL* **General comments:** Considered first line therapy Perform liver function tests before initiating therapy, at 4-6 and 12 weeks, and after each dose increase, then periodically (or per manufacturer's recommendations) To be used in conjunction with diet, exercise, & weight reduction in overweight patients Watch for myopathy, rhabdomyolysis Watch for drug interactions, especially with grapefruit juice and lovastatin, simvastatin, and atorvastatin Pregnancy Category X	**atorvastatin**	**LDL-C reduction < 45%** **Adult**: *Initial*: 10 or 20 mg/day *Usual*: 10-80 mg/day *Max*: 80 mg/day **LDL-C reduction > 45%** *Initial*: 40 mg/day *Usual*: 40-80 mg/day *Max*: 80 mg/day **Heterozygous Familial Hypercholesterolemia** **Children < 10 yrs:** not recommended **10-17 yrs:** *Initial*: 10 mg/day *Usual*: 10 mg/day *Max*: 20 mg/day	• If concomitant use with gembibrozil, the maximum dose should not exceed 10 mg/day • If concomitant use with clarithromycin, itraconazole, or protease inhibitors, the maximum dose should not exceed 20 mg/day
	Lipitor	*Tabs: 10 mg, 20 mg, 40 mg, 80 mg*	
	fluvastatin	**LDL-C reduction < 25%** **Adult:** *Initial*: 20 mg in evening *Usual*: 20-80 mg/day *Max*: 80 mg/day **LDL-C reduction > 25%** **Adult**: *Initial:* Lescol XL 80 mg in PM or 40 mg Lescol daily or twice daily *Usual:* 80 mg/day *Max:* 80 mg/day **Children**: not recommended	• Avoid in patients with substantial alcohol consumption • Avoid concomitant fibrates, cyclosporine • May be taken without regard to meals
	Lescol	*Tabs: 20 mg, 40 mg*	
	Lescol XL	*Ext. Rel: 80 mg*	

continued

LIPID LOWERING AGENTS

Class	Drug Generic name (Trade name®)	Dosage How supplied	Comments
	lovastatin	<u>**Cr Cl > 30mL/min**</u> **Adult**: *Initial*: 10-20 mg (evening) *Usual*: 10-80 mg/day in single or divided doses *Max*: 80 mg day (single or divided dose) <u>**Cr Cl < 30mL/min**</u> **Adult**: *Initial*: 10-20 mg/day *Usual*: 10-20 mg/day *Max*: 20 mg day <u>**Heterozygous Familial Hypercholesterolemia**</u> **Children < 10 yrs:** not recommended **10-17 yrs:** *Initial*: 10-20 mg/day *Usual*: 10-40 mg/day *Max*: 40 mg/day	• Take with evening meal • Patients on amiodarone or verapamil should not exceed 40 mg/day • Start with lower doses if patient on cyclosporin or danazol; do not exceed 20 mg/day • For patients on fibrates or high-dose niacin, do not exceed 20 mg/day
	Mevacor Altocor	*Tabs: 10 mg, 20 mg, 40 mg*	
	pravastatin	<u>**Normal Renal/Hepatic Function**</u> **Adult**: *Initial*: 10 mg/day *Usual*: 20-40 mg/day *Max*: 80 mg/day **Children < 8 yrs:** not recommended **8-13 yrs:** 20 mg/daily **14-18 yrs:** 40 mg/daily <u>**Impaired Renal/Hepatic Function**</u> **Adult**: *Initial*: 10 mg/day *Usual*: 20 mg/day *Max*: 20 mg/day	• May adjust dose after 4 weeks • Take at bedtime
	Pravachol	*Tabs: 10 mg, 20 mg, 40 mg, 80 mg*	

continued

LIPID LOWERING AGENTS

Class	Drug Generic name (Trade name®)	Dosage How supplied	Comments
	rosuvastatin	<u>**Cr Cl > 30mL/min**</u> **Adult**: *Initial*: 10 mg/day, *Usual*: 5-20 mg/day *Max*: 40 mg/day <u>**Cr Cl < 30mL/min**</u> **Adult**: *Initial*: 5 mg/day *Max*: 10 mg/day <u>**Heterozygous Familial Hypercholesterolemia**</u> **Children < 10 yrs:** not recommended **10-17 yrs:** *Initial*: 5-10 mg/day *Usual*: 5-20 mg/day *Max*: 20 mg/day	• May be taken without regard to meals • Maximum dose is reserved only for patients who do not achieve LDL-C goal • In Asian patients, initiate therapy at 5 mg /day • In patients taking cyclosporine, the maximum dose is 5 mg/day • In patients taking anti-viral agents, the maximum dose is 10 mg/day
	Crestor	*Tabs: 5 mg, 10 mg, 20 mg, 40 mg*	
	simvastatin	<u>**Normal risk of CHD event**</u> **Adult**: *Initial*: 20-40 mg/HS *Usual*: 5-80 mg/HS *Max*: 80 mg/HS <u>**High risk of CHD event**</u> **Adult:** *Initial*: 40 mg/HS *Usual*: 40-80 mg/HS *Max*: 80 mg/HS <u>**Heterozygous Familial Hypercholesterolemia**</u> **Children < 10 yrs:** not recommended **10-17 yrs:** *Initial*: 10 mg/HS *Usual*: 10-40 mg/HS *Max*: 40 mg/HS	• Dosage adjustments should be determined at intervals of 4 weeks or more • If concomitant use with gemfibrozil, the maximum dose of simvastatin should not exceed 10 mg/day • Start with lower doses if patient on cyclosporin or danazol; do not exceed 10 mg/day • Patients on amiodarone or verapamil should not exceed 20 mg/day • Patients on diltiazem should not exceed 40 mg/day
	Zocor	*Tabs: 5 mg, 10 mg, 20 mg, 40 mg, 80 mg*	

continued

LIPID LOWERING AGENTS

Class	Drug Generic name (Trade name®)	Dosage How supplied	Comments
Bile Acid Sequestrants *Bind bile acids in the intestine which prevents their absorption. These insoluble bile acid complexes are excreted in the feces*	**cholestyramine**	**Adult**: *Initial*: one packet with food or fluids 1-2 times a day *Usual*: 2-4 packets divided in 2 doses daily *Max*: 6 doses/day	• Pregnancy Category C • Do not administer with other medications • Use non-carbonated liquids for mixing
General comments In conjunction with diet, are used to decrease total cholesterol, LDL	Questran	*Carton: 60 pkts* *Can: 378 g*	
	Questran Light	*Carton: 60 pkts* *Can: 268 g*	
May prevent absorption of fat soluble vitamins A, D, E & K Watch for constipation, flatulence May reduce absorption of many oral medications	**colesevelam**	**Adult**: *Initial*: 3 tabs twice/day OR 1 pkt 3.75 g/day OR 1 pkt 1.875 g twice/day *Usual*: same as initial *Max*: same as initial **Children < 10 yrs:** not recommended **10-17 yrs:** Same as adult but use powder form	• Pregnancy Category B; but used with caution due to binding of other nutrients • If powder, mix in 4-8 ounces of water • Should be taken with meals • Contraindicated in patients with history of bowel obstruction • Contraindicated in patients with serum triglycerides > 500 mg/dL • Caution in patients with history of pancreatitis
	WelChol	*Tabs: 625 mg* *Pkt: 1.875 g, 3.75 g*	
	colestipol	**Adult**: *Initial*: 1 pkt OR 1 scoop/day OR 2-4 g/day *Usual*: 1-6 pkt or 1-6 scoops OR 2-16 g (either per day or divided doses) or *Max*: 6 pkt or 6 scoops or 16 g (either per day or divided doses) **Children**: not recommended	• Pregnancy Category B; but used with caution due to binding of other nutrients • Do not crush tablet formulation • Titrate dose upwards on weekly schedule to achieve max • Chronic use can lead to increased bleeding tendency (Vitamin K depletion)
	Colestid	*Carton: 30 pkt, 90 pkt* *Powder: 300 g, 500 g*	
	Colestipol	*Tab: 1 g*	

continued

LIPID LOWERING AGENTS

Class	Drug Generic name (Trade name®)	Dosage How supplied	Comments
Fibric Acids *Increase lipolysis and elimination of triglyceride rich particles from plasma. This results in lowering of triglycerides, LDL* **General comments** Gemfibrozil and statins concomitantly can produce rhabdomyolysis and acute renal failure Increases risk of gallstone formation Monitor liver function studies and glucose during therapy; both may be elevated	**gemfibrozil** Lopid	**Adult**: *Initial*: 1.2 g daily in 2 divided doses, 30 min AC *Usual*: same as initial *Max*: same as initial **Children**: not recommended *Tabs: 600 mg*	• Pregnancy Category C • Concomitant therapy with cerivastatin increases risk of myopathy and rhabdomyolysis • Avoid in patients with pre-existing gallbladder disease • Discontinue after 3 months if lipid response is inadequate • Avoid concomitant therapy with HMG-CoA reductase inhibitors
	fenofibrate TriCor	**Normal Triglycerides** **Adult**: *Initial*: 145 mg/day *Usual*: same as initial *Max*: same as initial **Elevated Triglycerides** *Initial*: 48 mg/day *Usual*: 48-145 mg/day *Max*: 145 mg/day **Children**: not recommended *Tabs: 48 mg, 145 mg*	• Pregnancy Category C • Contraindicated in patients with severe renal or hepatic dysfunction • Avoid in patients with pre-existing gallbladder disease • Caution in patients with coumarin-type anticoagulants • Adjust at 4-8 week intervals; discontinue after 2 months of max dose if not favorable lipid response
	Fenofibric acid Trilipix	**Mixed Hyperlipidemia** **Adult**: *Initial*: 135 mg/day *Usual*: same as initial *Max*: same as initial **Hypertriglyceridemia** **Adult**: *Initial*: 45 mg/day *Usual*: 45-135 mg/day *Max*: 135 mg/day **Renal Impairment** **Adult**: *Initial*: 45 mg/day *Usual*: 45 mg/day *Max*: 45 mg/day **Children**: not recommended *Caps: 45 mg, 135 mg*	• Pregnancy Category C • As mono therapy, targets severe hypertriglyceridemia • As combination therapy (with HMG-CoA reductase inhibitors, targets mixed hyperlipidemia • Contraindicated in patients on dialysis

continued

LIPID LOWERING AGENTS

Class	Drug Generic name (Trade name®)	Dosage How supplied	Comments
Niacin *Not well understood but thought to decrease hepatic VLDL production. VLDL is converted to LDL. Also, may decrease lipoprotein production in the liver; increases HDL* General comments Monitor liver function studies before initiation of treatment, at 6 & 12 weeks after treatment, with each dosage increase, and periodically Poorly tolerated. Causes flushing & hypotension. Take at bedtime with an aspirin to improve tolerability Monitor for myalgias & rhabdomyolysis	**niacin (nicotinic acid)** Niacor	**Adult**: *Initial*: 250 mg with evening meal; increase every 4-7 days until 1.5-2 g/day *Usual*: 1.5-3 g/day (may be in 3 divided doses) *Max*: 6 g/day **Children**: not recommended *Tabs: 500 mg*	• Pregnancy Category C • Upward titration of dose required • Avoid taking on empty stomach • **Do not interchange immediate release dosage form with extended release dosage form**
	niacin (nicotinic acid), extended release Niaspan	**Adult**: *Initial*: 500 mg/HS, weeks 1-4; then 1000 mg/HS weeks 5-8; then 1500 mg/HS weeks 9-12; then 2000 mg/HS weeks 13-16 *Usual*: 1000-2000 mg/HS *Max*: 2000 mg/HS **Children**: not recommended *Tabs: 500 mg, 750 mg, 1000 mg*	• Pregnancy Category C • Upward titration should not exceed 500 mg in a 4-week period • If therapy interrupted, resume on titration schedule • Females may require lower doses than males • Use with caution in patients with renal or hepatic dysfunction • **Do not interchange immediate release dosage form with extended release dosage form**
Cholesterol Absorption Inhibitor Inhibits absorption of cholesterol by the small intestine. Does not inhibit cholesterol synthesis (statins) or increase bile acid excretion	**ezetimibe** Zetia	**Adult**: *Initial*: 10 mg/day *Usual*: same as initial *Max*: same as initial **Children > 10 years of age:** *Initial*: 10 mg/day *Usual*: same as initial *Max*: same as initial *Tabs: 10 mg*	• Pregnancy Category C • Adjunct to diet alone or in combination with "statin" • No evidence of myopathy when used alone • Not necessary to monitor hepatic function unless patient on other therapy that requires monitoring • GI complaints are most common

PREGNANCY/LACTATION CONSIDERATIONS

- Cholesterol levels are usually elevated during pregnancy
- Treatment contraindicated

CONSIDERATIONS FOR SPECIAL POPULATIONS

- Elderly: Benefits seen with total cholesterol and LDL reduction
- Statins typically well tolerated by elderly
- Diabetics: Aggressive management of hyperlipidemia needed

CONSULTATION/REFERRAL

- Dietitian
- Refer to lipid specialist for children with hyperlipidemia not responsive to dietary and conservative measures

FOLLOW-UP

- Evaluate lipid values every 5 years starting at age 20 if normal values obtained
- After initiation of lipid lowering therapy, monitor lipids every 6-8 weeks until goal attained; then every 6-12 months to evaluate compliance

EXPECTED COURSE

- Depends on etiology and severity of disease
- 1% decrease in LDL value decreases CHD risk by 2%

POSSIBLE COMPLICATIONS

- Coronary artery disease
- Cerebrovascular disease
- Peripheral vascular disease
- Arteriosclerosis

STABLE ANGINA

(Angina Pectoris)

DESCRIPTION

A symptom that results when myocardial oxygen demand is greater than myocardial oxygen supply. Some patients may not be symptomatic. This is usually predictable with exertion and able to be relieved by rest or nitroglycerin.

ETIOLOGY

- Coronary artery disease
- Coronary artery vasospasm
- Coronary thrombosis
- Aortic stenosis/insufficiency

Women who have myocardial ischemia in the absence of significant coronary artery disease may have microvascular disease. Unfortunately, this is associated with a high degree of morbidity and mortality.

INCIDENCE

- Males > premenopausal females
- Males = Females after menopause
- Most common in fifties, sixties, seventies

RISK FACTORS

- Family history of coronary artery disease
- Hypertension
- Hypercholesterolemia
- Diabetes mellitus
- Tobacco/cocaine use
- Obesity
- Advancing age

TYPES OF ANGINA	
Classic angina	Heaviness, choking, pressure deep in the chest due to exertion, anxiety; relieved by rest and nitroglycerin
Prinzmetal's angina	Results from coronary artery vasospasm; occurs in atypical patterns
Unstable angina	Recent onset, or an increase in severity, frequency or duration from usual, symptoms at rest, or nocturnal symptoms

ASSESSMENT FINDINGS

- Change in symptoms warrants further investigation
- Heaviness, discomfort, pressure, pain, ache radiating to back, chest, arms, jaw, teeth
- May be precipitated by exercise, stress, cold temperature, ingestion of a heavy meal, smoking
- Pain/discomfort relieved after nitroglycerin administration
- Shortness of breath with or without activity
- Asymptomatic ("silent ischemia")
- Nausea
- Perspiration
- Palpitations

DIFFERENTIAL DIAGNOSIS

- Esophagitis/esophageal spasm
- Gastritis/peptic ulcer disease/GERD
- Pericarditis
- Pulmonary embolus
- Costochondritis
- Pneumothorax
- Chest wall syndrome
- Cholecystitis
- Treadmill exercise test (if stable)
- Stress radionuclide imaging
- Coronary angiography

DIAGNOSTIC STUDIES

- Electrocardiogram: may demonstrate ST segment changes
- Chest x-ray: new or worsening CHF
- Lipid level measurements: may demonstrate hyperlipidemia
- Echocardiogram if on medication affecting conduction, syncopal episode, dysrhythmia, new or worsening valvular disease

NONPHARMACOLOGIC MANAGEMENT

- Cardiac rehabilitation program if appropriate
- Modify coronary artery disease risk factors
- Adhere to antianginal medication schedule
- Stress management
- Consumption of low fat diet
- Smoking cessation
- Regular, aerobic exercise
- Attain/maintain ideal body weight
- Patient education regarding disease, treatment, lifestyle changes, reporting of changes in symptoms, etc.

PREVENTION

- Modify coronary artery disease risk factors
- Adhere to antianginal medication schedule
- Consumption of low fat diet
- Monitoring and control of hypertension, hyperlipidemia, and diabetes mellitus
- Smoking cessation
- Regular, aerobic exercise

STABLE ANGINA PHARMACOLOGIC MANAGEMENT

Combinations of these (ACE inhibitor, aspirin, β-blocker and statin) have shown to reduce the incidence of MI and other adverse ischemic events in patients with previous MI

Class	Drug Generic name (Trade name®)	Dosage How supplied	Comments
Nitrates *Most effective therapy for acute angina. Produces arterial and venous dilation by relaxing vascular smooth muscle* **General comments** Patients may develop tolerance; therefore, a nitrate free period should be considered May produce headaches Monitor for hypotension episodes or palpitations	**nitroglycerin**	**Acute Anginal Pain** **Adult:** *Initial*: 1 sublingual at onset; may repeat in 5 minutes. *Max*: 3 sublingual tabs over 15 minutes **-OR-** **Adult:** *Initial*: 1-2 sprays at onset; may repeat in 5 minutes *Max*: 3 sprays over 15 minutes **Prophylaxis of Angina Topical Patches** **Adult:** *Initial*: 0.2-0.4 mg/hr patch worn daily for up to 12 hours, then removed *Max*: 0.8 mg/hr patch worn daily for up to 12 hours, then removed **Prophylaxis of Angina Topical Ointment** **Adult:** *Initial*: ½ inch in AM and repeat in 6 hours *Max*: 2 inches in AM and repeat in 6 hours	• Pregnancy Category C • **ACUTE ANGINAL PAIN unrelieved after 15 minutes warrants additional follow up and evaluation in emergency care setting** • Individualize therapy for prophylaxis, advance as tolerated • Advise patients of potential for headaches, postural hypotension • Male patients should avoid concomitant use of erectile dysfunction products • Avoid abrupt cessation of prophylaxis use products • Sublingual spray may be used prior to activity with exertion
	Nitrostat (sublingual route)	*Tabs: 0.3 mg, 0.4 mg, 0.6 mg*	
	Nitrolingual (translingual spray)	*Spray: 0.4 mg/spray*	
	Nitro-Dur (topical patch)	*Patch: 0.1 mg/hr, 0.2 mg/hr, 0.3 mg/hr, 0.4 mg/hr, 0.6 mg/hr, 0.8 mg/hr*	
	Nitro-Bid (topical ointment)	*Oint: 15 mg/inch*	

continued

STABLE ANGINA PHARMACOLOGIC MANAGEMENT

Combinations of these (ACE inhibitor, aspirin, β-blocker and statin) have shown to reduce the incidence of MI and other adverse ischemic events in patients with previous MI

Class	Drug Generic name (Trade name®)	Dosage How supplied	Comments
Aspirin *Prevents platelet aggregation and exerts anti-inflammatory effect in vessels by inhibiting prostaglandin synthesis* **General comments** Observe for bleeding, tinnitus, gastric irritation Reduces morbidity and mortality for CV events	**acetylsalicylic acid (ASA)** Various generics	**Prophylaxis** **Adult**: *Initial*: 81 mg/day *Max*: 325 mg/day **Post Myocardial Infarction** *Initial*: 162-325 mg/day *Usual*: 75-162 mg/day *Max*: 325 mg/day *Tabs: 81 mg, 162 mg, 325 mg* *Caplets: 81 mg, 325 mg* *Gelcaps: 325 mg*	• Pregnancy Category D • Use in caution with patients with reactive airway disease (asthma) • Consider enteric coated in patients with prior gastric irritation • Avoid in patients with NSAID allergies • May need to reduce dose in severe hepatic or renal dysfunction
Angiotensin Converting Enzyme Inhibitors (ACEI) *Inhibit the action of angiotensin converting enzyme (ACE) which is responsible for conversion of angiotensin I to angiotensin II; Angiotensin II causes vasoconstriction & sodium retention. Prevents breakdown of bradykinin.* **General comments** First line agent End in "pril" Dry cough is common side effect; monitor for first dose hypotension, hyperkalemia, acute renal failure Angioedema is rare but more common in African-Americans Monitor for renal failure and worsening chronic heart failure	**captopril** Capoten	**For Patients NOT on Diuretics** **Adult**: *Initial*: 25 mg two or three times/day *Usual*: 20-40 mg/day *Max*: 450 mg/day **Children**: not recommended **For Patients On Diuretics** *Initial*: 6.25-12.5 mg two or three times/day *Usual*: 25-150 mg two or three times/day *Max*: 450 mg/day **For Patients with Renal Impairment (Glomerular Filtration < 30mL)** *Initial*: 6.25-12.5 mg two or three times/day *Usual*: same as initial *Tabs: 12.5 mg, 25 mg, 50 mg, 100 mg*	• Pregnancy Category D • Take 1 hour before meals and with diuretics • Adjust dose after 2 weeks to 50 mg three times/day • Patient must be under close supervision if on diuretic; can increase catopril to 100 mg two or three times/day

continued

STABLE ANGINA PHARMACOLOGIC MANAGEMENT

Combinations of these (ACE inhibitor, aspirin, β-blocker and statin) have shown to reduce the incidence of MI and other adverse ischemic events in patients with previous MI

Class	Drug Generic name (Trade name®)	Dosage How supplied	Comments
Preferred in patients with diabetes and CHF Avoid use in patients with bilateral renal artery stenosis	**lisinopril**	**For Patients NOT on Diuretics** **Adult**: *Initial*: 10 mg/day *Usual*: 20-40 mg/day *Max*: 80 mg/day **Children ≥ 6 yrs:** *Initial:* 0.07 mg/kg *Usual*: Individualize *Max*: 0.61 mg/kg - do not exceed adult dose **For Patients on Diuretics OR For Patients with Renal Impairment (Glomerular Filtration < 30mL)** **Adult:** *Initial*: 2.5 mg/day *Usual*: 2.5-5 mg/day *Max*: 5 mg/day **Children**: not recommended	• Pregnancy Category D • Recommend holding diuretics 3 days prior to starting, if appropriate for patient • Doses at 80 mg may not produce significantly greater effect compared to 40 mg
	Prinivil Zestril	*Tabs: 2.5 mg, 5 mg, 10 mg, 20 mg, 40 mg*	
	ramipril	**For Patients NOT on Diuretics** **Adult**: *Initial*: 2.5 mg/day for 7 days; 5 mg/day for 21 days; then 10 mg/day *Usual*: 2.5-20 mg/day (either as single or two doses) *Max*: 20 mg/day **Children**: not recommended	• Pregnancy Category D • Requires initial titration of dosage schedule • May increase lithium levels

continued

STABLE ANGINA PHARMACOLOGIC MANAGEMENT

Combinations of these (ACE inhibitor, aspirin, β-blocker and statin) have shown to reduce the incidence of MI and other adverse ischemic events in patients with previous MI

Class	Drug Generic name (Trade name®)	Dosage How supplied	Comments
		For Patients on Diuretics **OR** **For Patients with Renal Impairment (Cr Cl < 40 mL/min)** *Initial*: 1.25 mg/day for 7 days; 2.5 mg/day for 21 days; then 5 mg/day *Usual*: 2.5-5 mg/day (either as single or two doses) *Max*: 5 mg/day	
	Altace	*Caps 1.25 mg, 2.5 mg, 5 mg, 10 mg* *Tabs 1.25 mg, 2.5 mg, 5 mg, 10 mg*	
Cardio-selective β-Blockers *Decrease sympathetic stimulation by β-blockade in the heart* **General comments** Consider post-MI, in CHF, ischemic heart disease Should be avoided (or used cautiously) in patients with airway disease, heart block Should be used with caution in diabetics (may mask the symptoms of hypoglycemia) and in those with peripheral vascular disease	**atenolol**	**Adult**: *Initial*: 50 mg/day *Usual*: 50-100 mg/day *Max*: 200 mg/day **Children**: not recommended **Elderly or Patients with Renal Impairment** **Cr Cl 15-35 mL/min** *Initial*: 25 mg/day *Max*: 50 mg/day **Cr Cl < 15 mL/min** *Initial*: 25 mg/day *Max*: 25 mg/day	• Pregnancy Category D • **DO NOT ABRUPTLY STOP DRUG** • May titrate dose upwards after 1 week • Patients on dialysis should be monitored under hospital supervision for dosages given post treatment
	Tenormin	*Tabs: 25 mg, 50 mg, 100 mg*	
May cause exercise intolerance	**metoprolol succinate, extended release**	**Adult**: *Initial*: 100 mg/day *Usual*: 100-400 mg/day *Max*: 400 mg/day **Children**: not recommended	• Pregnancy Category C • **DO NOT ABRUPTLY STOP DRUG; must be tapered over 2 weeks** • **NOTE different dosage forms** • Individualize for patient effect • Advance dosage at weekly intervals

continued

STABLE ANGINA PHARMACOLOGIC MANAGEMENT

Combinations of these (ACE inhibitor, aspirin, β-blocker and statin) have shown to reduce the incidence of MI and other adverse ischemic events in patients with previous MI

Class	Drug Generic name (Trade name®)	Dosage How supplied	Comments
	Lopressor	*Ext. Rel. Tabs: 25 mg, 50 mg, 100 mg, 200 mg*	
	Toprol-XL	*Ext. Rel. Tabs: 25 mg, 50 mg, 100 mg, 200 mg*	
	metoprolol tartrate	**Adult**: *Initial:* 100 mg/day (single or divided dose) *Usual:* 100-400 mg/day (single or divided dose) *Max*: 400 mg/day (single or divided dose) **Children**: not recommended	• Pregnancy Category C • **DO NOT ABRUPTLY STOP DRUG; must be tapered over 2 weeks** • **NOTE different dosage forms** • Individualize for patient effect • Advance dosage at weekly intervals • **Should be given with meals**
	Lopressor	*Ext. Rel. Tabs: 25 mg, 50 mg, 100 mg, 200 mg*	
	Toprol	*Ext. Rel. Tabs: 25 mg, 50 mg, 100 mg, 200 mg*	
Non-Cardioselective β-blockers *Block stimulation of both β1 (heart) and β2 (lungs) receptors causing decreased heart rate, blood pressure, and cardiac output (β1) as well as decreased central motor activity, inhibition of renin release from the kidneys, reduction of norepinephrine from neurons, and mild bronchoconstriction (β2)* **General comments** End in "lol" Contraindicated in patients with bronchoconstrictive disease (i.e,, asthma, COPD, etc.)	**nadolol**	**Adult**: *Initial*: 20-40 mg/day *Usual*: 40-80 mg/day *Max*: 320 mg/day **Children**: not recommended **Special Dosing Schedule in Renal Impairment** *Initial*: 20 mg **Cr Cl > 50**: 24 hours **Cr Cl 31-50**: 24-36 hours **Cr Cl 10-30**: 24-48 hours **Cr Cl < 10**: 40-60 hours	• Pregnancy Category C • **DO NOT ABRUPTLY STOP DRUG; may take 2 weeks to withdraw drug while patient undergoes close monitoring** • Individualize therapy • May be taken without regard to meals • Note dosing schedule for renal dysfunction
	Corgard	*Tabs: 20 mg, 40 mg, 80 mg, 120 mg, 160 mg*	
	Visken	*Tabs: 5 mg, 10 mg*	

continued

STABLE ANGINA PHARMACOLOGIC MANAGEMENT

Combinations of these (ACE inhibitor, aspirin, β-blocker and statin) have shown to reduce the incidence of MI and other adverse ischemic events in patients with previous MI

Class	Drug Generic name (Trade name®)	Dosage How supplied	Comments
Cautious use in diabetics because of masking signs and symptoms of hypoglycemia (tachycardia, blood pressure changes) Nonspecific β-blockade helpful in patients with tremors, anxiety and migraine headaches	**propranolol**	<u>**Immediate Release**</u> **Adult**: *Initial*: 10-20 mg (divided into 2 or 3 doses/day) *Usual*: 160-240 mg/day (divided into 2 or 3 doses/day) *Max*: 320 mg/day (divided into 2 or 3 doses/day) <u>**Extended Release**</u> **Adult**: *Initial*: 80 mg/day *Usual*: 120-160 mg/day *Max*: 640 mg/day	• Pregnancy Category C • **DO NOT ABRUPTLY STOP DRUG; withdraw product over several weeks** • **Ext. Release form has different kinetics, CANNOT switch between dosage forms on a 1:1 mg basis** • Titrate to symptoms; titration may vary from a few days to several weeks • Do not crush or chew tablets • Contraindicated with thioridazine
	Inderal	*Tabs: 10 mg, 20 mg, 40 mg, 60 mg, 80 mg*	
	Inderal LA	*Ext. Rel. Cap: 60 mg, 80 mg, 120 mg, 160 mg*	
Calcium Channel Blockers Dihydropyridine (DHP) *Inhibit movement of calcium ions across the cell membrane and vascular smooth muscle which depress myocardial contractility and increase cardiac blood flow*	**amlodipine besylate**	**Adult**: *Initial*: 5 mg/day *Usual*: 5-10 mg/day *Max*: 10 mg/day **Elderly, renal or hepatic patients:** *Initial*: 2.5 mg/day	• Pregnancy Category C • Titrate for effect; increase doses at 7-14 day intervals; must reassess patient after each titration
	Norvasc	*Tabs: 2.5 mg, 5 mg, 10 mg*	
<u>General comments</u> End in suffix "pine" Does not cause bradycardia Monitor for hypotension and worsening of CHF, ankle edema	**felodipine**	**Adult**: *Initial*: 2.5-5 mg/day *Usual*: 2.5-10 mg/day *Max*: 10 mg/day **Elderly or hepatic patients:** *Initial*: 2.5 mg/day **Children**: not recommended	• Pregnancy Category C • Titrate for effect; increase dose after minimum of 2 week interval • Do not crush or chew tablets • Bioavailability affected by meals; should take on empty stomach
	Plendil	*Ext. Rel. Tabs: 2.5 mg, 5 mg, 10 mg*	

continued

STABLE ANGINA PHARMACOLOGIC MANAGEMENT

Combinations of these (ACE inhibitor, aspirin, β-blocker and statin) have shown to reduce the incidence of MI and other adverse ischemic events in patients with previous MI

Class	Drug Generic name (Trade name®)	Dosage How supplied	Comments
Good choice in diabetics with proteinuria, patients with ISH (isolated systolic hypertension) for migraine prophylaxis and in patients with stable angina Serious drug interactions with grapefruit juice Long acting DHP calcium channel blockers preferred for isolated systolic hypertension	**nifedipine**	**Immediate Release** **Adult**: *Initial*: 10 mg three times/day *Usual*: 10-20 mg three times/day *Max*: 120 mg/day **Extended Release** **Adult**: *Initial*: 30-60 mg/day *Usual*: 30-60 mg/day *Max*: 90 mg/day **Children**: not recommended	• Pregnancy Category C • Individualize treatment; advance doses at 1-2 week intervals • Take on empty stomach • Do not crush or chew extended release formulations • Must be withdrawn slowly if discontinued • If moving from immediate release to extended release, use nearest equivalency
	Procardia (immediate release)	*Caps: 10 mg, 20 mg*	
	Procardia XL (extended release)	*Ext. Rel. Tabs: 30 mg, 60 mg, 90 mg*	
Calcium Channel Blockers: Non-Dihydropyridine (Non-DHP) *Inhibit movement of calcium ions across the cell membrane and vascular smooth muscle which depress myocardial contractility and increase cardiac blood flow* **General comments** Watch for conduction defects Decreases heart rate Use cautiously or avoid with use of β-blockers Monitor for worsening of CHF, hypotension, bradycardia, constipation	**diltiazem**	**Immediate Release** **Adult**: *Initial*: 30 mg four times/day *Usual*: 180-360 mg/day *Max*: 360 mg/day* **Children**: not recommended **Extended Release** **Adult**: *Initial*: 120-180 mg/day *Usual*: 240-360 mg/day *Max*: 360-480 mg/day* **See specific drug manufacturer for maximum dose limits*	• Pregnancy Category C • Available in multiple formulations (tablets and capsules) and strengths • Individualize therapy; titrate immediate release at 1-2 DAY intervals; titrate extended release at 1-2 WEEK intervals • Start with lowest dose possible, especially in elderly • Do not crush or chew • Incidence of side effects increases with dose increases
	Cardizem	*Tabs: 30 mg, 60 mg, 90 mg, 120 mg*	
	Cardizem LA	*Ext. Rel. Tabs: 120 mg, 180 mg, 240 mg, 300 mg, 360 mg, 420 mg*	
	Cardizem CD	*Ext. Rel. Caps: 120 mg, 180 mg, 240 mg, 300 mg, 360 mg*	

continued

STABLE ANGINA PHARMACOLOGIC MANAGEMENT

Combinations of these (ACE inhibitor, aspirin, β-blocker and statin) have shown to reduce the incidence of MI and other adverse ischemic events in patients with previous MI

Class	Drug Generic name (Trade name®)	Dosage How supplied	Comments
Consider in patients with atrial fibrillation with rapid ventricular response, in patients with angina, and in diabetics with proteinuria	Dilacor XR Tiazac	*Ext. Rel. Caps: 120 mg, 180 mg, 240 mg* *Ext. Rel. Caps: 120 mg, 180 mg, 240 mg, 300 mg, 360 mg, 420 mg*	
Serious drug interactions with grapefruit juice	**verapamil**	<u>**Immediate Release**</u> **Adult**: *Initial*: 80-120 mg three times/ day *Usual*: 80-120 mg three times/ day *Max*: 120 mg three times/day* <u>**Renal Impairment**</u> *Initial*: 40 mg three times/day *Usual*: 80-120 mg three times/ day *Max*: 120 mg three times/day* **Children**: not recommended <u>**Extended Release**</u> **Adult:** *Initial*: 180 mg/day *Usual*: 240-360 mg/day *Max*: 360-480 mg/day* *Refer to specific product for additional guidelines	• Pregnancy Category C • Use extended release formulations as for HTN control • Available in multiple formulations (tablets and capsules) and strengths. Refer to specific product for additional guidelines • Individualize therapy; titrate at bi-weekly intervals • **Elderly or small stature people may require lower starting dose**
	Calan (immediate release) Covera HS (Give at bedtime)	*Tabs: 40 mg, 80 mg, 120 mg* *Ext. Rel. Tabs: 120 mg, 240 mg*	

continued

STABLE ANGINA PHARMACOLOGIC MANAGEMENT

Combinations of these (ACE inhibitor, aspirin,β-blocker and statin) have shown to reduce the incidence of MI and other adverse ischemic events in patients with previous MI

Class	Drug Generic name (Trade name®)	Dosage How supplied	Comments
HMG-CoA Reductase Inhibitors ("Statins") *Inhibit HMG-CoA, the enzyme which is partly responsible for cholesterol synthesis; decrease total cholesterol, LDL, minimal increase in HDL* **General comments** Considered first line therapy Perform liver function tests before initiating therapy, at 4-6 and 12 wks, and after each dose increase, then periodically, or per manufacturer's recommendations To be used in conjunction with diet, exercise, & weight reduction in overweight patients Watch for myopathy, rhabdomyolysis Watch for drug interactions, especially with grapefruit juice and lovastatin, simvastatin, and atorvastatin Pregnancy Category X	**atorvastatin**	**LDL-C reduction < 45%** **Adult**: *Initial*: 10 or 20 mg/day *Usual*: 10-80 mg/day *Max*: 80 mg/day **LDL-C reduction > 45%** *Initial*: 40 mg/day *Usual*: 40-80 mg/day *Max*: 80 mg/day **Heterozygous Familial Hypercholesterolemia** **Children < 10 yrs:** not recommended **10-17 yrs:** *Initial*: 10 mg/day *Usual*: 10 mg/day *Max*: 20 mg/day	• Pregnancy Category X • If concomitant use with gembibrozil, the maximum dose should not exceed 10 mg/day • If concomitant use with clarithromycin, itraconazole, or protease inhibitors, the maximum dose should not exceed 20 mg/day
	Lipitor	*Tabs: 10 mg, 20 mg, 40 mg, 80 mg*	
	fluvastatin	**LDL-C reduction < 25%** **Adult:** *Initial*: 20 mg in evening *Usual*: 20-80 mg/day *Max*: 80 mg/day **LDL-C reduction > 25%** **Adult:** *Initial*: Lescol XL 80 mg in PM or 40 mg Lescol daily or twice daily *Usual*: 80 mg/day *Max*: 80 mg/day **Children**: not recommended	• Pregnancy Category X • Avoid in patients with substantial alcohol consumption • Avoid concomitant fibrates, cyclosporine • May be taken without regard to meals
	Lescol	*Tabs: 20 mg, 40 mg*	
	Lescol XL	*Ext. Rel.: 80 mg*	

continued

STABLE ANGINA PHARMACOLOGIC MANAGEMENT

Combinations of these (ACE inhibitor, aspirin, β-blocker and statin) have shown to reduce the incidence of MI and other adverse ischemic events in patients with previous MI

Class	Drug Generic name (Trade name®)	Dosage How supplied	Comments
	lovastatin	<u>**Cr Cl > 30mL/min**</u> **Adult**: *Initial*: 10-20 mg (evening) *Usual*: 10-80 mg/day in single or divided doses *Max*: 80 mg day (single or divided dose) <u>**Cr Cl < 30mL/min**</u> **Adult**: *Initial*: 10-20 mg/day *Usual*: 10-20 mg/day *Max*: 20 mg day <u>**Heterozygous Familial Hypercholesterolemia**</u> **Children < 10 yrs:** not recommended **10-17 yrs:** *Initial*: 10-20 mg/day *Usual*: 10-40 mg/day *Max*: 40 mg/day	• Pregnancy Category X • Take with evening meal • Patients on amiodarone or verapamil should not exceed 40 mg/day • Start with lower doses if patient on cyclosporin or danazol; do not exceed 20 mg/day • For patients on fibrates or high-dose niacin, do not exceed 20 mg/day
	Mevacor Altocor	*Tabs: 10 mg, 20 mg, 40 mg*	
	pravastatin	<u>**Normal Renal/Hepatic Function**</u> **Adult**: *Initial*: 10 mg/day *Usual*: 20-40 mg/day *Max*: 80 mg/day **Children < 8 yrs:** not recommended **8-13 yrs:** 20 mg/daily **14-18 yrs:** 40 mg/daily <u>**Impaired Renal/Hepatic Function**</u> **Adult**: *Initial*: 10 mg/day *Usual*: 20 mg/day *Max*: 20 mg/day	• Pregnancy Category X • May adjust dose after 4 weeks • Take at bedtime
	Pravachol	*Tabs: 10 mg, 20 mg, 40 mg, 80 mg*	

continued

STABLE ANGINA PHARMACOLOGIC MANAGEMENT

Combinations of these (ACE inhibitor, aspirin, β-blocker and statin) have shown to reduce the incidence of MI and other adverse ischemic events in patients with previous MI

Class	Drug Generic name (Trade name®)	Dosage How supplied	Comments
	rosuvastatin	**Cr Cl > 30 mL/min** **Adult**: *Initial*: 10 mg/day, *Usual*: 5-20 mg/day *Max*: 40 mg/day **Cr Cl < 30 mL/min** **Adult:** *Initial*: 5 mg/day *Max*: 10 mg/day **Heterozygous Familial Hypercholesterolemia** **Children < 10 yrs:** not recommended **10-17 yrs:** *Initial*: 5-10 mg/day *Usual*: 5-20 mg/day *Max*: 20 mg/day	• Pregnancy Category X • May be taken without regard to meals • Maximum dose is reserved only for patients who do not achieve LDL-C goal • In Asian patients, initiate therapy at 5 mg /day • In patients taking cyclosporine, the maximum dose is 5 mg/day • In patients taking anti-viral agents, the maximum dose is 10 mg/day
	Crestor	*Tabs: 5 mg, 10 mg, 20 mg, 40 mg*	
	simvastatin	**Normal risk of CHD event** **Adult**: *Initial*: 20-40 mg/HS *Usual*: 5-80 mg/HS *Max*: 80 mg/HS **High risk of CHD event** **Adult:** *Initial*: 40 mg/HS *Usual*: 40-80 mg/HS *Max*: 80 mg/HS **Heterozygous Familial Hypercholesterolemia** **Children <10 yrs:** not recommended **10-17 yrs:** *Initial*: 10 mg/HS *Usual*: 10-40 mg/HS *Max*: 40 mg/HS	• Pregnancy Category X • Dosage adjustments should be determined at intervals of 4 weeks or more • If concomitant use with gembibrozil, the maximum dose of simvastatin should not exceed 10 mg/day • Start with lower doses if patient on cyclosporin or danazol; do not exceed 10 mg/day • Patients on amiodarone or verapamil should not exceed 20 mg/day • Patients on diltiazem should not exceed 40 mg/day
	Zocor	*Tabs: 5 mg, 10 mg, 20 mg, 40 mg, 80 mg*	

CONSULTATION/REFERRAL

- Refer to cardiologist/emergency department for initial symptoms or symptoms which increase in intensity, severity, duration
- For suspected myocardial infarction, give aspirin and transfer to nearest emergency facility

FOLLOW-UP

- Depends on frequency and severity of symptoms
- Patients with stable angina should be clinically assessed every 4-6 months for the first year; then at least annually and for any change in symptoms

EXPECTED COURSE

- Depends on severity of disease, age, gender, and left ventricular function

POSSIBLE COMPLICATIONS

- Myocardial infarction
- Chronic heart failure
- Arrhythmias
- Cardiac arrest
- Death

ACUTE CORONARY SYNDROME (ACS)

DESCRIPTION

A set of closely related disorders resulting in atheromatous plaque disruption within the coronary arteries and subsequent intravascular clot formation. Myocardial ischemia results that are sufficient to cause damage to the cardiac musculature.

ACS CLASSIFICATIONS
Unstable angina (UA)
Non-ST segment MI (NSTEMI)
ST segment MI (STEMI)

ETIOLOGY

- Coronary thrombosis (plaque rupture)
- Coronary artery vasospasm

INCIDENCE

- 1.8 million hospital admissions annually
- Males > Females under age 70 years; then Males = Females

RISK FACTORS

- Family history of premature CAD (prior to age 60 years)
- Hyperlipidemia
- Age (men over 40 and post-menopausal women)
- Cigarette smoking
- Hypertension
- Sedentary lifestyle
- Diabetes mellitus
- Stressful lifestyle

ASSESSMENT FINDINGS

- Ache, pain, tightness, discomfort, or pressure in chest, arm(s), jaw, teeth, epigastrium or neck usually lasting longer than 20 minutes; often unrelieved by nitroglycerin
- Escalating severity of angina
- Nausea, vomiting, diaphoresis
- Weakness, syncope
- Feeling of impending doom
- Hypertension/hypotension
- Silent (occurs about 20% of the time in diabetics, women, the elderly)

DIFFERENTIAL DIAGNOSIS

- Esophageal spasm
- Gastritis
- Pericarditis
- Costochondritis
- Pulmonary emboli
- Anxiety

DIAGNOSTIC STUDIES

- Troponin I: detectable 3-6 hrs after MI (if negative, consider repeating at 8-12 hours), peaks at 16 hrs, declining levels over 9-10 days (best marker of cardiac damage, more sensitive and specific than CK MB)
- Electrocardiogram: may show elevation/depression ST segment; presence of Q waves
- CK-MB isoenzymes: presence in serum indicative of myocardial infarction
- Coagulation studies: PT & INR
- Chest x-ray: helps identify cardiomegaly, CHF, and pulmonary diseases which may mimic or exacerbate cardiac disease
- Angiography: demonstrates narrowed coronary artery by atherosclerotic lesion
- Echocardiogram: 2D and M mode
- Others: CBC, glucose, metabolic and lipid panels, TSH, and as indicated by history

PREVENTION

- Modify coronary artery disease risk factors
- Consumption of low fat diet
- Smoking cessation
- Regular, aerobic exercise
- Stress reduction/management
- Aspirin daily
-

NONPHARMACOLOGIC MANAGEMENT

- Re-establish coronary perfusion via angiographic/surgical means ASAP
- Low sodium, low fat diet
- Patient education regarding disease, treatment, lifestyle changes, medications
  - ◊ Anticoagulants/antiplatelets: precautions for bleeding
  - ◊ "Cardiac cocktail" (ACEI, ASA, beta blocker, statin)
  - ◊ Blood pressure lowering
  - ◊ Lipid-lowering medications: GI side effects of nausea, vomiting and diarrhea

PHARMACOLOGIC MANAGEMENT

- Acute Phase:
  - ◊ Intravenous thrombolytic drugs
  - ◊ Heparin, aspirin, other anticoagulants
  - ◊ Nitrates
  - ◊ β-blockers
  - ◊ Antiarrhythmics
  - ◊ Oxygen
  - ◊ Analgesics
- Post-MI:
  - ◊ β-blockers or calcium channel blockers
  - ◊ ACE inhibitors
  - ◊ "Statins" and/or fibrates or niacin for lipid abnormalities
  - ◊ Nitrates as needed
  - ◊ Anticoagulants/antiplatelets

POST-MI PHARMACOLOGIC MANAGEMENT

Combinations of these (ACE inhibitors, aspirin, B-blocker and statin) have shown to reduce adverse ischemic events in patients with previous MI.

Class	Drug Generic name (Trade name®)	Dosage How supplied	Comments
Nitrates *Most effective therapy for acute angina. Produces arterial and venous dilation by relaxing vascular smooth muscle* **General comments** Patients may develop tolerance; therefore, a nitrate free period should be considered May produce headaches Monitor for hypotension episodes or palpitations	**nitroglycerin**	**Acute Anginal Pain** **Adult:** *Initial*: 1 sublingual at onset; may repeat in 5 minutes. *Max*: 3 sublingual tabs over 15 minutes **-OR-** **Adult:** *Initial*: 1-2 sprays at onset; may repeat in 5 minutes *Max*: 3 sprays over 15 minutes **Prophylaxis of Angina Topical Patches** **Adult:** *Initial*: 0.2-0.4 mg/hr patch worn daily for up to 12 hours, then removed *Max*: 0.8 mg/hr patch worn daily for up to 12 hours, then removed **Prophylaxis of Angina Topical Ointment** **Adult:** *Initial*: ½ inch in AM and repeat in 6 hours *Max*: 2 inches in AM and repeat in 6 hours	• Pregnancy Category C • **ACUTE ANGINAL PAIN unrelieved after 15 minutes warrants additional follow up and evaluation in emergency care setting** • Individualize therapy for prophylaxis, advance as tolerated • Advise patients of potential for headaches, postural hypotension • Male patients should avoid concomitant use of erectile dysfunction products • Avoid abrupt cessation of prophylaxis use products • Sublingual spray may be used prior to activity with exertion
	Nitrostat (sublingual route)	*Tabs: 0.3 mg, 0.4 mg, 0.6 mg*	
	Nitrolingual (translingual spray)	*Spray: 0.4 mg/spray*	
	Nitro-Dur (topical patch)	*Patch: 0.1 mg/hr, 0.2 mg/hr, 0.3 mg/hr, 0.4 mg/hr, 0.6 mg/hr, 0.8 mg/hr*	
	Nitro-Bid (topical ointment)	*Oint: 15 mg/inch*	

continued

POST-MI PHARMACOLOGIC MANAGEMENT

Combinations of these (ACE inhibitors, aspirin, B-blocker and statin) have shown to reduce adverse ischemic events in patients with previous MI.

Class	Drug Generic name (Trade name®)	Dosage How supplied	Comments
Angiotensin Converting Enzyme Inhibitors (ACEI) *Inhibit the action of angiotensin converting enzyme (ACE) which is responsible for conversion of angiotensin I to angiotensin II; Angiotensin II causes vasoconstriction & sodium retention. Prevents breakdown of bradykinin.* First line agent End in "pril" Dry cough is common side effect; monitor for first dose hypotension, hyperkalemia, acute renal failure Angioedema is rare but more common in African-Americans Monitor for renal failure and worsening chronic heart failure Preferred in patients with diabetes and CHF Avoid use in patients with bilateral renal artery stenosis	**captopril**	**For Patients NOT on Diuretics** **Adult**: *Initial*: 25 mg two or three times/day *Usual*: 20-40 mg/day *Max*: 450 mg/day **Children**: not recommended	• Pregnancy Category D • Take 1 hour before meals and with diuretics • Adjust dose after 2 weeks to 50 mg three times/day
		For Patients On Diuretics *Initial*: 6.25-12.5 mg two or three times/day *Usual*: 25-150 mg two or three times/day *Max*: 450 mg/day	• Patient must be under close supervision if on diuretic; can increase catopril to 100 mg two or three times/day
		For Patients with Renal Impairment (Glomerular Filtration < 30mL) *Initial*: 6.25-12.5 mg two or three times/day	
	Capoten	*Tabs: 12.5 mg, 25 mg, 50 mg, 100 mg*	
	lisinopril	**For Patients NOT on Diuretics** **Adult**: *Initial*: 10 mg/day *Usual*: 20-40 mg/day *Max*: 80 mg/day **Children:≥ 6 yrs:** *Initial:* 0.07 mg/kg *Usual*: same as initial *Max*: 0.61 mg/kg - do not exceed max adult dose	• Pregnancy Category D • Recommend holding diuretics 3 days prior to starting, if appropriate for patient • Doses at 80 mg may not produce significantly greater effect compared to 40 mg

continued

POST-MI PHARMACOLOGIC MANAGEMENT

Combinations of these (ACE inhibitors, aspirin, B-blocker and statin) have shown to reduce adverse ischemic events in patients with previous MI.

Class	Drug Generic name (Trade name®)	Dosage How supplied	Comments
		For Patients on Diuretics **OR** **For Patients with Renal Impairment (Glomerular Filtration < 30mL)** **Adult:** *Initial*: 2.5 mg/day *Usual*: 2.5-5 mg/day *Max*: 5 mg/day **Children**: not recommended	
	Prinivil Zestril	*Tabs: 2.5 mg, 5 mg, 10 mg, 20 mg, 40 mg*	
	ramipril	**For Patients NOT on Diuretics** **Adult**: *Initial*: 2.5 mg/day for 7 days; 5 mg/day for 21 days; then 10 mg/day *Usual*: 2.5-20 mg/day (either as single or two dose doses) *Max*: 20 mg/day **Children**: not recommended **For Patients on Diuretics** **OR** **For Patients with Renal Impairment (Cr Cl < 40 mL/min)** *Initial*: 1.25 mg/day for 7 days; 2.5 mg/day for 21 days; then 5 mg/day *Usual*: 2.5-5 mg/day (either as single or two doses) *Max*: 5 mg/day	• Pregnancy Category D • Requires initial titration of dosage schedule • May increase lithium levels
	Altace	*Caps: 1.25 mg, 2.5 mg, 5 mg, 10 mg* *Tabs: 1.25 mg, 2.5 mg, 5 mg, 10 mg*	

continued

POST-MI PHARMACOLOGIC MANAGEMENT

Combinations of these (ACE inhibitors, aspirin, B-blocker and statin) have shown to reduce adverse ischemic events in patients with previous MI.

Class	Drug Generic name (Trade name®)	Dosage How supplied	Comments
Cardio-selective β-Blockers *Decrease sympathetic stimulation by β-blockade in the heart* **General comments** Consider post-MI, in CHF, ischemic heart disease Should be avoided (or used cautiously) in patients with airway disease, heart block Should be used with caution in diabetics (may mask the symptoms of hypoglycemia) and in those with peripheral vascular disease May cause exercise intolerance	**atenolol**	**Adult**: *Initial* 50 mg/day *Usual*: 50-100 mg/day *Max*: 200 mg/day **Children**: not recommended **Elderly or Patients with Renal Impairment** **Cr Cl 15-35 mL/min** *Initial*: 25 mg/day *Max*: 50 mg/day **Cr Cl < 15 mL/min** *Initial*: 25 mg/day *Max*: 25 mg/day	• Pregnancy Category D • **DO NOT ABRUPTLY STOP DRUG** • May titrate dose upwards after 1 week • Patients on dialysis should be monitored under hospital supervision for dosages given post treatment
	Tenormin	*Tabs: 25 mg, 50 mg, 100 mg*	
	metoprolol succinate, extended release	**Adult**: *Initial:* 100 mg/day *Usual:* 100-400 mg/day *Max*: 400 mg/day **Children**: not recommended	• Pregnancy Category C • **DO NOT ABRUPTLY STOP DRUG; must be tapered over 2 weeks** • **NOTE different dosage forms** • Individualize for patient effect • Advance dosage at weekly intervals
	Lopressor	*Ext. Rel. Tabs: 25 mg, 50 mg, 100 mg, 200 mg*	
	Toprol-XL	*Ext. Rel. Tabs: 25 mg, 50 mg, 100 mg, 200 mg*	
	metoprolol tartrate	**Adult**: *Initial:* 100 mg/day (single or divided dose) *Usual:* 100-400 mg/day (single or divided dose) *Max:* 400 mg/day (single or divided dose) **Children**: not recommended	• Pregnancy Category C • **DO NOT ABRUPTLY STOP DRUG; must be tapered over 2 weeks** • **NOTE different dosage forms** • Individualize for patient effect • Advance dosage at weekly intervals • **Should be given with meals**

continued

POST-MI PHARMACOLOGIC MANAGEMENT

Combinations of these (ACE inhibitors, aspirin, B-blocker and statin) have shown to reduce adverse ischemic events in patients with previous MI.

Class	Drug Generic name (Trade name®)	Dosage How supplied	Comments
	Lopressor	*Tabs: 25 mg, 50 mg* *100 mg, 200 mg*	
	Toprol	*Tabs: 25 mg, 50 mg* *100 mg, 200 mg*	
Non-Cardioselective β-blockers *Block stimulation of both β1 (heart) and β2 (lungs) receptors causing decreased heart rate, blood pressure, and cardiac output (β1) as well as decreased central motor activity, inhibition of renin release from the kidneys, reduction of norepinephrine from neurons, and mild bronchoconstriction (β2)* **General comments**	**nadolol**	**Adult**: *Initial*: 20-40 mg/day *Usual*: 40-80 mg/day *Max*: 160-240 mg/day **Children**: not recommended **Special Dosing Schedule in Renal Impairment** *Initial*: 20 mg **Cr Cl > 50**: 24 hours **Cr Cl 31-50**: 24-36 hours **Cr Cl 10-30**: 24-48 hours **Cr Cl < 10**: 40-60 hours	• Pregnancy Category C • **DO NOT ABRUPTLY STOP DRUG; may take 2 weeks to withdraw drug while patient undergoes close monitoring** • Individualize therapy • May be taken without regard to meals • Note dosing schedule for renal dysfunction
End in "lol"	Corgard	*Tabs: 20 mg, 40 mg, 80 mg, 120 mg, 160 mg*	
Contraindicated in patients with bronchoconstrictive disease (i.e,, asthma, COPD, etc.)	Visken	*Tabs: 5 mg, 10 mg*	
Cautious use in diabetics because of masking signs and symptoms of hypoglycemia (tachycardia, blood pressure changes) Nonspecific β-blockade helpful in patients with tremors, anxiety and migraine headaches	**propranolol**	**Immediate Release** **Adult**: *Initial*: 10-20 mg (divided into 2 or 3 doses/day) *Usual*: 160-240 mg/day (divided into 2 or 3 doses/day) *Max*: 320 mg/day (divided into 2 or 3 doses/day) **Extended Release** **Adult**: *Initial*: 80 mg/day *Usual*: 160-240 mg/day *Max*: 640 mg/day	• Pregnancy Category C • **DO NOT ABRUPTLY STOP DRUG; withdraw product over several weeks** • **Ext. Release form has different kinetics, CANNOT switch between dosage forms on a 1:1 mg basis** • Titrate for effective; titration may vary from a few days to several weeks • Do not crush or chew tablets • Contraindicated with thioridazine
	Inderal	*Tabs: 10 mg, 20 mg, 40 mg, 60 mg, 80 mg*	
	Inderal LA	*Ext. Rel. Caps: 60 mg, 80 mg, 120 mg, 160 mg*	

continued

POST-MI PHARMACOLOGIC MANAGEMENT

Combinations of these (ACE inhibitors, aspirin, B-blocker and statin) have shown to reduce adverse ischemic events in patients with previous MI.

Class	Drug Generic name (Trade name®)	Dosage How supplied	Comments
Calcium Channel Blockers Dihydropyridine (DHP) *Inhibit movement of calcium ions across the cell membrane and vascular smooth muscle which depress myocardial contractility and increase cardiac blood flow* <u>General comments</u> End in suffix "pine" Does not cause bradycardia Monitor for hypotension and worsening of CHF, ankle edema Good choice in diabetics with proteinuria, patients with ISH (isolated systolic hypertension) for migraine prophylaxis and in patients with stable angina Serious drug interatctions with grapefruit juice Long acting DHP calcium channel blockers preferred for isolated systolic hypertension	**amlodipine besylate**	**Adult**: *Initial*: 5 mg/day *Usual*: 5-10 mg/day *Max*: 10 mg/day **Elderly, renal or hepatic patients:** *Initial*: 2.5 mg/day	• Pregnancy Category C • Titrate for effect; increase doses at 7-14 day intervals; must reassess patient after each titration
	Norvasc	*Tabs: 2.5 mg, 5 mg, 10 mg*	
	felodipine	**Adult**: *Initial*: 2.5-5 mg/day *Usual*: 2.5-10 mg/day *Max*: 10 mg/day **Elderly or hepatic patients:** *Initial*: 2.5 mg/day **Children**: not recommended	• Pregnancy Category C • Titrate to symptoms; increase dose after minimum of 2 week interval • Do not crush or chew tablets • Bioavailability affected by meals; should take on empty stomach
	Plendil	*Ext. Rel. Tabs: 2.5 mg, 5 mg, 10 mg*	
	nifedipine	<u>**Immediate Release**</u> **Adult**: *Initial*: 10 mg three times/day *Usual*: 10-20 mg three times/day *Max*: 120 mg/day <u>**Extended Release**</u> *Initial*: 30-60 mg/day *Usual*: 30-60 mg/day *Max*: 90 mg/day **Children**: not recommended	• Pregnancy Category C • Individualize treatment; advance doses at 1-2 week intervals • Take on empty stomach • Do not crush or chew extended release formulations • Must be withdrawn slowly if discontinued • If moving from immediate release to extended release, use nearest equivalency
	Procardia (immediate release)	*Caps: 10 mg, 20 mg*	
	Procardia XL (extended release)	*Ext. Rel. Tabs: 30 mg, 60 mg, 90 mg*	

continued

POST-MI PHARMACOLOGIC MANAGEMENT

Combinations of these (ACE inhibitors, aspirin, B-blocker and statin) have shown to reduce adverse ischemic events in patients with previous MI.

Class	Drug Generic name (Trade name®)	Dosage How supplied	Comments
Calcium Channel Blockers: Non-Dihydropyridine (Non-DHP) *Inhibit movement of calcium ions across the cell membrane and vascular smooth muscle which depress myocardial contractility and increase cardiac blood flow* **General comments** Watch for conduction defects Decreases heart rate Use cautiously or avoid with use of β-blockers Monitor for worsening of CHF, hypotension, bradycardia, constipation Consider in patients with atrial fibrillation with rapid ventricular response, in patients with angina, and in diabetics with proteinuria Serious drug interactions with grapefruit juice	**diltiazem**	**Immediate Release** **Adult**: *Initial:* 30 mg four times/day *Usual:* 180-360 mg/day *Max:* 360 mg/day* **Children**: not recommended **Extended Release** **Adult**: *Initial:* 120-180 mg/day *Usual:* 240-360 mg/day *Max:* 360-480 mg/day* **See specific drug manufacturer for maximum dose limits*	• Pregnancy Category C • Available in multiple formulations (tablets and capsules) and strengths • Individualize therapy; titrate immediate release at 1-2 DAY intervals; titrate extended release at 1-2 WEEK intervals • Start with lowest dose possible, especially in elderly • Do not crush or chew • Incidence of side effects increases with dose increases
	Cardizem	*Tabs: 30 mg, 60 mg, 90 mg, 120 mg*	
	Cardizem LA	*Ext. Rel. Tabs: 120 mg, 180 mg, 240 mg, 300 mg, 360 mg, 420 mg*	
	Cardizem CD	*Ext. Rel. Caps: 120 mg, 180 mg, 240 mg, 300 mg, 360 mg*	
	Dilacor XR	*Ext. Rel. Caps: 120 mg, 180 mg, 240 mg*	
	Tiazac	*Ext. Rel. Caps: 120 mg, 180 mg, 240 mg, 300 mg, 360 mg, 420 mg*	
	verapamil	**Immediate Release** **Adult**: *Initial*: 80-120 mg three times/day *Usual*: 80-120 mg three times/day *Max*: 120 mg three times/day*	• Pregnancy Category C • Use extended release formulations for HTN control • Available in multiple formulations (tablets and capsules) and strengths. Refer to specific product for additional guidelines • Individualize therapy; titrate at bi-weekly intervals • **Elderly or small stature people may require lower starting dose**

continued

POST-MI PHARMACOLOGIC MANAGEMENT

Combinations of these (ACE inhibitors, aspirin, B-blocker and statin) have shown to reduce adverse ischemic events in patients with previous MI.

Class	Drug Generic name (Trade name®)	Dosage How supplied	Comments
		Renal Impairment *Initial*: 40 mg three times/day *Usual*: 80-120 mg three times/day *Max*: 120 mg three times/day* **Children**: not recommended **Extended Release** **Adult:** *Initial*: 180 mg/day *Usual*: 240-360 mg/day *Max*: 360-480 mg/day* *Refer to specific product for additional guidelines	
	Calan (immediate release)	*Tabs: 40 mg, 80 mg, 120 mg*	
	Covera HS (Give at bedtime)	*Ext. Rel. Tabs: 120 mg, 240 mg*	
Aspirin *Prevents platelet aggregation and exerts anti-inflammatory effect in vessels by inhibiting prostaglandin synthesis* **General comments** Observe for bleeding, tinnitus, gastric irritation Reduces morbidity and mortality for CV events	**acetylsalicylic acid (ASA)**	**Prophylaxis** **Adult**: *Initial*: 81 mg/day *Max*: 325 mg/day **Post Myocardial Infarction** *Initial*: 162-325 mg/day *Usual*: 75-162 mg/day *Max*: 325 mg/day	• Pregnancy Category D • Use in caution with patients with reactive airway disease (asthma) • Consider enteric coated in patients with prior gastric irritation • Avoid in patients with NSAID allergies • May need to reduce dose in severe hepatic or renal dysfunction
	Various generics	*Tabs: 81 mg, 162 mg, 325 mg* *Caplets: 81 mg, 325 mg* *Gelcaps: 325 mg*	

continued

POST-MI PHARMACOLOGIC MANAGEMENT

Combinations of these (ACE inhibitors, aspirin, B-blocker and statin) have shown to reduce adverse ischemic events in patients with previous MI.

Class	Drug Generic name (Trade name®)	Dosage How supplied	Comments
HMG-CoA Reductase Inhibitors ("Statins") *Inhibit HMG-CoA, the enzyme which is partly responsible for cholesterol synthesis; decrease total cholesterol, LDL, minimal increase in HDL* **General comments** Considered first line therapy Perform liver function tests before initiating therapy, at 4-6 and 12 wks, and after each dose increase, then periodically, or per manufacturer's recommendations To be used in conjunction with diet, exercise, & weight reduction in overweight patients Watch for myopathy, rhabdomyolysis Watch for drug interactions, especially with grapefruit juice and lovastatin, simvastatin, and atorvastatin Pregnancy Category X	**atorvastatin**	**LDL-C reduction < 45%** **Adult**: *Initial*: 10 or 20 mg/day *Usual*: 10-80 mg/day *Max*: 80 mg/day **LDL-C reduction > 45%** *Initial*: 40 mg/day *Usual*: 40-80 mg/day *Max*: 80 mg/day **Heterozygous Familial Hypercholesterolemia** **Children < 10 yrs:** not recommended **10-17 yrs:** *Initial*: 10 mg/day *Usual*: 10 mg/day *Max*: 20 mg/day	• If concomitant use with gembibrozil, the maximum dose should not exceed 10 mg/day • If concomitant use with clarithromycin, itraconazole, or protease inhibitors, the maximum dose should not exceed 20 mg/day
	Lipitor	*Tabs: 10 mg, 20 mg, 40 mg, 80 mg*	
	fluvastatin	**LDL-C reduction < 25%** **Adult:** *Initial*: 20 mg in evening *Usual*: 20-80 mg/day *Max*: 80 mg/day **LDL-C reduction > 25%** **Adult:** *Initial*: Lescol XL 80 mg in PM or 40 mg Lescol daily or twice daily *Usual*: 80 mg/day *Max*: 80 mg/day **Children**: not recommended	• Avoid in patients with substantial alcohol consumption • Avoid concomitant fibrates, cyclosporine • May be taken without regard to meals
	Lescol Lescol XL	*Tabs: 20 mg, 40 mg* *Ext. Rel. Tabs: 80 mg*	

continued

POST-MI PHARMACOLOGIC MANAGEMENT

Combinations of these (ACE inhibitors, aspirin, B-blocker and statin) have shown to reduce adverse ischemic events in patients with previous MI.

Class	Drug Generic name (Trade name®)	Dosage How supplied	Comments
	lovastatin	**<u>Cr Cl > 30 mL/min</u>** **Adult**: *Initial*: 10-20 mg (evening) *Usual*: 10-80 mg/day in single or divided doses *Max*: 80 mg/day (single or divided dose) **<u>Cr Cl < 30 mL/min</u>** **Adult**: *Initial*: 10-20 mg/day *Usual*: 10-20 mg/day *Max*: 20 mg/day **<u>Heterozygous Familial Hypercholesterolemia</u>** **Children < 10 yrs:** not recommended **10-17 yrs:** *Initial*: 10-20 mg/day *Usual*: 10-40 mg/day *Max*: 40 mg/day	• Take with evening meal • Patients on amiodarone or verapamil should not exceed 40 mg/day • Start with lower doses if patient on cyclosporin or danazol; do not exceed 20 mg/day • For patients on fibrates or high-dose niacin, do not exceed 20 mg/day
	Mevacor Altocor	*Tabs: 10 mg, 20 mg, 40 mg*	
	pravastatin	**<u>Normal Renal/Hepatic Function</u>** **Adult**: *Initial*: 10 mg/day *Usual*: 20-40 mg/day *Max*: 80 mg/day **Children < 8 yrs:** not recommended **8-13 yrs:** 20 mg/daily **14-18 yrs:** 40 mg/daily **<u>Impaired Renal/Hepatic Function</u>** **Adult**: *Initial*: 10 mg/day *Usual*: 20 mg/day *Max*: 20 mg/day	• May adjust dose after 4 weeks • Take at bedtime
	Pravachol	*Tabs: 10 mg, 20 mg, 40 mg, 80 mg*	

continued

POST-MI PHARMACOLOGIC MANAGEMENT

Combinations of these (ACE inhibitors, aspirin, B-blocker and statin) have shown to reduce adverse ischemic events in patients with previous MI.

Class	Drug Generic name (Trade name®)	Dosage How supplied	Comments
	rosuvastatin	**Cr Cl > 30 mL/min** **Adult**: *Initial*: 10 mg/day *Usual*: 5-20 mg/day *Max*: 40 mg/day **Cr Cl < 30 mL/min** **Adult:** *Initial*: 5 mg/day *Max*: 10 mg/day **Heterozygous Familial Hypercholesterolemia** **Children < 10 yrs:** not recommended **10-17 yrs:** *Initial*: 5-10 mg/day *Usual*: 5-20 mg/day *Max*: 20 mg/day	• May be taken without regard to meals • Maximum dose is reserved only for patients who do not achieve LDL-C goal • In Asian patients, initiate therapy at 5 mg /day • In patients taking cyclosporine, the maximum dose is 5 mg/day • In patients taking anti-viral agents, the maximum dose is 10 mg/day
	Crestor	*Tabs: 5 mg, 10 mg, 20 mg, 40 mg*	
	simvastatin	**Normal risk of CHD event** **Adult**: *Initial*: 20-40 mg/HS *Usual*: 5-80 mg/HS *Max*: 80 mg/HS **High risk of CHD event** **Adult:** *Initial*: 40 mg/HS *Usual*: 40-80 mg/HS *Max*: 80 mg/HS **Heterozygous Familial Hypercholesterolemia** **Children < 10 yrs:** not recommended **10-17 yrs:** *Initial*: 10 mg/HS *Usual*: 10-40 mg/HS *Max*: 40 mg/HS	• Dosage adjustments should be determined at intervals of 4 weeks or more • If concomitant use with gembibrozil, the maximum dose of simvastatin should not exceed 10 mg/day • Start with lower doses if patient on cyclosporin or danazol; do not exceed 10 mg/day • Patients on amiodarone or verapamil should not exceed 20 mg/day • Patients on diltiazem should not exceed 40 mg/day
	Zocor	*Tabs: 5 mg, 10 mg, 20 mg, 40 mg, 80 mg*	

CONSULTATION/REFERRAL

- Immediate referral to nearest emergency department (give aspirin stat, O_2, nitroglycerin, and transport)

FOLLOW-UP

- Per cardiologist
- Encourage participation in cardiac rehab program

EXPECTED COURSE

- Dependent on severity, underlying coronary artery disease, age, response time to emergency facility

POSSIBLE COMPLICATIONS

- Death
- Chronic heart failure
- Dysrhythmias
- Left ventricular aneurysm, thrombus
- DVT, pulmonary embolism
- Mitral regurgitation
- Ventricular rupture
- Acute mitral regurgitation

VARICOSE VEINS

DESCRIPTION

Veins in which valves become incompetent and allow blood flow in the reverse direction resulting in dilated, tortuous, elongated veins

ETIOLOGY

- Faulty valves at the saphenofemoral junction (valvular reflux)
- Previous deep venous thrombophlebitis (DVT)
- Pregnancy
- Obesity
- Prolonged standing
- Ascites

INCIDENCE

- Females > Males (5:1)
- 20% of U.S. adults

RISK FACTORS

- Female gender
- Prolonged standing
- Pregnancy
- Family history
- Constrictive garments (e.g., girdles, knee-high stockings)

ASSESSMENT FINDINGS

- Leg aching/burning/cramping/itching
- Fatigue
- Orthostatic edema
- Visibly dilated and tortuous veins in lower extremities
- Symptoms may be worse during menses or at end of day

DIFFERENTIAL DIAGNOSIS

- Peripheral neuritis (diabetic or alcoholic neuropathy)
- Lumbar nerve root compression or irritation
- Deep vein thrombosis
- Osteoarthritis of the hip
- Arterial insufficiency

DIAGNOSTIC STUDIES

- Usually none except inspection
- Trendelenburg test: demonstrates retrograde blood flow past incompetent saphenous valves (leg is lifted above level of heart to empty vein, then leg is quickly lowered to observe refilling; the more quickly the veins refill, the more likely severe disease)
- Duplex ultrasound, venous Doppler study

PREVENTION

- Leg elevation when symptomatic
- Support hose
- Avoid restrictive clothing (e.g., knee-high stockings, girdles)

NONPHARMACOLOGIC MANAGEMENT

- Support hose (best if applied before getting out of bed)
- Avoid long periods of standing in one place
- Surgical ligation and stripping
- Endovenous saphenous vein obliteration (shorter recovery time than ligation and stripping)
- Weight loss if obese
- Patient education regarding standing, use of support hose, etc.

PHARMACOLOGIC MANAGEMENT

- Usually none unless sclerotherapy is used (sclerosant is injected into intracapillary region)

PREGNANCY/LACTATION CONSIDERATIONS

- Support hose recommended
- Nonpharmacologic management as described above

CONSULATION/REFERRAL

- Usually none needed
- Surgeon for recurrent, painful varicosities

FOLLOW-UP

- Usually none needed except to reinforce patient education

POSSIBLE COMPLICATIONS

- Edema
- Venous stasis ulcers
- Pigmentation
- Phlebitis

DEEP VEIN THROMBOPHLEBITIS
(DVT)

DESCRIPTION

The presence of blood clot(s) in the venous system of the extremities or the pelvis which may migrate to the lung

ETIOLOGY

Hypercoagulable states	Oral contraceptive use Blood dyscrasias Malignant tumors (particularly prostate cancer) Pregnancy
Stasis	Postoperative period Postpartum Pregnancy
Trauma	Injury to the epithelium of the vein Hypercoagulability Stasis
Septic states	Especially from the placement of an indwelling catheter in a vein

INCIDENCE

- Males > Females (1.2:1)
- Mean age is 60 years
- Causes 50,000 deaths per year

RISK FACTORS

- Immobility; especially travel > 4 hours
- Malignancy
- Trauma, especially crush injuries
- Obesity
- Pregnancy with hypertension, eclampsia
- Increasing age
- Oral contraceptive use; hormone replacement therapy
- Smoking
- Postoperative status
- Placement of an indwelling catheter

ASSESSMENT FINDINGS

- Asymptomatic; especially initially

- Pain, warmth, erythema, tenderness, swelling of effected limb
- Possible swelling without tenderness of the limb
- Palpable cord over the involved vein (reflects a thrombosed vein)
- Positive Homan sign (calf pain with dorsiflexion of the foot); low sensitivity and specificity

DIFFERENTIAL DIAGNOSIS

- Muscle strain or tear
- Lymph obstruction
- Cellulitis
- Baker's cyst
- Superficial thrombophlebitis
- Venous insufficiency

DIAGNOSTIC STUDIES

- Physical exam only 30% accurate for diagnosis
- D-dimer (highly sensitive, but not specific)
- Ultrasound: inability to compress affected venous segment is diagnostic of thrombus
- Contrast venography
- CBC: elevated white count in sepsis
- PT, aPTT, INR, renal function tests
- Consider PSA in men over age 50 years (DVT often sentinel event for malignancy)

DVT CRITERIA	
Active cancer within 6 months	+1
Paralysis or immobilization of lower extremity	+1
Recent bedridden >3 days or major surgery within 4 weeks	+1
Tenderness/cord along vein	+1
Entire leg swollen	+1
Calf circumference >3 cm vs other leg	+1
Alternative diagnosis likely	-2
INTERPRETATION	
High probability	+3
Moderate probability	+1 to +2
Low probability	0

Source: Wells Criteria for DVT, 1997

PREVENTION

- Depends on etiology
- Minimize or eliminate risk factors as described above

NONPHARMACOLOGIC MANAGEMENT

- Hospitalization required for acute DVT for anticoagulation therapy (heparin or IV unfractionated heparin until patient is transitioned to warfarin)
- Filter device (umbrellas) inserted in vena cava
- Surgical removal of very large clots
- Patient education regarding disease, treatment, etc.

PHARMACOLOGIC MANAGEMENT

- Uncomplicated DVT: low molecular weight heparin
- Complicated DVT: Heparin, unfractionated heparin, or low molecular weight heparin
- Maintenance: warfarin
- Thrombolytics (second line agents)
- Antibiotics if sepsis is suspected

PREGNANCY/LACTATION CONSIDERATIONS

- Warfarin (teratogenic) contraindicated
- Heparin is a large molecule and does not cross the placenta
- Warfarin safe with breast-feeding

CONSULTATION/REFERRAL

- Refer to specialist for DVT, septic thrombophlebitis, hypercoagulable states

FOLLOW-UP

- Patient usually on oral anticoagulation therapy for 3-12 months depending on etiology
- Compression stockings capable of 30-40 mm compression worn for at least one year

EXPECTED COURSE

- Good prognosis for aseptic thrombophlebitis
- Superficial thrombophlebitis is generally not associated with DVT
- Pulmonary embolism more likely if thigh veins are involved; less likely if calf veins are involved

POSSIBLE COMPLICATIONS

- Pulmonary embolism from DVT
- Sepsis

PERIPHERAL ARTERIAL DISEASE (PAD)
(Arteriosclerosis obliterans)

DESCRIPTION

A systemic disease which leads to impedance of arterial blood flow in the lower extremities. The upper extremities can be involved, but this is not usual

ETIOLOGY

Arterial atheromatous plaques develop in vessels of the lower extremities secondary to systemic atherosclerosis

INCIDENCE

- 20% of patients older than 70 years have PAD, 5% of these patients are symptomatic
- Males > Females (2:1)

RISK FACTORS

- Cigarette smoking (a major risk factor)
- Advancing age (age > 40 years)
- Hyperlipidemia
- Hypertension
- Diabetes mellitus
- Obesity
- Family history

ASSESSMENT FINDINGS

- Intermittent claudication (earliest manifestation): pain in legs with exercise; relief with rest (usually within 2-5 minutes)
- 50% of patients with PAD are asymptomatic
- Pain, ache, cramp, or tired feeling in extremity, foot, hip, thigh, or buttocks with exercise/activity (narrowed lumen produces characteristic pain distal to site)
- Lack of hair growth on lower legs
- Thickened toenails
- Pain at rest (signifies severe disease)
- Diminished or absent pulse distal to the lesion
- Bruits in abdominal, femoral or popliteal areas
- Pale, cool extremities
- Dependent rubor (signifies severe disease)
- Prolonged capillary fill time

DIFFERENTIAL DIAGNOSIS

- Varicose veins
- Spinal stenosis
- Thromboangiitis obliterans (Buerger's Disease): seen in young, male smokers
- Lumbar disk disease
- DVT

DIAGNOSTIC STUDIES

- Gold standard is contrast angiography (MR angiography is highly sensitive for location of lesions)
- Duplex ultrasound and Doppler color-flow imaging to identify location of lesions
- Ankle-brachial index (ABI) is the ratio of the ankle systolic BP divided by the brachial systolic pressure measured by a Doppler probe
  - ◊ Normal: 0.9-1.2
  - ◊ 0.4-0.9 usually indicates claudication
  - ◊ < 0.4 usually indicates severe disease
  - ◊ Segmental blood pressure measurements if ABI abnormal: expect reduction in pressure

PREVENTION

- Eliminate/minimize risk factors as described above

NONPHARMACOLOGIC MANAGEMENT

- Lifestyle modifications for smoking cessation, improving status of diabetes, hypertension, and hyperlipidemia
- Exercise, stop when it hurts, but start again when relieved (exercise training, especially walking or bicycle riding, shown to be beneficial in symptom relief; regression of relief if exercise stopped) Recommend walking 3x weekly for 30-60 minutes; improves quality of life
- Prophylactic foot care
- Percutaneous transluminal angioplasty (PTA) for isolated, short lesions with or without stent placement
- Bypass surgery is gold standard for extensive disease
- Patient education regarding disease, treatment options, etc.

PERIPHERAL ARTERIAL DISEASE PHARMACOLOGIC MANAGEMENT

Class	Drug Generic name (Trade name®)	Dosage How supplied	Comments
Anti-platelet *Inhibits platelet aggregation and produces mild vasodilation*	**cilostazol** Pletal	**Adult**: *Initial*: 100 mg twice daily (either before meals or 2 hours after) *Usual*: 100 mg twice daily (either before meals or 2 hours after) *Max*: 100 mg twice daily (either before meals or 2 hours after) **Children**: not recommended *Tabs: 50 mg, 100 mg*	• Pregnancy Category C • Contraindicated in patients with chronic heart failure • Contraindicated in patients with hemostatic disorders • Caution in patients with hepatic or renal impairment • Reduce dose if patient takes CYP3A4 or CYP2C19 inhibitors
Blood Viscosity *Reducer mechanism is unclear but thought to reduce blood viscosity*	**pentoxifylline** Trental	**Adult**: *Initial*: 400 mg three times daily with meals *Usual*: 400 mg three times daily with meals *Max*: 400 mg three times daily with meals **Children**: not recommended *Tabs: 400 mg*	• Pregnancy Category C • If digestive or central nervous system effects seen, reduce daily dose to 800 mg • Monitor for hypotension, arrhythmias, and angina • Avoid in patients with known xanthine intolerance

To prevent claudication: pentoxifylline, cilostazol. Avoid beta blockers: may worsen claudication. Neither nitrates nor anticoagulant therapy have proven helpful.

CONSULTATION/REFERRAL

- Refer to vascular surgeon for persistent symptoms or moderate or severe ischemia
- Refer if exercise and meds have not helped after 3-6 months (75% of patients will improve on this regimen)
- Refer all nonhealing ulcers

FOLLOW-UP

- As dictated by patient condition

EXPECTED COURSE

- Mild disease may be managed conservatively
- PTA has 95% success rates in iliac vessels
- Lower rates in thigh and calf vessels
- Poor prognosis for diabetics and smokers
- High incidence of coronary disease, stroke, and CHF in patients with arteriosclerosis obliterans

POSSIBLE COMPLICATIONS

- Amputation
- Intractable pain
- Immobility
- Ischemia → necrosis → gangrene

CONGENITAL HEART DISEASE
(CHD)

DESCRIPTION

Disease of the cardiovascular system that occurs prenatally and becomes evident at birth, infancy, or young adulthood. May be cyanotic or acyanotic disorders.

ETIOLOGY

- Multifactorial and too complex to identify a specific factor

INCIDENCE

- 8-10 per 1000 births
  - ◊ 33% have critical symptoms
  - ◊ 33% have symptoms in childhood
  - ◊ 33% have no symptoms
- 8-10% of CHD is due to or associated with chromosomal abnormalities
- Overall Males > Females
- Most common CHD is ventricular septal defect (30%)
- Patent ductus arteriosus (PDA) and atrial septal defect (ASD) more common in females
- Coarctation of the aorta, tetralogy of Fallot, and transposition of the great vessels are more common in males

RISK FACTORS

- Family history
- Premature birth
- Maternal exposure to alcohol, coxsackie B, cytomegalovirus, influenza, isotretinoin, lithium, mumps, rubella, thalidomide, x-ray exposure during pregnancy, or other substances
- Associated with some chromosomal abnormalities (trisomy 21, 13, 18)
- Maternal age over 40 years
- Prenatal or perinatal fetal distress
- CHD in other siblings

TYPES OF CONGENITAL HEART DISEASE	
Acyanotic diseases	Atrial septal defect (ASD) Atrioventricular septal defect Ventricular septal defect (VSD) Patent ductus arteriosus (PDA)
Cyanotic diseases	Transposition of the great vessels (arteries) Tetralogy of Fallot Tricuspid atresia
Obstructive lesions	Aortic stenosis Pulmonic stenosis Coarctation of the aorta

ASSESSMENT FINDINGS

SUMMARY OF MURMURS		
Murmur	Timing	Characteristics
Atrial septal defect (ASD)	Mid-systolic ejection	Asymptomatic early in life Accentuation of tricuspid valve closure Wide, fixed S2 Arterial pulses = bilaterally Grade I-III/VI harsh Easy fatigability Prone to respiratory infections May have delayed growth and development

continued

SUMMARY OF MURMURS		
Murmur	Timing	Characteristics
Atrioventricular septal defect	Systolic and mid-diastolic	Frequent respiratory infections Delayed growth and development, poor weight gain Widely split S_2 Usually diagnosed in first year of life; often associated with trisomy 21
Ventricular septal defect (VSD)	Holosystolic	Frequent respiratory symptoms Easy fatigability Delayed growth and development; poor weight gain Chronic heart failure frequently present; S_3 audible Grade II-VI/VI murmur depending on severity Palpable left sternal border thrill
Patent ductus arteriosus (PDA)	Systolic and diastolic	Poor weight gain Diaphoretic during feedings May present as soft, localized at left clavicle Murmur progresses to harsh, continuous, rumbling murmur Bounding pulses
Transposition of the great arteries	Systolic and diastolic	Cyanosis Chronic heart failure (CHF) Large for gestational age, but delayed growth and development
Tetralogy of Fallot	Systolic ejection	Cynaosis CHF "Tet" spells; cyanotic episodes precipitation by crying, feeding, other activities Poor growth and development Squatting after exertion Easy fatigability Pale skin, poor turgor, clubbing Grade III-VI/VI harsh, murmur at 2nd ICS, left sternal border, with a thrill
Tricuspid atresia	Holosystolic	Cyanosis Tachycardia Grade III-VI/VI harsh, murmur at left sternal border Poor growth, development, poor feeding, easy fatigability
Aortic stenosis	Systolic ejection	Grade III or IV/VI harsh murmur at upper right sternal border, right neck, apex Weak peripheral pulses Easy fatigability CHF
Pulmonic stenosis	Mid to late systolic ejection	Cyanosis CHF Grade III-IV/VI harsh, murmur heard at the upper left sternal border, transmission into both lungs, left neck
Coarctation of the aorta	Systolic	Decreased blood pressure in lower extremities (upper extremity hypertension, lower extremity hypotension) Diminished pulses in lower extremities compared to upper extremities

DIFFERENTIAL DIAGNOSIS

- Innocent heart murmur
- Pulmonary disease
- Cyanotic vs. acyanotic disease
- Metabolic abnormalities
- Thyrotoxicosis
- Dysrhythmias

DIAGNOSTIC STUDIES

- Chest x-ray
- Electrocardiogram
- Echocardiogram
- Arterial blood gases
- Angiographic studies

PREVENTION

- Elimination of maternal risk factors when possible

NONPHARMACOLOGIC MANAGEMENT

- Depends on severity
- Activity restriction
- Surgical repair
- Patient/family education regarding disease, treatment, prognosis, etc.

PHARMACOLOGIC MANAGEMENT

- PDA: indomethacin (Indocin®) helps constrict and close PDA. Administered during neonatal period
- Transposition of the great arteries: prostaglandin E1 to delay closure of the ductus until surgery

CONSULTATION/REFERRAL

- Innocent murmurs need no referral
- Refer to cardiologist all murmurs which are not innocent

FOLLOW-UP

- Depends on severity, age, and type of defect
- Careful attention to murmur at each visit; consider referral to pediatric cardiologist for changes in murmur

EXPECTED COURSE

- Many congenital heart defects are amenable to surgery
- Depending on severity, many may be medically managed
- Small VSD may close spontaneously during childhood

POSSIBLE COMPLICATIONS

- Cyanosis with hypoxemia
- Delayed growth and development
- Shortened lifespan
- Death

HEART MURMURS

DESCRIPTION

The sound detected when there is turbulent blood flow through the heart or the great vessels.

ETIOLOGY

Organic	Due to cardiovascular disease
Functional	Disturbances produced within the cardiovascular system but which are due to other causes (e.g., anemia, thyrotoxicosis, pregnancy)
Innocent Murmurs	Disturbances which may or may not be cardiac in origin, but no cardiac disease is recognized as the cause

INCIDENCE

- 30%-50% of children on random auscultation will have an innocent murmur
- True rates of congenital and acquired murmurs are unknown
- Systolic murmurs during the 3rd trimester of pregnancy are very common

RISK FACTORS

- Age (very common in children, elderly)
- Fever
- Anemia
- Pregnancy
- Thyrotoxicosis
- Hypertension
- Rigid carotid arteries
- Myocardial infarction
- Atrial tumor or thrombus (usually causes "tumor flop")
- Congenital heart disease
- Valvular disease

ASSESSMENT OF MURMURS

Timing	Systolic or diastolic, position in systole or diastole (early, mid, late, pan)
Site	Point of maximal intensity, point of propagation
Loudness	(see Grading of Murmurs)
Quality	Blowing, harsh, musical, soft
Shape	Decrescendo, crescendo, plateau, diamond

GRADING OF MURMURS

Grade 1	Barely audible with intense concentration
Grade 2	Faint, but audible immediately
Grade 3	Moderately loud, no thrill palpable
Grade 4	Loud with a palpable thrill
Grade 5	Very loud, audible with part of the stethoscope off the chest, thrill palpable
Grade 6	Audible without a stethoscope on the chest wall, thrill palpable

ASSESSMENT FINDINGS

Summary of Innocent Murmurs:

- *Still's Venous Hum*
  - ◊ Most frequently detected in children and adolescents
  - ◊ Soft, short, systolic, no other evidence of abnormality
- *Systolic Ejection*
  - ◊ May be musical or vibratory (e.g., Stills's)
  - ◊ Able to alter by maneuvers (e.g., standing, lying, deep respiration, posture change); diminishes when in supine position
  - ◊ Varies in loudness from visit to visit
  - ◊ Does not affect growth and development
  - ◊ Left lower sternal border (LLSB) or pulmonic area are most common sites
  - ◊ Normal S_1 and S_2, normal vital signs

SUMMARY OF SYSTOLIC MURMURS		
Murmur	**Timing**	**Characteristics**
Aortic stenosis	Systolic ejection (mid systole)	Most frequently heard in elderly patients Heard best in 2nd intercostal space (ICS) to the right of the sternum Sound radiates to right clavicle and transmitted to both carotid arteries Systolic thrill may be present
Hypertrophic obstructive cardiomyopathy (HOCM)	Late systolic	Best heard at the lower left sternal border Increases with Valsalva maneuver, standing Crescendo/decrescendo murmur Usually does not radiate to neck, but biphasic carotid pulse
Pulmonic stenosis	Mid systolic	Mitral valve prolapse may not produce murmurs (mid to late systolic cycle) Mitral regurgitation is holosystolic Best heard at apex of heart with patient in left lateral decubitus position Radiates toward left axilla Varies in intensity
Tricuspid regurgitation	Systolic	Best heard at left lower sternal border, over the xiphoid, sometimes over the liver Increases in intensity with inspiration
Mitral valve insufficiency	Systolic	Best heard at apex of heart with patient in left lateral decubitus position Radiates toward left axilla Varies in intensity
Tricuspid regurgitation	Systolic	Best heard at left lower sternal border, over the xiphoid, sometimes over the liver Increases in intensity with inspiration Regurgitant "v" waves in the neck veins
Ventricular septal defect	Holosystolic	Holosystolic murmur Best heard at left sternal border, 4th ICS Often harsh The greater the gradient, the louder the murmur

SUMMARY OF DIASTOLIC MURMURS (Always considered abnormal) (Tend to be softer than systolic murmurs. Best heard with the bell of the stethoscope because low pitched.)		
Murmur	**Timing**	**Characteristics**
Mitral stenosis	Mid-diastolic	Low-pitched apical murmur Best heard after mild exercise and patient in left lateral decubitus position May be isolated to the apex Does not radiate
Tricuspid stenosis	Early diastolic	Best heard in the 4th or 5th ICS left of the sternum, xiphoid, or apex Increased in duration and intensity by exercise, inspiration, sitting forward Decrescendo murmur
Aortic regurgitation	Early diastolic	Blowing, high-pitched, decrescendo murmur Best heard at left sternal border and toward the apex
Pulmonic regurgitation	Diastolic	High-pitched decrescendo murmur Radiates to apex Heard loudest at 2nd ICS at sternal border

SUMMARY OF CONTINUOUS MURMURS	
Examples	**Characteristics**
Patent ductus arteriosus (PDA)	Heard throughout systole and diastole Equal bounding pulses
Coarctation of the aorta	Weak femoral pulses

DIFFERENTIAL DIAGNOSIS

- Systolic vs. diastolic vs. continuous murmurs
- Pulmonary disease

DIAGNOSTIC STUDIES

- Electrocardiogram
- Chest x-ray
- Doppler echocardiography
- Angiography

PREVENTION

- Depends on etiology
- Avoidance/elimination of risk factors listed above

NONPHARMACOLOGIC MANAGEMENT

- Surgical repair (palliative)
- Patient and family education regarding disease, treatment options, etc.

PHARMACOLOGIC MANAGEMENT

- Depends on etiology

PREGNANCY/LACTATION CONSIDERATIONS

- Murmurs due to high flow state of pregnancy usually require no intervention
- Pathological murmurs present prior to pregnancy should be managed by obstetrician/cardiologist

CONSULTATION/REFERRAL

- Evaluation and follow up by cardiologist

FOLLOW-UP

- Depends on severity and etiology

EXPECTED COURSE

- Murmurs associated with pregnancy disappear when pregnancy ends (2-6 weeks after delivery)
- Innocent murmurs of childhood disappear as child matures
- Other murmurs may be managed medically or surgically depending on severity
- Consider antibiotic prophylaxis prior to dental procedures or tooth cleaning for non-innocent murmurs (specific guidelines available online American Heart Association, www.aha.org)

POSSIBLE COMPLICATIONS

- Exercise intolerance
- Chronic heart failure
- Thrombotic events
- Hypoxia

RHEUMATIC FEVER

DESCRIPTION

An inflammatory disease that develops in about 1-3% of children who have untreated infection with Group A β-streptococcal infections. This can affect the heart, joints, skin, and central nervous system.

ETIOLOGY

- Untreated Group A β-streptococcal infections of the upper airways (e.g., pharyngitis, sinusitis)

INCIDENCE

- 1-3% of untreated Streptococcal infections in U.S.; resurgence since the mid-1980s
- Most frequently occurs in 5-17 year olds
- Recurrences are common
- Males = females

RISK FACTORS

- Untreated/incompletely treated Group A β-streptococcal infections

ASSESSMENT FINDINGS

- History of pharyngitis 2-4 weeks prior to onset of symptoms
- Modified Jones criteria used to diagnose patient: 2 major or 1 major and 2 minor criteria must be present as well as evidence of recent streptococcal infection

Major Criteria

- Carditis: 65% have with murmurs
- Polyarthritis: 75%
- Chorea: 15%
- Erythema marginatum: 5% (macular rash with an erythematous border)
- Subcutaneous nodules: 5-10%

Minor Criteria

- Fever (101-104°F or 38.3-40.0°C)
- Arthralgias (cannot use if arthritis was a major criteria)
- Previous rheumatic fever
- Elevated ESR, C-reactive protein
- Prolonged PR interval demonstrated on electrocardiogram

DIFFERENTIAL DIAGNOSIS

- Streptococcal reactive arthritis
- Juvenile rheumatoid arthritis
- Systemic lupus erythematosus
- Lyme disease
- Kawasaki syndrome
- Carditis
- Huntington's chorea
- Congenital heart defects/innocent murmurs
- Septic arthritis

DIAGNOSTIC STUDIES

- Throat culture
- ESR, C-reactive protein: monitors rebounds of inflammation
- ASO titer: identifies streptococcal antibodies
- Electrocardiogram
- Chest x-ray
- CBC with differential

PREVENTION

- Prompt treatment of Group A β-streptococcal pharyngitis

NONPHARMACOLOGIC MANAGEMENT

- Supportive therapy
- Bedrest during acute episode of carditis
- Limited physical activity in patients with carditis
- Patient education regarding disease, treatment, etc.

PHARMACOLOGIC MANAGEMENT

- Treat streptococcal infection: Penicillin preferred (may use erythromycin or first-generation cephalosporin depending on severity of penicillin allergy; sulfadiazine second line)
- Prednisone (2 mg/kg/d; 60 mg/kg/d max) for carditis with cardiomegaly for 2 weeks, then taper
- Aspirin (80-100 mg/kg/d in children; 4-8 g/d in adults, for 4-6 weeks after steroid taper); treat until symptoms are absent and ESR and CRP are normal; treats inflammation if no cardiomegaly present
- Potential risk of Reye's syndrome with aspirin use in children; use with caution
- Prophylactic treatment with penicillin (1.2 million units IM monthly preferred; oral Pen VK 250 mg twice daily alternative to monthly injections) for patients with carditis until at least age 21 years, possibly for life
- Prophylactic treatment with penicillin for patients without carditis minimally for 5 years after initial attack or until age 18 years; some sources recommend until age 21 years

CONSULTATION/REFERRAL

- Refer new cases to cardiologist as soon as suspected or diagnosed

FOLLOW-UP

- Cardiology referral and follow-up for patients with carditis
- For patients without carditis, assess closely for first 2-3 weeks to assess for carditis

EXPECTED COURSE

- Depends on severity
- Acute phase lasts 2-6 weeks
- 90% of symptoms resolved by 12 weeks

POSSIBLE COMPLICATIONS

- Chronic heart failure
- Recurrent rheumatic fever
- Endocarditis
- Valvular or myocardial disease

KAWASAKI SYNDROME
(Mucocutaneous Lymph Node Syndrome)

DESCRIPTION

An acute, febrile, self limited disease of young children characterized by vasculitis, especially in the medium sized vessels, and multisystem involvement; leading cause of acquired heart disease in children.

ETIOLOGY

- Unknown

INCIDENCE

- Most children are < 4 years old
- Average age of patients is 2.3 years
- Most prevalent in Japan
- 10 cases/100,000 non-Asian children
- 33 cases/100,000 Asian children

RISK FACTORS

- History of Kawasaki syndrome increases risk of recurrence
- Siblings of Japanese offspring have 10-fold risk

ASSESSMENT FINDINGS

Acute (1-2 weeks)

- High fever (103-105°F or 39-41°C) for at least 5 days unresponsive to antibiotics
- Oral mucosal lesions may last 1-2 weeks
- Perineal rash
- Non-tender cervical adenopathy (1.5 cm or > may be unilateral)
- Painful rash and edema of the feet
- Diagnosis requires fever for 5 days and 4 of these criteria:
    - ◊ Edema or erythema of the hands and feet
    - ◊ Conjunctival injection (bilateral)
    - ◊ Cervical adenopathy
    - ◊ Rash (non vesicular and polymorphous)
    - ◊ Exudative pharyngitis, diffuse oral erythema, strawberry tongue, crusting of lips and mouth

Subacute (2-8 weeks after onset)

- Without treatment: desquamation of palms, feet, periungual area, perineal area, coronary artery aneurysms, joint aches and pains
- Acute myocardial infarction may be seen
- Pancarditis
- Diarrhea, jaundice, hepatosplenomegaly
- Aseptic meningitis
- Sterile pyuria

DIFFERENTIAL DIAGNOSIS

- Infection with other Group A streptococcal organisms
- Infection with Staphylococcal scalded skin syndrome
- Measles
- Epstein-Barr virus, Adenovirus, roseola
- Toxic shock syndrome
- Rocky Mountain spotted fever
- Stevens-Johnson syndrome
- Juvenile rheumatoid arthritis

DIAGNOSTIC STUDIES

- CBC: rule out sepsis; leukocytosis
- Anemia: normocytic, normochromic
- Elevated platelet count: 50% have greater than 450,000 mm3
- Erythrocyte sedimentation rate (ESR): > 100 mm/hour
- C-reactive protein: positive
- Electrocardiogram: prolonged PR intervals, decreased QRS voltage, arrhythmias
- Chest x-ray: dilated heart, pleural effusion
- Echocardiogram: effusion, coronary aneurysms
- Pyuria/mild proteinuria

NONPHARMACOLOGIC MANAGEMENT

- Comfort measures
- Bedrest and limited physical activity
- Isolation of patients not necessary
- Patient education regarding disease, treatment, prognosis, etc.

PHARMACOLOGIC MANAGEMENT

- Intravenous immunoglobulins (IVIG) may shorten acute phase and thought to decrease risk of coronary artery aneurysms
- IVIG administration
- Aspirin: 80-100 mg/kg/d in 4 doses; decreased (3-5 mg/kg/d) over the next 6-8 weeks
- Potential risk of Reye's syndrome with aspirin use in children; use with caution
- If coronary aneurysms form: aspirin or other antiplatelet agents

CONSULTATION/REFERRAL

- Consult pediatric cardiologist immediately for suspected cases

FOLLOW-UP

- Depends on severity
- Per cardiologist

EXPECTED COURSE

- Acute phase lasts 1-2 weeks from onset of symptoms
- Subacute phase lasts 2-8 weeks after onset (gradual improvement during this phase)
- Convalescent phase lasts months to years depending on severity

POSSIBLE COMPLICATIONS

- Myocardial infarction
- Development and rupture of coronary artery aneurysms
- Myocardial dysfunction
- Heart failure

References

Baumer, J. H., Love, S. , Gupta, A. K., Haines, L., Maconochie, I. K., & Dua, J. S. . (2009). Salicylate for the treatment of kawasaki disease in children. Cochran Database of Systematic Reviews., Art. No. CD004175.

Bickley, L.S., & Szilagyi, P.G. (2008). Bates' guide to physical examination and history taking (10th ed.). Philadelphia: Lippincott Williams & Wilkins.

Bonow, R. O., Carabello, B. A., Chatterjee, K., de Leon, A. C., Jr., Faxon, D. P., Freed, M. D., . . . Shanewise, J. S. (2008). 2008 focused update incorporated into the acc/aha 2006 guidelines for the management of patients with valvular heart disease: A report of the american college of cardiology/american heart association task force on practice guidelines (writing committee to revise the 1998 guidelines for the management of patients with valvular heart disease): Endorsed by the society of cardiovascular anesthesiologists, society for cardiovascular angiography and interventions, and society of thoracic surgeons. Circulation, 118(15), e523-661. doi: 10.1161/CIRCULATIONAHA.108.190748

Burns, C.E., Brady, M.A., Blosser, C., Starr, N.B., & Dunn, A.M. (2009). Pediatric primary care: A handbook for nurse practitioners (4th ed.). Philadelphia: W.B. Saunders.

Carapetis, J. R., Steer, A. C., Mulholland, E. K., & Weber, M. (2005). The global burden of group a streptococcal diseases. Lancet Infect Dis, 5(11), 685-694. doi: 10.1016/S1473-3099(05)70267-X

Cherry, D. K., Hing, E., Woodwell, D. A., & Rechtsteiner, E. A. (2008). National ambulatory medical care survey: 2006 summary. Natl Health Stat Report(3), 1-39.

Chiesa, R., Marone, E. M., Limoni, C., Volonte, M., & Petrini, O. (2007). Chronic venous disorders: Correlation between visible signs, symptoms, and presence of functional disease. Journal of Vascular Surgery, 46(2), 322-330. doi: 10.1016/j.jvs.2007.04.030

Chobanian, A. V., Bakris, G. L., Black, H. R., Cushman, W. C., Green, L. A., Izzo, J. L., Jr., . . . Roccella, E. J. (2003). The seventh report of the joint national committee on prevention, detection, evaluation, and treatment of high blood pressure: The jnc 7 report. JAMA, 289(19), 2560-2572. doi: 10.1001/jama.289.19.2560

Coy, V. (2005). Genetics of essential hypertension. Journal of the American Academy of Nurse Practitioners, 17(6), 219-224. doi: 10.111/j.1745-7599.2005.0036.x

Crowther, M., & McCourt, K. (2005). Venous thromboembolism: A guide to prevention and treatment. Nurse Practitioner, 30(8), 26-29, 32-24, 39-43; quiz 44-25. doi: 00006205-200508000-00006 [pii]

Cutler, J. A., Sorlie, P. D., Wolz, M., Thom, T., Fields, L. E., & Roccella, E. J. (2008). Trends in hypertension prevalence, awareness, treatment, and control rates in United States adults between 1988-1994 and 1999-2004. Hypertension, 52(5), 818-827. doi: 10.1161/HYPERTENSIONAHA.108.113357

Dickstein, K., Cohen-Solal, A., Filippatos, G., McMurray, J. J., Ponikowski, P., Poole-Wilson, P. A., . . . Zamorano, J. L. (2008). Esc guidelines for the diagnosis and treatment of acute and chronic heart failure 2008: The task force for the diagnosis and treatment of acute and chronic heart failure 2008 of the european society of cardiology. Developed in collaboration with the heart failure association of the esc (hfa) and endorsed by the european society of intensive care medicine (esicm). European Heart Journal, 29(19), 2388-2442. doi: 10.1093/eurheartj/ehn309

Domino, F., Baldor, R., Golding, J., Grimes, J., & Taylor, J. (2011). The 5-minute clinical consult 2011. Philadelphia: Lippincott Williams & Wilkins.

Drug facts and comparisons. (2010). St. Louis: Wolters Kluwer Health. Facts & Comparisons.

Duprez, D. A. (2007). Pharmacological interventions for peripheral artery disease. Expert Opin Pharmacother, 8(10), 1465-1477. doi: 10.1517/14656566.8.10.1465

Ernst, D. , & Lee, A. (2010). Nurse practitioners prescribing reference. New York: Haymarket Media Publication.

Executive summary of the third report of the national cholesterol education program (ncep) expert panel on detection, evaluation, and treatment of high blood cholesterol in adults (adult treatment panel iii). (2001). JAMA, 285(19), 2486-2497. doi: jsc10094 [pii]

Fedder, D. O., Koro, C. E., & L'Italien, G. J. (2002). New national cholesterol education program iii guidelines for primary prevention lipid-lowering drug therapy: Projected impact on the size, sex, and age distribution of the treatment-eligible population. Circulation, 105(2), 152-156.

Ferri, F. . (2010). Ferri's 2010 clinical advisor. Philadelphia: Mosby Elsevier.

Fuster, V., Ryden, L. E., Cannom, D. S., Crijns, H. J., Curtis, A. B., Ellenbogen, K. A., . . . Zamorano, J. L. (2006). Acc/aha/esc 2006 guidelines for the management of patients with atrial fibrillation--executive summary: A report of the american college of cardiology/american heart association task force on practice guidelines and the european society of cardiology committee for practice guidelines (writing committee to revise the 2001 guidelines for the management of patients with atrial fibrillation). Journal of the American College of Cardiology, 48(4), 854-906. doi: 10.1016/j.jacc.2006.07.009

Gibbons, R. J., Abrams, J., Chatterjee, K., Daley, J., Deedwania, P. C., Douglas, J. S., . . . Williams, S. V. (2003). Acc/aha 2002 guideline update for the management of patients with chronic stable angina--summary article: A report of the american college of cardiology/american heart association task force on practice guidelines (committee on the management of patients with chronic stable angina). Journal of the American College of Cardiology, 41(1), 159-168. doi: S0735109702028486 [pii]

Gohel, M. S., Barwell, J. R., Taylor, M., Chant, T., Foy, C., Earnshaw, J. J., . . . Poskitt, K. R. (2007). Long term results of compression therapy alone versus compression plus surgery in chronic venous ulceration (eschar): Randomised controlled trial. BMJ, 335(7610), 83. doi: 10.1136/bmj.39216.542442.BE

Grundy, S. M., Cleeman, J. I., Merz, C. N., Brewer, H. B., Jr., Clark, L. T., Hunninghake, D. B., . . . Stone, N. J. (2004). Implications of recent clinical trials for the national cholesterol education program adult treatment panel iii guidelines. Circulation, 110(2), 227-239. doi: 10.1161/01.CIR.0000133317.49796.0E

Hahn, R. G., Knox, L. M., & Forman, T. A. (2005). Evaluation of poststreptococcal illness. American Family Physician, 71(10), 1949-1954.

Hankey, G. J., Norman, P. E., & Eikelboom, J. W. (2006). Medical treatment of peripheral arterial disease. JAMA, 295(5), 547-553. doi: 10.1001/jama.295.5.547

Hanna, I. R., & Wenger, N. K. (2005). Secondary prevention of coronary heart disease in elderly patients. American Family Physician, 71(12), 2289-2296.

Hunt, S. A., Abraham, W. T., Chin, M. H., Feldman, A. M., Francis, G. S., Ganiats, T. G., . . . Yancy, C. W. (2009). 2009 focused update incorporated into the acc/aha 2005 guidelines for the diagnosis and management of heart failure in adults: A report of the american college of cardiology foundation/american heart association task force on practice guidelines: Developed in collaboration with the international society for heart and lung transplantation. Circulation, 119(14), e391-479. doi: 10.1161/CIRCULATIONAHA.109.192065

Jones, R. H., & Carek, P. J. (2008). Management of varicose veins. American Family Physician, 78(11), 1289-1294.

Kearney, P. M., Blackwell, L., Collins, R., Keech, A., Simes, J., Peto, R., . . . Baigent, C. (2008). Efficacy of cholesterol-lowering therapy in 18,686 people with diabetes in 14 randomised trials of statins: A meta-analysis. Lancet, 371(9607), 117-125. doi: 10.1016/S0140-6736(08)60104-X

Kelechi, T. J. (2005). Chronic venous insufficiency. Advance for Nurse Practitioners, 13(7), 31-34.

Lambing, A. (2005). Clearing the way: Treating venous thomboembolism and deep vein thrombosis. Advance for Nurse Practitioners, 13(6), 24-30.

Major outcomes in high-risk hypertensive patients randomized to angiotensin-converting enzyme inhibitor or calcium channel blocker vs diuretic: The antihypertensive and lipid-lowering treatment to prevent heart attack trial (allhat). (2002). JAMA, 288(23), 2981-2997. doi: joc21962 [pii]

Mancia, G., De Backer, G., Dominiczak, A., Cifkova, R., Fagard, R., Germano, G., . . . Zanchetti, A. (2007). 2007 esh-esc practice guidelines for the management of arterial hypertension: Esh-esc task force on the management of arterial hypertension. Journal of Hypertension, 25(9), 1751-1762. doi: 10.1097/HJH.0b013e3282f0580f

Marriott, H. J. . (1993). Bedside cardiac diagnosis. Philadelphia: J. B. Lippincott.

Montori, V. M., Devereaux, P. J., Adhikari, N. K., Burns, K. E., Eggert, C. H., Briel, M., . . . Guyatt, G. H. (2005). Randomized trials stopped early for benefit: A systematic review. JAMA, 294(17), 2203-2209. doi: 10.1001/jama.294.17.2203

Newburger, J. W., Takahashi, M., Gerber, M. A., Gewitz, M. H., Tani, L. Y., Burns, J. C., . . . Taubert, K. A. (2004). Diagnosis, treatment, and long-term management of kawasaki disease: A statement for health professionals from the committee on rheumatic fever, endocarditis, and kawasaki disease, council on cardiovascular disease in the young, american heart association. Pediatrics, 114(6), 1708-1733. doi: 10.1542/peds.2004-2182

Nicolucci, A. (2008). Aspirin for primary prevention of cardiovascular events in diabetes: Still an open question. JAMA, 300(18), 2180-2181. doi: 10.1001/jama.2008.625

Thomas-Kvidera, D. (2005). Heart failure from diastolic dysfunction related to hypertension: Guidelines for management. Journal of the American Academy of Nurse Practitioners, 17(5), 168-175. doi: 10.111/j.1745-7599.2005.0028.x

United States Preventive Services Task Force. (2008). Screening for lipid disorders in adults Retrieved from www.ahrq.gov/clinic/uspstf08/lipid/lipidrs.htm

Wells, P. S., Anderson, D. R., Rodger, M., Forgie, M., Kearon, C., Dreyer, J., . . . Kovacs, M. J. (2003). Evaluation of d-dimer in the diagnosis of suspected deep-vein thrombosis. New England Journal of Medicine, 349(13), 1227-1235. doi: 10.1056/NEJMoa023153

Wilson, W., Taubert, K. A., Gewitz, M., Lockhart, P. B., Baddour, L. M., Levison, M., . . . Durack, D. T. (2007). Prevention of infective endocarditis: Guidelines from the american heart association: A guideline from the american heart association rheumatic fever, endocarditis, and kawasaki disease committee, council on cardiovascular disease in the young, and the council on clinical cardiology, council on cardiovascular surgery and anesthesia, and the quality of care and outcomes research interdisciplinary working group. Circulation, 116(15), 1736-1754. doi: 10.1161/CIRCULATIONAHA.106.183095

2

DERMATOLOGIC DISORDERS

Dermatologic Disorders

Acne Vulgaris 87

Actinic Keratosis 92

Atopic Dermatitis 95

Bacterial Infections of the Skin 100

Burns 104

*Cafe' au lait Spots 107

Cat Scratch Fever 108

Cellulitis 109

*Common Benign Pediatric Skin Lesions 113

Contact Dermatitis 114

Diaper Dermatitis 119

Fifth Disease 121

*Hand Foot and Mouth Disease 122

*Herpangina 123

Herpes Zoster 124

Hidradenitis Suppurativa 127

Impetigo 128

Lyme Disease 130

Oral Candidiasis 132

Paronychia 134

Pediculosis 137

Pityriasis Rosea 139

Psoriasis 142

*Roseola, Exanthem Subitum 143

*Rubella 144

*Rubeola 146

Scabies 147

*Scarlet Fever 149

Seborrheic Dermatitis 150

Skin Cancer 152

Spider/Insect Bites and Stings 154

Tinea Infections 158

*Varicella 162

Warts 163

References 166

** Denotes pediatric diagnosis*

Dermatologic Disorders

ACNE VULGARIS
(Acne)

DESCRIPTION

Inflammatory disorder of the androgen-dependent sebaceous glands in which excessive amounts of sebum are produced which can lead to comedones, pustules, papules, and scarring.

ETIOLOGY

- Increase in androgen production, especially during puberty; but may have normal androgen production with hypersensitivity
- Increased rate of keratin production which blocks movement of sebum out of the cell
- Presence of bacteria (*Propionibacterium acnes)* which increase inflammatory response

ASSESSMENT FINDINGS

- **Whiteheads** (closed comedones) are noninflammatory papules which result from blockage at the follicle neck
- **Blackheads** (open comedones) are noninflammatory papules which result from blockage at the follicle mouth. Black color is from oxidized melanin.
- ***P. acnes*** instrumental in inflammation

INCIDENCE

- Adolescences (virtually 100% are affected)
- Females > Males in adolescence
- Males may be more severely affected
- Improves in summer

RISK FACTORS

- Family history: 50% have family history of acne
- Adolescence (nearly 100% are affected at some point)
- Caucasians
- Oil-based cosmetics
- Touching face and skin with hands
- Skin contact with chin straps, shoulder pads, telephone receiver
- Hot, humid climates
- Worsens with stress, menses

Males often have later onset and worse severity. Females often have worsening prior to menses.

CHARACTERISTICS OF ACNE			
	Comedonal Acne	**Inflammatory Acne**	**Nodulocystic**
Age	Pre-teens and early adolescence	Adolescence and early 20s	Adolescence
Clinical Findings	Whiteheads (closed comedones)	Pustules Papules, minimal scarring Mild inflammation	Nodules, cysts Moderate to severe inflammation
Infection with *P. acnes*	Not usually	Usually	Usually

Areas most commonly affected are face, anterior and posterior chest, upper arms, and shoulders.

DIFFERENTIAL DIAGNOSIS

- Acne rosacea
- Folliculitis
- Kertosis pilaris
- Folliculitis barbae
- Occupational exposure to grease, tar, or other agents

DIAGNOSTIC STUDIES

- Usually none are indicated

PREVENTION

- Avoid occupational irritants
- Good hand-face hygiene
- Frequent cleansing of the skin and area (too frequent cleansing may lead to irritation)
- Rapid treatment if inflammatory and cystic to prevent scarring
- Avoid anabolic steroids

Dermatologic Disorders

NONPHARMACOLOGIC MANAGEMENT

- Avoid rubbing the skin with hands; avoid occluding the skin with materials like face creams, oily topical preparations (e.g., suntan lotion)
- Choose oil free or water based cosmetics
- Cleanse affected area twice daily with mild soap to decrease oil accumulation
- Avoid picking or squeezing lesions
- Reassure patient that acne may take months to improve, but usually will show improvement in 4 weeks
- Moderate sun exposure may help
- Address psychosocial concerns of patient
- Discuss stress management if stress precipitates outbreaks
- Counsel regarding good nutrition (there is no evidence that fatty foods, chocolate, etc. cause acne)

Prescribing Strategy

Comedonal acne: topical retinoid

Mild mixed papular/pustular acne: topical retinoid plus topical antimicrobial, +/- benzoyl peroxide

Moderate mixed papular/pustular acne: oral antibiotic plus topical retinoid +/- benzoyl peroxide

Nodulocystic: oral antibiotic plus topical retinoid plus benzoyl peroxide

PHARMACOLOGIC MANAGEMENT

Dry or sensitive skin: cream
Oily skin: gel or solution
Hairy area (scalp, eyebrows): lotion

ACNE PHARMACOLOGIC MANAGEMENT

Class	Drug Generic name (Trade name®)	Dosage How supplied	Comments
Topical Retinoids **Tretinoin** General comments Retinoids are used to accelerate turnover of keratin plugs and decreases comedone formation Preferred in patients with comedonal acne or as an adjunct with more severe acne forms	**adapalene** Differin	**Adult and > 12 years:** apply daily at bedtime after washing *Gel 0.1%, 0.3% : 45 g* *Cream 0.1% : 45 g*	• Pregnancy Category C • Do not use on broken skin; Avoid mucus membranes • Caution with other photosensitizing agents (tetracyclines, thiazides, sulfonamides, fluroquinolones) • Redness, dryness, scaling of skin treated with retinoid is common in the first 2-4 weeks
	tazarotene	**Adult and > 12 years:** apply thin film 0.1% at bedtime	• Pregnancy Category X • Women of childbearing potential: begin during normal menses • Cleanse affected skin gently, pat dry, apply thin film • Do not use on broken skin; Avoid mucus membranes • Caution with other photosensitizing agents (tetracyclines, thiazides, sulfonamides, fluroquinolones)

continued

ACNE PHARMACOLOGIC MANAGEMENT

Class	Drug Generic name (Trade name®)	Dosage How supplied	Comments
	Tazorac	*Gel: 30 g, 100 g* *Cream: 15 g, 30 g, 60 g*	• Do not use over > 20% of body • Common side effects: desquamation, burning, stinging in treated areas
	tretinoin topical Retin-A	**Adult**: apply sparingly to affected areas at bedtime	• Pregnancy Category C • Wash face and allow to dry for 20 minutes before applying tretinoin • If amount applied to skin does not disappear in at least 60 seconds, too much is being applied • Do not use on broken skin; Avoid mucus membranes • Caution with other photosensitizing agents (tetracyclines, thiazides, sulfonamides, fluroquinolones) • Common side effects: desquamation, burning, stinging in treated areas • Within 2 weeks: peeling, redness to treated areas • 3-6 weeks: new blemishes (continue to use) • Improvement may not be seen before 12 weeks
Topical Anti-Microbials *decrease number of anaerobic bacteria by oxidizing bacterial proteins in the sebaceous follicles*	**benzoyl peroxide topical** Benzac Wash	**Adult and Children > 12 years:** initial daily wash, may increase to 2-3 times daily as tolerated *Wash 5%: 4 oz, 8 oz; 10%: 8 oz*	• Pregnancy Category C • Avoid eyes, mucous membranes, • Do not use on broken skin • May bleach fabric, hair • Common side effects are drying and erythema of treated areas • Avoid unnecessary sun exposure and use sunscreen
Topical Antibiotics	**clindamycin topical** Clindagel 1%	**Adult and Children > 12 years:** Apply thin film once daily *60 mL applicator bottle*	• Pregnancy Category B • Contraindicated in clindamycin allergic patients • Common side effect is dry skin • Wash affected area, pat dry, apply topical clindamycin
	sulfacetamide topical Klaron	**Adult and Children > 12 years:** Apply thin film twice daily *4 oz. bottle*	• Pregnancy Category C • Contraindicated in sulfa allergic individuals • Monitor for hypersensitivities to sulfa including Stevens Johnson syndrome, toxic epidermal necrolysis, blood dyscrasias

continued

ACNE PHARMACOLOGIC MANAGEMENT

Class	Drug Generic name (Trade name®)	Dosage How supplied	Comments
	erythromycin topical	**Adult and Children > 12 years**: Apply to affected areas twice daily after washing with warm water and patting skin dry	• Pregnancy Category C • Common side effects peeling, erythema, oiliness, and burning sensation to treated areas • Avoid mucus membranes
	Erythra-Derm	*60 mL bottle*	
Combination Agents	**erythromycin/benzoyl peroxide**	**Adult and Children > 12 years**: Apply to cleansed skin twice daily	• Pregnancy Category C • Requires thorough mixing by the patient immediately prior to each use • Wash skin gently, rinse with warm water, pat dry, apply to affected areas • May bleach hair, skin, fabrics • Limit exposure to sunlight and use sunscreen • Addition of benzoyl peroxide decreases risk of resistance to erythromycin
	Benzamycin Pak (erythromycin 3% + benzoyl peroxide 5%)	*60 pouches per carton*	
	clindamycin/benzoyl peroxide	**Adult and Children > 12 years:** Apply twice daily to affected areas after the skin has been gently washed, rinsed with warm water, and patted dry.	• Pregnancy Category C • May bleach hair, skin, fabrics • Limit exposure to sunlight and use sunscreen • Addition of benzoyl peroxide decreases risk of resistance to clindamycin
	Benzaclin (clindamycin 1% + benzoyl peroxide 5%)	*6 g plastic jars*	
Systemic Antibiotics *improve inflammatory acne by inhibiting growth of P.acne* **General comments** Oral antibiotics are used to treat patients with moderate to severe acne All oral antibiotics may make birth control pills less effective	**minocycline**	**Adult and Children ≥ 12 years**: 200 mg once then 100 mg every 12 hours *Alternate*: 100-200 mg once, then 50 mg 4 times	• Pregnancy Category D • Can cause vertigo, skin discoloration and a lupus like syndrome • Increases risk of photosensitivity • Do not administer to age < 8 years old • Potential interactions with anticoagulants, ergots, antacids containing aluminum, calcium, magnesium or iron • Take with a full glass of liquid • May take with or without food • No consensus on length of time to continue oral antibiotics to treat acne but less than 6 months. Discontinue as acne improves
	Minocin	*Caps: 50 mg, 100 mg*	

continued

ACNE PHARMACOLOGIC MANAGEMENT

Class	Drug Generic name (Trade name®)	Dosage How supplied	Comments
	doxycycline	**Adult and Children > 12 years:** 100 mg every 12 hours for one day, then 100 mg daily	• Pregnancy Category D • Increases risk of photosensitivity • Do not administer to age < 8 years old • Potential interactions with anticoagulants, ergots, antacids containing aluminum, calcium, magnesium or iron • Take with a full glass of liquid • May take with or without food • No consensus on length of time to continue oral antibiotics to treat acne but less than 6 months. Discontinue as acne improves
	Doryx	*Del Rel. Caps: 75 mg, 100 mg* *Del Rel Tabs: 75 mg, 100 mg, 150 mg*	
Oral Contraceptives **General comments** Acne therapy is considered for women who have moderate to severe acne that has been unresponsive to other therapies Use in females ≥ 15 years who have achieved menarche Cigarette smoking increases the risk of serious cardiovascular side effects; risk increases with age	**progestin plus estrogen**	**Adult and Children ≥ 15 years of age:** 1 tab PO daily: start day one of menstrual cycle on first Sunday after onset of menses Alternate: Take first pill on first day of menstrual cycle and continue daily taking at the same time each day	• Pregnancy Category X • Cigarette smoking increases the risk of serious cardiovascular side effects; risk increases with age • Contraindicated in females with thrombophlebitis or thromboembolic disorders, severe hypertension, valvular heart disease, diabetes with vascular involvement, headaches with focal neurologic symptoms, prolonged immobilization, hepatic dysfunction, known or suspected pregnancy
	Ortho tri-cyclen 28	*Tablet dispenser with 28 tablets*	
	progestin plus estrogen	**Adult and Children ≥ 15 years of age:** 1 tab PO daily: start day one of menstrual cycle on first Sunday after onset of menses Alternate: Take first pill on first day of menstrual cycle and continue daily taking at the same time each day	• Pregnancy Category X • Monitor for hyperkalemia • Recommend taking at the same time each day • Contraindicated in females with thrombophlebitis or thromboembolic disorders, severe hypertension, valvular heart disease, diabetes with vascular involvement, headaches with focal neurologic symptoms, prolonged immobilization, hepatic dysfunction, known or suspected pregnancy
	Yaz	*Packages of 3 BLISTER packs*	

Dermatologic Disorders

Acne often worsens in the first 2 weeks of treatment.

PREGNANCY/LACTATION CONSIDERATIONS

- Do not use tetracycline in breastfeeding women or pregnant patients
- Erythromycin may be safely used during pregnancy; topical preferred over systemic
- Pregnancy may cause remission or exacerbation of acne
- Some oral antibiotics may reduce effectiveness of oral contraceptives

CONSULTATION/REFERRAL

- Severe acne
- Unresponsive acne
- Scar management

FOLLOW-UP

- Monthly visits until adequate response achieved

EXPECTED COURSE

- 4-6 weeks before improvement can be seen
- Treatment may last for months or years
- Gradual improvement as adolescence progresses

POSSIBLE COMPLICATIONS

- Scarring
- Damage to self-image and self-esteem

ACTINIC KERATOSIS (AK)

DESCRIPTION

Premalignant skin lesion identified on sun-exposed areas of the skin; these are usually more easily felt than seen and are considered precursors of squamous cell carcinoma (SCC).

ETIOLOGY

- Short wave UV light (UVB)

INCIDENCE

- Common in middle-aged and older adults

RISK FACTORS

- Sun exposure
- Common in fair skinned individuals
- More common in males

ASSESSMENT FINDINGS

- Round or oval shaped
- Flesh colored, red, pink, brown or black
- May be papules or plaques and are rough when palpated
- Size varies from 0.25-2.0 cm; usually < 1 cm

DIFFERENTIAL DIAGNOSIS

- Squamous cell carcinoma
- Warty lesions
- Solar lentigo
- Malignant melanoma
- Basal cell carcinoma
- Squamous cell carcinoma

DIAGNOSTIC STUDIES

- Usually made on clinical presentation because of the characteristic appearance and presentation
- Skin biopsy

PREVENTION

- Liberal use of sunscreen during sun exposure
- Encourage routine sunscreen applied twice daily for 7 months to prevent further AK development

PHARMACOLOGIC MANAGEMENT

- Topical fluorouracil (FU) twice daily for 3-6 weeks destroys most AKs for up to 12 months
- Topical imiquimod 5% cream 3 times weekly for up to 2 months (helpful for small lesions but more expensive than FU)
- Topical tretinoin or tazarotene to enhance efficacy of topical FU

ACTINIC KERATOSIS PHARMACOLOGIC MANAGEMENT

Class	Drug Generic name (Trade name®)	Dosage How supplied	Comments
Antineoplastic/ Antimetabolite	**fluorouracil**	**Adult:** Twice daily with fingertips and wash hands afterwards *Usual*: 2-6 weeks	• Pregnancy Category X • Fluorouracil is contraindicated in women who are or may become pregnant • Apply with non-metallic applicator, clean fingertips, or gloved fingers in an amount sufficient to cover the lesions. If unprotected fingers are used to apply fluorouracil, wash hands immediately afterward
	Fluoroplex	*Cream 1%: 30 g*	
	Carac	Apply once daily to skin, up to 4 weeks *Cream 0.5%: 30 g*	• Pregnancy Category X • Wash and dry area. Wait 10 minutes before applying product • Do not occlude • Wash hands well after use
	Efudex	Apply twice daily for 2-4 weeks *Solution 2%, 5%: 10 mL, 25 mL* *Cream: 40 g*	• Pregnancy Category X • Apply twice daily until erosion occurs (usually 2-4 weeks) • Biopsy unresponsive lesions • Avoid exposure to UV light after use
Topical Imiquimod 5%	**imiquimod**	**Adult:** Apply twice weekly for 16 weeks	• Pregnancy Category C • Apply prior to sleep and leave on the skin for approximately 8 hours, then remove by washing the area with mild soap and water • Do not occlude • Avoid mucus membranes
	Aldara	*Box: 12 packets of single use*	
Topical Anti-inflammatory Agents	**diclofenac**	**Adult:** Apply twice daily for 60-90 days	• Pregnancy Category B • Avoid sun exposure • Contraindicated in aspirin allergy • Avoid concomitant use of systemic NSAIDs
	Solaraze	*Gel: 100 g*	

continued

ACTINIC KERATOSIS PHARMACOLOGIC MANAGEMENT

Class	Drug Generic name (Trade name®)	Dosage How supplied	Comments
Photosensitizing Agents	**aminolevulinic acid HCl**	**Adult:** One application of solution and one dose of illumination per treatment site per 8 week treatment session	• Pregnancy Category C • Photodynamic therapy for actinic keratoses with LEVULAN KERASTICK for Topical Solution is a two stage process involving a) application of Topical Solution, followed 14 to 18 hours later by b) illumination with blue light using the BLU-U Blue Light Photodynamic Therapy Illuminator. The second visit, for illumination, must take place in the 14-18 hour window following application. • Multiple possible drug interactions. Check compatibility prior to prescribing.
	Levulan	*Solution: packs of 6 individual use or individual single dose*	
	Metvixia	Treatment is a multistage process 7 days apart, with debriding, application, occlusive dressing for 3 hours, removal of dressing and cream, illumination *Cream: 2 g*	• Pregnancy Category C • Contraindicated with peanut and almond sensitivities; allergy to porphyrins • During 3 hours with cream on, avoid sunlight or bright light exposure, wear protective hat

CONSULTATION/REFERRAL

- Dermatologist if AKs appear with frequency
- Refer for malignancy associated with AK (i.e. Squamous Cell Carcinoma)

FOLLOW-UP

- Depends on frequency of appearance of AKs and whether there is associated malignancy

EXPECTED COURSE

- Excellent

POSSIBLE COMPLICATIONS

- Squamous cell carcinoma or basal cell carcinoma

ATOPIC DERMATITIS
(Eczema)

DESCRIPTION

Chronic, pruritic skin eruption with acute exacerbations appearing in characteristic sites. Eczema is often used interchangeably with atopic dermatitis, but the word eczema describes acute symptoms associated with atopic dermatitis.

Commonly seen in patients with other atopic illnesses (e.g., asthma, allergic rhinitis).

ETIOLOGY

- Multifactorial: genetic, physiological, immunologic and environmental factors

INCIDENCE

- Effects almost 10% of children
- Almost half of affected infants have initial symptoms by 6 months of age
- Begins after 2 months of age, resolves by 3 years
- 90% have remission by puberty
- Males = Females
- More common in Asians and African-Americans

RISK FACTORS

- Family history of atopic diseases
- Skin Infections
- Stress
- Temperature extremes
- Contact with irritating substances (wearing new clothing prior to washing)

ASSESSMENT FINDINGS

- General: pruritus, erythema, dry skin, facial erythema, infraorbital folds (Dennie-Morgan folds)

Infants:
- Lesions on flexural surfaces of arms, legs, on trunk, face (especially cheeks)
- Lesions are erythematous and papular
- Vesicles may ooze, form crusts

Children:
- Lesions common in wrists, ankles and flexural surfaces
- Presence of scales and plaques; lichenification occurs from scratching

Adults:
- Flexural surfaces are common sites, dorsa of the hands and feet
- Often reappears in adulthood after absence since childhood
- Lichenification and scaling are typical

DIFFERENTIAL DIAGNOSIS

- Contact dermatitis
- Seborrheic dermatitis
- Scabies
- Psoriasis

DIAGNOSTIC STUDIES

- Usually none needed
- Skin biopsy to rule out other skin disorders
- 80% of patients may have eosinophilia during episodes of disease activity

PREVENTION

- Prevent dry skin (liberal use of emollients is essential for good control)
- Avoid any known precipitating factors (stress, wool clothing, fragrance-free detergents, etc.)

NONPHARMACOLOGIC MANAGEMENT

- Limit bathing (do not use hot water) to avoid further drying of skin
- Superfatted soaps are best
- Prevent skin trauma (sunburns, etc.)
- Soak for 20 minutes in warm water before applying emollient (when possible)
- Wet compresses (Burow's solution) if lesions are weeping or oozing
- Patient education regarding disease process, self-care, and precipitating factors

PHARMACOLOGIC MANAGEMENT

- Topical corticosteroids (creams are preferred) are the mainstay of therapy (use lowest potency which controls symptoms)
- Antihistamines (oral and topical) for itching
- Emollients 2-3 times per day or as needed to correct dry skin (Eucerin®, Lubriderm®, Cetaphil®, Vaseline®)
- Oral corticosteroids may be used for severe cases. Due to the chronic nature of this disease, this should be reserved and only used in short bursts
- Intralesional steroid injections

ATOPIC DERMATITIS PHARMACOLOGIC MANAGEMENT

Pediatric patients may be more susceptible to topical corticosteroid-induced HPA axis suppression than older patients because of larger skin surface area to body weight ratio. Limit use to lowest effect potency and time.

Class	Drug Generic name (Trade name®)	Dosage How supplied	Comments
Low Potency Steroids *exert their anti-inflammatory effect through mechanical, chemical, microbiological and immunological means*	**alclometasone dipropionate 0.05%**	**Adult:** apply thin film, massage in 2-3 times/day **Children > 1 year**: same as adult	• Pregnancy Category C • For external use only • Do not use longer than 3 weeks • No adjustment in dosage needed for geriatric patients
<u>General comments</u>	Aclovate	*Cream, oint: 15 g, 45 g, 60 g*	
Use lowest potency that produces desired effect			
Skin atrophy and changes in skin color are possible with long term use	**fluocinolone acetonide 0.01%**	**Adult**: thin film 2-4 times daily **Children**: Pediatric dosing not available	• Pregnancy Category C • For external use only • Do not use longer than 3 weeks • No adjustment in dosage needed for geriatric patients
Areas with greatest absorption of steroid are the face, groin, and axillae. Consider lowest potency steroids in these areas	Synalar solution	*Cream/oint: 15 g, 60 g* *Solution: 20 mL, 60 mL*	
Systemic absorption is usually minimal, but broken skin will absorb significantly more steroid	**hydrocortisone base or acetate 0.5%**	**Adult and Children > 2 years:** apply thin film 2-4 times daily	• Pregnancy Category C • For external use only • Do not use longer than 3 weeks
Topical steroids will worsen skin infections	Cortisporin cream Hytone ointment U-cort cream Vytone cream	*Cream/Oint: 1 oz, 2 oz*	

continued

ATOPIC DERMATITIS PHARMACOLOGIC MANAGEMENT

Pediatric patients may be more susceptible to topical corticosteroid-induced HPA axis suppression than older patients because of larger skin surface area to body weight ratio. Limit use to lowest effect potency and time.

Class	Drug Generic name (Trade name®)	Dosage How supplied	Comments
Medium Potency Steroids *exert their anti-inflammatory effect through mechanical, chemical, microbiological, and immunological means*	**triamcinolone acetonide 0.025%**	**Adult**: apply thin film 2-4 times daily **Children**: Pediatric dosing not available	• Pregnancy Category C • Intended for external use only • Use caution in use longer than 2 weeks, may change skin pigmentation
General comments Use lowest potency that produces desired effect Skin atrophy and changes in skin color are possible with long term use Areas with greatest absorption of steroid are the face, groin, and axillae. Consider lowest potency steroids in these areas Topical steroids will worsen skin infections	Aristocort cream Kenalog cream, lotion, ointment	*Cream 0.025% and 0.1%: 15 g, 60 g; 0.5%, 15 g; 0.1%: 15 g, 60 g* *Kenalog also in lotion: 60 mL* *Oint: 15 g, 60 g*	
	desoximetasone 0.05%	**Adult**: apply thin film twice a day **Children**: Pediatric dosing not available	• Pregnancy Category C • Intended for topical use only • Use caution in use longer than 2 weeks, may change skin pigmentation
	Topicort LP cream	*Cream/gel: 15 g, 60 g* *Oint: 60 g*	
	flurandrenolide 0.025%	**Adult**: apply every 12 hours **Children**: Pediatric dosing not available	• Pregnancy Category C • Intended for topical use only • Use caution in use longer than 2 weeks, may change skin pigmentation
	Cordran	*Cream/oint: 30 g, 60 g*	
	fluticasone propionate 0.05%	**Adult**: apply thin film twice a day **Children > 3 months**: Apply a thin film once or twice daily	• Pregnancy Category C • Intended for topical use only • Use in pediatric patients for more than 4 weeks of use has not been established • No dosage adjustment recommended for geriatric patients
	Cutivate	*Cream: 15 g, 30 g, 60 g* *Lotion: 60 mL, 120 mL*	
	hydrocortisone valerate 0.2%	**Adult**: apply thin film 2-3 times daily **Children**: Pediatric dosing not available	• Pregnancy Category C • Intended for topical use only • Use caution in use longer than 2 weeks, may change skin pigmentation
	Westcort	*Cream/oint: 15 g, 45 g, 60 g*	

continued

ATOPIC DERMATITIS PHARMACOLOGIC MANAGEMENT

Pediatric patients may be more susceptible to topical corticosteroid-induced HPA axis suppression than older patients because of larger skin surface area to body weight ratio. Limit use to lowest effect potency and time.

Class	Drug Generic name (Trade name®)	Dosage How supplied	Comments
	mometasone furoate 0.1%	**Adult**: apply thin film daily **Children > 2 years**: apply sparingly once daily to affected areas	• Pregnancy Category C • Intended for topical use only • Use caution in use longer than 2 weeks, may change skin pigmentation • DO NOT USE WITH AN OCCLUSIVE DRESSING
	Elocon	*Cream/oint: 15 g, 45 g* *Lotion: 30 mL, 60 mL*	
	triamicinolone acetonide 0.1%	**Adult**: apply thin film 3-4 times daily **Children**: Pediatric dosing not available	• Pregnancy Category C • Intended for topical use only • Use caution with use longer than 2 weeks, may change skin pigmentation
	Aristocort A cream, oint; Kenalog cream, lotion	*Cream/oint: 15 g, 60 g* *Lotion: 6 mL, 15 mL*	
High Potency Corticosteroids *exert their anti-inflammatory effect through mechanical, chemical, microbiological, and immunological means* <u>General comments</u> Use lowest potency that produces desired effect Skin atrophy and changes in skin color are possible with long term use Areas with greatest absorption of steroid are the face, groin, and axillae. Consider lowest potency steroids in these areas Topical steroids will worsen skin infections Do not use more than 50 g/week	**amcinonide 0.1%**	**Adult**: thin film 2-3 times daily **Children**: Pediatric dosing not available	• Pregnancy Category C • Intended for topical use only • Use caution with use longer than 2 weeks, may change skin pigmentation
	Cyclocor	*Cream/oint: 15 g, 30 g, 60 g* *Lotion: 30 mL, 60 mL*	
	betamethasone dipropionate 0.05%	**Adult and children > 12 years**: apply thin film 1-2 times daily *Max*: 2 consecutive weeks	• Pregnancy Category C • Intended for topical use only • Use caution with use longer than 2 weeks, may change skin pigmentation • **Studies demonstrate HPA axis suppression in some children** • No dosage adjustment recommended for geriatric patients
	Diprolene AF	*Oint/cream: 15 g, 50 g* *Lotion: 30 mL, 60 mL*	
	desoximetasone 0.05%	**Adult**: apply thin film twice a day **Children**: Pediatric dosing not available	• Pregnancy Category C • Intended for topical use only • Use caution with use longer than 2 weeks, may change skin pigmentation • **Studies demonstrate HPA axis suppression in some children**
	Topicort gel 0.25% Topicort cream, oint	*Cream/gel: 15 g, 60 g* *Ointment: 60 g*	

continued

ATOPIC DERMATITIS PHARMACOLOGIC MANAGEMENT

Pediatric patients may be more susceptible to topical corticosteroid-induced HPA axis suppression than older patients because of larger skin surface area to body weight ratio. Limit use to lowest effect potency and time.

Class	Drug Generic name (Trade name®)	Dosage How supplied	Comments
Super High Potency *exert their anti-inflammatory effect through mechanical, chemical, microbiological, and immunological means* __General comments__ Use lowest potency that produces desired effect Skin atrophy and changes in skin color are possible with long term use Areas with greatest absorption of steroid are the face, groin, and axillae. Consider lowest potency steroids in these areas Topical steroids will worsen skin infections Do not use more than 50 g/week	**betamethasone dipropionate augmented 0.05%** Diprolene	**Adult and children > 12 years**: apply thin film 1-2 times daily *Max*: 2 consecutive weeks *Oint/cream: 15 g, 50 g* *Lotion: 30 mL, 60 mL*	• Pregnancy Category C • Intended for topical use only • Use caution with use longer than 2 weeks, may change skin pigmentation • **Studies demonstrate HPA axis suppression in some children** • No dosage adjustment recommended for geriatric patients
	clobetasol propionate 0.05% Temovate	**Adult and children ≥ 16 years**: apply thin film twice a day *Max*: 50 g/week *Cream/Oint: 15 g, 30 g, 45 g, 60 g* *Soln: 50 mL* *Scalp emollient: 50 mL*	• Pregnancy Category C • Intended for topical use only • Use caution with use longer than 2 weeks, may change skin pigmentation • **Studies demonstrate HPA axis suppression in some children** • No dosage adjustment recommended for geriatric patients
	flurandrenolide 4 mcg/sq cream Cordran tape	**Adult**: apply every 12 hours *Tape: 3" x 24" and 3" x 80"; Patch: 2" x 3"; Oint/cream 0.05%: 30 g, 60 g* *Lotion: 15 mL, 60 mL*	• Pregnancy Category C • Intended for topical use only • Use caution with use longer than 2 weeks, may change skin pigmentation • Change tape every 12 hours
	halobetasol propionate 0.05% Ultravate	**Adult and children > 12 years**: apply thin layer twice a day *Max*: 50 g/week *Cream/Oint: 15 g, 45 g*	• Pregnancy Category C • Intended for topical use only • Use caution with use longer than 2 weeks, may change skin pigmentation • Do not use with occlusive dressings • No dosage adjustment recommended for geriatric patients

BACTERIAL INFECTIONS OF THE SKIN
(Folliculitis, Furunculosis, Carbunculosis)

Dermatologic Disorders

DESCRIPTION

Folliculitis	Superficial infection/irritation of the hair follicles. Lesions consist of a pustular or inflammatory nodule which surrounds the hair follicle
Furunculosis (boils)	Deep infection of the hair follicle. The nodule becomes a pustule which contains necrotic tissue and purulent exudate. Neck, face, buttocks, waistline and breasts are common areas
Carbunculosis (a cluster of furuncles)	Deep suppurative lesion with extension into the subcutaneous area. The nape of the neck and posterior thigh are common areas

ETIOLOGY

- Folliculitis, Furunculosis, Carbunculosis: *Staphylococcus aureus* is the most common causative organism; consider MRSA (methicillin resistant Staph *aureus*) as a very common outpatient pathogen
- Hot tub folliculitis: *Pseudomonas aeruginosa*

INCIDENCE

Folliculitis	Very common in all age groups Tends to recur frequently
Furunculosis (boils)	Common in teenagers & adults Tends to be recurrent
Carbunculosis (a cluster of furuncles)	Males > females Common in at-risk populations (e.g., patients with chronic diseases, the elderly, the immunocompromised)

RISK FACTORS

- *Folliculitis*: poor hygiene, shaving, tight jeans
- *Furunculosis*: adolescence, prior furunculosis, crowded quarters, poor hygiene, diabetes
- *Carbunculosis*: chronic disease, diabetes, alcoholism, advancing age

ASSESSMENT FINDINGS

Folliculitis	Superficial pustule, hair easily removed, mild erythema, inflammation
Furunculosis (boils)	Pustular lesion with central necrosis and a core of purulent exudate, pain, inflammation, and erythema; sometimes spontaneous drainage, but may need incision and drainage
Carbunculosis (a cluster of furunculosis)	Cluster of furunculosis, slow development, fever, local sloughing of tissues, drainage from multiple openings, pain; usually requires incision and drainage

Skin lesions are painful and more common in areas where skin rubs against other skin.

DIFFERENTIAL DIAGNOSIS

- ***Folliculitis:*** pseudofolliculitis, furunculosis
- ***Furunculosis:*** folliculitis, carbunculosis, hidradenitis suppurativa
- ***Carbunculosis:*** cystic acne, epidermal cyst, folliculitis, hidradenitis suppurativa

DIAGNOSTIC STUDIES

- ***Folliculitis:*** usually none
- ***Furunculosis:*** usually none; may culture for frequent recurrences
- ***Carbunculosis:*** culture

PREVENTION

- Good hygiene
- For recurrent, severe infections

◊ Culture nares, skin, axilla
◊ Use povidone-iodine (Betadine®) or chlorhexidine 2% (Hibiclens®) for full body showers daily for 1-3 weeks (may cause severe drying of skin)
◊ WARNING: Hibiclens® can cause eye damage!
◊ Change towels and sheets daily
◊ Frequent hand washing
◊ Avoid heat, friction

NONPHARMACOLOGIC MANAGEMENT

Folliculitis

◊ Warm, moist compresses intermittently
◊ Allow spontaneous drainage (excision may cause spread)
◊ Frequent hand washing

Furunculosis

◊ Warm moist compresses intermittently for pain and to promote spontaneous drainage
◊ Good hygiene and preventive measures listed above
◊ Possible incision and drainage
◊ Consider culture and sensitivity

Carbunculosis

◊ Good hygiene and preventive measures listed above
◊ Warm moist compresses intermittently
◊ Possible incision and drainage
◊ Packing will promote drainage if wound is deep
◊ Strongly consider culture and sensitivity; especially if immunocompromised or diabetic

PHARMACOLOGIC MANAGEMENT

Folliculitis

◊ Treatment with an oral antibiotic usually not indicated
◊ May use 5% benzoyl peroxide or a topical antibiotic (mupirocin)
◊ Mupirocin (Bactroban®)
Apply three times a day
Not for use < 2 months age
Ointment: 22 g
Cream: 15 g, 20 g OR
◊ Retapamulin (Altabax®)
> 9 months: apply thin film twice daily
Ointment: 5 g, 10 g, 15 g

Furunculosis

◊ Systemic antibiotics do not shorten the duration, but consider for lesions in the facial area; empirically treated with a first-generation cephalosporin; consider TMPS or minocycline for MRSA

Carbunculosis

◊ Systemic antibiotics (consider first generation cephalosporin: or TMPS for MRSA)
◊ Warm moist compresses intermittently
◊ Consider a combination of oral and topical antibiotics may hasten infection eradication

BACTERIAL SKIN INFECTIONS PHARMACOLOGIC MANAGEMENT

If MRSA is the suspected or identified organism, in addition to an oral agent, consider chlorhexidine 2% washes daily for at least 7 days or until infection resolved; and mupirocin ointment in anterior nares 3 times daily or twice daily for 5-7 days.

Class	Drug Generic name (Trade name®)	Dosage How supplied	Comments
First Generation Cephalosporins *inhibit cell wall synthesis by bacteria* **General comments** More effective against rapidly reproducing organisms with cell walls Monitor for hypersensitivity reactions: rash, urticaria, angioedema and pruritis	**cephalexin**	**Adult**: 1-4 g daily in divided doses PO every 6-12 hours *Max*: 4 g/24 hours *Alternate*: 500 mg PO every 12 hours **Children > 1 year of age**: 25-50 mg/kg/day PO divided every 6-12 hours *Max*: 4 g/24 hours *Alternate*: 25-50 mg/kg/day PO divided every 12 hours *Max*: 4 g/24 hours	• Pregnancy Category B • **DO NOT USE IN PATIENTS WHO HAD HIVES OR ANAPHYLAXIS TO PENICILLIN** • Dosage reduction needed for renal impairment • Give without regard to meals • PT should be monitored in patients at risk: renal or hepatic impairment, poor nutritional state • After mixing suspension, store in refrigerator for up to 14 days

continued

BACTERIAL SKIN INFECTIONS PHARMACOLOGIC MANAGEMENT

If MRSA is the suspected or identified organism, in addition to an oral agent, consider chlorhexidine 2% washes daily for at least 7 days or until infection resolved; and mupirocin ointment in anterior nares 3 times daily or twice daily for 5-7 days.

Class	Drug Generic name (Trade name®)	Dosage How supplied	Comments
	Keflex	*Caps: 250 mg, 500 mg, 750 mg* *Susp: 125 mg/5 mL, 250 mg/5 mL*	
	cefadroxil	**Adult:** 1 g daily in single or 2 divided doses for 10 days **Children**: 30 mg/kg/day in a single or 2 divided doses for 10 days *Max*: 1 g/day	• Pregnancy Category B • **DO NOT USE IN PATIENTS WHO HAD HIVES OR ANAPHYLAXIS TO PENICILLIN** • Dosage reduction needed for renal impairment • No dosage reduction needed for geriatric patients
	Duricef	*Caps: 500 mg, 1000 mg* *Tablets: 1000 mg* *Susp: 250 mg/5 mL, 500 mg/5 mL*	
Sulfa Agents *block synthesis of folic acid by bacteria and thus inhibit bacterial replication* **General Comment** Consider for MRSA infections of the skin	**sulfamethoxazole (SMZ) - trimethoprim (TMP)**	**Adult:** one DS or 2 regular strength tabs twice daily for 10-14 days **Children > 2 mos.:** give 8 mg/kg/day of trimethoprim and 40 mg/kg/day of sulfamethoxazole in 2 divided doses daily *Max***:** do not exceed max adult dose	• Pregnancy Category C • Avoid use during pregnancy • Hypersensitivity reactions like Stevens-Johnson syndrome, toxic epidermal necrolysis and blood dyscrasias have been associated with sulfa use • Photosensitivity may occur with these drugs
	Bactrim Septra	*Tabs: 400 mg SMZ- 80 mg TMP* *Susp: 200 mg SMZ- 40 mg TMP/5 mL*	
	Bactrim DS	*Tabs: 800 mg SMZ-160 mg TMP*	

continued

BACTERIAL SKIN INFECTIONS PHARMACOLOGIC MANAGEMENT

If MRSA is the suspected or identified organism, in addition to an oral agent, consider chlorhexidine 2% washes daily for at least 7 days or until infection resolved; and mupirocin ointment in anterior nares 3 times daily or twice daily for 5-7 days.

Class	Drug Generic name (Trade name®)	Dosage How supplied	Comments
Miscellaneous Antibiotics	**clindamycin**	**Adult**: 150-300 mg PO every six hours daily *Alternate*: 300-450 mg PO every 6 hours daily **Children**: 8-16 mg/kg/day in 3-4 divided doses *Max*: Do not exceed max adult dose	• Pregnancy Category B • Consider for MRSA infections of the skin • Clostridium difficile associated diarrhea has been associated with severe colitis. Reserve for serious infections where less toxic antimicrobial agents are not warranted
	Cleocin	*Caps: 75 mg, 150mg, 300 mg*	• Higher doses are associated with greater incidence of side effects • Cautious use in patients with colitis. • Take with a big glass of water. • Monitor geriatric patients more closely since diarrhea may be more severe
	rifampin	**Adult**: 300 mg twice daily **Children**: 10-20 mg/kg/day in 2 divided doses *Max*: 600 mg/day	• Pregnancy Category C • Consider for MRSA infections of the skin • **DO NOT USE AS MONOTHERAPY**
	Rifadin Rimactane	*Caps: 150 mg, 300 mg*	• Can produce hepatic dysfunction Do not use in patients with hepatic dysfunction. Teach patient to report signs of jaundice, dark urine, etc. • Can interact with many medications, check compatibility prior to prescribing
	linezolid	**Adult and ≥ 12 years with MRSA**: 600 mg every 12 hours for 10-14 days **Children 5-11 years**: 10 mg/kg every 8 hours for 10-14 days *Max*: not to exceed 600 mg/ dose	• Pregnancy Category C • Consider for MRSA infections of the skin • **USE ONLY FOR COMPLICATED SKIN INFECTIONS** • Do not use in patient taking an MAO inhibitor or within 2 weeks of the last dose • Monitor for potential increases in blood pressure; do not use in patients with uncontrolled hypertension • Do not administer in pateitst taking SSRIs, TCAs, triptans, meperidine, or buspirone

continued

BACTERIAL SKIN INFECTIONS PHARMACOLOGIC MANAGEMENT

If MRSA is the suspected or identified organism, in addition to an oral agent, consider chlorhexidine 2% washes daily for at least 7 days or until infection resolved; and mupirocin ointment in anterior nares 3 times daily or twice daily for 5-7 days.

Class	Drug Generic name (Trade name®)	Dosage How supplied	Comments
	Zyvox	*Tabs: 400 mg, 600 mg* *Susp: 100 mg/5 mL available in 240 mL bottles*	• Myelosuppression can occur Monitor with CBC at least weekly • Monitor for lactic acidosis (recurrent nausea, vomiting) • Monitor for peripheral and optic neuropathy • May be taken without regard to food, but avoid foods high in tyramine while taking linezolid

CONSULTATION/REFERRAL

- Consider referral for furunculosis on face, scalp, and neck
- Consider referral for immunocompromised individuals, diabetics, others with chronic diseases

FOLLOW-UP

- Depends on severity and comorbid conditions

EXPECTED COURSE

- Complete resolution expected
- Recurrences are common
- For recurrences, consider nasal/skin carriage of organism

POSSIBLE COMPLICATIONS

- Cellulitis
- Sepsis
- Scarring

BURNS

DESCRIPTION

Injury to skin and tissues caused by chemicals, thermal energy, radiation or electricity.

ETIOLOGY

- Excessive sun exposure
- Flames or hot water most common
- Electrical wires, lightning
- Chemical splashes: acids or bases

INCIDENCE

- Common
- Splashes and flames are most common causes
- Leading cause of death in children
- Hot water burns are common means of abuse

RISK FACTORS

- Occupational exposure to chemicals
- Carelessness
- Age: very young and elderly have skin that is very susceptible to injury
- Hot water heaters set too high, especially in the elderly
- Improper use of sunscreens
- Insensitivity (e.g., diabetes mellitus, paralysis)

ASSESSMENT FINDINGS

- *Partial thickness*: first and second degree burns
- *Full thickness:* third degree burns
- General distribution of burns may indicate source
- Straight burn lines may indicate child abuse (bilaterally symmetrical on extremities)
- Adults: flame burns more common
- Children: scald burns more common
- Geriatric burns heal more slowly

Degrees of Burns and Differentiation	
Burns	**Appearance**
Partial Thickness **First-degree (superficial layers of epidermis)**	Redness Tenderness No blisters Skin blanches with pressure
Partial Thickness **Second degree (epidermal injury with blister formation)**	Redness Tenderness Presence of blisters
Full Thickness **Third degree (destruction of all skin elements)**	Charred, leathery appearance of skin Skin may be white with red edges Very little tenderness

Rule of Nines

- Each upper extremity: 9%
- Each lower extremity: 18% adult, 14% child
- Anterior trunk: 18%
- Posterior trunk: 18%
- Head and neck: 10% adult, 18% child

Estimate percent body surface area injured.

TRANSFER TO BURN CENTER

- 2nd or 3rd degree burns > 10% body surface area (BSA) in children or older adults
- 2nd degree burns > 20% BSA and full-thickness burns > 5% BSA in any age range

DIFFERENTIAL DIAGNOSIS

- Chemical vs. electrical vs. thermal vs. solar
- Scalded skin syndrome
- Toxic epidermal necrolysis

DIAGNOSTIC STUDIES

- Usually none indicated for first- or second-degree burns of limited area
- Culture and sensitivity if infected
- EKG, urine myoglobin, creatine kinase isoenzymes if electrical burn

PREVENTION

- Liberal sunscreen use
- In children, limit access to electrical cords, wires, chemicals, etc.
- Parental supervision
- Use of home smoke detectors and plan for evacuation of home in case of fire
- Knowledge of proper use of home fire extinguishers
- Set home water heaters < 120° F

NONPHARMACOLOGIC MANAGEMENT

- Do not apply ice to burns. Apply room temperature water or saline only in the first 15 minutes after injury. May use a mild soap
- Remove clothing, jewelry, over and around burned areas
- Flush chemical burns with cool water for 30 minutes to 2 hours depending on substance and severity
- Remove blistered skin after rupturing blisters
- Clean and redress burn 1-2 times/day (frequency dependent on severity)
- Good nutrition during convalescence

BURNS PHARMACOLOGIC MANAGEMENT

Class	Drug Generic name (Trade name®)	Dosage How supplied	Comments
Antimicrobial *Broad coverage against gram positive and negative organisms, and yeast*	**silver sulfadiazine** Silvadene	**Adult and > 2 months:** Cover burn area with cream once to twice daily to a thickness of 1/16 inch *Jars: 50 g, 400 g, 1000 g* *Tubes: 20 g, 85 g*	• Pregnancy Category B; avoid near term and in premature infants related to possibility of kernicterus • Contraindicated in sulfa allergy • Cleanse and debride burn (if appropriate) before applying • Continue applying to burn until satisfactory healing has occurred • Silver may inactivate topical proteolytic enzymes used in conjunction to treat burn • Monitor silver levels if drug is applied to extensive areas of the body • Monitor for leukopenia
	bacitracin Various generics OTC	**Adult**: Cleanse affected area and apply small amount 1 to 3 times daily *Ointment: 28 g*	• No information available on use in pediatric patients or during pregnancy • Ointments are preferred for burns involving the face • For external use only

CONSULTATION/REFERRAL

- Refer all burns not considered minor to specialist: second-degree burns > 20% of body, all third-degree burns, burns of the eyes, hands, face, feet, or perineum, lightening burns, electrical burns, burns over joints
- Child/elderly protection for suspected abuse

FOLLOW-UP

- Most burns are minor and can be managed on an outpatient basis
- Depends on severity and age of patient, but follow-up 1-3 days and until resolved

EXPECTED COURSE

- First degree burns resolve without complications
- Second degree burns resolve in about 2 weeks

POSSIBLE COMPLICATIONS

- Bacterial secondary infection (usually Gram negative organisms)
- Scarring

CAFE' AU LAIT SPOTS

DESCRIPTION

Brown, macular lesions which are almost always benign, but are also present in neurofibromatosis, a neurocutaneous syndrome.

ETIOLOGY

- An increase in the amount of melanin found within the melanocytes

INCIDENCE

- Common

RISK FACTORS

- Unknown
- Possible family history

ASSESSMENT FINDINGS

- Well marginated light brown macules usually < 1.5 cm in diameter
- Usually less than 5 lesions present
- If > 5 lesions are present that are >5 mm, suggests neurofibromatosis
- If 6 or more lesions are >15 mm in postpubertal child, strongly suggests neurofibromatosis
- Lesions may increase in size and number as person ages

DIFFERENTIAL DIAGNOSIS

- Freckles
- Neurofibromatosis

DIAGNOSTIC STUDIES

- Usually none indicated

NONPHARMACOLOGIC MANAGEMENT

- Patient education about regular examination of skin, reporting of changes to health care provider
- Measure and diagram location of lesions for identifying changes in lesions

CONSULTATION/REFERRAL

- Refer for suspected neurofibromatosis

FOLLOW-UP

- Annual visits to evaluate lesions

EXPECTED COURSE

- Benign course, no malignant changes expected
- Lesions may grow in size and number as patient ages

POSSIBLE COMPLICATIONS

- Neurofibromatosis

CAT SCRATCH FEVER

DESCRIPTION

Subacute lymphadenitis following contact with a cat (99% of the time), usually from a scratch.

ETIOLOGY

- *Bartonella henselae*
- No person-to-person transmission

INCIDENCE

- 24,000 cases annually in the U.S.
- Most common in people < 21 years

RISK FACTORS

- Contact with a cat, (a scratch is the most usual means of inoculation) most often a kitten. Animals are usually described as "well"

ASSESSMENT FINDINGS

- Mild symptoms of malaise, anorexia, aches, headache, and occasionally fever
- Erythematous, crusty papule (2-6 mm in diameter) 3-10 days after inoculation
- Unilateral lymphadenopathy evident within 1-2 weeks of scratch
- Nodes are tender and firm for several weeks

DIFFERENTIAL DIAGNOSIS

- Hodgkin's and non-Hodgkin's lymphoma
- Kawasaki disease

DIAGNOSTIC STUDIES

- Culture of primary papule
- Direct fluorescence antibody testing for detection of antibodies to *B. henselae*
- Cat scratch antigen skin test when diagnosis is uncertain

PREVENTION

- Cleanse cat scratches as soon as possible after they occur
- Supervise children around animals

NONPHARMACOLOGIC MANAGEMENT

- Treatment is symptomatic usually
- Local heat to painful nodes
- Limit vigorous activity
- Possible biopsy of node

PHARMACOLOGIC MANAGEMENT

- Analgesics
- Antibiotic treatment in immunocompromised: azithromycin; but antibiotic treatment controversial: will resolve in 2-6 months without treatment
- No clear evidence that antibiotic treatment improves outcomes

PREGNANCY/LACTATION CONSIDERATIONS

- Pregnant women should maintain cautious contact with cats, especially litter boxes

CONSULTATION/REFERRAL

- Consult physician for immunocompromised patients or patients with lymphadenopathy of uncertain origin

FOLLOW-UP

- Usually none needed
- Individualize follow up for severe cases or in immunocompromised patients

EXPECTED COURSE

- Usually benign without any complications within 2 weeks of onset of symptoms; complete resolution may take up to 2 months

POSSIBLE COMPLICATIONS

- Chronic lymphadenopathy
- Encephalitis/encephalopathy
- Erythema nodosum

CELLULITIS

DESCRIPTION

Acute, spreading infection of the skin and its subcutaneous structures.

ETIOLOGY

- Group A *Streptococcus*
- *Staphylococcus aureus*
- MRSA
- *Haemophilus influenza* (more common in children and often associated with an upper respiratory infection)
- Other organisms depending on cause

INCIDENCE

- Unknown
- Facial (periorbital) cellulitis common in children, elderly

Cellulitis usually affects the extremities or head.

RISK FACTORS

- Prior trauma
- Untreated, undertreated furunculosis
- Burns
- Diabetes mellitus
- Upper respiratory infection in children
- Immunocompromised state

ASSESSMENT FINDINGS

- Most common sites are lower legs and face (face is common site in children)
- Erythema
- Warmth
- Edema
- Pain
- Fever
- Lymphadenopathy

DIFFERENTIAL DIAGNOSIS

- Gout
- Erysipelas (superficial cellulitis)
- Contact dermatitis
- Ruptured Baker's cyst
- Thrombophlebitis

DIAGNOSTIC STUDIES

- Culture and sensitivity, yield is low (45%) even if good culture)
- CBC: mild leukocytosis with a shift to the left
- Blood culture if sepsis suspected
- ESR: elevated
- Imaging studies if osteomyelitis suspected

PREVENTION

- Good skin hygiene, especially when there is a break in the skin
- Avoid swimming when skin abrasion present
- Early treatment of upper respiratory infections

NONPHARMACOLOGIC MANAGEMENT

- Elevation of extremity to help prevent edema
- Moist heat for pain relief

PHARMACOLOGIC MANAGEMENT

- Antibiotic specific for organism if culture obtained
- Consider penicillin initially. If allergic, consider first generation cephalosporin or macrolide, unless MRSA is suspected

CELLULITIS PHARMACOLOGIC MANAGEMENT

If MRSA is the suspected or identified organism, in addition to an oral agent, consider chlorhexidine 2% washes daily for at least 7 days or until infection resolved; and mupirocin ointment in anterior nares 3 times daily or twice daily for 5-7 days.

Class	Drug Generic name (Trade name®)	Dosage How supplied	Comments
First Generation Cephalosporins *inhibit cell wall synthesis by bacteria* General comments More effective against rapidly reproducing organisms with cell walls Monitor for hypersensitivity reactions: rash, urticaria, angioedema and pruritis Consider for MSSA infections of the skin; do not use for suspected MRSA infections	**cephalexin**	**Adult**: 1-4 g daily in divided doses PO every 6-12 hours *Max*: 4 g/24 hours *Alternate*: 500 mg PO every 12 hours **Children > 1 year of age**: 25-50 mg/kg/day PO divided every 6-12 hours *Max*: 4 g/24 hours *Alternate*: 25-50 mg/kg/day PO divided every 12 hours *Max*: 4 g/24 hours	• Pregnancy Category B • **DO NOT USE IN PATIENTS WHO HAD HIVES OR ANAPHYLAXIS TO PENICILLIN** • Dosage reduction needed for renal impairment • Give without regard to meals • PT should be monitored in patients at risk: renal or hepatic impairment, poor nutritional state • After mixing suspension, store in refrigerator for up to 14 days
	Keflex	*Caps: 250 mg, 500 mg, 750 mg* *Susp: 125 mg/5 mL, 250 mg/5 mL*	
	cefadroxil	**Adult**: 1 g daily in single or divided doses twice daily for 10 days **Children**: 30 mg/kg/day in a single or 2 divided doses for 10 days *Max*: 1 g/day	• Pregnancy Category B • **DO NOT USE IN PATIENTS WHO HAD HIVES OR ANAPHYLAXIS TO PENICILLIN** • Dosage reduction needed for renal impairment • No dosage reduction needed for geriatric patients
	Duricef	*Caps: 500 mg, 1000 mg* *Tablets: 1000 mg* *Susp: 250 mg/5 mL, 500 mg/5 mL*	
Sulfa Agents *block synthesis of folic acid by bacteria and thus inhibit bacterial replication* General comment Consider for MRSA infections of the skin	**sulfamethoxazole (SMZ) - trimethoprim (TMP)**	**Adult:** one DS or 2 regular strength tabs twice daily for 10-14 days **Children > 2 mos.:** give 8 mg/kg/day of trimethoprim and 40 mg/kg/day of sulfamethoxazole in 2 divided doses daily *Max***:** do not exceed max adult dose	• Pregnancy Category C • Avoid use during pregnancy • Hypersensitivity reactions like Stevens-Johnson syndrome, toxic epidermal necrolysis and blood dyscrasias have been associated with sulfa use • Photosensitivity may occur with these drugs
	Bactrim Septra	*Tabs: 400 mg SMZ- 80 mg TMP* *Susp: 200 mg SMZ- 40 mg TMP/5 mL*	

continued

CELLULITIS PHARMACOLOGIC MANAGEMENT

If MRSA is the suspected or identified organism, in addition to an oral agent, consider chlorhexidine 2% washes daily for at least 7 days or until infection resolved; and mupirocin ointment in anterior nares 3 times daily or twice daily for 5-7 days.

Class	Drug Generic name (Trade name®)	Dosage How supplied	Comments
	Bactrim DS	*Tabs: 800 mg SMZ-160 mg TMP*	
Miscellaneous Antibiotics	**clindamycin**	**Adult**: 150 mg-300 mg PO every six hours daily *Alternate*: 300-450 mg PO every 6 hours daily **Children**: 8-16 mg/kg/day in 3-4 divided doses *Max*: Do not exceed max adult dose	• Pregnancy Category B • Consider for MRSA infections of the skin • *Clostridium difficile* associated diarrhea has been associated with severe colitis. Reserve for serious infections where less toxic antimicrobial agents are not warranted
	Cleocin	*Caps: 75, 150, 300 mg*	• Higher doses are associated with greater incidence of side effects • Cautious use in patients with colitis • Take with a big glass of water • Monitor geriatric patients more closely since diarrhea may be more severe
	rifampin	**Adult**: 300 mg twice daily **Children**: 10-20 mg/kg/day in 2 divided doses *Max*: 600 mg/day	• Pregnancy Category C • Consider for MRSA infections of the skin • **DO NOT USE AS MONOTHERAPY**
	Rifadin Rimactane	*Caps: 150 mg, 300 mg*	• Can produce hepatic dysfunction. Do not use in patients with hepatic dysfunction. Teach patient to report signs of jaundice, dark urine, etc. • Can interact with many medications, check compatibility prior to prescribing

continued

Dermatologic Disorders

CELLULITIS PHARMACOLOGIC MANAGEMENT

If MRSA is the suspected or identified organism, in addition to an oral agent, consider chlorhexidine 2% washes daily for at least 7 days or until infection resolved; and mupirocin ointment in anterior nares 3 times daily or twice daily for 5-7 days.

Class	Drug Generic name (Trade name®)	Dosage How supplied	Comments
	linezolid	**Adult and ≥ 12 years with MRSA**: 600 mg every 12 hours for 10-14 days **Children 5-11 years**: 10 mg/kg every 8 hours for 10-14 days *Max*: not to exceed 600 mg/ dose	• Pregnancy Category C • Consider for MRSA infections of the skin • **USE ONLY FOR COMPLICATED SKIN INFECTIONS** • Do not use in patients taking an MAO inhibitor or within 2 weeks of the last dose • Monitor for potential increases in blood pressure; do not use in patients with uncontrolled hypertension • Do not administer in patients taking SSRIs, TCAs, triptans, meperidine, or buspirone • Myelosuppression can occur. Monitor with CBC at least weekly • Monitor for lactic acidosis (recurrent nausea, vomiting) • Monitor for peripheral and optic neuropathy • May be taken without regard to food, but avoid foods high in tyramine while taking linezolid
	Zyvox	*Tabs: 400 mg, 600 mg* *Susp: 100 mg/5 mL available in 240 mL bottles*	

CONSULTATION/REFERRAL

- Consider referral for infections of the face, scalp, or neck; or if sepsis is suspected
- Consider referral for patients with chronic illnesses or who are immunocompromised

FOLLOW-UP

- 48 hours after initial treatment and then as patient condition indicates

Consider MRSA if patient not responding to penicillin or cephalosporin in first 48 hours after treatment.

EXPECTED COURSE

- Complete resolution expected with appropriate treatment

POSSIBLE COMPLICATIONS

- Septicemia/bacteremia
- Meningitis (from facial cellulitis in children) and cavernous sinus thrombosis
- Superinfection with gram negative organisms

COMMON, BENIGN PEDIATRIC SKIN LESIONS
(Mongolian Spots, Hemangiomas, Milia, Freckles)

DESCRIPTION

These skin lesions are variations from normal and are of no particular physical significance, but may be of cosmetic importance to parents/patients.

ETIOLOGY

Mongolian spots: dermal pigmented cells
Hemangiomas: dilation of capillaries
Milia: superficial cysts filled with keratin
Freckles: epidermal cells which contain an increased amount of pigment

INCIDENCE

- Very common
- Patient education regarding permanency of lesion

RISK FACTORS

- Unknown for most lesions
- Maybe familial (Mongolian spots, freckles)
- Fair skinned, blue-eyed individuals (freckles)
- Ultraviolet (UV) light exposure (freckles)

ASSESSMENT FINDINGS

Mongolian spots

◊ Blue-black macular lesion (may be mistaken for bruising)

◊ Prevalent in lumbosacral area of African-Americans, Native Americans, Hispanics, and Asians

◊ Usually disappear by 3 years of age

Hemangiomas

◊ Raised

◊ Cavernous: appear bluish, located deep beneath the skin, not present at birth, appear within a few months of life and then disappear before the end of the first decade of life

◊ Capillary (strawberry hemangiomas): bright red vascular overgrowth, elevated, vary in size

◊ Flat

  * Port-wine stains: dark red to deep purple lesions present at birth, frequently found on the face, do not fade with time

Milia

◊ White papules found on the forehead, face, chin, and cheeks of infants

◊ 1-2 mm in size

◊ Disappear a few weeks after birth

◊ May appear on palate, referred to as Epstein's pearls

Freckles

◊ Light brown macules present in large numbers on skin exposed to UV light

DIFFERENTIAL DIAGNOSIS

- Mongolian spots: bruises, child abuse
- Hemangiomas: other types of vascular nevi
- Milia: molluscum contagiosum
- Freckles: measles

DIAGNOSTIC STUDIES

- Usually none indicated

PREVENTION

- Unknown

NONPHARMACOLOGIC MANAGEMENT

- Reassure parents that these are benign lesions
- Laser treatment for port-wine stains

CONSULTATION/REFERRAL

- Dermatologist for questionable lesions

EXPECTED COURSE

- Benign lesions
- Course as described in assessment findings

CONTACT DERMATITIS

DESCRIPTION

Acute inflammation of the skin due to contact with an external substance or object that produces irritation (irritant dermatitis); or may be due to a delayed hypersensitivity reaction in individuals who were previously sensitized to an agent (allergic contact dermatitis).

ETIOLOGY

- Chemical irritants: nickel, turpentine, soaps, detergents (usually produce immediate discomfort)
- Plants (rhus-urushiol): poison ivy or oak (delayed hypersensitivity reaction produce discomfort within 4-12 hours)
- Other chemicals: antibiotics (neomycin), adhesives

INCIDENCE

- Common

RISK FACTORS

- Family history
- Continued contact with an offending substance: plants, chemicals, soaps

Fluid in blister NOT able to spread reaction.

- Topical drugs: neomycin, thimerosal, paraben
- Occupation: gloves; especially latex

ASSESSMENT FINDINGS

- Redness, itching, bullae, and/or surrounding erythema
- Lines of demarcation with sharp borders (allergic dermatitis from plants)
- Papules and/or vesicles
- Scaling, crusting, or oozing
- Initially, the dermatitis may be limited to the site of contact, but may later spread
- Palms and soles less likely to exhibit reaction
- Thin skin areas may be more sensitive (e.g., antecubital space, eyelids, genitalia)

DIFFERENTIAL DIAGNOSIS

- Seborrheic dermatitis
- Eczema
- Herpes simplex if appearance vesicular

DIAGNOSTIC STUDIES

- Usually none needed if history indicates obvious cause
- Patch test with offending substance

PREVENTION

- Avoid contact with offending substance
- Use protective items when contact possible with allergic substance (e.g., gloves, long sleeves)

NONPHARMACOLOGIC MANAGEMENT

- Avoid contact with offending substance
- If contact with substance occurs, wash skin immediately (within 15 minutes) with soap and water and rinse liberally
- Soaks with Burow solution (aluminum acetate and water 1:40 dilution), saline solution (1 tsp/pint of water)
- Soaks with cool water may help burning and/or irritation
- Tepid bath may help with pruritus
- Emollients to prevent drying if chronic inflammation
- Monitor for bacterial secondary infection

PHARMACOLOGIC MANAGEMENT

- Corticosteroids: topical, oral and/or injectable
- 3 factors affect potency of topical corticosteroids: steroid, concentration, and vehicle (vehicle = lotion, cream, etc.)
- Absorption increases based on the vehicle: lotion < cream < gel < ointment
- Calamine lotion for itching
- Moisture barrier: zinc oxide
- Antihistamine: topical and/or oral
- Topical or oral antibiotics if secondarily infected

CONTACT DERMATITIS PHARMACOLOGIC MANAGEMENT

Pediatric patients may be more susceptible to topical corticosteroid-induced HPA axis suppression than older patients because of larger skin surface area to body weight ratio. Limit use to lowest effect potency and time.

Class	Drug Generic name (Trade name®)	Dosage How supplied	Comments
Low Potency Steroids *exert their anti-inflammatory effect through mechanical, chemical, microbiological and immunological means*	**alclometasone dipropionate 0.05%**	**Adult:** apply thin film, massage in 2-3 times/day **Children > 1 year**: same as adult	• Pregnancy Category C • For external use only • Do not use longer than 3 weeks • No adjustment in dosage needed for geriatric patients
General comments Use lowest potency that produces desired effect	Aclovate	*Cream/oint: 15 g, 45 g, 60 g*	
Skin atrophy and changes in skin color are possible with long term use Areas with greatest absorption of steroid are the face, groin, and axillae. Consider lowest potency steroids in these areas	**fluocinolone acetonide 0.01%**	**Adult**: thin film 2-4 times daily **Children**: Pediatric dosing not available	• Pregnancy Category C • For external use only • Do not use longer than 3 weeks • No adjustment in dosage needed for geriatric patients
	Synalar solution	*Cream/oint: 15 g, 60 g* *Solution: 20 mL, 60 mL*	
Systemic absorption is usually minimal, but broken skin will absorb significantly more steroid	**hydrocortisone base or acetate 0.5%**	**Adult and Children > 2 years:** apply thin film 2-4 times daily	• Pregnancy Category C • For external use only • Do not use longer than 3 weeks
Topical steroids will worsen skin infections	Cortisporin cream Hytone ointment U-cort cream Vytone cream	*Cream/Oint: 1 oz, 2 oz.*	
Medium Potency Steroids *exert their anti-inflammatory effect through mechanical, chemical, microbiological, and immunological means*	**triamcinolone acetonide 0.025%**	**Adult**: apply thin film 2-4 times daily **Children**: Pediatric dosing not available	• Pregnancy Category C • Intended for external use only • Use caution in use longer than 2 weeks, may change skin pigmentation
General comments Use lowest potency that produces desired effect Skin atrophy and changes in skin color are possible with long term use Areas with greatest absorption of steroid are the face, groin, and axillae. Consider lowest potency steroids in these areas Topical steroids will worsen skin infections	Aristocort cream Kenalog cream, lotion, ointment	*Cream: 0.025% and 0.1%, 15 g, 60 g; 0.5%, 15 g; 0.1%, 15 g , 60 g* *Kenalog lotion: 60 mL* *Oint: 15 g, 60 g*	

continued

Dermatologic Disorders

Dermatologic Disorders

CONTACT DERMATITIS PHARMACOLOGIC MANAGEMENT

Pediatric patients may be more susceptible to topical corticosteroid-induced HPA axis suppression than older patients because of larger skin surface area to body weight ratio. Limit use to lowest effect potency and time.

Class	Drug Generic name (Trade name®)	Dosage How supplied	Comments
	desoximetasone 0.05%	**Adult**: apply thin film twice a day **Children**: Pediatric dosing not available	• Pregnancy Category C • Intended for topical use only • Use caution in use longer than 2 weeks, may change skin pigmentation
	Topicort LP	*Cream/gel: 15 g, 60 g* *Oint: 60 g*	
	flurandrenolide 0.025%	**Adult**: apply every 12 hours **Children**: Pediatric dosing not available	• Pregnancy Category C • Intended for topical use only • Use caution in use longer than 2 weeks, may change skin pigmentation
	Cordran	*Cream/oint: 30 g, 60 g*	
	fluticasone propionate 0.05%	**Adult**: apply thin film twice a day **Children > 3 months**: Apply a thin film once or twice daily	• Pregnancy Category C • Intended for topical use only • Use in pediatric patients for more than 4 weeks of use has not been established • No dosage adjustment recommended for geriatric patients
	Cutivate	*Cream: 15 g, 30 g, 60 g* *Lotion: 120 ml*	
	hydrocortisone valerate 0.2%	**Adult**: apply thin film 2-3 times daily **Children**: Pediatric dosing not available	• Pregnancy Category C • Intended for topical use only • Use caution in use longer than 2 weeks, may change skin pigmentation
	Westcort	*Cream/oint: 15 g, 45 g, 60 g*	
	mometasone furoate 0.1%	**Adult**: apply thin film daily **Children > 2 years**: apply sparingly once daily to affected areas	• Pregnancy Category C • Intended for topical use only • Use caution in use longer than 2 weeks, may change skin pigmentation • DO NOT USE WITH AN OCCLUSIVE DRESSING
	Elocon	*Cream/oint: 15 g, 45 g* *Lotion: 30 mL, 60 mL*	

continued

CONTACT DERMATITIS PHARMACOLOGIC MANAGEMENT

Pediatric patients may be more susceptible to topical corticosteroid-induced HPA axis suppression than older patients because of larger skin surface area to body weight ratio. Limit use to lowest effect potency and time.

Class	Drug Generic name (Trade name®)	Dosage How supplied	Comments
	triamicinolone acetonide 0.1%	**Adult**: apply thin film 3-4 times daily **Children**: pediatric dosing not available	• Pregnancy Category C • Intended for topical use only • Use caution with using longer than 2 weeks, may change skin pigmentation
	Aristocort A cream, oint; Kenalog cream, lotion	*Cream/oint: 15 g, 60 g* *Lotion: 15 mL, 60 mL*	
High Potency Corticosteroids *exert their anti-inflammatory effect through mechanical, chemical, microbiological, and immunological means* **General comments** Use lowest potency that produces desired effect Skin atrophy and changes in skin color are possible with long term use Areas with greatest absorption of steroid are the face, groin, and axillae. Consider lowest potency steroids in these areas Topical steroids will worsen skin infections Do not use more than 50 g/week	**amcinonide 0.1%**	**Adult**: thin film 2-3 times daily **Children**: pediatric dosing not available	• Pregnancy Category C • Intended for topical use only • Use caution with using longer than 2 weeks, may change skin pigmentation
	Cyclocor	*Cream/oint: 15 g, 30 g, 60 g* *Lotion: 30 mL, 60 mL*	
	betamethasone dipropionate 0.05%	**Adult and children > 12 years**: apply thin film 1-2 times daily *Max*: 2 consecutive weeks	• Pregnancy Category C • Intended for topical use only • Use caution with using longer than 2 weeks, may change skin pigmentation • **Studies demonstrate HPA axis suppression in some children** • No dosage adjustment recommended for geriatric patients
	Diprolene AF	*Oint/cream: 15 g, 50 g* *Lotion: 30 mL, 60 mL*	
	desoximetasone 0.05%	**Adult**: apply thin film twice a day **Children**: pediatric dosing not available	• Pregnancy Category C • Intended for topical use only • Use caution with using longer than 2 weeks, may change skin pigmentation • **Studies demonstrate HPA axis suppression in some children**
	Topicort	*Cream/0.25% gel: 15 g, 60 g* *Ointment: 60 g*	
Super High Potency *exert their anti-inflammatory effect through mechanical, chemical, microbiological, and immunological means* **General comments** Use lowest potency that produces desired effect	**betamethasone dipropionate augmented 0.05%**	**Adult and children > 12 years**: apply thin film 1-2 times daily *Max*: 2 consecutive weeks	• Pregnancy Category C • Intended for topical use only • Use caution with using longer than 2 weeks, may change skin pigmentation • **Studies demonstrate HPA axis suppression in some children** • No dosage adjustment recommended for geriatric patients
	Diprolene	*Oint/cream: 15 g, 50 g* *Lotion: 30 mL, 60 mL*	

continued

Dermatologic Disorders

CONTACT DERMATITIS PHARMACOLOGIC MANAGEMENT

Pediatric patients may be more susceptible to topical corticosteroid-induced HPA axis suppression than older patients because of larger skin surface area to body weight ratio. Limit use to lowest effect potency and time.

Class	Drug Generic name (Trade name®)	Dosage How supplied	Comments
Skin atrophy and changes in skin color are possible with long term use Areas with greatest absorption of steroid are the face, groin, and axillae. Consider lowest potency steroids in these areas Topical steroids will worsen skin infections Do not use more than 50 g/week	**clobetasol propionate 0.05%**	**Adult and children ≥ 16 years**: apply thin film twice a day *Max*: 50 g/week	• Pregnancy Category C • Intended for topical use only • Use caution with use longer than 2 weeks, may change skin pigmentation • **Studies demonstrate HPA axis suppression in some children** • No dosage adjustment recommended for geriatric patients
	Temovate cream, gel, oint, scalp, emollient	*Cream/Oint: 15 g, 30 g, 45 g, 60 g* *Soln: 50 mL* *Scalp emollient: 50 mL*	
	flurandrenolide 4 mcg/sq cream	**Adult**: apply every 12 hours	• Pregnancy Category C • Intended for topical use only • Use caution with use longer than 2 weeks, may change skin pigmentation • Change tape every 12 hours
	Cordran	*Tape: 3" x 24" and 3" x 80"; Patch: 2" x 3";* *Oint/cream 0.05%: 30 g, 60 g* *Lotion: 15 mL, 60 mL*	
	halobetasol propionate 0.05%	**Adult and children > 12 years**: apply thin layer twice a day *Max*: 50 g/week	• Pregnancy Category C • Intended for topical use only • Use caution with use longer than 2 weeks, may change skin pigmentation • Do not use with occlusive dressings • No dosage adjustment recommended for geriatric patients
	Ultravate	*Cream/Oint: 15 g, 45 g*	

PREGNANCY/LACTATION CONSIDERATIONS

- Prudent use of medications

CONSULTATION/REFERRAL

- Dermatologist for slow to respond lesions
- Allergist if offending substance unable to be identified

FOLLOW-UP

- Depends on severity
- Consider follow up within 24 hours if systemic reaction has occurred

EXPECTED COURSE

- Self-limited

POSSIBLE COMPLICATIONS

- Secondary bacterial infection
- More severe subsequent reactions

DIAPER DERMATITIS
(Diaper Rash)

DESCRIPTION

Inflamed skin found in the diaper area.

ETIOLOGY

- Irritant contact dermatitis
- Candidal infection
- Atopic dermatitis
- Seborrheic dermatitis

INCIDENCE

- Common
- Males = Females
- Common pediatric problem and in incontinent geriatric population

RISK FACTORS

- Prolonged contact with soiled/wet diaper
- Waterproof diapers
- Hot and humid climates
- Family history of dermatitis
- Diarrhea
- Recent treatment with oral antibiotics

ASSESSMENT FINDINGS

Irritant Contact Dermatitis	Chapped skin Rarely involves skin creases Dusky red rash
Candidal Diaper Rash	Bright beefy rash Satellite lesions visible Excoriated skin Often involves skin creases
Atopic Diaper Dermatitis	Excoriated skin Weeping, crusting lesions Not usually in skin creases
Seborrheic Dermatitis	Patches or plaques may be present Dusky red appearance Other sites of seborrheic dermatitis often present (scalp, eyebrows) Usually found within skin creases

DIFFERENTIAL DIAGNOSIS

- Dermatitis: atopic vs. seborrheic vs. contact
- Candidiasis

DIAGNOSTIC STUDIES

- Usually none needed
- KOH preparation if possible fungal etiology

PREVENTION

- Key to prevention is good hygiene
- Change diapers frequently
- Avoid use of baby powder (retains moisture in creases)

NONPHARMACOLOGIC MANAGEMENT

- Leave dermatitis open to air as much as possible
- Change diapers frequently
- Treat at earliest sign of rash
- Cleanse skin with milk soap, pat dry, allow to air dry as long as possible after cleaning
- Avoid waterproof diapers, waterproof pants

CONSULTATION/REFERRAL

- Child/elder protection if neglect is suspected

FOLLOW-UP

- Every 3-4 days if not improving

EXPECTED COURSE

- Resolution with proper treatment in 4-7 days

POSSIBLE COMPLICATIONS

- Secondary bacterial or yeast infections
- Two or more types of dermatitis may exist concurrently

DIAPER DERMATITIS PHARMACOLOGICAL MANAGEMENT

Class	Drug Generic name (Trade name®)	Dosage How supplied	Comments
Skin Barrier *Acts as skin protection*	**zinc oxide**	Apply liberally with each diaper change (especially at night or times when exposure to wet diapers may be prolonged)	• For external use only • Not intended for deep or puncture wounds, animal bites, or serious burns
	Various names	*Tubes:* Multiple sizes	
Antifungals *Medications that have fungistatic and fungicidal properties*	**econozole nitrate 1%**	*Candidiasis* infections Apply twice daily for a 2 week period	• Pregnancy Category C • Intended for topical use only
	Spectazole	*Cream: 15 g, 30 g, 85 g*	
	nystatin	Apply sparingly 2 times a day	• Pregnancy Category C • Intended for topical use only • Moist lesions are best treated with powder form
	Mycostatin	*Cream: 30 g* *Powder: 15 g*	
Low Potency Corticosteroids	**alclometasone dipropionate 0.05%**	Children > 1 year Apply sparingly 2-3 times/day	• Pregnancy Category C • Do not use longer than 3 weeks
	Aclovate	*Cream: 15 g, 45 g, 60 g* *Oint: 15 g, 45 g, 60 g*	
	fluocinolone acetonide 0.01%	Apply 2-4 times/day	• Pregnancy Category D • Do not use longer than 4 weeks
	Synalar	*Cream: 15 g, 60 g* *Oint: 15 g, 60 g*	
	hydrocortisone base or acetate, 0.5% - 1%	Apply 2-4 times a day	• Pregnancy Category C
	Various trade names	*Cream, ointments*	
	triamcinolone acetonide 0.025%	Apply thin film 2-4 times/day	• Pregnancy Category C • Can be occluded • Store at room temperature
	Various trade names	*Cream: 15 g, 80 g* *Ointments*	
Combination Products	**triamcinolone acetonide 0.1% (Triamcinolone + Nystatin)**	Apply sparingly 2 times a day	• Pregnancy Category C • Maximum 25 days of use • Contraindicated in varicella lesions • Do not occlude
	Various trade names	*Cream: 15 g, 30 g, 60 g*	

FIFTH DISEASE
(Erythema Infectiosum, Slapped-Cheek Disease)

DESCRIPTION

A common viral infection characterized by an eruptive rash. Since it was the fifth disease described with an eruptive rash, it was named "Fifth Disease".

ETIOLOGY

- Parvovirus B19

INCIDENCE

- Most common in 4-12 year olds
- Also occurs in infants and adults
- Most common in late spring

RISK FACTORS

- Incubation period is 4-28 days (average = 16 days)
- Contact with a person before the rash erupts (communicable period ends when rash erupts)
- Nasal secretions and aerosolized respiratory droplets are means of transmission

ASSESSMENT FINDINGS

- Prodrome: low-grade fever, malaise, sore throat, lethargy (lasts 1-4 days)
- Rash
  - ◊ First phase often appears first on cheeks of face: intense red rash with circumoral pallor; hence the name "slapped-cheek disease"
  - ◊ Second phase of rash spreads to body and extremities over next few days: (macular and lacy appearing, rash blanches)
  - ◊ Final phase of rash may be pruritic and itch more intensely with exercise, sun exposure, emotional distress or bathing (can last up to 21 days)
  - ◊ Palms and soles may be affected: pruritic (lasts 7-20 days)
  - ◊ Children may return to school during the rash phase if fever free for 24 hours
  - ◊ Adults may have arthralgias and/or arthritis

POSSIBLE COMPLICATIONS

- Seizures due to high fever (5-10% of children)
- Aseptic meningitis (rare)

Presence of rash indicates patient is no longer infectious.

DIFFERENTIAL DIAGNOSIS

- Rubella
- Enterovirus
- Lupus
- Drug rashes
- Other viral exanthems

DIAGNOSTIC STUDIES

- Usually none; diagnosis is made clinically
- B19 specific IgM (confirms acute infection)
- B19 specific IgG (confirms past infection)

PREVENTION

- Avoid exposure to persons with known infections
- Danger to fetus is primarily severe anemia due to RBC destruction and aplasia
- Pregnant women should avoid close contact with aplastic Parvo B19 patients because they are highly contagious

Prompt referral to maternal-fetal specialist if pregnant woman infected with parvovirus B19.

NONPHARMACOLOGIC MANAGEMENT

- Supportive care
- Rest

PHARMACOLOGIC MANAGEMENT

- No specific treatment
- Analgesics if needed - do not use aspirin due to risk of Reye's Syndrome

PREGNANCY/LACTATION CONSIDERATIONS

- Rash in pregnant women should be assessed for possible Parvo B19 infection
- Infection during pregnancy is associated with a

- 10% fetal death (greatest threat is before 34th week gestation)
- There is no indication for routine exclusion in the work place if known infected personnel are present
- Fetal ultrasound and α-fetoprotein testing can help assess fetal damage if documented infection and exposure have taken place

CONSULTATION/REFERRAL

- Obstetrician/maternal-fetal specialist for known exposure
- Consider referral for immunocompromised patients

FOLLOW-UP

- Usually none needed

EXPECTED COURSE

- Rash may last up to 3 weeks
- Rash may fade, intensify depending on temperature, sunlight, exercise

POSSIBLE COMPLICATIONS

- Arthritis: adults more prone; may begin 2-3 weeks after onset of symptoms
- Aplastic crisis: may occur in patients with sickle cell or other types of anemias
- Fetal hydrops

HAND-FOOT-AND-MOUTH DISEASE

DESCRIPTION

This is a highly contagious viral illness similar to herpangina, but the characteristic lesions appear on the buccal mucosa, palate, palms of the hands, soles of the feet and buttocks.

ETIOLOGY

- Coxsackie A 16 (most common)
- Other Coxsackie viruses
- Other enteroviruses

INCIDENCE

- Common in children under 5 years
- Occurs in late summer and fall

RISK FACTORS

- Contact with oral, fecal, or respiratory secretions of infected persons (highly contagious)

ASSESSMENT FINDINGS

- Low-grade fever
- Malaise
- Abdominal pain
- 25% have enlarged anterior cervical nodes or submandibular nodes
- Oral manifestations may be small, red papules on the tongue and buccal mucosa which progress to ulcerative vesicles on an erythematous base which ulcerates
- Exanthem is rarely pruritic and may occur on the palms, soles, arms, legs, buttocks, fingers, and toes

DIFFERENTIAL DIAGNOSIS

- Herpangina
- Aphthous stomatitis
- Stevens-Johnson syndrome

DIAGNOSTIC STUDIES

- Usually none needed (diagnosis made from history and examination)

PREVENTION

- Avoid exposure to known infected persons
- Good hygiene
- Good hand washing

NONPHARMACOLOGIC MANAGEMENT

- Maintain hydration and provide cool liquids frequently
- Avoid spicy foods
- Rest
- Return to clinic if no improvement in 3-4 days
- Treatment is symptomatic

PHARMACOLOGIC MANAGEMENT

- Analgesics for pain and fever
- Topical antihistamine/anesthetic (aluminum hydroxide/magnesium hydroxide gel with diphenhydramine) applied to painful lesions (relief is short-lived)
- Topical lidocaine is NOT recommended because it can be absorbed from mucous membranes and may be toxic (adult & child fatalities reported)

CONSULTATION/REFERRAL

- Rarely needed because condition is self-limiting
- Refer for dehydration

FOLLOW-UP

- Usually none needed

EXPECTED COURSE

- Resolution within 7 days of onset

POSSIBLE COMPLICATIONS

- Myocarditis (extremely rare)
- Meningitis, encephalitis

HERPANGINA

DESCRIPTION

Viral infection that causes fever and multiple vesicles and ulcerations on the posterior third of the mouth that involves the soft palate, uvula, tonsils, and pharynx.

ETIOLOGY

- Coxsackie A (most common) and B virus (rarely)
- Rarely Echovirus

INCIDENCE

- Occurs in outbreaks during the summer and fall in children 3 months to 16 years; occurs year round in tropical climates

RISK FACTORS

- Contact with saliva of infected persons

ASSESSMENT FINDINGS

- High fever
- Severe throat pain which can cause impairment of fluid intake
- 1-2 mm grey-white vesicles surrounded by an erythematous halo (before ulceration occurs) on the anterior 2/3 of the mouth
- Drooling
- Coryza
- Anorexia
- Malaise
- Irritability
- Gastrointesinal symptoms: diarrhea, emesis

DIFFERENTIAL DIAGNOSIS

- Hand-foot-mouth disease
- Herpes simplex
- Gingivostomatitis
- Drug reaction

DIAGNOSTIC STUDIES

- Usually none needed; diagnosed on clinical presentation
- Consider viral cultures of lesions (rarely performed)
- Consider quick streptococcal test

PREVENTION

- Avoid exposure to oral secretions of infected persons
- Good hygiene
- Good hand washing

NONPHARMACOLOGIC MANAGEMENT

- Maintain hydration and provide cool liquids frequently
- Avoid spicy foods
- Rest
- Teach parents to return to office with child if no improvement in 3-4 days
- Treatment is symptomatic

PHARMACOLOGIC MANAGEMENT

- Analgesics for fever and throat pain
- Consider topical anesthetic but cautious use in young children
- Mouthwash: 1% diphenhydramine in 50% attapulgite (Kaopectate)

CONSULTATION/REFERRAL

- None usually needed
- Refer for severe dehydration

FOLLOW-UP

- None usually needed

Virus may be shed for several weeks in feces. Therefore, children are allowed to return to daycare/school after they have been fever-free for 24 hours and drooling has stopped.

EXPECTED COURSE

- Ulcerations heal/resolve in 3-6 days
- Resolution usually by day 7

POSSIBLE COMPLICATIONS

- Unusual

HERPES ZOSTER
(SHINGLES)

DESCRIPTION

A reactivation of the varicella-zoster virus (chickenpox virus) that has lain dormant in nerve cells. This involves the skin of a single dermatome or less commonly, several dermatomes.

ETIOLOGY

- Varicella-zoster virus

INCIDENCE

- 215/100,000 annually
- Higher incidence in the elderly, neonates, and immunocompromised patients
- Rarely occurs in children unless immunocompromised

RISK FACTORS

- Advancing age
- Biologic stress
- Majority of patients have no risk factors
- Immunocompromised status
- Emotional stress
- Treatment of a malignancy
- Spinal surgery or spinal radiation

ASSESSMENT FINDINGS

Prodrome

◊ Itching
◊ Burning
◊ Photophobia
◊ Fever, headache, malaise

Acute Phase

◊ Dermatomal rash erupts over 3-4 days: expect unilateral
◊ Fever, malaise, headache
◊ Maculopapular rash which progresses to grouped vesicles on an erythematous base, and then pustules in 3-4 days. Successive crops of

vesicles may appear for a week.
- ◊ Pain, possibly severe

Convalescent Phase
- ◊ Within 2-3 weeks, rash resolves
- ◊ Pain
- ◊ May be prolonged in elderly and immunocompromised patients
  Postherpetic neuralgia (pain longer than 1 month after rash has resolved) common in the elderly, may last for months

DIFFERENTIAL DIAGNOSIS

- Other viral infections: coxsackievirus, herpes simplex virus, varicella
- Contact dermatitis
- Herniated disc
- Poison ivy
- Early HIV

DIAGNOSTIC STUDIES

- Usually none needed
- Consider HIV testing, screening for diabetes if patient is young or has multiple eruptions across several dermatomes
- Direct immunofluorescence of viral exudate

PREVENTION

- None at this time if < 60 years
- Zostavax® recommended by CDC as a single dose given at > 60 years of age
- Elderly, neonates, and immunocompromised should avoid persons with known shingles until lesions have crusted over

Zostavax®, the immunization to prevent shingles, is a live virus. Consequently, it is contraindicated in immunocompromised patients. It can be given regardless of a prior episode of shingles.

NONPHARMACOLOGIC MANAGEMENT

- Wet compresses of Domeboro solution several times per day
- Avoid contact with known patients if member of high-risk group (they can develop chickenpox)

Patients who have shingles are not able to transmit shingles to other susceptible patients. They may only transmit the chickenpox virus to susceptible patients. A patient cannot be infected with shingles from another patient who has shingles.

PHARMACOLOGIC MANAGEMENT

Treatment of post herpetic neuralgia:
- Capsaicin cream (Zostrix®): available OTC, only use on intact skin
- Gabapentin (Neurontin®): start at 300 mg daily, titrate to pain relief or 1.8 g per day
- Amitriptylline: off label use but commonly used for long term pain control
- Pregabalin (Lyrica®): start at 75 mg twice daily, titrate up (see manuf directions for dosing)
- Lidoderm patch 5%: provides relief of pain topically; lidocaine can be absorbed systemically

HERPES ZOSTER PHARMACOLOGIC MANAGEMENT

Class	Drug Generic name (Trade name®)	Dosage How supplied	Comments
Antiviral Agents *inhibit viral DNA synthesis and thus viral DNA replication* **General comment** Initiate at earliest sign of zoster infection. Most effective when started within 48-72 hours of onset of rash	**acyclovir**	**Adult**: 800 mg every 4 hours orally, 5 times daily for 7-10 days	• Pregnancy Category B • Dosage adjustment recommended for patients with renal impairment • No data on treatment initiated after 72 hours • Geriatric patients (> 65 years): more likely to have nausea, vomiting, and dizziness than younger patients

continued

HERPES ZOSTER PHARMACOLOGIC MANAGEMENT

Class	Drug Generic name (Trade name®)	Dosage How supplied	Comments
	Zovirax	*Tabs: 200 mg, 400 mg, 800 mg* *Susp: 200 mg/5 mL*	• Geriatric patients more likely to have renal or CNS adverse events (somnolence, hallucinations, confusion, and coma)
	famciclovir Famvir	**Adult >18 years**: 500 mg every 8 hours for 7 days *Tabs: 125 mg, 250 mg, 500 mg*	• Pregnancy Category B • Efficacy not established for disseminated zoster or zoster in immunocompromised patients • No increased adverse events in older patients but caution if decreased hepatic, renal or cardiac function
	valacyclovir Valtrex	**Adult**: 1 g every 8 hr for 7 days *Caplets: 500 mg, 1000 mg*	• Pregnancy Category B • Can be given without regard to meals • Cautious use in geriatric patients with or without impaired renal function • Dosage adjustment needed for renal impairment • Ensure adequate hydration • Geriatric patients more likely to have renal or CNS adverse events (somnolence, hallucinations, confusion, and coma) • No significant drug interactions

The advantage of treating with oral antiviral agents within 48-72 hours is probable faster resolution of rash and symptoms; prevention or minimization of post herpetic neuralgia.

PREGNANCY/LACTATION CONSIDERATIONS

- Acyclovir, famciclovir, and valacyclovir are all pregnancy category B drugs

CONSULTATION/REFERRAL

- Urgent consultation of ophthalmologist for dermatomes involving the eye
- Consider referral to infectious disease for neonatal or immunocompromised patients

FOLLOW-UP

- Usually recheck in 3-5 days after diagnosis, then in 1-2 weeks

EXPECTED COURSE

- Resolution of acute phase usually 14-21 days
- Postherpetic neuralgia may last for months

POSSIBLE COMPLICATIONS

- Postherpetic neuralgia
- Superinfection of skin lesions
- Cranial nerve syndromes, especially if the facial or ophthalmic nerves are involved
- Guillain-Barré syndrome
- Corneal ulceration

HIDRADENITIS SUPPURATIVA

DESCRIPTION

Inflammation of apocrine glands of the skin that produce tender, cyst-like abscesses. Common sites are the axilla, groin, trunk, and the scalp. They tend to recur because sinus tracts develop and acute abscesses develop and often drain.

ETIOLOGY

- Blockage of the apocrine glands leading to rupture of the ducts

INCIDENCE

- Common from late puberty to age 40 years
- More common in females
- Rare in children, rare after menopause

RISK FACTORS

- Obesity
- Diabetes mellitus
- African-American females
- Female gender
- Hyperandrogenism

ASSESSMENT FINDINGS

- Cyst like abscesses
- Most frequent places of occurrence: axilla, groin, and anus
- Pain
- Warmth
- Erythema
- Discharge
- Papules, nodules (1-3 cm)
- Fluctuance (a wave-like impulse felt on palpation) in larger lesions

Boils may exacerbate at time of menses.

DIFFERENTIAL DIAGNOSIS

- Furunculosis
- Carbunculosis
- Lymphadenitis/lympahdenopathy

DIAGNOSTIC STUDIES

- Culture and sensitivity of lesion exudate, though often no organism is isolated
- Infections are usually polymicrobial and a deep culture is required to collect organisms

PREVENTION

- Avoid constrictive clothing; especially tight jeans
- Weight loss if indicated
- Good hygiene

NONPHARMACOLOGIC MANAGEMENT

- Aspirate; culture and sensitivity
- Incision and drainage
- Good hygiene
- Avoid antiperspirants (if lesion is in axilla) or other irritants
- Rest
- Moist heat
- Surgical excision for large persistent lesions

PHARMACOLOGIC MANAGEMENT

- Systemic antibiotics not curative; relapse almost always results, base treatment on culture results
- Consider treating initially with first or second generation cephalosporin or sulfa drug if MRSA is likely pathogen
- Topical clindamycin
- Topical application around nostrils helpful in reducing spread

PREGNANCY/LACTATION CONSIDERATIONS

- Do not use tetracycline in pregnant or lactating women

CONSULTATION/REFERRAL

- Consider referral for large lesions and slow healing lesions

FOLLOW-UP

- Depends on severity and patient condition

EXPECTED COURSE

- Rare spontaneous resolution
- Lesions may take a month or more to heal

POSSIBLE COMPLICATIONS

- Scarring
- Recurrences may take years to heal

IMPETIGO

DESCRIPTION

Superficial infection of the skin which begins as small superficial vesicles which rupture and form honey-colored crusts.

> **Superficial infections are usually treated with topical agents unless they span a large surface area; then, oral agents are usually more economical.**

ETIOLOGY

- *Staphylococcus aureus* (predominant organism)
- Group A β-hemolytic *Streptococcus* (presents in 10-20% of cases)

INCIDENCE

- Common
- Most prevalent in ages 2-5 years
- Summer and fall

RISK FACTORS

- Residing in warm, humid climates
- Insect bites, minor cuts
- Infected family member
- Direct contact with lesions
- Poor hygiene

ASSESSMENT FINDINGS

- 1-2 mm vesicles which rupture
- Honey-colored crusts
- Weeping shallow red ulcer
- Common on mouth, face, nose, or site of insect bites or trauma

DIFFERENTIAL DIAGNOSIS

- Chickenpox
- Folliculitis
- Herpes simplex
- Insect bites
- Dermatitis

DIAGNOSTIC STUDIES

- Usually none required

PREVENTION

- Good hygiene
- Good hand washing, especially by household members

NONPHARMACOLOGIC MANAGEMENT

- Washing of lesions 2-3 times per day
- Good hygiene
- Good hand washing, especially by household members

PHARMACOLOGIC MANAGEMENT

- Topical is preferred: mupirocin ointment (Bactroban®) Apply three times a day
  Not for use <2 months age
  Ointment: 22 g; Cream: 15 g, 20 g OR
  Retapamulin (Altabax®)
  > 9 months: apply thin film twice daily
  Ointment: 5 g, 10 g, 15 g
- First or second-generation cephalosporin for large area of infection; may consider macrolide if unable to use penicillin or cephalosporin
- Some resistance to erythromycin encountered in U.S., dicloxacillin (Dynapen®) may be substituted

IMPETIGO PHARMACOLOGIC MANAGEMENT

If MRSA is the suspected or identified organism, in addition to an oral agent, consider chlorhexidine 2% washes daily for at least 7 days or until infection resolved; and mupirocin ointment in anterior nares 3 times daily or twice daily for 5-7 days.

Class	Drug Generic name (Trade name®)	Dosage How supplied	Comments
Topical Antibiotic Ointments	**mupirocin**	**Adult and children ≥ 2 months:** Apply a small amount to the affected area three times daily for 10 days	• Inadequate studies available to indicate a pregnancy category; use only if clearly needed • Not formulated for mucosal surfaces (use nasal specific mupirocin for treatment in nares) • Not for ophthalmic use • Re-evaluate if no improvement in 3-5 days
	Bactroban	*Ointment: 22 g* *Ointment: generic available* *Cream: 15 g, 30 g*	
First Generation Cephalosporins *inhibit cell wall synthesis by bacteria* **General comments** More effective against rapidly reproducing organisms with cell walls Monitor for hypersensitivity reactions: rash, urticaria, angioedema and pruritis Consider for MSSA infections of the skin; do not use for suspected MRSA infections	**cephalexin**	**Adult**: 1-4 g daily in divided doses PO every 6-12 hours *Max*: 4 g/24 hours *Alternate*: 500 mg PO every 12 hours **Children > 1 year of age**: 25-50 mg/kg/day PO divided every 6-12 hours *Max*: 4 g/24 hours *Alternate*: 25-50 mg/kg/day PO divided every 12 hours *Max*: 4 g/24 hours	• Pregnancy Category B • **DO NOT USE IN PATIENTS WHO HAD HIVES OR ANAPHYLAXIS TO PENICILLIN** • Dosage reduction needed for renal impairment • Give without regard to meals • PT should be monitored in patients at risk: renal or hepatic impairment, poor nutritional state • After mixing suspension, store in refrigerator for up to 14 days
	Keflex	*Caps: 250 mg, 500 mg, 750 mg* *Susp: 125 mg/5 mL* *250 mg/5 mL*	
	cefadroxil	**Adult**: 1 g daily in single or divided doses twice daily for 10 days **Children**: 30 mg/kg/day in a single or 2 divided doses for 10 days *Max*: 1 g/day	• Pregnancy Category B • **DO NOT USE IN PATIENTS WHO HAD HIVES OR ANAPHYLAXIS TO PENICILLIN** • Dosage reduction needed for renal impairment • No dosage reduction needed for geriatric patients
	Duricef	*Caps: 500 mg, 1000 mg* *Tablets: 1000 mg* *Susp: 250 mg/5 mL, 500 mg/5 mL*	

CONSULTATION/REFERRAL

- None usually needed
- Consider secondary cause if infection slow to resolve

FOLLOW-UP

- Usually none needed (because complete resolution within 7-10 days)
- If no improvement in 48 hours, culture and sensitivity

May restrict athletic participation until clear.

EXPECTED COURSE

- Complete resolution 7-10 days with treatment

POSSIBLE COMPLICATIONS

- Ecthyma: entire epidermis is infected, crusts are dark-colored
- Poststreptococcal acute glomerulonephritis
- Cellulitis

LYME DISEASE

DESCRIPTION

Multisystem infection transmitted by a tick. Disease ranges in severity from mild to severe.

ETIOLOGY

- *Borrelia burgdorferi* is the spirochete transmitted by the Ixodid tick

INCIDENCE

- 4.4/100,000 population
- States with highest prevalence: Connecticut, New York, New Jersey, Pennsylvania, Rhode Island, Wisconsin, Maryland, Minnesota but is found in almost every state in the U.S.

RISK FACTORS

- Exposure to the bite of infected ticks during May to October
- Exposure to outdoors, hunting, hiking, camping, or living in wooded areas

Transmission cannot occur if tick has attached < 48 hours. Treatment is not necessary if attachment has been < 48 hours.

ASSESSMENT FINDINGS

Early Lyme Disease (Stage 1)	Asymptomatic Erythema migrans (60-80%) Headache, malaise Fever Myalgias and arthralgias
Early Disseminated Lyme Disease-Stage 2 (days to weeks later)	Erythema migrans Aseptic meningitis, iritis Heart block, pericarditis Orchitis Hepatitis Arthritis of the large joints
Chronic Persistent Lyme Disease (Stage 3)	Aches and pains of the joints (especially knees) and soft tissues Neurological impairment (memory loss, dementia, confusion, difficulty concentrating, peripheral neuropathies) Iritis, optic neuritis

DIFFERENTIAL DIAGNOSIS

- Arthritis
- Multiple sclerosis
- Parkinson's disease
- Ophthalmic disorders
- JRA
- STARI (Southern Tick-associated rash illness)
- Viral disorders
- Systemic lupus erythematosus

DIAGNOSTIC STUDIES

- ELISA for *Borrelia burgdorferi* antibodies
- Lumbar puncture for neuro symptoms
- ELISA of CSF for *Borrelia burgdorferi* antibodies

PREVENTION

- Teach patients to protect themselves from ticks while in potentially tick-infested areas (e.g., wearing of clothing that protects ankles)
- Use of insect repellents
- Self-examination after exposure in tick infested areas
- Prompt removal of ticks with tweezers
- May consider prophylactic treatment (within 72 hours of bite) with single dose of 200 mg doxycycline if tick bite occurs in highly endemic area

NONPHARMACOLOGIC MANAGEMENT

- Self-examination for ticks; examination of backs of ears and neck
- Remove ticks by using tweezers and grasping the tick as near to the skin as possible. Do not twist! Do not use a lighted match on the tick.
- Examine area for remaining tick parts. Attempt to remove. Occasionally there can be a local reaction to remaining parts.
- Teach patient that to contract Lyme disease, tick must be infected and remain in place for at least 24 hours

PHARMACOLOGIC MANAGEMENT

Stage 1	doxycycline (Vibramycin®) 100 mg twice a day on day one, then daily for 14-21 days OR amoxicillin for 14-21 days; 875 mg PO twice daily cefuroxime (Ceftin®) 500 mg twice daily for 14 days
Stage 2 (no CSF involvement)	doxycycline OR amoxicillin for 14-21 days; short course (one week) of steroids may help joint pains
Stage 2 (CSF involvement)	ceftriaxone (Rocephin®) OR cefotaxime (Claforan®) OR penicillin G for 21-28 days
Stage 3	doxycycline OR amoxicillin for 28 days; if oral treatment fails, intravenous ceftriaxone (Rocephin®) OR cefotaxime (Claforan®) OR penicillin G for 14-21 days

- Do not use doxycycline in children <9 years; amoxicillin is preferred
- Erythromycin for patients unable to tolerate PCN or tetracycline
- IV antibiotics required for treatment of Stage 3

Erythema migrans in a patient who has visited a Lyme Disease endemic area is sufficient for prophylactic treatment.

PREGNANCY/LACTATION CONSIDERATIONS

- Do not use doxycycline during pregnancy or during breastfeeding
- *Borrelia burgdorferi* can cross the placenta, therefore, treat with intravenous antibiotics
- Oral contraceptives may be less effective if tetracycline is taken

CONSULTATION/REFERRAL

- Refer patients with cardiac or neurological involvement
- Consult obstetrician for pregnant patients

FOLLOW-UP

- Depends on stage and severity

- Follow up for Stage 2 and 3 patients may be months to years

EXPECTED COURSE

- Stage 1 infection responds well to antibiotics
- Stages 2 and 3 have a variable response and depend on the severity

POSSIBLE COMPLICATIONS

- Persistent neurological symptoms
- Persistent arthralgias and myalgias
- Heart block

ORAL CANDIDIASIS
(Thrush)

DESCRIPTION

Fungal infection of the mucus membranes of the mouth which may involve the throat, esophagus, trachea, and angles of the mouth.

ETIOLOGY

- Usually *Candida albicans*: normal flora of the mouth that flourishes under warm, moist, and glucose-rich environment

INCIDENCE

- Most common in newborns, infants, and elderly, and immunocompromised patients

RISK FACTORS

- Age extremes (very young and very old)
- Recent antibiotic use
- Use of inhaled steroids
- Immunocompromised status
- Presence of chronic disease(s)

ASSESSMENT FINDINGS

- White oral plaques on an erythematous base
- May have concurrent diaper candidiasis

DIFFERENTIAL DIAGNOSIS

- Geographic tongue
- Leukoplakia
- Stomatitis
- Other yeasts

DIAGNOSTIC STUDIES

- Usually none indicated
- 10% KOH wet prep: demonstrates pseudohyphae and spores
- Culture
- Consider tests to rule out HIV and/or diabetes in patients with recurrent candidiasis

PREVENTION

- Discourage thumb sucking to prevent spread to nails
- Oral hygiene

NONPHARMACOLOGIC MANAGEMENT

- See Prevention

ORAL CANDIDIASIS PHARMACOLOGIC MANAGEMENT

Class	Drug Generic name (Trade name®)	Dosage How supplied	Comments
Oral Antifungal Agents	**Nystatin oral suspension**	**Infants**: 2 mL (200,000 units) four times daily. Place half in each side of mouth and avoid feeding for 5-10 minutes **Children and Adult:** 4-6 mL (400,000-600,000 units) four times daily (one half dose in each side of mouth). Retain in mouth as long as possible before swallowing	• Pregnancy Category C • Continue treatment for at least 48 hours after perioral symptoms have disappeared • **NOT FOR USE IN SYSTEMIC MYCOSES** • Well tolerated even with prolonged use • Shake well before using
	Nystatin suspension Various generics	*Susp: 60 mL, 473 mL*	
	clotrimazole troche	**Adult and children > 3 years**: One troche five times per day for 14 days	• Pregnancy Category C • Administer as a lozenge to dissolve in mouth • Periodic assessment of liver function suggested, especially if pre-existing hepatic disease • **NOT FOR USE IN SYSTEMIC MYCOSES**
	Mycelex	*Troches: 10 mg*	

PREGNANCY/LACTATION CONSIDERATIONS

- Exercise good hygiene of lactating mother's nipples if baby has thrush
- Do not prophylactically treat mother (controversial)

CONSULTATION/REFERRAL

- Consult physician for disease which persists
- Consult physician for HIV-positive or other immunocompromised patients

FOLLOW-UP

- Usually none needed if resolution occurs by 2 weeks
- Return if thrush worsens while on medication or if unresolved after 2 weeks

EXPECTED COURSE

- Usually resolves with appropriate treatment
- Frequently recurs

POSSIBLE COMPLICATIONS

- Systemic infection (rare)

PARONYCHIA

DESCRIPTION

Skin surrounding finger (nail folds) or toenails becomes infected/inflamed. May be acute or chronic.

ETIOLOGY

- *Staphylococcus aureus* (most common pathogen)
- *Streptococcus* sp. (less common)
- *Pseudomonas* sp. (less common)
- *Candida albicans* (chronic paronychia)

Pseudomonas infections produce a green nail.

INCIDENCE

- Common all ages
- Increased incidence in diabetics
- Female > Male 3:1

RISK FACTORS

- Trauma to finger, nailbed
- Poorly managed diabetes
- Trauma to skin around nail or ingrown nails
- Nail biting, thumb-sucking
- Frequent and continuous wet hands: certain occupations (e.g., hairdressers, dishwashers) are at high risk

ASSESSMENT FINDINGS

- Nail fold separates from nail plate
- Pain around skin of nail plate
- Erythema, tenderness around nail plate
- Changes in nail plate or nail

DIFFERENTIAL DIAGNOSIS

- Psoriasis
- Herpetic whitlow

DIAGNOSTIC STUDIES

- Usually none
- KOH for suspected fungal infection
- Consider Gram stain

PREVENTION

- Avoid long term contact with moisture to hands
- Wear gloves to wash dishes
- Adequate glycemic control in diabetics

Make certain that patient has an up to date tetanus immunization.

NONPHARMACOLOGIC MANAGEMENT

- Keep fingers from moist conditions
- Warm compresses or soaks for acute infection
- Incision and drainage if abscess present
- Possible nail removal if severe

Vinegar/water soaks: 1:1 solution for fingertip soaks 3-4 times daily. Use this as an adjunct or as primary therapy for paronychia.

PARONYCHIA PHARMACOLOGIC MANAGEMENT

Class	Drug Generic name (Trade name®)	Dosage How supplied	Comments
Topical Antibiotic Ointments	**mupirocin** Bactroban	**Adult and children ≥ 2 months:** Apply a small amount to the affected area three times daily for 10 days *Ointment: 22 g* *Ointment: generic available* *Cream: 15 g, 30 g*	• Inadequate number of studies available to indicate a pregnancy category; use only if clearly needed • Not formulated for mucosal surfaces (use nasal specific mupirocin for treatment in nares) • Not for ophthalmic use • Re-evaluate if no improvement in 3-5 days
First Generation Cephalosporins *inhibit cell wall synthesis by bacteria* General comments More effective against rapidly reproducing organisms with cell walls Monitor for hypersensitivity reactions: rash, urticaria, angioedema and pruritis Consider for MSSA infections of the skin; do not use for suspected MRSA infections	**cephalexin** Keflex	**Adult**: 1-4 g daily in divided doses PO every 6-12 hours *Max*: 4 g/24 hours *Alternate*: 500 mg PO every 12 hours **Children > 1 year of age**: 25-50 mg/kg/day PO divided every 6-12 hours *Max*: 4 g/24 hours *Alternate*: 25-50 mg/kg/day PO divided every 12 hours *Max*: 4 g/24 hours *Caps: 250 mg, 500 mg, 750 mg* *Susp: 125 mg/5 mL, 250 mg/5 mL*	• Pregnancy Category B • **DO NOT USE IN PATIENTS WHO HAD HIVES OR ANAPHYLAXIS TO PENICILLIN** • Dosage reduction needed for renal impairment • Give without regard to meals • PT should be monitored in patients at risk: renal or hepatic impairment, poor nutritional state • After mixing suspension, store in refrigerator for up to 14 days
	cefadroxil Duricef	**Adult**: 1 g daily in single or divided doses twice daily for 10 days **Children**: 30 mg/kg/day in a single or 2 divided doses for 10 days *Max*: 1 g/day *Caps: 500 mg, 1000 mg* *Tablets: 1000 mg* *Susp: 250 mg/5 mL, 500 mg/5 mL*	• Pregnancy Category B • **DO NOT USE IN PATIENTS WHO HAD HIVES OR ANAPHYLAXIS TO PENICILLIN** • Dosage reduction needed for renal impairment • No dosage reduction needed for geriatric patients

continued

PARONYCHIA PHARMACOLOGIC MANAGEMENT

Class	Drug Generic name (Trade name®)	Dosage How supplied	Comments
Lincosamide Antibiotic General comments Use for *E. coli* or suspected anaerobes	**clindamycin** Cleocin	**Adult**: 300 mg PO every six hours daily **Children**: 10 mg/kg/day in 3 divided doses *Max*: Do not exceed max adult dose *Caps: 75 mg, 150 mg, 300 mg*	• Pregnancy Category B • *Clostridium difficile* associated diarrhea has been associated with severe colitis. Reserve for serious infections where less toxic antimicrobial agents are not warranted • Higher doses are associated with greater incidence of side effects • Cautious use in patients with colitis • Take with a big glass of water • Monitor geriatric patients more closely since diarrhea may be more severe
Extended Spectrum Penicillin *inhibits cell wall synthesis of Gram positive bacteria (Staph, Strep) and are most effective against organisms with rapidly dividing cell walls* General comments Use for *E. coli* or suspected anaerobes	**amoxicillin/clavulanic acid (as potassium)** Augmentin Augmentin EX	**Adult:** One 875 mg tablet every 12 hours for 10 days **Children**: 45 mg/kg/d in 2 divided doses every 12 hours for 10 days (Must use 200 mg/5 mL susp or 400 mg/5 mL susp for this regimen) - do not exceed max adult dose *Tabs: 875 mg* *Chew tabs: 400-57 mg* *Susp: 250-62.5 mg/5 mL; 75 mL, 100 mL, 150 mL* *Susp: 600-42.9 mg/5 mL; 75 mL*	• Pregnancy Category B • **DO NOT USE IN PATIENTS WHO HAD HIVES OR ANAPHYLAXIS TO PENICILLIN** • Two 500 mg amoxicillin/clavulanic acid tablets are NOT equivalent to one 1000 mg amoxicillin/clavulanic acid tablet • Do not substitute Augmentin 200 mg/5 mL and 400 mg/5 mL suspensions for Augmentin ES-600 These are NOT interchangeable • Take with meals to minimize gastrointestinal side effects • Contraindicated in severe renal impairment (Cr Cl < 30 mL/min), dialysis, or history of Augmentin associated cholestatic jaundice/ hepatic dysfunction • Chewtabs contain phenylalanine

CONSULTATION/REFERRAL

- Urgent referral for felon (abscess of the fingertip pulp)
- Dermatologist for infection/inflammation which does not resolve after routine treatment

FOLLOW-UP

- Recheck as needed by patient condition

EXPECTED COURSE

- Nails grow slowly, complete resolution when nail plate is effected may take weeks to months

POSSIBLE COMPLICATIONS

- Nail loss
- Thickening and hardening of nail
- Subungual abscess

PEDICULOSIS
(Lice)

DESCRIPTION

An infestation of the body, head, or pubic area by lice.

ETIOLOGY

- Lice are ectoparasites which feed on human blood. Nits are the eggs laid by the females which may survive up to 3 weeks when removed from the human host

Head lice: *Pediculus humanus capitis*
Body lice: *Pediculus humanus corporis*
Pubic lice: *Phthirus pubis*

INCIDENCE

- Head and body lice are more common in children
- Pubic lice are more common in adults
- Females > Males
- Head lice unusual in African American patients

RISK FACTORS

***Head lice:* crowded conditions, sharing of hats, combs, etc.; poor hygiene is NOT a risk factor**
***Body lice:* poor hygiene, infrequent laundering of clothes (lice live and multiply in the seams of clothing), crowded conditions, contact with infected bed linen, towels, clothing etc.**
***Pubic lice:* sexual contact with an infected person**

ASSESSMENT FINDINGS

Head lice
- ◊ Itching, prickly sensation on the scalp
- ◊ "Dandruff that moves"
- ◊ Nits are tiny, white spheres (<1 mm long) which are attached to the hair shaft and are immovable. They are found in greater numbers than adult lice
- ◊ Back of head, neck, and behind ears are common places of attachment because these are warmer areas of the hair

Body lice
- ◊ Pruritus
- ◊ Papules 2-4 mm in diameter
- ◊ Skin of the axilla, trunk, and groin are common sites of attachment

Pubic lice
- ◊ Pruritus ani
- ◊ Nits found at the base of pubic hair shafts
- ◊ Inflammation in groin area, adenopathy
- ◊ Macular rash in area of infestation
- ◊ Commonly found in pubic hair but may be spread to other hairy parts of the body

Incubation period is about one month.

DIFFERENTIAL DIAGNOSIS

- Lice vs. mite infestation
- Dandruff

DIAGNOSTIC STUDIES

- Wood's lamp
  - ◊ Live nits fluoresce white
  - ◊ Empty nits fluoresce gray
  - ◊ Identification of live lice

PREVENTION

- Launder clothes in hot water
- Good hygiene
- Washing/not sharing combs, hats, bed linens, towels, etc.

NONPHARMACOLOGIC MANAGEMENT

- Patient education about means of transmission and mechanism to break life cycle
- Consider use of petrolatum or mayonnaise (suffocation therapy) directly to hair and left on overnight with a showercap. Consider using 3-4 days in succession
- Nit removal: soak hair in equal parts water & white vinegar for at least 15 minutes
- Careful monitoring/treatment by parents and school personnel after lice discovered

Empty nits will remain on hair shafts for months after eradication.

PHARMACOLOGIC MANAGEMENT

Head lice

- ◊ 1% permethrin (Nix®): most effective treatment because it exerts effect for up to 2 weeks after application; apply to dry hair for 10 minutes, then wash
- ◊ Synergized pyrethrins: 0.33% piperonyl butoxide 4% (Rid®) (Apply to dry hair for 10 minutes, wash off)
- ◊ Malathion 0.5% lotion (Ovide®) to affected areas for 8-12 hours, then wash (effective because of ability to kill eggs)
- ◊ Frequently need repeat treatments

Body lice

- ◊ Same as for head lice
- ◊ Pyrethrins may have greatest effectiveness

Pubic lice

- ◊ Synergized pyrethrins: piperonyl butoxide (Rid®)
- ◊ 1% permethrin (Nix®): most effective treatment
- ◊ Alternative treatment: lindane (Kwell®), avoid use in pregnant women and infants

DO NOT USE ANY MEDICATION LISTED ABOVE FOR EYELASH INFESTATION!

- ◊ Manual removal of nits necessary
- ◊ May use petroleum jelly 3-4 times per day for a week

Avoid pyrethrins in patients with ragweed allergy. This may exacerbate it!

PREGNANCY/LACTATION CONSIDERATIONS

- Preferred: permethrin, pyrethrins or malathion (all Category B)
- Lindane (Kwell®): avoid use in pregnant women due to potential neurotoxic effects and seizure potential

CONSULTATION/REFERRAL

- School personnel
- Parents
- Consult dermatologist for lice unresponsive to treatment

FOLLOW-UP

- Recheck for live head lice after treatment. Do not allow re-admission to school if live lice are present. Children may return to school after treatment even if nits are present

If first line treatment does not eradicate infestation, use malathion. It is effective in killing eggs.

EXPECTED COURSE

- Complete resolution if appropriate treatment and other measures taken

POSSIBLE COMPLICATIONS

- Spread of pubic lice to other areas of the body
- Check for STDs if pubic lice present
- Bacterial secondary infections from scratching

PITYRIASIS ROSEA

DESCRIPTION

Idiopathic self-limiting skin disorder characterized by papulosquamous lesions distributed over the trunk and extremities.

ETIOLOGY

- Unknown; may be viral or autoimmune

INCIDENCE

- Common
- Males = Females
- Occurs in all age groups, but most common in ages 10-35 years

RISK FACTORS

- None known

ASSESSMENT FINDINGS

- *"Herald patch"* on trunk resembles tinea corporis and precedes the generalized rash (present 40-76% of the time)
- Generalized rash usually begins 1-2 weeks after the appearance of the herald patch
- *Salmon-colored oval plaques* 1-10 cm in diameter and with fine scales
- *"Collarette" of loose scales* along the border of the plaques
- Oval shaped lesions appear parallel to each other on the trunk, hence the term, *"Christmas tree"* pattern rash
- Mild pruritus; occasional reports of severe pruritus
- In children, lesions may be more papular and on face and distal extremities

DIFFERENTIAL DIAGNOSIS

- Tinea corporis, versicolor
- Viral exanthems
- Drug rash
- Secondary syphilis

DIAGNOSTIC STUDIES

- None usually needed
- Syphilis serology strongly suggested since secondary syphilis can present in this manner
- KOH if fungal infection suspected

NONPHARMACOLOGIC MANAGEMENT

- Lukewarm oatmeal bath to relieve itching
- Reassurance that condition is self-limiting
- Good hygiene to prevent bacterial secondary infections

PHARMACOLOGIC MANAGEMENT

- Antipruritics (topical): Calamine lotion®
- Oral antihistamines: hydroxyzine (Atarax®); any non-sedating (loratadine, fexofenadine)

CONSULTATION/REFERRAL

- Dermatologist if questionable diagnosis

FOLLOW-UP

- Usually none needed
- Resolution usually 2-6 weeks

EXPECTED COURSE

- Benign course, resolution in 1-14 weeks

POSSIBLE COMPLICATIONS

- Secondary bacterial infection from scratching

PITYRIASIS ROSEA PHARMACOLOGIC MANAGEMENT

Class	Drug Generic name (Trade name®)	Dosage How supplied	Comments
Topical Anti-pruritics *This is a skin protectant containing calaime 8% and zinc oxide 8%* **General comments** For topical use only Avoid eyes This product has not been reviewed and approved by the FDA	**calamine** Various generics	Apply liberally to affected areas *Bottles: Multiple sizes*	• Pregnancy category not available • Shake well before applying • All available OTC
First Generation Antihistamines **General comments** Avoid simultaneous use of CNS depressants Care when driving or engaging in activities that require attention Most available over the counter This product has not been reviewed and approved by the FDA	**diphenhydramine** Benadryl	**Adult**: 25-50 mg every 4-6 hr *Max*: 300 mg/day **Children < 6 yr**: individualize **Children 6-12 yr**: 12.5-25 mg every 4-6 hr *Max*: 150 mg/day *Tabs: 25 mg* *Chew tabs: 12.5 mg* *Liquid: 12.5 mg/5 mL* *Injection: 50 mg/mL*	• Pregnancy Category B • Cautious use in patients with glaucoma, difficulty urinating due to an enlarged prostate gland, COPD • Avoid alcohol within 6 hour of taking • May cause profound drowsiness in some patients
	hydroxyzine Vistaril Atarax	**Adult**: 25 mg 3-4 times daily **Children < 6 yr**: 50 mg daily in divided doses **Children > 6 yr**: 50-100 mg daily in divided doses *Caps: 25 mg, 50 mg* *Suspension: 4 oz, 1 pt, 25 mg/5 mL*	• Pregnancy Category C • Unable to establish safety during pregnancy • May produce drowsiness in any dose. Appropriate care advised • If used in geriatric patients, should administer a low dose and monitor carefully, sedation and fall risk increased
Second Generation Antihistamines **General comment** Does not typically produce drowsiness (except cetirizine) and usually dosed once daily	**cetirizine** Zyrtec	**Adult and Children > 12 years**: 5-10 mg daily **Children 6-11 years**: 5-10 mg based on symptom relief **Children 2-5 years**: 2.5 mg daily or twice daily *Tabs: 10 mg;* *Chew tabs: 5 mg, 10 mg* *Syrup: 4 oz, 1 mg/mL*	• Pregnancy Category B • Caution regarding activities requiring mental alertness, produces drowsiness because of its affinity for H1 receptors • Dosage adjustment needed for ages 77 and older, renal and hepatic impairment • Take without regard to food • Consider taking in the evening

continued

PITYRIASIS ROSEA PHARMACOLOGIC MANAGEMENT

Class	Drug Generic name (Trade name®)	Dosage How supplied	Comments
	levocetirizine	**Adult and children ≥ 12 years**: 5 mg once daily in the evening **Children 6-11 years**: 2.5 mg once daily in the evening **Children 6 months to 5 years**: 1.25 mg once daily in the evening	• Pregnancy Category B • Adjust dose for renal impairment; contraindicated in children 6 months to 11 years with renal impairment • Avoid engaging in activities requiring mental alertness • Avoid concurrent use alcohol or CNS depressants
	Xyzal	*Tabs: 5 mg scored* *Oral solution: 0.5 mg/mL*	
	fexofenadine	**Adult and Children > 12 years:** 180 mg daily or 60 mg twice daily **Children 6 months -11 years**: 30 mg twice daily **Children 6 months – 2 years**: 15 mg twice daily	• Pregnancy Category C • Shake bottle well before use • Reduce dose for renal impairment • Allegra ODT contains phenylalanine (other Allegra products do not) • Avoid aluminum and magnesium containing antacids • Less effective if taken with fruit juices; therefore, take with water • Do not expect sedation
	Allegra	*Tab: 30 mg, 60 mg, 180 mg* *ODT tab: 30 mg* *Susp: 6 mg/mL; 300 mL*	
	loratadine	**Adult and Children > 6 years**: 10 mg daily **Children 2-5 yrs**: 5 mg once daily	• Pregnancy Category B • Children use chew tabs or syrup • Adjustment needed for renal or hepatic impairment • Do not expect sedation
	Claritin	*Syrup: 1 mg/mL* *Chew tabs: 5 mg* *RediTabs: 10 mg*	
	desloratadine	**Adult**: 5 mg daily **Children 6 mos-11 mos**: 1 mg (2 mL) daily **Children 1-5 yrs:** 1.25 mg (2.5 mL) daily **Children 6-11 yrs**: 2.5 mg (5 mL) daily	• Pregnancy Category C • Children use RediTabs or syrup • Do not expect sedation
	Clarinex	*Tabs: 5 mg;* *RediTabs: 2.5 mg; 5 mg* *Syrup: 0.5 mg/mL*	

PSORIASIS

DESCRIPTION

A chronic, pruritic, inflammatory skin disorder characterized by rapid proliferation of epidermal cells. Expect frequent remissions and exacerbations.

There are several variants, but the most common form occurs with plaque type lesions.

ETIOLOGY

- Unknown, but family history present in one-third of cases
- **β**-hemolytic streptococcal infections in children (acute guttate psoriasis)

INCIDENCE

- 1/1000 persons in U.S.
- Males = Females
- Mean age of onset 33 years; usually occurs prior to age 46 years; earlier onset in females

RISK FACTORS

- Streptococcal infection
- Family history
- Stress
- Diabetes, metabolic syndrome, obesity
- Local trauma or irritation

ASSESSMENT FINDINGS

- Silvery, white scales on erythematous base
- Pruritus
- Common distribution to elbows, knees, scalp
- May also appear on eyebrows, ears, trunk
- Nails may be pitted in 50% of patients
- Positive Auspitz sign (pinpoint bleeding occurs when lesions are scraped)

DIFFERENTIAL DIAGNOSIS

- Scalp: Seborrheic dermatitis
- Trunk: Pityriasis rosea, tinea corporis (guttate psoriasis)
- Candidal infections
- Contact dermatitis
- Eczema

DIAGNOSTIC STUDIES

- Usually diagnosed on history and physical exam
- Biopsy if diagnosis uncertain
- May order streptococcal swab if guttate psoriasis is suspected
- KOH to rule out fungal infection
- ESR, CRP: elevated
- If joint involvement: rheumatoid factor (negative)

PREVENTION

- Avoid sunburn which may precipitate exacerbations
- Avoid known precipitants
- Avoid sudden withdrawal of steroids
- Avoid stimulating drugs: ACE inhibitors, **β**-blockers, NSAIDs, penicillin, salicylates, sulfonamides, tetracyclines

NONPHARMACOLOGIC MANAGEMENT

- Warm soaks to remove thickened plaques
- Solar radiation, ultraviolet radiation
- Oatmeal bath for itching
- Wet dressings (Burow's solution) for itching

PHARMACOLOGIC MANAGEMENT

- Keep skin well hydrated with an emollient as needed (Eucerin, Lubriderm, Cetaphil, etc.)
- Topical steroids (*Refer to topical corticosteroid table Contact Dermatitis, page 115*): consider plastic occlusion in adults and older children (with caution) to hasten resolution; increases skin penetration 10-fold
- For scalp: use strong potency steroid in alcohol base
- Face, intertriginous areas: low potency steroid cream
- Plaques: initial treatment with high potency steroid cream or ointment
- Limit use of high and super high potency steroids to < 2 weeks
- Intralesional steroid injections

- Tar solutions alone or in combination with topical steroids
- Salicylic acid gel or ointment as a keratolytic agent
  - ◊ Ultraviolet lamps and sunlight in conjunction with topical agents
- Systemic treatments: Methotrexate, Etanercept (Enbrel®), cyclosporin, Acitretin used for severe cases

May need multiple medications to treat: if one does not work, try another or add another from a different medication class.

PREGNANCY/LACTATION CONSIDERATIONS

- Ultraviolet radiation may be safest
- Avoid coal tar preparations, systemic steroids if possible

CONSULTATION/REFERRAL

- Dermatologist for severe cases and those that are slow to respond to treatment

FOLLOW-UP

- Individualize per patient

EXPECTED COURSE

- Chronic disease: Remissions and exacerbations are expected
- May be refractory to treatment

POSSIBLE COMPLICATIONS

- Thinning of skin, striae due to topical steroids
- Rebound after steroids are withdrawn

Avoid exacerbations when withdrawing steroids by using a lower potency steroid for a few days before discontinuing steroid completely.

ROSEOLA, EXANTHEM SUBITUM

DESCRIPTION

A viral illness characterized by 3-5 days of high fever with a sudden disappearance of fever and the appearance of a blanching maculopapular rash lasting 1-2 days.

Infection is usually self-limited and without sequela.

ETIOLOGY

- Human herpes virus 6 (HHV-6)
- Roseola-like illnesses are associated with other types of viruses

INCIDENCE

- Very common in daycare attendees and preschool age (usually prior to 3 years of age)
- Most common age is 6 months to 3 years

Suspect roseola infection if young child presents with high fever and roseola is known to be occurring in the community. Common in spring and fall.

RISK FACTORS

- Contact with saliva/feces of a roseola patient during the fever phase (most contagious) or during the 5-15 day incubation period

ASSESSMENT FINDINGS

- Sudden onset of fever up to 104°F (40°C) for 3-5 days
- Child does not seem as ill as degree of fever would indicate
- Signs of mild upper respiratory infection may be present
- Sudden disappearance of fever and appearance of non-pruritic, maculopapular rash on neck and trunk and spreading to extremities

- Rash blanches with pressure
- Lymphadenopathy in cervical and posterior auricular regions
- Tympanic membrane inflammation is common

DIFFERENTIAL DIAGNOSIS

- Other viral illnesses
- Antibiotic rash
- Streptococcal rash

DIAGNOSTIC STUDIES

- Usually none needed
- HHV-6-IgM: diagnostic for acute illness but not needed unless diagnosis questionable

PREVENTION

- Avoid contact with respiratory secretions of infected persons

NON-PHARMACOLOGIC MANAGEMENT

- Supportive care
- Cooling measures for elevated temperatures

PHARMACOLOGIC MANAGEMENT

- Analgesics/antipyretics
- Do not use aspirin due to risk of Reye's syndrome

CONSULTATION/REFERRAL

- Consult pediatrician/infectious disease specialist if disease follows atypical course

FOLLOW-UP

- Usually none needed

EXPECTED COURSE

- Benign and self-limited
- Child may return to daycare as soon as afebrile

RUBELLA

(German Measles, Three Day Measles, Third Disease)

DESCRIPTION

Acute viral infection of childhood (and adults) that may occur in two different forms:

- Acquired: mild viral exanthem
- Congenital: may induce abortion, congential defects if exposed during pregnancy

ETIOLOGY

- Rubivirus, a member of the Togaviridae family of viruses

INCIDENCE

- < 1,000 cases annually are reported
- Late winter and spring likely for outbreaks
- Congenital rubella syndrome occurs rarely
- Infection rates are highest for persons 5-9 years; but may affect any age
- Fetal infection if exposed during the first trimester is 50-80%
- Fetal infection if exposed during the second trimester is 10-20%
- Fetal infection if exposed during the third trimester is >60%

RISK FACTORS

- Lack of vaccination and subsequent exposure to viral particles by airborne transmission
- Incubation period is 7-21 days
- Most contagious when rash is erupting

ASSESSMENT FINDINGS

Acquired (postnatal)

- ◊ Mild catarrhal symptoms, conjunctivitis
- ◊ Low-grade fever
- ◊ Occipital lymph nodes are most commonly involved and are essentially diagnostic
- ◊ Lymphadenopathy: postauricular, posterior cervical
- ◊ Possible splenomegaly
- ◊ Maculopapular rash (1-4 mm) which starts on the face and spreads to chest, usually lasts about 3 days
- ◊ Possible desquamation
- ◊ In adults and adolescents, arthralgia and arthritis common

Congenital

- ◊ Premature delivery
- ◊ Fetal demise
- ◊ Low birth weight
- ◊ Eye defects: cataracts, glaucoma, retinopathy
- ◊ Cardiac defects: patent ductus arteriosus, atrial and ventricular septal defects, coarctation of the aorta, pulmonic stenosis
- ◊ Nervous system defects: mental retardation, psychomotor retardation, encephalitis, autism, deafness
- ◊ Endocrine defects: thyroid disorders, diabetes mellitus, precocious puberty
- ◊ Hematological defects: splenomegaly, thrombocytopenia, heapatitis

DIFFERENTIAL DIAGNOSIS

- Scarlet fever
- Roseola/Fifth disease
- Drug reactions
- Other viral exanthems

DIAGNOSTIC STUDIES

- Viral cultures from throat or urine (not usually needed)
- Rubella antibodies: titer of 1:10 or higher usually considered immune

PREVENTION

- Routine immunization at 12-15 months, then age 4-6 years
- Do not immunize patients during pregnancy
- Communicable in breast-milk

NONPHARMACOLOGIC MANAGEMENT

- Supportive care

PHARMACOLOGIC MANAGEMENT

- Usually none needed
- May use NSAIDs for arthralgias
- Acetaminophen for fever

PREGNANCY/LACTATION CONSIDERATIONS

- Pregnancy avoided for 1 month after vaccination
- Vaccine virus may be communicable through breast milk

CONSULTATION/REFERRAL

- Obstetrician for suspected exposure during pregnancy
- Refer for complications
- Report all cases to local public health authorities

FOLLOW-UP

- Individualize per patient

EXPECTED COURSE

- 50% of infections are asymptomatic
- Infection in early pregnancy has worse outcomes than those associated with infection after the 20th week

POSSIBLE COMPLICATIONS

- As described above for congenitally acquired infants
- Arthritis and arthralgia (common in adults)
- Encephalitis
- Bleeding (more common in children)

RUBEOLA
(Measles, Nine Day Measles, First Disease)

DESCRIPTION

Acute, highly contagious viral disease with a characteristic rash. Associated with a significant degree of morbidity and mortality worldwide.

ETIOLOGY

- Morbillivirus of the family Paramyxoviridae

INCIDENCE

- Outbreaks occurred in 1989-1990 (mortality and significant morbidity occurred)
- Since 1990, drastic decrease in incidence
- Isolated outbreaks occur most commonly in persons unvaccinated, but CDC no longer considers this endemic

RISK FACTORS

- Lack of immunization (MMR given at 12-15 months of age)
- Waiting rooms (up to 45% of known exposures have occurred here) with an infected patient (spread by microaerosolized respiratory droplets)
- Incubation period is 10-12 days from exposure to onset of symptoms
- Patients are contagious from 1-2 days prior to onset of symptoms until 4 days after appearance of the rash

ASSESSMENT FINDINGS

Prodromal stage (2-3 days before rash)
- ◊ Upper respiratory infection symptoms
- ◊ Fever up to 104°F (40°C)
- ◊ The 3-Cs: croupy cough, coryza, conjunctivitis
- ◊ Presence of Koplik's spots (2-3 mm gray-white raised lesions on buccal mucosa) is pathognomonic
- ◊ Malaise

Rash phase (the more severe the rash, the more severe the illness)
- ◊ Emergence of maculopapular rash and elevation of temperature up to 104.7°F (40.5°C) occur simultaneously
- ◊ Pharyngitis, cervical lymphadenopathy and splenomegaly often accompany rash
- ◊ Rash appears on forehead and behind the ears initially
- ◊ Over the first 24 hours, rash spreads to face, neck, and arms
- ◊ Next 24 hours rash spreads to trunk and thighs, hips
- ◊ Rarely rash can become hemorrhagic leading to fatality
- ◊ After 3-4 days, rash begins to clear and may leave a brownish discoloration and scaling

DIFFERENTIAL DIAGNOSIS

- Roseola
- Scarlet fever
- Other viral rashes
- Drug rashes
- Kawasaki Disease
- Stevens-Johnson syndrome

DIAGNOSTIC STUDIES

- Measles specific IgM titers (usually detectable 3 days after onset of rash; do not measure prior to this time)
- Substantial rise (4-fold) in IgG titers between acute and convalescent phase (7 days after rash onset)

All cases of suspected measles must be reported to public health department.

PREVENTION

- Routine vaccination at 12-15 months, then age 4-6 years
- Respiratory isolation until 4 days after rash appears. Exception: isolate immunocompromised patients for the entire illness
- Vaccination with live virus within 72 hours after exposure can provide protection
- Immunoglobulin if given within 6 days after exposure

NONPHARMACOLOGIC MANAGEMENT

- Antipyretic measures
- Oral fluids
- Antitussives
- Room humidification

PHARMACOLOGIC MANAGEMENT

- Water miscible vitamin A for children 6 months to 2 years in developing countries has been shown to decrease morbidity and mortality (not routinely given in U.S. unless child is hospitalized or has risk factors for complications)
- Children 6-12 months: 100,000 IU as one dose
- Children > 12 months: 200,000 IU as one dose

Vitamin A deficiency predisposes patient to keratitis and subsequent vision complications.

PREGNANCY/LACTATION CONSIDERATIONS

- During pregnancy there is significant increase in fetal morbidity and mortality
- Immunoglobulin recommended for susceptible pregnant women who have been in contact with known rubeola patient

CONSULTATION/REFERRAL

- Report to local health department
- Consider referral for all severe cases, pregnant women, and immunocompromised patients

FOLLOW-UP

- Individualize for each patient

EXPECTED COURSE

- Mild to severe symptoms depending on age and immune status of patient

POSSIBLE COMPLICATIONS

- Otitis media (most common, 5-15%)
- Bronchopneumonia (5-10%)
- Pneumonitis (immunocompromised patients)
- Diarrhea
- Keratitis
- Encephalitis (rare)
- Laryngotracheitis

SCABIES

DESCRIPTION

Infection of human skin by mites

ETIOLOGY

- Infection with *Sarcoptes scabiei*, a human skin mite

INCIDENCE

- Common
- Usually infects children and young adults

RISK FACTORS

- Crowded living conditions
- Skin-to-skin contact with infected patients or infected bedding, cloth furniture, etc.
- Immunocompromised patients

Incubation may be 3-6 weeks.

ASSESSMENT FINDINGS

- Itching (more noticeable at nighttime, can be severe)
- Small itching blisters in a thin line
- Mite burrows between finger webbing, feet, wrists, axilla, scrotum, penis, waist, and or buttocks; rarely effect the head
- Scaling
- Erythema
- Vesicles, papules
- Vesicles and papules more common on soles and palms in infants
- Mite may be recovered from the burrow

Itching occurs because of a delayed hypersensitivity reaction with mite feces, saliva, or eggs.

PREVENTION

- Treat all intimate contacts, household contacts, roommates, etc.
- Maintain good personal hygiene
- Launder clothes often
- Wash hands

DIFFERENTIAL DIAGNOSIS

- Atopic dermatitis
- Contact dermatitis
- Insect bites
- Psychogenic causes

DIAGNOSTIC STUDIES

- Examination of the skin with a magnifying lens
- Burrow ink test (apply a drop of black ink to the rash, then wash off with alcohol, the burrow will remain stained)
- Recovery of mite from the burrow using a 25 gauge needle or #15 surgical blade, visualize microscopically

The visible dark spot at the end of the burrow is the mite. This may be extracted as evidence of infection. Inability to extract mite does not exclude diagnosis.

NONPHARMACOLOGIC MANAGEMENT

- Wash all clothing, bedding, towels, etc. used within the last 4 days
- Wash toys used prior to treatment and during treatment
- Carpets, floors do NOT need special treatment under usual circumstances

Items that cannot be laundered (pillow) can be placed in sealed bag for 3-5 days to kill mites.

SCABIES PHARMACOLOGIC MANAGEMENT

Class	Drug Generic name (Trade name®)	Dosage How supplied	Comments
Topical Scabicides *inhibit nerve cell function in the mites/ lice producing paralysis and death of the mite/louse* **General comments** Must treat all household members and sexual contacts at the same time Clothing, bedding, cloth furniture must be treated to kill eggs and mites; permethrin spray available	**permethrine 5%** **Elimite** Various generics	**Adult and infants > 2 months:** Thoroughly massage permethrin cream, 5% into the skin from the head to the soles of the feet. Remove cream by shower or bath after 8-14 hours *60 g tube*	• Pregnancy Category B • Adults are rarely infested but infants and elderly are more likely. In these populations, massage cream into hairline, neck, temple, and forehead • Treatment may occasionally exacerbate itching • One application usually curative • Itching is common

PREGNANCY/LACTATION CONSIDERATIONS

- Lindane (Kwell®) should be used cautiously (if at all) in pregnancy due to the potential neurotoxic effects and potential for convulsions
- Permethrin is a category B

CONSULTATION/REFERRAL

- Consider referral to dermatologist for cases resistant to treatment

FOLLOW-UP

- Recheck patient if itching is persistent

EXPECTED COURSE

- Resolution begins in 24-48 hours after treatment
- Geriatric patients may itch more severely than other patients
- Itching may prevail beyond infectious period up to 4 weeks. This is due to antigenic reaction to dead

mites and debris which is present under the skin. This does not indicate persistent infection

POSSIBLE COMPLICATIONS

- Bacterial secondary infections

SCARLET FEVER
(Scarlatina)

DESCRIPTION

Childhood disease characterized by sore throat, fever, and a scarlet "sandpaper" rash.

ETIOLOGY

- Group A β-hemolytic *Streptococcus pyogenes* that produces an erythrogenic toxin

INCIDENCE

- Ages 6-12 years are most common
- Males = Females

RISK FACTORS

- Age 6-12 years
- Wound infection
- Burns

ASSESSMENT FINDINGS

- Sore throat
- Headache
- Fever and chills
- Vomiting
- Erythematous tonsils usually covered with an exudate; pharynx may have exudate as well
- Petechiae on palate
- White coating on tongue which sheds by day 2 or 3 and leaves a "strawberry" tongue with shiny red papillae
- Fine sandpaper rash begins on chest and axillae, then appears on abdomen and extremities; blanches with pressure
- Pastia's lines present (transverse red streaks in skin folds of antecubital space, abdomen, and axillae)
- Desquamation from face which proceeds over trunk and finally to hands and feet

DIFFERENTIAL DIAGNOSIS

- Pharyngitis: non scarlatina
- Measles
- Rubella
- Drug rash
- Viral exanthems
- Toxic shock syndrome
- Scalded skin syndrome

DIAGNOSTIC STUDIES

- Throat culture
- Rapid streptococcal test: diagnostic if positive; if negative, confirm with laboratory culture
- Antistreptolysin O (ASO) confirms infection but not helpful for diagnosis

Throat culture needed prior to treatment. Antibiotic therapy prior to throat culture usually results in negative culture.

PREVENTION

- Avoid contact with respiratory secretions of infected person
- Prophylactic penicillin NOT recommended after exposure to scarlet fever
- Antibiotic started within 10 days after onset effective in preventing rheumatic fever
- Antibiotic does not completely eliminate possibility of glomerulonephritis

NONPHARMACOLOGIC MANAGEMENT

- Supportive care
- Maintain hydration status

PHARMACOLOGIC MANAGEMENT

- Antipyretics for fever
- Penicillin is drug of choice
- Cephalosporins acceptable
- Erythromycin or advanced macrolides for penicillin allergic patients (climbing rates of resistance)

Tetracyclines and sulfonamides should not be used to treat Streptococcal infections.

CONSULTATION/REFERRAL

- Refer for sequella

FOLLOW-UP

- Individualize per patient

EXPECTED COURSE

- Excellent prognosis after appropriate treatment

POSSIBLE COMPLICATIONS

- Sinusitis
- Otitis media
- Rheumatic fever (virtually eliminates risk if treated within 10 days of infection)
- Glomerulonephritis (can occur even with treatment of *Streptococcus* if nephrogenic strain of *Streptococcus* caused infection)

Streptococcal organisms can persist on toothbrushes and dental appliances for up to 15 days. Re-infection can occur unless thoroughly cleansed.

SEBORRHEIC DERMATITIS
(Cradle Cap, Seborrhea)

DESCRIPTION

Chronic, superficial disorder affecting the hairy areas of the body where many sebaceous glands are present (e.g., scalp, eyebrows, face).

ETIOLOGY

- Multifactorial: genetics, environment
- *Malassezia sp.* thought to be a causative agent
- *D. folliculorum* (mite) may play a role

INCIDENCE

- Common throughout lifespan
- Males > Females

RISK FACTORS

- Flares occur with emotional stress
- Family history
- Parkinson's disease
- HIV infection (early cutaneous manifestation)

ASSESSMENT FINDINGS

- *Infants:*
  - ◊ Mild disease presents as fine, white or yellow greasy scale on an erythematous base (usually resolves by 1 year of age)
  - ◊ Severe disease presents as dull, red plaques with thick white or yellow scale on an erythematous base
  - ◊ "Cradle cap" when occurs on scalp
  - ◊ Diaper rash
  - ◊ Axillary rash
  - ◊ Mild erythema
  - ◊ Usually resolves by 8-12 months
- *Adults:*
  - ◊ Greasy, scaling rash
  - ◊ Commonly found in scalp, eyebrows, nasolabial area, ear canals, upper back/anterior chest
  - ◊ Erythema
  - ◊ Rash is usually symmetrical and bilateral
  - ◊ No loss of hair

DIFFERENTIAL DIAGNOSIS

- Atopic dermatitis
- Dandruff
- Acne rosacea
- Psoriasis
- Candidal infection
- Tinea capitis

DIAGNOSTIC STUDIES

- Usually none
- Consider biopsy if diagnosis is in question or if resistant to treatment

NONPHARMACOLOGIC MANAGEMENT

- Exposure to sunlight
- Shampoo frequently (for scalp lesions)
- Apply warm peanut, olive or mineral oil in PM to help remove thick scale, wash off in AM with shampoo (may use soft bristle brush to loosen scale)

PHARMACOLOGIC MANAGEMENT

- *Scalp*
  - ◊ Ketoconazole shampoo (Nizoral®) twice weekly for clearance, then once weekly or every other week for maintenance
  - ◊ Ciclopirox 1% shampoo twice weekly
  - ◊ Topical steroid gel (start with hydrocortisone 1% and increase as needed) massaged into scalp 2-3 times per week (use if not responsive to OTC agents); taper steroid after resolution
- *Face*
  - ◊ 1% hydrocortisone cream (thin layer, short term-less than one week)
- *Ears and scalp margin*
  - ◊ Fluorinated hydrocortisone cream (short term use only)
- *Eyelids*
  - ◊ Cleanse with dilute baby shampoo using a cotton swab
  - ◊ 1% ophthalmic hydrocortisone preparation
- *Other areas*
  - ◊ Antiseborrheic shampoo
  - ◊ Low potency hydrocortisone cream

SEBORRHEIC DERMATITIS PHARMACOLOGIC MANAGEMENT

Class	Drug Generic name (Trade name®)	Dosage How supplied	Comments
Antiseborrheic shampoos	**selenium sulfide 2.5%**	**Adult and ≥ 12 years**: massage into wet scalp, rinse after 3 mins; repeat 2 times weekly	• Pregnancy Category C • See dermatologist for severe cases or cases which are unresponsive to therapy; 2 treatments per week are usually sufficient
	Selsum Blue OTC (1%)	*Shampoo/lotion: 4 oz.*	
	Capitrol Shampoo 2%	**Adult**: massage into wet scalp, rinse after 3 mins; repeat 2 times weekly **Children**: not recommended *Shampoo: 4 oz.*	• Pregnancy Category C • Avoid contact with eyes. If this occurs, flush with cool water • Improvement usually seen by 14 days of use
	fluocinolone	**Adult**: up to 1 oz. on scalp daily, rinse after 5 mins **Children**: not recommended	• Pregnancy Category C • Use for brief periods or under close medical supervision in patients with evidence of pre-existing skin atrophy and elderly patients
	Capex Shampoo	*Shampoo: 6 oz.*	

CONSULTATION/REFERRAL

- Dermatologist for severe cases or cases which are unresponsive to therapy

FOLLOW-UP

- Individualize for patients

EXPECTED COURSE

- In infants, usually resolves by 8 months of age
- In adults, expect remissions and unpredictable exacerbations

POSSIBLE COMPLICATIONS

- Striae from use of fluorinated corticosteroids, especially if used on face
- Skin atrophy

SKIN CANCER

DESCRIPTION

Malignant tumors of the skin arising from various skin layers. *Squamous Cell Carcinoma* (SCC): epithelial tumors arising from the keratinocytes of the epidermis. *Basal Cell Carcinoma* (BCC): tumors arising from the basal cell layer of the skin appendages. *Malignant Melanoma* (MM): tumors arising from malignant degeneration of cells in the melanocytic system.

ETIOLOGY

- Almost always due to overexposure of the skin to ultraviolet rays

INCIDENCE

- Squamous cell: 20% of all skin cancers
- Basal cell: 1,000,000 cases annually (most common skin cancer)
- Malignant melanoma: < 5% of all skin cancers

RISK FACTORS

- Exposure to ultraviolet rays, thermal burns, or radiation
- Fair skin; blondes and redheads
- Light blue or green eye color
- Improper and infrequent use of sunscreen
- Blistering sunburn in adolescence
- Intense, episodic sun exposure
- Living in sunny climates
- Family history of skin cancer

ASSESSMENT FINDINGS

- *Squamous cell carcinoma* (SCC)
  - ◊ Common on sun exposed areas of the skin
  - ◊ Lower lip is common location in smokers
  - ◊ Nodule has indistinct margins; surface is firm, scaly, irregular and may bleed easily
  - ◊ Lesions may be red, tan, brown, pearly gray; may exhibit crusting, ulceration, erosion or scaliness
- *Basal cell carcinoma* (BCC)
  - ◊ Common in 40 to 60 year olds but incidence is increasing in younger age groups
  - ◊ Males more common than females but incidence is increasing in females
  - ◊ Most common sites are head and neck (80% of cases); 20% on lower extremities
  - ◊ Common appearance is pearly domed nodule with overlying telangiectatic vessels; may be a plaque, may be a papule; later in pathogenesis may see central ulceration and crusting
- *Malignant melanoma*
  - ◊ Usual age is early forties
  - ◊ ABCDE characteristics of any lesion:

A = asymmetry
B = border is irregular
C = color variegation
D = diameter > 6 mm (size of pencil eraser)
E = elevation above level of skin

7 Point System for Identifying Malignant Melanoma

3 Major Features:
Change in size, color, or shape of lesion

4 Minor Features:
Presence of inflammation, bleeding or crusting, sensation, diameter > 6 mm

- ◊ Hypo or hyperpigmentation, bleeding, scaling, texture, or size change of an existing mole or lesion
- ◊ Common in Caucasians on back, anterior lower leg
- ◊ Common in African Americans on nails, hands, and feet

DIFFERENTIAL DIAGNOSIS

- Basal cell vs. squamous cell vs. malignant melanoma
- Actinic keratosis
- Seborrheic keratosis
- Dysplastic nevi

DIAGNOSTIC STUDIES

- Removal of lesion
- Surgical biopsy

PREVENTION

- Actinic keratosis is a scaly patch of red or brown skin which often becomes SCC
- Avoidance of sun exposure
- Frequent total body skin examination every 3-6 months after diagnosis of melanoma
- Teach importance of avoidance of sunlight at peak hours, use of sunscreen to patients, especially adolescents
- Hats, long sleeve shirts while exposed to sunlight

NONPHARMACOLOGIC MANAGEMENT

- Surgical biopsy
- Surgical removal of lesion
- Lymph node excision in melanoma

PHARMACOLOGIC MANAGEMENT

- Chemotherapy/immunotherapy for melanoma

PREGNANCY/LACTATION CONSIDERATIONS

- Melanoma may be spread to the fetus via the placenta
- Melanoma patients are encouraged to wait two years after no evidence of malignancy before attempting pregnancy

CONSULTATION/REFERRAL

- Dermatologist
- Surgeon

FOLLOW-UP

- By dermatologist or surgeon
- Skin exams every 3-6 months by professional
- Self-exam once monthly, report any changes in lesions or appearance of new lesions to health care professional

EXPECTED COURSE

- Squamous cell: may metastasize
- Basal cell: slow-growing, rarely metastasizes; often there is recurrence within 5 years at another site
- Malignant melanoma: accounts for over 60% of skin cancer deaths, metastasizes to any organ

POSSIBLE COMPLICATIONS

- Metastatic spread
- Local recurrence
- Disfigurement

SPIDER/INSECT BITES AND STINGS

DESCRIPTION

The injection of venom or another substance by a bee, wasp, ant, mosquito, flea, tick, or spider which can produce local or systemic hypersensitivity.

ETIOLOGY

- *Bees/wasps/ants:* local or systemic hypersensitivity reaction
- *Mosquitoes/fleas:* local or systemic hypersensitivity reaction
- *Ticks*: blood is sucked by the female tick and toxin may be injected which enables disease transmission
- *Spiders/scorpions/caterpillars*: venom injected can be necrotizing, hemolytic; reaction can be local, systemic, or both

INCIDENCE

- *Bees/wasps*: common
- *Mosquitoes/fleas:* most common insect bite; seasonal pattern of incidence
- *Ticks*: common in spring and early summer
- *Spiders/caterpillars:* common, bites from most spiders are harmless, but the brown recluse, black widow, and hobo spiders can cause local as well as systemic reactions

RISK FACTORS

- Human contact with grasses, weeds, bushes, or dark, cool areas where insects inhabit
- Residence in parts of the U.S. where certain insects or spiders are indigenous
- Previous bite by same insect or spider
- Wearing of bright-colored clothes or scented perfumes, cosmetics, lotions, soaps, etc.
- Improper protective clothing while exposed to insects or spiders

Patients who are very young, elderly, immunocompromised, or who have history of allergic reactions are at highest risk for negative consequences from insect bites/stings.

ASSESSMENT FINDINGS

- Bees/wasps
    - ◊ Local redness
    - ◊ Pruritus
    - ◊ Pain
    - ◊ Edema
    - ◊ Cellulitis
    - ◊ Anaphylaxis in susceptible individuals
- Mosquitoes/fleas
    - ◊ Urticarial wheal
    - ◊ Itching
    - ◊ Central punctum
    - ◊ Secondary bacterial infection (impetigo)
- Ticks
    - ◊ Presence of tick (which may go undetected for several days)
    - ◊ Erythematous halo
    - ◊ Pruritus if tick body parts remain under the skin
- Spiders/caterpillars
    - ◊ Punctate marks on the skin
    - ◊ Severe burning, stinging at site when bite occurs
    - ◊ Severe pain, swelling, burning, stinging for several hours after bite
    - ◊ Necrosis locally
    - ◊ Abdominal pain (black widow spider bite)
    - ◊ Local reaction can progress to systemic reaction in certain individuals; characterized by fever, chills, aches, rash, nausea, vomiting, diarrhea, cramps, shock

DIFFERENTIAL DIAGNOSIS

- Bites/stings from harmless insects/spiders vs. poisonous insects/spiders
- Contact dermatitis
- Cellulitis
- Allergic reaction
- Poison ivy/oak
- Acute abdomen (black widow spider bite)

DIAGNOSTIC STUDIES

- Usually none indicated
- CBC, eosinophilia, possible leukocytosis
- Culture and sensitivity if secondarily infected

PREVENTION

- *See* Risk Factors
- Minimize contact with environments likely to harbor insects/spiders

NONPHARMACOLOGIC MANAGEMENT

- Remove stinger
- Firmly grasp tick with forceps or tweezers to remove (do not attempt to burn tick)
- Cool compresses for itching/edema
- Elimination of fleas from home environment
- Elevation of extremity for severe edema
- Application of ice to spider bites. **Avoid application of heat!**
- Examination of unprotected body parts after exposure to potential tick infested areas
- Possible debridement

PHARMACOLOGIC MANAGEMENT

- *Oral* antipruritics/antihistamines/analgesics/steroids
- *Topical* - antipruritics/antihistamines/corticosteroids
- Application of insect repellents (may be absorbed systemically). Apply with caution in pediatric and elderly patients
- Tetanus prophylaxis for spider bites
- Analgesics for spider bites
- Topical/systemic antibiotics for secondarily infected bites (*Refer to Furunculosis, Carbunculosis and Cellulitis antibiotic tables, page 101*)
- Preloaded syringe of epinephrine for patients with potential for anaphylactic reaction
- Short course of steroids for severe local reactions which extend beyond two joints
- Anti-venoms

Dermatologic Disorders

SPIDER BITES AND STINGS PHARMACOLOGIC MANAGEMENT

Class	Drug Generic name (Trade name®)	Dosage How supplied	Comments
Topical Anti-pruritics *This is a skin protectant containing calaime 8% and zinc oxide 8%*	**calamine**	Apply liberally to affected areas	• Shake well before applying • All available OTC
General comments For topical use only Avoid eyes This product has not been reviewed and approved by the FDA	Various generics	*Bottles: Multiple sizes*	
First Generation Antihistamines	**diphenhydramine**	**Adult**: 25-50 mg every 4-6 hr *Max*: 300 mg/day **Children < 6 yrs**: individualize **Children 6-12 yr:** 12.5-25 mg every 4-6 hr *Max*: 150 mg/day	• Pregnancy Category B • Cautious use in patients with glaucoma, difficulty urinating due to an enlarged prostate gland, COPD • Avoid alcohol within 6 hours of taking • May cause profound drowsiness in some patients
General comments Avoid simultaneous use of CNS depressants Care when driving or engaging in activities that require attention Most available over the counter	Benadryl	*Tabs: 25 mg; Chew tabs: 12.5 mg; Liquid: 12.5 mg/ 5 mL Injection: 50 mg/mL*	

continued

SPIDER BITES AND STINGS PHARMACOLOGIC MANAGEMENT

Class	Drug Generic name (Trade name®)	Dosage How supplied	Comments
	hydroxyzine	**Adult**: 25 mg 3-4 times daily **Children < 6 yrs**: 50 mg daily in divided doses **Children > 6 yrs**: 50-100 mg daily in divided doses	• Unable to establish safety during pregnancy • May produce drowsiness in any dose. Appropriate care advised • If used in geriatric patients, should administer a low dose and monitor carefully
	Vistaril Atarax	*Caps: 25 mg; 50 mg* *Suspension: 25 mg/5 mL; available in 4 oz; 1 pt.*	
Second Generation Antihistamines <u>**General comment**</u> Does not typically produce drowsiness (except cetirizine) and usually dosed once daily	**cetirizine**	**Adult and Children > 12 years**: 5-10 mg daily **Children 6-11 years**: 5-10 mg based on symptom relief **Children 2-5 years**: 2.5 mg daily or twice daily	• Pregnancy Category B • Caution regarding activities requiring mental alertness, produces drowsiness because of its affinity for H1 receptors • Dosage adjustment needed for ages 77 and older, renal and hepatic impairment • Take without regard to food • Consider taking in the evening
	Zyrtec	*Tabs: 10 mg* *Chew tab: 5 mg; 10 mg* *Syrup: 1 mg/ mL; 4 oz. bottle*	
	levocetirizine	**Adult and children ≥ 12 years**: 5 mg once daily in the evening **Children 6-11 years**: 2.5 mg once daily in the evening **Children 6 months to 5 years**: 1.25 mg once daily in the evening	• Pregnancy Category B • Adjust dose for renal impairment; contraindicated in children 6 months to 11 years with renal impairment • Avoid engaging in activities requiring mental alertness • Avoid concurrent use alcohol or CNS depressants
	Xyzal	*Tabs: 5 mg scored* *Oral solution: 0.5 mg/mL*	
	fexofenadine	**Adult and Children > 12 years:** 180 mg daily or 60 mg twice daily **Children 6 months -11 years**: 30 mg twice daily **Children 6 months – 2 years**: 15 mg twice daily	• Pregnancy Category C • Shake bottle well before use • Reduce dose for renal impairment • Allegra ODT contains phenylalanine (other Allegra products do not) • Avoid aluminum and magnesium containing antacids • Less effective if taken with fruit juices; therefore, take with water • Do not expect sedation
	Allegra	*Tab: 30 mg, 60 mg, 180 mg* *ODT tab: 30 mg* *Susp: 6 mg/mL in 300 mL*	
	loratadine	**Adult and Children > 6 years**: 10 mg daily **Children 2-5 yrs**: 5 mg once daily	• Pregnancy Category B • Children use chew tabs or syrup • Adjustment needed for renal or hepatic impairment • Do not expect sedation

continued

SPIDER BITES AND STINGS PHARMACOLOGIC MANAGEMENT

Class	Drug Generic name (Trade name®)	Dosage How supplied	Comments
	Claritin	*Syrup: 1 mg/mL* *Chewtabs: 5 mg* *RediTabs: 10 mg*	
	desloratadine	**Adult**: 5 mg daily **Children 6-11 mos**: 1 mg (2 mL) daily **Children 1-5 yrs:** 1.25 mg (2.5 mL) daily **Children 6-11 yrs**: 2.5 mg (5 mL) daily	• Pregnancy Category C • Children use RediTabs or syrup • Do not expect sedation
	Clarinex	*Tabs: 5 mg* *RediTabs: 2.5 mg; 5 mg* *Syrup: 0.5 mg/mL*	
Epinephrine *acts on the alpha and beta adrenergic receptors. It causes bronchial smooth muscle relaxation, decreases vasodilation, improves pruritis, urticaria, and angioedema* **General comment** Epinephrine is the drug of choice for emergency treatment of allergic reactions	**epinephrine**	**Adult**: (use for patients > 66 lbs) 0.3 mg IM in thigh, repeat if needed **Children**: (use for patients 15-65 lbs.) 0.15 mg IM in thigh, may repeat if needed Use other forms if < 0.15 is needed	• Instruct patient on use when prescribed • The needle emerges through the orange cap. Place the cap against thigh for injection. After injection, about 85% of the medication remains in the auto-injector. This indicates correct administration • There are no absolute contraindications • Proceed immediately to an emergency department after using • Visualize epinephrine solution periodically for particulate matter • Discard if present or for any discoloration • Instruct patient to carry at all times • Store at room temperature and keep away from direct sunlight
	EpiPen EpiPenJr	*Auto-injector: 0.3 mg* *Auto-injector: 0.15 mg*	

CONSULTATION/REFERRAL

- **Do not delay treatment!** Reactions usually take place within 2-60 minutes
- Emergency department for severe reactions
- Surgeon/dermatologist for severe local reactions
- Consider referral for severe reaction in the very young and very old

Most deaths secondary to anaphylaxis occur 30-60 minutes after the bite or sting.

FOLLOW-UP

- Individualize by severity

EXPECTED COURSE

- Depends on type of bite, type of reaction, age of patient

POSSIBLE COMPLICATIONS

- Anaphylactic reactions possible and are more likely to occur in patients who have been previously sensitized
- Secondary bacterial infections
- Increased intensity of reactions with subsequent bites

TINEA INFECTIONS
(RINGWORM)

DESCRIPTION

Fungal infections affecting various parts of the body.

ETIOLOGY

- *Trichophyton* sp.: most common
- *Microsporum* sp.
- *Epidermophyton* sp.: causative agent for some tinea cruris and tinea pedis infections
- *Pityrosporum* sp.: causative agent for tinea versicolor

INCIDENCE

- Common
- More prevalent in summer months, warm climates

RISK FACTORS

Tinea capitis

◊ Daycare age group
◊ Contact with infected items (e.g., combs, brushes, hats)
◊ Poor hygiene

Tinea corporis

◊ Close contact with animals
◊ Warm climates
◊ Obesity
◊ Prolonged use of topical steroids
◊ Immunocompromised state

Tinea cruris

◊ Wearing wet clothing
◊ Excessive sweating
◊ Obesity
◊ Prolonged use of topical steroids
◊ Immunocompromised state

Tinea pedis

◊ Occlusive footwear
◊ Damp footwear
◊ Prolonged use of topical steroids
◊ Immunocompromised state

Tinea versicolor

◊ Hot, humid climates
◊ Wearing wet clothing
◊ Prolonged use of topical steroids
◊ Immunocompromised state

ASSESSMENT FINDINGS

Tinea capitis
- ◊ Round patchy scales on scalp
- ◊ Occasionally alopecia will develop
- ◊ Most commonly found in pediatric patients

Tinea corporis
- ◊ Rash
- ◊ Pruritus
- ◊ Well-circumscribed, red, plaque usually found on the trunk
- ◊ May occur in groups of 3 or more

Tinea cruris
- ◊ Pruritus
- ◊ Well marginated half-moon plaques in the groin and/or upper thighs
- ◊ May take on eczematous appearance from chronic scratching
- ◊ Does not affect the scrotum or penis
- ◊ May appear as vesicles
- ◊ Rare in pediatric patients before puberty

Tinea pedis
- ◊ Itching in interdigital spaces
- ◊ Maceration in affected areas
- ◊ Scaling
- ◊ Can affect the sole and arch
- ◊ Elderly more susceptible

Tinea versicolor
- ◊ Well-marginated lesions of varying colors (white, red, brown); hence the name "versicolor"
- ◊ Rare itching
- ◊ Common in axilla, shoulders, chest, back (sebum rich areas)

DIFFERENTIAL DIAGNOSIS

- *Tinea capitis:* alopecia areata, psoriasis, seborrhea, trichotillomania
- *Tinea corporis:* pityriasis rosea, psoriasis, atopic dermatitis
- *Tinea cruris:* candidiasis, intertrigo, psoriasis
- *Tinea pedis:* intertrigo, dyshidrosis, psoriasis
- *Tinea versicolor:* pityriasis alba, vitiligo

DIAGNOSTIC STUDIES

- KOH scraping
- Wood's lamp exam (some tinea will not fluoresce, most forms of tinea capitis will not fluoresce)

PREVENTION

- Good personal hygiene
- Identification and treatment of infected humans and pets (tinea capitis and corporis)
- Remove wet clothes as soon as possible
- Dry between toes after showering and bathing
- Avoid direct contact with surfaces in public bathing facilities

NONPHARMACOLOGIC MANAGEMENT

Tinea capitis
- ◊ Good hygiene
- ◊ Consider monitoring liver function tests for treatment with griseofulvin or another oral antifungal
- ◊ Teach patients to wear sunscreen and minimize sun exposure because of increased photosensitivity when taking griseofulvin
- ◊ Treat family members and infected pets
- ◊ Shaving of head is not necessary for treatment

Tinea corporis
- ◊ Good hygiene
- ◊ Avoid contact with lesions

Tinea cruris
- ◊ Keep area as dry as possible
- ◊ Do not scratch

Tinea pedis
- ◊ Dry between toes
- ◊ Trim dead skin

Tinea versicolor
- ◊ Keep area as dry as possible

TINEA INFECTIONS PHARMACOLOGIC MANAGEMENT

Class	Drug Generic name (Trade name®)	Dosage How supplied	Comments
Tinea Capitis	**griseofulvin**	**Adult:** 500 mg daily *Max*: 1 g daily **Children 30-50 pounds:** 125-250 mg daily **Children > 50 pounds:** 250-500 mg daily	• Pregnancy Category C • Usually requires treatment for 4-6 weeks • Take with a high fat meal to improve absorption • Contraindicated in patients with porphyria, hepatic dysfunction • Derived from penicillin so theoretically possible for reaction in penicillin sensitive patients, though no reports • Avoid exposure to sunlight • May reduce the efficacy of oral contraceptives
	Grifulvin V Various generics	*Tabs: 100 mg, 500 mg* *Susp: 125 mg/5 mL*	
Tinea Corporis/Cruris/ Pedis	**econazole**	**Adult**: Apply to cover area once daily	• Pregnancy Category C • Treat for at least 2 weeks; if no improvement, reassess diagnosis • Tinea pedis: TREAT 4 WEEKS • Information on pediatric dosing is not available • Do not use vaginally
<u>General comments</u> To prevent relapse, use 1 week after apparent resolution	Spectazole Various generics	*Cream: 15 g, 30 g, 85 g*	
Keep skin clean, dry, and expose to air and light when possible to speed resolution	**ketoconazole 2%**	**Adult**: Apply once daily to cover the affected and immediate surrounding area	• Pregnancy Category C • Treat at least 2 weeks; if no improvement, reassess diagnosis • Tinea pedis: TREAT 6 WEEKS • Safety and efficacy in children has not been established • Do not use vaginally
Many antifungals available, all have specific indications for fungal infections	Various generics	*Cream: 15 g, 30 g, 60 g*	
	terbinafine	**Adult and children > 12 years**: wash affected skin with soap and water and dry completely before applying	• Pregnancy Category B • Pregnancy information not available • Treat for at least 2 weeks; if no improvement, reassess diagnosis • Information on pediatric dosing is not available • Do not use vaginally
	Lamisil	*Cream: various sizes*	
Tinea Versicolor	**ketoconazole 2% shampoo**	**Adult**: Apply the shampoo to damp skin of the affected area and a wide margin surrounding affected area. Leave in place for 5 minutes, rinse off with water. One application should be sufficient	• Pregnancy Category C • Treatment of infection my not result in immediate normalization of pigment to skin. May take several months • Keep away from eyes and mucous membranes
	Nizoral shampoo	*4 ounce plastic bottle*	

continued

TINEA INFECTIONS PHARMACOLOGIC MANAGEMENT

Class	Drug Generic name (Trade name®)	Dosage How supplied	Comments
	Selenium sulfide 2.25% shampoo	**Adult**: Apply to affected areas and lather with a small amount of water. Allow to remain on skin for 10 minutes, then rinse thoroughly. Repeat daily for 7 days.	• Pregnancy Category C • Pediatric information not available • May cause skin irritation, increase in normal hair loss • Keep away from eyes and mucous membranes
	Various generics	*180 mL bottle*	

PREGNANCY/LACTATION CONSIDERATIONS

- Oral antifungals are contraindicated in pregnancy

CONSULTATION/REFERRAL

- Dermatologist for cases which are not responsive to treatment

FOLLOW-UP

- If on oral anti-fungal medication, consider liver function tests; recheck after 2 weeks and then in 6 weeks
- Recheck as needed for conditions requiring topical therapy

EXPECTED COURSE

Tinea capitis
- ◊ Will resolve completely in about 4 weeks with appropriate treatment

Tinea corporis
- ◊ Complete resolution in 1-2 weeks following treatment

Tinea cruris
- ◊ Complete resolution in 1-2 weeks with appropriate treatment

Tinea pedis
- ◊ Symptoms become controlled, but cure never occurs
- ◊ Frequent recurrences

Tinea versicolor
- ◊ Frequent recurrences, especially during springtime

POSSIBLE COMPLICATIONS

Tinea capitis
- ◊ Possible permanent alopecia and/or scarring

Tinea corporis
- ◊ Bacterial secondary infection from scratching

Tinea cruris
- ◊ Bacterial secondary infection

Tinea pedis
- ◊ Frequent recurrences

Tinea versicolor
- ◊ None

VARICELLA
(Chickenpox)

DESCRIPTION

A highly contagious viral illness characterized by the development of pruritic vesicles and papules on the skin, scalp and less commonly, on mucus membranes.

ETIOLOGY

- Varicella-zoster virus (VZV), a herpesvirus

Virus establishes latency in the dorsal root ganglia. Reactivation results in "shingles".

INCIDENCE

- Common, but becoming less prevalent with the advent of the varicella vaccine
- Peak age is 5-9 years, but any age susceptible
- Outbreaks from January to May

RISK FACTORS

- No prior history of varicella, no vaccination
- Immunocompromised status

Incubation for varicella is about 2 weeks. Patients are infectious to others for 2 days BEFORE the appearance of the rash AND until all lesions have crusted.

ASSESSMENT FINDINGS

Prodrome
- ◊ Fever
- ◊ Malaise
- ◊ Anorexia, abdominal pain
- ◊ Headache

Rash Phase
- ◊ Crops of lesions begin on trunk, become vesicles, then scabs in 6-10 hours
- ◊ Successive crops appear over the next several days
- ◊ Lesions may be found on any mucosal membrane: mouth, larynx, vagina

DIFFERENTIAL DIAGNOSIS

- Other viral illnesses
- Other herpetic illnesses
- Impetigo
- Contact dermatitis

DIAGNOSTIC STUDIES

- Usually none indicated except in pregnant women

PREVENTION

- Vaccination
  - ◊ 12 months to 12 years old: given as single immunization (70-90% efficacy)
  - ◊ 13 years and older: two vaccinations 4-8 weeks apart (70% efficacy)
- Most contagious period is 2 days prior to appearance of rash and up to crusting of ALL lesions; therefore, keep infected individuals at home until lesions have crusted
- Passive immunization with VZIG (Varicella-zoster immune globulin) within 4 days of exposure for immunocompromised individuals
- If unable to administer VZIG within timeframe, consider acyclovir to decrease duration and time of viral shedding (recommended for high risk individuals)

NONPHARMACOLOGIC MANAGEMENT

- Supportive therapy
- Good hygiene to prevent bacterial secondary infections
- Cut fingernails short in young children to decrease incidence of bacterial infections from scratching
- Tepid bath, oatmeal bath for itching

PHARMACOLOGIC MANAGEMENT

- Supportive therapy: skin protectant such as calamine topical
- Antipyretics: DO NOT GIVE ASPIRIN due to increased risk of Reye's syndrome with varicella patients
- Antiviral agents: consider in adolescents, adults,

high risk patients to decrease viral shedding, duration of fever
- Acyclovir (2-16 year olds): 20 mg/kg/dose (max. 800 mg/dose), four times daily for 5 days; Adults: 800 mg, 5 times daily for 5 days
- Famciclovir (adults): 500mg three times daily for 7-10 days
- Valaciclovir (adults): 1g three times daily for 7-10 days

Infection in adults is more likely to produce serious illness.

PREGNANCY/LACTATION CONSIDERATIONS

- Do not vaccinate pregnant women
- In pregnant women who have never had chickenpox or immunization, avoid contact with recently vaccinated individuals for 6 weeks
- Fetal infection following maternal infection is 25%
- Increased incidence of pneumonia in women infected during pregnancy
- Congenital malformations seen in 5% of infants if mother was infected during the first or second trimester

CONSULTATION/REFERRAL

- Consider referral for infected newborns, immunocompromised patients, pregnant women, or severe cases

FOLLOW-UP

- Usually none needed if disease follows normal course
- If complications develop, individualize follow-up

EXPECTED COURSE

- Complete resolution in 2-3 weeks
- Lifelong immunity conferred after disease

POSSIBLE COMPLICATIONS

- Bacterial secondary infections
- Pneumonia (most common in adults and the elderly)
- Encephalitis (rare)
- Reye's syndrome (rare)
- Disseminated infection

WARTS

DESCRIPTION

Painless, benign skin tumors.

ETIOLOGY

- Human papillomavirus (HPV)
- Different genotypes cause different warts
  - ◊ Common wart: verruca vulgaris
  - ◊ Plantar wart: verruca plantaris

INCIDENCE

- Common, approximately 7-10% of population in U.S.
- Occurs in children and young adults predominantly
- Females > Males

RISK FACTORS

- Skin trauma
- Contact with wart exudate after treatment
- Immunocompromised state

ASSESSMENT FINDINGS

- Common wart: rough surface, elevated, flesh-colored papules
- Plantar wart: rough, flat surface, flesh-colored, can attain size of up to 2-3 cm in diameter; usually located on sole of foot
- Black dots seen in the middle of the wart are thrombosed capillaries

More commonly found on hands and feet because these areas are more subject to trauma.

DIFFERENTIAL DIAGNOSIS

- Molluscum contagiosum
- Seborrheic keratoses
- Corns
- Squamous cell, basal cell carcinomas
- Condyloma lata

DIAGNOSTIC STUDIES

- Usually none needed

PREVENTION

- Avoid contact with wart exudate from self (auto-inoculation) and others by covering wart
- Avoid skin trauma

NONPHARMACOLOGIC MANAGEMENT

- Paring and debridement of wart prior to any treatment
- Soaking of wart in warm water to soften and moisten it
- Occlude the wart with waterproof tape for one week, leave open to air for 8-12 hours, then re occlude for one week. This creates an environment that is not conducive to growth. Best used for periungual warts
- Cryotherapy
- Excision

PHARMACOLOGIC MANAGEMENT

- There are no ideal treatments
- Many topical keratolytic preparations are available OTC. They must be applied for up to 12 weeks (Duofilm, Occlusal-HP, Trans-Ver-Sal)

Most warts will spontaneously regress in about 2 years.

Warts resistant to treatment should be biopsied. Verrucous carcinoma can appear like a common wart.

CONSULTATION/REFERRAL

- Dermatologist or surgeon for removal if large or if possibility of scarring is likely
- Refer all warts unresponsive to treatment

FOLLOW-UP

- Usually none needed

EXPECTED COURSE

- Resolution with or without treatment

No single treatment for warts is considered superior to another.

POSSIBLE COMPLICATIONS

- Scarring
- Auto-inoculation
- Nail deformity

References

Alberta, L., Sweeney, S.M., & Wiss, K. (2005). Diaper dye dermatitis. Pediatrics, 116(3), e450-452. doi: 116/3/e450 [pii] 10.1542/peds.2004-2066

American Academy of Pediatrics. (2009a). Group a streptococcal infections. In L. K. Pickering (Ed.), Red book: 2009 report of the committee on infectious diseases (pp. 616). Elk Grove Village, IL: American Academy of Pediatrics.

American Academy of Pediatrics. (2009b). Herpes simplex. In L. K. Pickering (Ed.), Red book: 2009 report of the committee on infectious diseases (28th ed., pp. 363). Elk Grove Village, IL: American Academy of Pediatrics

American Academy of Pediatrics. (2009c). Human herpesvirus 6 (including roseola) and 7. In L. K. Pickering (Ed.), Red book: 2009 report of the committee on infectious diseases (28th ed., pp. 378). Elk Grove Village, IL: American Academy of Pediatrics

American Academy of Pediatrics. (2009d). Measles. In L. K. Pickering (Ed.), Red book: 2009 report of the committee on infectious diseases (pp. 444). Elk Grove Village, IL: American Academy of Pediatrics.

American Academy of Pediatrics. (2009e). Red book: 2009 report of the committee on infectious diseases (28th ed.). Elk Grove Village, IL: American Academy of Pediatrics.

Balkrishnan, R., Camacho, F. T., Pearce, D. J., Kulkarni, A. S., Spencer, L., Fleischer, A. B., Jr., & Feldman, S. R. (2005). Factors affecting prescription of ultra-high potency topical corticosteroids in skin disease: An analysis of us national practice data. The Journal of Drugs in Dermatology, 4(6), 699-706.

Belsito, D. V. (2005). Occupational contact dermatitis: Etiology, prevalence, and resultant impairment/disability. Journal of the American Academy of Dermatology, 53(2), 303-313. doi: S019096220500914X [pii]

Borkowski, S. (2004). Diaper rash care and management. Pediatric Nursing, 30(6), 467-470.

Brantsch, K. D., Meisner, C., Schonfisch, B., Trilling, B., Wehner-Caroli, J., Rocken, M., & Breuninger, H. (2008). Analysis of risk factors determining prognosis of cutaneous squamous-cell carcinoma: A prospective study. Lancet Oncol, 9(8), 713-720. doi: S1470-2045(08)70178-5 [pii]

Bratton, R. L., Whiteside, J. W., Hovan, M. J., Engle, R. L., & Edwards, F. D. (2008). Diagnosis and treatment of lyme disease. Mayo Clinic Proceedings, 83(5), 566-571.

Burgess, I. F. (2009a). Current treatments for pediculosis capitis. Current Opinion in Infectious Diseases, 22(2), 131-136.

Burgess, I. F. (2009b). Head lice. Clinical Evidence (Online), 2009. doi: 1703 [pii]

Burns, C.E., Brady, M.A., Blosser, C., Starr, N.B., & Dunn, A.M. (2009). Pediatric primary care: A handbook for nurse practitioners (4th ed.). Philadelphia: W.B. Saunders.

Cantwell, M. M., Murray, L. J., Catney, D., Donnelly, D., Autier, P., Boniol, M., . . . Gavin, A. T. (2009). Second primary cancers in patients with skin cancer: A population-based study in northern ireland. British Journal of Cancer, 100(1), 174-177. doi: 10.1038/sj.bjc.6604842

Chen, J., Ruczinski, I., Jorgensen, T. J., Yenokyan, G., Yao, Y., Alani, R., . . . Alberg, A. J. (2008). Nonmelanoma skin cancer and risk for subsequent malignancy. Journal of the National Cancer Institute, 100(17), 1215-1222. doi: 10.1093/jnci/djn260

Chosidow, O. (2006). Clinical practices. Scabies. New England Journal of Medicine, 354(16), 1718-1727. doi: 10.1056/NEJMcp052784

Chuh, A. A., Dofitas, B. L., Comisel, G. G., Reveiz, L., Sharma, V., Garner, S. E., & Chu, F. (2007). Interventions for pityriasis rosea. Cochrane Database Syst Rev(2), CD005068. doi: 10.1002/14651858.CD005068.pub2

Clayman, G. L., Lee, J. J., Holsinger, F. C., Zhou, X., Duvic, M., El-Naggar, A. K., . . . Lippman, S. M. (2005). Mortality risk from squamous cell skin cancer. Journal of Clinical Oncology, 23(4), 759-765. doi: 10.1200/JCO.2005.02.155

Daum, R. S. (2007). Clinical practice. Skin and soft-tissue infections caused by methicillin-resistant staphylococcus aureus. New

England Journal of Medicine, 357(4), 380-390. doi: 10.1056/NEJMcp070747

de Haen, M., Spigt, M. G., van Uden, C. J., van Neer, P., Feron, F. J., & Knottnerus, A. (2006). Efficacy of duct tape vs placebo in the treatment of verruca vulgaris (warts) in primary school children. Archives of Pediatrics and Adolescent Medicine, 160(11), 1121-1125. doi: 10.1001/archpedi.160.11.1121

DeAngelis, Y. M., Gemmer, C. M., Kaczvinsky, J. R., Kenneally, D. C., Schwartz, J. R., & Dawson, T. L., Jr. (2005). Three etiologic facets of dandruff and seborrheic dermatitis: Malassezia fungi, sebaceous lipids, and individual sensitivity. Journal of Investigative Dermatology. Symposium Proceedings, 10(3), 295-297. doi: 10.1111/j.1087-0024.2005.10119.x

Domino, F., Baldor, R., Golding, J., Grimes, J., & Taylor, J. (2011). The 5-minute clinical consult 2011. Philadelphia: Lippincott Williams & Wilkins.

Drago, F., Broccolo, F., & Rebora, A. (2009). Pityriasis rosea: An update with a critical appraisal of its possible herpesviral etiology. Journal of the American Academy of Dermatology, 61(2), 303-318. doi: 10.1016/j.jaad.2008.07.045

Drug facts and comparisons. (2010). St. Louis: Wolters Kluwer Health. Facts & Comparisons.

Elewski, B. E., Caceres, H. W., DeLeon, L., El Shimy, S., Hunter, J. A., Korotkiy, N., . . . Friedlander, S. F. (2008). Terbinafine hydrochloride oral granules versus oral griseofulvin suspension in children with tinea capitis: Results of two randomized, investigator-blinded, multicenter, international, controlled trials. Journal of the American Academy of Dermatology, 59(1), 41-54. doi: 10.1016/j.jaad.2008.02.019

Ernst, D., & Lee, A. . (2010). Nurse practitioners prescribing reference. New York: Haymarket Media Publication.

Factor, S.H., Levine, O.S., Schwartz, B., Harrison, L.H., Farley, M.M., McGeer, A., & Schuchat, A. (2003). Invasive group a streptococcal disease: Risk factors for adults. Emerging Infectious Diseases, 9(8), 970-977.

Feldman, S. R. (2006). Tachyphylaxis to topical corticosteroids: The more you use them, the less they work? Clinics in Dermatology, 24(3), 229-230; discussion 230. doi: 10.1016/j.clindermatol.2005.09.003

Florin, T. A., Zaoutis, T. E., & Zaoutis, L. B. (2008). Beyond cat scratch disease: Widening spectrum of bartonella henselae infection. Pediatrics, 121(5), e1413-1425. doi: 10.1542/peds.2007-1897

Gehrig, K. A., & Warshaw, E. M. (2008). Allergic contact dermatitis to topical antibiotics: Epidemiology, responsible allergens, and management. Journal of the American Academy of Dermatology, 58(1), 1-21. doi: 10.1016/j.jaad.2007.07.050

Gilbert, D.N., Moellering, R.C., Eliopoulos, G.M., & Saag, M.S. (Eds.). (2010). The sanford guide to antimicrobial therapy 2010 (40 ed.). Sperryville, VA: Antimicrobial Therapy.

Glazenburg, E. J., Wolkerstorfer, A., Gerretsen, A. L., Mulder, P. G., & Oranje, A. P. (2009). Efficacy and safety of fluticasone propionate 0.005% ointment in the long-term maintenance treatment of children with atopic dermatitis: Differences between boys and girls? Pediatric Allergy and Immunology, 20(1), 59-66. doi: 10.1111/j.1399-3038.2008.00735.x

Gonzalez, U., Seaton, T., Bergus, G., Jacobson, J., & Martinez-Monzon, C. (2007). Systemic antifungal therapy for tinea capitis in children. Cochrane Database Systemic Reviews(4), CD004685. doi: 10.1002/14651858.CD004685.pub2

Graft, D. F. (2006). Insect sting allergy. Medical Clinics of North America, 90(1), 211-232. doi: 10.1016/j.mcna.2005.08.006

Harpaz, R., Ortega-Sanchez, I. R., & Seward, J. F. (2008). Prevention of herpes zoster: Recommendations of the advisory committee on immunization practices (acip). MMWR Recomm Rep, 57(RR-5), 1-30; quiz CE32-34. doi: rr5705a1 [pii]

He, L., Zhang, D., Zhou, M., & Zhu, C. (2008). Corticosteroids for preventing postherpetic neuralgia. Cochrane Database Systemic Reviews(1), CD005582. doi: 10.1002/14651858.CD005582.pub2

Hebert, A. A., Friedlander, S. F., & Allen, D. B. (2006). Topical fluticasone propionate lotion does not cause hpa axis suppression. Journal of Pediatrics, 149(3), 378-382. doi: 10.1016/j.jpeds.2006.05.008

Heininger, U, & Seward, JF. (2006). Varicella. Lancet, 368(9544), 1365-1376. doi: 10.1016/S0140-6736(06)69561-5

Hernandez, R. G., & Cohen, B. A. (2006). Insect bite-induced hypersensitivity and the scratch principles: A new approach to papular urticaria. Pediatrics, 118(1), e189-196. doi: 10.1542/peds.2005-2550

Heymann, W. R. (2007). Oral contraceptives for the treatment of acne vulgaris. Journal of the American Academy of Dermatology, 56(6), 1056-1057. doi: 10.1016/j.jaad.2007.01.027

Hoppa, E., & Bachur, R. (2007). Lyme disease update. Current Opinion in Pediatrics, 19(3), 275-280. doi: 10.1097/MOP.0b013e3280e1269a

Impetigo, folliculitis, furunculosis, and carbuncles. (2010). Up to Date. Retrieved from

Kabra, SK, Lodha, R, & Hilton, DJ. (2008). Antibiotics for preventing complications in children with measles. Cochrane Database Syst Rev(3), CD001477. doi: 10.1002/14651858.CD001477.pub3

Kagan, R. J., Yakuboff, K. P., Warner, P., & Warden, G. D. (2005). Surgical treatment of hidradenitis suppurativa: A 10-year experience. Surgery, 138(4), 734-740; discussion 740-731. doi: 10.1016/j.surg.2005.06.053

Kalb, R. E., Bagel, J., Korman, N. J., Lebwohl, M. G., Young, M., Horn, E. J., & Van Voorhees, A. S. (2009). Treatment of intertriginous psoriasis: From the medical board of the national psoriasis foundation. Journal of the American Academy of Dermatology, 60(1), 120-124. doi: 10.1016/j.jaad.2008.06.041

Keogh-Brown, M. R., Fordham, R. J., Thomas, K. S., Bachmann, M. O., Holland, R. C., Avery, A. J., . . . Harvey, I. (2007). To freeze or not to freeze: A cost-effectiveness analysis of wart treatment. British Journal of Dermatology, 156(4), 687-692. doi: 10.1111/j.1365-2133.2007.07768.x

Kimberlin, D. W., & Whitley, R. J. (2007). Varicella-zoster vaccine for the prevention of herpes zoster. New England Journal of Medicine, 356(13), 1338-1343. doi: 10.1056/NEJMct066061

Kolokotronis, A, & Doumas, S. (2006). Herpes simplex virus infection, with particular reference to the progression and complications of primary herpetic gingivostomatitis. Clinical Microbiology and Infection, 12(3), 202-211. doi: 10.1111/j.1469-0691.2005.01336.x

Lam, J., Krakowski, A. C., & Friedlander, S. F. (2007). Hidradenitis suppurativa (acne inversa): Management of a recalcitrant disease. Pediatric Dermatology, 24(5), 465-473. doi: 10.1111/j.1525-1470.2007.00544.x

Landau, M, & Krafchik, BR. (1999). The diagnostic value of cafè-au-lait macules. Journal of the American Academy of Dermatology, 40(6 Pt 1), 877-890; quiz 891-872. doi: S0190-9622(99)70075-7 [pii]

Lebwohl, M., Clark, L., & Levitt, J. (2007). Therapy for head lice based on life cycle, resistance, and safety considerations. Pediatrics, 119(5), 965-974. doi: 10.1542/peds.2006-3087

Lee, R. A., Yoon, A., & Kist, J. (2007). Hidradenitis suppurativa: An update. Advances in Dermatology, 23, 289-306.

Leone, P. A. (2007). Scabies and pediculosis pubis: An update of treatment regimens and general review. Clinical Infectious Diseases, 44 Suppl 3, S153-159. doi: 10.1086/511428

Love, W. E., Bernhard, J. D., & Bordeaux, J. S. (2009). Topical imiquimod or fluorouracil therapy for basal and squamous cell carcinoma: A systematic review. Archives of Dermatology, 145(12), 1431-1438. doi: 10.1001/archdermatol.2009.291

Lyme disease-United States, 2003-2005. (2007). MMWR. Morbidity and Mortality Weekly Report, 56, 573-576.

Megged, O, Yinnon, AM, Raveh, D, Rudensky, B, & Schlesinger, Y. (2006). Group a streptococcus bacteraemia: Comparison of adults and children in a single medical centre. Clinical Microbiology and Infection, 12(2), 156-162. doi: CLM1311 [pii] 10.1111/j.1469-0691.2005.01311.x

Menter, A., & Griffiths, C. E. (2007). Current and future management of psoriasis. Lancet, 370(9583), 272-284. doi: 10.1016/S0140-6736(07)61129-5

Menter, A., Korman, N. J., Elmets, C. A., Feldman, S. R., Gelfand, J. M., Gordon, K. B., . . . Bhushan, R. (2010). Guidelines of care for the management of psoriasis and psoriatic arthritis: Section 5. Guidelines of care for the treatment of psoriasis with

Dermatologic Disorders

phototherapy and photochemotherapy. Journal of the American Academy of Dermatology, 62(1), 114-135. doi: 10.1016/j.jaad.2009.08.026

Mertens, D. M., Jenkins, M. E., & Warden, G. D. (1997). Outpatient burn management. Nursing Clinics of North America, 32(2), 343-364.

Monafo, W. W. (1996). Initial management of burns. New England Journal of Medicine, 335(21), 1581-1586. doi: 10.1056/NEJM199611213352108

Mounsey, A. L., Matthew, L. G., & Slawson, D. C. (2005). Herpes zoster and postherpetic neuralgia: Prevention and management. American Family Physician, 72(6), 1075-1080.

Muller, M. J., & Herndon, D. N. (1994). The challenge of burns. Lancet, 343(8891), 216-220. doi: S0140-6736(94)90995-4 [pii]

Naldi, L., & Rebora, A. (2009). Clinical practice. Seborrheic dermatitis. New England Journal of Medicine, 360(4), 387-396. doi: 10.1056/NEJMcp0806464

Nguyen, HQ, Jumaan, AO, & Seward, JF. (2005). Decline in mortality due to varicella after implementation of varicella vaccination in the United States. New England Journal of Medicine, 352(5), 450-458. doi: 10.1056/NEJMoa042271

Nunley, KS, Gao, F, Albers, AC, Bayliss, SJ, & Gutmann, DH. (2009). Predictive value of cafè au lait macules at initial consultation in the diagnosis of neurofibromatosis type 1. Archives of Dermatology, 145(8), 883-887. doi: 10.1001/archdermatol.2009.169

Orion, E., Marcos, B., Davidovici, B., & Wolf, R. (2006). Itch and scratch: Scabies and pediculosis. Clinics in Dermatology, 24(3), 168-175. doi: 10.1016/j.clindermatol.2005.11.001

Ozcan, H., Seyhan, M., & Yologlu, S. (2007). Is metronidazole 0.75% gel effective in the treatment of seborrhoeic dermatitis? A double-blind, placebo controlled study. European Journal of Dermatology, 17(4), 313-316. doi: 10.1684/ejd.2007.0206

Parish, L. C., Jorizzo, J. L., Breton, J. J., Hirman, J. W., Scangarella, N. E., Shawar, R. M., & White, S. M. (2006). Topical retapamulin ointment (1%, wt/wt) twice daily for 5 days versus oral cephalexin twice daily for 10 days in the treatment of secondarily infected dermatitis: Results of a randomized controlled trial. Journal of the American Academy of Dermatology, 55(6), 1003-1013. doi: 10.1016/j.jaad.2006.08.058

Perry, RT, & Halsey, NA. (2004). The clinical significance of measles: A review. Journal of Infectious Diseases, 189 Suppl 1, S4-16. doi: 10.1086/377712

Prevention of varicella: Recommendations of the advisory committee on immunization practices (acip). Centers for disease control and prevention. (1996). MMWR Recomm Rep, 45(RR-11), 1-36.

Quaedvlieg, P. J., Tirsi, E., Thissen, M. R., & Krekels, G. A. (2006). Actinic keratosis: How to differentiate the good from the bad ones? European Journal of Dermatology, 16(4), 335-339.

Richardson, M, Elliman, D, Maguire, H, Simpson, J, & Nicoll, A. (2001). Evidence base of incubation periods, periods of infectiousness and exclusion policies for the control of communicable diseases in schools and preschools. Pediatric Infectious Disease Journal, 20(4), 380-391.

Richter, SS, Heilmann, KP, Beekmann, SE, Miller, NJ, Miller, AL, Rice, CL, . . . Doern, GV. (2005). Macrolide-resistant streptococcus pyogenes in the United States, 2002-2003. Clinical Infectious Diseases, 41(5), 599-608. doi: 10.1086/432473

Rimon, A., Hoffer, V., Prais, D., Harel, L., & Amir, J. (2008). Periorbital cellulitis in the era of haemophilus influenzae type b vaccine: Predisposing factors and etiologic agents in hospitalized children. Journal of Pediatric Ophthalmology and Strabismus, 45(5), 300-304.

Sampathkumar, P., Drage, L. A., & Martin, D. P. (2009). Herpes zoster (shingles) and postherpetic neuralgia. Mayo Clinic Proceedings, 84(3), 274-280. doi: 10.4065/84.3.274

Scheinfeld, N. (2005). Diaper dermatitis: A review and brief survey of eruptions of the diaper area. Amreican Journal of Clinical Dermatology, 6(5), 273-281. doi: 651 [pii]

Severino, M., Bonadonna, P., & Passalacqua, G. (2009). Large local reactions from stinging insects: From epidemiology to management. Curr Opin Allergy Clin Immunol, 9(4), 334-337. doi: 10.1097/ACI.0b013e32832d0668

Shaw, J., & Body, R. (2005). Best evidence topic report. Incision and drainage preferable to oral antibiotics in acute paronychial nail infection? Emergency Medicine Journal, 22(11), 813-814. doi: 10.1136/emj.2005.030163

Shin, HT. (2005). Diaper dermatitis that does not quit. Dermatology Therapy, 18(2), 124-135. doi: DTH05013 [pii] 10.1111/j.1529-8019.2005.05013.x

Strauss, J. S., Krowchuk, D. P., Leyden, J. J., Lucky, A. W., Shalita, A. R., Siegfried, E. C., . . . Bhushan, R. (2007). Guidelines of care for acne vulgaris management. Journal of the American Academy of Dermatology, 56(4), 651-663. doi: 10.1016/j.jaad.2006.08.048

Sugerman, DE, Barskey, AE, Delea, MG, Ortega-Sanchez, IR, Bi, D, Ralston, KJ, . . . Lebaron, CW. (2010). Measles outbreak in a highly vaccinated population, san diego, 2008: Role of the intentionally undervaccinated. Pediatrics, 125(4), 747-755. doi: 10.1542/peds.2009-1653

Tang, M. L., Osborne, N., & Allen, K. (2009). Epidemiology of anaphylaxis. Curr Opin Allergy Clin Immunol, 9(4), 351-356. doi: 10.1097/ACI.0b013e32832db95a

Treatment of lyme disease. (2007). Medical Letter on Drugs and Therapeutics, 49(1263), 49-51.

Venna, S. S., Lee, D., Stadecker, M. J., & Rogers, G. S. (2005). Clinical recognition of actinic keratoses in a high-risk population: How good are we? Archives of Dermatology, 141(4), 507-509. doi: 10.1001/archderm.141.4.507

Vetter, R. S., & Isbister, G. K. (2008). Medical aspects of spider bites. Annual Review of Entomology, 53, 409-429. doi: 10.1146/annurev.ento.53.103106.093503

Wareham, D. W., & Breuer, J. (2007). Herpes zoster. BMJ, 334(7605), 1211-1215. doi: 10.1136/bmj.39206.571042.AE

Weinmann, S, Chun, C, Mullooly, JP, Riedlinger, K, Houston, H, Loparev, VN, . . . Seward, JF. (2008). Laboratory diagnosis and characteristics of breakthrough varicella in children. Journal of Infectious Diseases, 197 Suppl 2, S132-138. doi: 10.1086/522148

Wenner, R., Askari, S. K., Cham, P. M., Kedrowski, D. A., Liu, A., & Warshaw, E. M. (2007). Duct tape for the treatment of common warts in adults: A double-blind randomized controlled trial. Archives of Dermatology, 143(3), 309-313. doi: 10.1001/archderm.143.3.309

Wharton, M. (1996). The epidemiology of varicella-zoster virus infections. Infectious Disease Clinics of North America, 10(3), 571-581.

Yan, A. C. (2006). Current concepts in acne management. Adolescent Medicine Clinic, 17(3), 613-637; abstract x-xi. doi: 10.1016/j.admecli.2006.06.014

3

EAR, NOSE, AND THROAT DISORDERS

Ear, Nose, and Throat Disorders

Hearing Loss 175

Mastoiditis 177

Otitis Externa 178

Otitis Media 180

Vertigo 187

Allergic Rhinitis 190

Common Cold 194

Epistaxis 197

Influenza 198

Sinusitis 202

Epiglottitis 211

Infectious Mononucleosis 212

Peritonsillar Abscess (Quinsy) 214

Pharyngitis/Tonsillitis 215

References *221*

HEARING LOSS

DESCRIPTION

Partial or complete hearing loss. Three types:

- Conductive (CHL): involving the external auditory canal or the middle ear
- Sensorineural (SNHL): involving the inner ear or the 8th cranial nerve
- Components of both conductive and sensorineural

Any sudden hearing loss is a medical emergency. Patient requires ENT referral immediately.

ETIOLOGY

Conductive:

- Anything that can occlude or mechanically block sound from traveling through the external auditory canal or the middle ear

Sensorineural:

- Anything that prevents sound from traveling through the inner ear or prevents the 8th cranial nerve from functioning

Type	Cause
Conductive	Cerumen impaction Tympanic membrane perforation Fluid (serous otitis media) Tympanosclerosis
Sensorineural	Acoustic neuroma Ménière's Disease Ototoxic drugs (ASA, gentamicin) Injury due to noise Viral (especially after mumps) Presbycusis (related to aging)

INCIDENCE

- > 20 times more common in adults than children
- SNHL more common in the elderly

RISK FACTORS

- Chronic allergic conditions-CHL
- Conditions which cause eustachian tube obstruction-CHL
- Heredity-CHL
- Use of ototoxic drugs-SNHL
- Aging (presbycusis)-SNHL
- Exposure to loud noise-SNHL
- Syphilis-SNHL
- Congenital rubella infection-SNHL

ASSESSMENT FINDINGS

- Hard of hearing
- Tinnitus
- Dizziness
- Withdrawal from group discussions and social activities

DIFFERENTIAL DIAGNOSIS

- Conductive hearing loss
- Sensorineural hearing loss
- Conductive and sensorineural hearing losses

DIAGNOSTIC STUDIES

- Audiometry: used to quantify hearing loss
- Tuning fork tests: tuning forks with frequencies of 256, 512, 1024, and 2048 Hz are used
- Whisper test: evaluates patient's gross hearing ability

Presbycusis is the term used to describe hearing loss related to aging.

Weber Test **Confirms result of Rinne and tests for lateralization of sound**	**Rinne Test** **Normal is AC** > BC***	**Results**
Tone heard louder in affected ear	**Tone heard louder in affected ear** **BC > AC**	**Conductive hearing loss (cerumen impaction, otitis media, otosclerosis)**
Tone heard louder in unaffected ear	**AC > BC** **BC = AC**	**Sensorineural hearing loss (inner ear infections, trauma, aging, exposure to loud noise)**

***AC = air conduction* **BC = bone conduction*

PREVENTION

- Avoid loud noise exposure (e.g., guns, loud music, occupational exposure)
- Use of earplugs when exposed to loud noises
- Treat upper respiratory infections and monitor for ear problems
- Minimize exposure to ototoxic medications ("mycin" often associated with ototoxicity)
- Avoid flying or diving if upper respiratory infection is present to prevent rupture of tympanic membrane

NONPHARMACOLOGIC MANAGEMENT

- Removal of cerumen with warm water
- Development of lip reading skills for untreatable forms of hearing loss
- Hearing aid when appropriate

PHARMACOLOGIC MANAGEMENT

- Agents used to soften ear wax if cerumen impaction
- Antibiotics if appropriate to treat otitis media

CONSULTATION/REFERRAL

- ENT for any conductive problem which does not respond after initial treatment
- ENT for any sensorineural hearing loss
- ENT for any sudden hearing loss
- Audiologist for hearing evaluation/hearing aid

FOLLOW-UP

- Depends on etiology, but for conductive hearing loss problems, follow up needed to insure resolution of problem

EXPECTED COURSE

- Sensorineural hearing loss usually unresponsive to treatment
- Conductive hearing losses usually improve with treatment or no progression of loss

POSSIBLE COMPLICATIONS

- Depends on etiology of problem
- Middle ear problems may progress to chronic problems
- Permanent hearing loss from loud noise exposure
- Delayed speech in young children

MASTOIDITIS

DESCRIPTION

A bacterial infection of the mastoid antrum and cells that can be asymptomatic or life-threatening. Usually is a result of untreated or under treated acute otitis media.

ETIOLOGY

- *Streptococcus pneumoniae,* other *Strep sp.*
- Group A β-hemolytic *Streptococcus*
- *H. influenza, M. catarrhalis*
- *S. aureus*
- *Pseudomonas aeruginosa*

RISK FACTORS

- Age < 2 years
- Cholesteatoma (from chronic mastoiditis)
- Recurrent or persistent otitis media
- Immunocompromised state
- Untreated/undertreated otitis media

ASSESSMENT FINDINGS

- Persistent, throbbing otalgia
- Bulging TM (normal in 10% of patients)
- Fever
- Postauricular swelling and tenderness
- Auricular protrusion (pinna displaced laterally and inferiorly)
- Possible creamy, profuse otorrhea since TM perforation often precedes mastoiditis
- Possible hearing loss

Suspect mastoiditis when symptoms of acute otitis media persist beyond 2 weeks even if TM appears normal. Refer immediately to ENT.

DIFFERENTIAL DIAGNOSIS

- Severe otitis externa
- Neoplasm of the mastoid bone
- Parotitis or mumps (swelling is over the parotid vs. preauricular area)
- Cellulitis

DIAGNOSTIC STUDIES

- CBC: demonstrates leukocytosis
- Middle ear aspirate
- Mastoid radiographs: demonstrates clouding of air cells

PREVENTION

- Early treatment of otitis media
- Early identification of cholesteatoma

NONPHARMACOLOGIC MANAGEMENT

- Keep ear dry
- Water precautions
- Myringotomy to drain middle ear (refer)
- Myringotomy

PHARMACOLOGIC MANAGEMENT

- Antibiotics (usually intravenous) on basis of most likely organisms until cultures are known
- Topical antibiotics
- Analgesics for pain
- Antipyretics for fever

CONSULTATION/REFERRAL

- ENT referral for myringotomy, hospitalization, intravenous antibiotic management
- Neurologist or ENT for suspected meningitis

FOLLOW-UP

- Depends on patient condition and age, but weekly follow-up after discharge
- Post-infection follow-up needed with audiograms to assess hearing loss

EXPECTED COURSE

- Depends on severity of infection, but prognosis is good if proper therapy initiated early

POSSIBLE COMPLICATIONS

- Meningitis
- Intracranial abscess
- Facial nerve paralysis

OTITIS EXTERNA
(Swimmer's Ear)

DESCRIPTION

An infection of the external auditory canal producing much inflammation, itching, and/or pain.

ETIOLOGY

Bacterial	Fungal
Pseudomonas (most common pathogen) Staphylococcus Streptococcus	Aspergillus (most common fungal pathogen) Candida albicans

INCIDENCE

- More common in summer months

RISK FACTORS

- Swimming
- Hearing aid use
- Diabetes mellitus
- Hot, humid climates
- Trauma to external canal (cotton swab use, foreign objects)
- Not drying ears after showering or profuse perspiration

ASSESSMENT FINDINGS

- Otalgia/conductive hearing loss
- Edema and redness in the external auditory canal
- Itching in the external auditory canal
- Purulent discharge in external canal
- Tragal and/or pinna pain
- Normal tympanic membrane

DIFFERENTIAL DIAGNOSIS

- Wisdom tooth eruption
- Temporomandibular joint disease
- Tympanic membrane rupture
- Foreign body
- Hearing loss

DIAGNOSTIC STUDIES

- Culture of discharge (usually not necessary)

PREVENTION

- Avoid prolonged ear exposure to warm, humid conditions
- Dry ears after showering and swimming
- Do not place objects in the ear which may cause trauma to the external auditory canal (cotton swab, paper clips, matches, toothpicks)
- Treat ear infections aggressively
- 2% acetic acid (50:50 solution with water) drops after swimming (helps restore acidic pH of ear)
- Treat eczema before it effects the external auditory canal
- Teach methods of prevention

NONPHARMACOLOGIC MANAGEMENT

- Thorough cleansing of the external auditory canal
- Use of cotton ear wick to facilitate passage of medication into an edematous, painful ear canal

CONSULTATION/REFERRAL

- Consider referral to ENT if evidence of systemic involvement (fever)
- Refer to ENT for response to therapy

OTITIS EXTERNA PHARMACOLOGIC MANAGEMENT

Class	Drug Generic name (Trade name®)	Dosage How supplied	Comments
Antibacterial with/ without steroid General comments Installation of cold fluids in the ear can cause dizziness. To minimize dizziness, warm suspension by holding bottle in hand for 1-2 minutes Patients should lie with the affected ear upward to instill drops. Maintain position for 5 minutes to facilitate penetration of drops into canal. A wick may be useful to facilitate entry of the medication in edematous canal. Change once every 24 hours	**ciprofloxacin + hydrocortisone** Cipro HC Otic	**Adult and Children > 1 year**: 3 drops twice daily for 7 days *Soln: 10 mL with dropper*	• Pregnancy Category C • Do not use if the tympanic membrane is perforated or tympanostomy tubes are in place. These drops are not sterile • Contraindicated in viral infections of the external canal
	ciprofloxacin 0.3% and dexamethasone 0.1% Ciprodex Otic	**Adults and Children > 6 months**: 4 drops twice daily for 7 days *Soln: 7.5 mL*	• Pregnancy Category C • This product is sterile and can be used in patients with tympanostomy tubes or patients with otitis externa • Contraindicated in viral infections of the external canal
	Neomycin sulfate 3.5 mg, polymyxin b sulfate 10000 units and hydrocortisone 10 mg/mL Cortisporin	**Adults:** 4 drops 3- 4 times daily *Max*: 10 days **Children 2-16 years:** 3 drops three to four times daily *Max*: 10 days *Soln: 10 mL*	• Pregnancy Category C • Can produce permanent hearing loss due to cochlear damage • **DO NOT USE IN PATIENTS WITH PERFORATED TYMPANIC MEMBRANE** • Neomycin can cause cutaneous sensitization. Monitor for reaction
	ofloxacin solution Floxin Otic	**Adults and Children ≥ 13 years**: 10 drops once daily for 7 days **Children 6 months- 13 years**: 5 drops once daily for 7 days *Soln: 5 mL, 10 mL*	

ENT Disorders

FOLLOW-UP

- Usually none

EXPECTED COURSE

- Improvement in 24-48 hours with treatment
- Resolution in a few days

POSSIBLE COMPLICATIONS

- Cellulitis/chondritis
- Infection at contiguous bone

OTITIS MEDIA

DESCRIPTION

Two types:

- *Acute otitis media* (AOM) is a sudden onset of middle ear effusion and signs or symptoms of local or systemic illness
- *Otitis media with effusion* (OME) is fluid accumulation in the middle ear without evidence of infection; also called a middle ear effusion (MEE)

ETIOLOGY

Acute otitis media:

- Bacteria/viruses

Etiologic Agents
Viruses: 15-44%
***Streptococcus pneumoniae*: 20-35%**
***H. influenzae*: 20-30%**
***Moraxella catarrhalis*: 15%**
Group A β-hemolytic *Streptococcus*: 15%
***S. aureus*: 12%**

Otitis media with effusion:

- Probably due to incomplete resolution of AOM or eustachian tube obstruction

INCIDENCE

- More common in winter months
- Most common in 6 months to 3 years
- Lowest incidence in breast fed babies

RISK FACTORS

- Daycare attendance
- Craniofacial abnormalities
- Upper respiratory infection
- Allergic rhinitis
- Second hand cigarette smoke
- First episode of AOM <12 months old
- Bottle feeding while in supine position

ASSESSMENT FINDINGS

Acute otitis media:

- Ear pain and irritability
- Decreased tympanic membrane (TM) mobility (observed using pneumatic otoscopy)
- Distorted landmarks
- Displaced light reflex
- Dull, opaque TM
- Possible bulging TM
- Fever
- GI symptoms (nausea, vomiting)
- Diminished hearing
- Pulling on ear
- Dizziness

Otitis media with effusion:

- Usually asymptomatic
- Dull TM
- Decreased mobility
- Visible air-fluid interface
- Visible air bubbles
- Diminished hearing

A diagnosis of acute otitis media requires a history of acute onset of signs and symptoms, presence of middle ear effusion, and signs and symptoms of middle ear inflammation.

DIFFERENTIAL DIAGNOSIS

- Otitis externa may present like AOM with TM rupture
- Tumors (cholesteatoma)
- Referred pain from jaw or teeth

Crying may cause the TM to appear red on examination.

DIAGNOSTIC STUDIES

- Pneumatic otoscopy
- Tympanometry to measure TM compliance
- Consider referral for tympanocentesis to obtain culture (rarely performed)

PREVENTION

- Breastfeeding
- Avoid cigarette smoke exposure
- Do not put baby to sleep in horizontal position with bottle

- Antibiotic prophylaxis for recurrent AOM (controversial)

NONPHARMACOLOGIC MANAGEMENT

- Local heat
- Myringotomy
- Swallowing to help the eustachian tube ventilate
- Patient and family education regarding treatment, disease, comfort measures, etc.

PHARMACOLOGIC MANAGEMENT

Antibiotics do NOT relieve pain in the first 24 hours!

- Analgesics (i.e., acetaminophen, ibuprofen, otalgic drops) - Antipyrine/benzocaine (Auralgan® Otic); Adult/child: 2-4 drops every 1-2 hours prn pain, Solution: 14 mL

OTITIS MEDIA PHARMACOLOGIC MANAGEMENT

American Academy of Pediatrics encourages symptomatic treatment (without antibiotics) initially if the diagnosis of otitis media is uncertain (or there is mild disease) and the child is > 6 months old. If antibiotics are used, the initial antibacterial agent for most children is amoxicillin (for children who are not penicillin allergic). The starting dosage of amoxicillin is recommended at 80-90 mg/kg/day in divided doses. This exceeds the FDA approved dosage for otitis media. There are no antibiotics with specific approval for use in adults for otitis media. It seems reasonable to use the same antibiotics for adults that are used for children. These have been incorporated into this table.

Class	Drug Generic name (Trade name®)	Dosage How supplied	Comments
Oral Antibiotics **Penicillin** *Inhibits cell wall synthesis of Gram positive bacteria (Staph, Strep) and are most effective against organisms with rapidly dividing cell walls* General comments Indicated for infections caused by penicillinase-sensitive microorganisms Generally well tolerated; watch for hypersensitivity reactions Clavulanate broadens spectrum of coverage Consider amoxicillin/ clavulanate if failure after 48-72 hrs. Give in divided doses	**amoxicillin** Amoxil	**Adult**: *Usual:* 875 mg every 12 hours for 5-7 days *Alternate:* 1000-2000 mg every 12 hours for 5-7 days **Children 2 months to 12 years:** *Usual:* 80-90 mg/kg/day in divided doses; max dose should not exceed adult dose *Alternative:* 45 mg/kg/d in divided doses *Alternative:* < 3 months: 30 mg/kg/day in divided doses *Capsules: 250 mg 500 mg* *Tabs: 500 mg, 875 mg* *Suspension: 250 mg/5 mL; 400 mg/5 mL* *Pediatric drops: 50 mg/mL*	• Pregnancy Category B • Amoxicillin is not stable in the presence of beta lactamase producing organisms • Considered first line agent in most cases unless patient has had antibiotic exposure in the last 90 days
	amoxicillin/clavulanate	**Adult**: *Usual*: One 875 mg tablet every 12 hours for 10 days *Alternate*: One 500 mg tablet every 12 hours for 10 days *Alternate*: Two 1000 mg tablets every 12 hours for 10 days	• Pregnancy Category B • Use first line if patient has severe illness, has had antibiotic exposure in the last 90 days • Two 500 mg amoxicillin/ clavulanic acid tablets are NOT equivalent to one 1000 mg amoxicillin/clavulanic acid tablet

continued

ENT Disorders

OTITIS MEDIA PHARMACOLOGIC MANAGEMENT

American Academy of Pediatrics encourages symptomatic treatment (without antibiotics) initially if the diagnosis of otitis media is uncertain (or there is mild disease) and the child is > 6 months old. If antibiotics are used, the initial antibacterial agent for most children is amoxicillin (for children who are not penicillin allergic). The starting dosage of amoxicillin is recommended at 80-90 mg/kg/day in divided doses. This exceeds the FDA approved dosage for otitis media. There are no antibiotics with specific approval for use in adults for otitis media. It seems reasonable to use the same antibiotics for adults that are used for children. These have been incorporated into this table.

Class	Drug Generic name (Trade name®)	Dosage How supplied	Comments
	Augmentin XR Augmentin ES Various generics	*Tabs: XR 1000 mg amoxicillin, 62.5 mg clavulanic acid;* *Also: 250 mg, 500 mg, 875 mg* *Chew tab: amoxicillin 125 mg, Clavulanic acid 31.25 mg* *Suspension: (based on amoxil dose) 125 mg/5 mL, 200 mg/5 mL, 250 mg/5 mL, 400 mg/5 mL*	• Do not substitute Augmentin 200mg/5 mL and 400 mg/5 mL suspensions for Augmentin ES-600. These are NOT interchangeable • Children: Base dose on amoxicillin component
Second generation Cephalosporins *Not stable in the presence of beta lactamase producers*	**cefuroxime**	**Adult**: 250-500 mg twice daily **Children**: 250 mg twice daily for 10 days	• **DO NOT USE IN PATIENTS WHO HAD HIVES OR ANAPHYLAXIS TO PENICILLIN** • Consider ceftriaxone (Rocephin®) if failure after 48-72 hours
	Ceftin	*Tab: 250 mg, 500 mg* *Suspension: 125 mg/5 mL; 250 mg/5 mL*	
Third generation Cephalosporins *Inhibit cell wall synthesis* *Stable in the presence of beta lactamase producers*	**cefpodoxime**	**Adult**: 200-400 mg every 12hr for 7-10 days **Children 2 mo-12 yr:** 5 mg/kg every 12 hr for 5-10 days *Max*: 400 mg/dose	• **DO NOT USE IN PATIENTS WHO HAD HIVES OR ANAPHYLAXIS TO PENICILLIN** • Consider ceftriaxone (Rocephin®) if failure after 48-72 hours
	Vantin	*Tabs: 100 mg and 200 mg* *Suspension: 50 mg/5 mL; 100 mg/5 mL*	
	cefdinir	**Adult**: 300 mg every 12 h for 10 days **Children**: **6 mo-12 yr**: 7 mg/kg every 12 hr or 14 mg/kg daily for 10 days *Max*: 300 mg/dose	

continued

OTITIS MEDIA PHARMACOLOGIC MANAGEMENT

American Academy of Pediatrics encourages symptomatic treatment (without antibiotics) initially if the diagnosis of otitis media is uncertain (or there is mild disease) and the child is > 6 months old. If antibiotics are used, the initial antibacterial agent for most children is amoxicillin (for children who are not penicillin allergic). The starting dosage of amoxicillin is recommended at 80-90 mg/kg/day in divided doses. This exceeds the FDA approved dosage for otitis media. There are no antibiotics with specific approval for use in adults for otitis media. It seems reasonable to use the same antibiotics for adults that are used for children. These have been incorporated into this table.

Class	Drug Generic name (Trade name®)	Dosage How supplied	Comments
	Omnicef	*Tabs: 300 mg* *Suspension: 125 mg/5 mL; 250 mg/5 mL*	
	ceftriaxone	**Children**: 50 mg/kg/day given IM *Max*: should not exceed 1000 mg/dose	• DO NOT USE IN PATIENTS WHO HAD HIVES OR ANAPHYLAXIS TO PENICILLIN • Given for children with AOM unresponsive to initial or second antibacterial therapy • 3 day course has higher efficacy than 1 day-regimen
	Rocephin	*250 mg, 500 mg, 1 g vials*	
Extended Spectrum Macrolides *Inhibit protein synthesis by binding to the 50S ribosomal subunit* <u>**General comments**</u> Contraindicated in a ketolide or related allergy	**azithromycin**	**Adults**: 500 mg daily for 3 days **Children**: 6 mo: 30 mg/kg as single dose *Max*: 1.5 grams *Alternative*: 10 mg/kg daily for 3 days, Max: 500 mg daily *Alternative*: 10 mg/kg on day one, followed by 4 days of 5 mg/kg *Max*: Day 1: 500 mg; *Max*: Day 2-5: 250 mg	• First line for penicillin allergic (Type I allergic reaction) • Consider clindamycin, if failure after 48-72 hours • Avoid concomitant use of aluminum or magnesium containing antacids • Cautious use if renal or hepatic impairment • Hypersensitivity reactions may recur after initial successful symptomatic treatment
	Zithromax	*Tabs: 250 mg, 500 mg* *Suspension: 100 mg/5 mL, 200 mg/5 mL*	
	clarithromycin	**Adults**: 250-500 mg every 12 hr for 7-14 days **Children > 6 mo:** 7.5 mg/kg every 12 hours *Max*: 500 mg/dose	
	Biaxin	*Tab: 250 mg, 500 mg* *Suspension: 125 mg/5 mL; 250 mg/5 mL*	

continued

OTITIS MEDIA PHARMACOLOGIC MANAGEMENT

American Academy of Pediatrics encourages symptomatic treatment (without antibiotics) initially if the diagnosis of otitis media is uncertain (or there is mild disease) and the child is > 6 months old. If antibiotics are used, the initial antibacterial agent for most children is amoxicillin (for children who are not penicillin allergic). The starting dosage of amoxicillin is recommended at 80-90 mg/kg/day in divided doses. This exceeds the FDA approved dosage for otitis media. There are no antibiotics with specific approval for use in adults for otitis media. It seems reasonable to use the same antibiotics for adults that are used for children. These have been incorporated into this table.

Class	Drug Generic name (Trade name®)	Dosage How supplied	Comments
Lincosamide *For use in serious susceptible infections where less toxic antibiotics are not effective or appropriate*	**clindamycin**	**Adult**: 150-300 mg every 6 hours for 5-10 days More serious infection: 300-450 mg every 6 hours for 5-10 days **Children**: 8-16 mg/kg/day in divided doses for 5-10 days *Max:* should not exceed adult dose *More serious infection*: 16-20 mg/kg/day in divided doses for 5-10 days *Max*: should not exceed adult dose	• Only use if other antibiotics have been unsuccessful • Use in patients with initial bacterial failure who are penicillin/cephalosporin allergic with Type I reaction; consider use in patients who failed therapy with ceftriaxone (used in conjunction with tympanocentesis) • Cautious use in patients with hepatic, renal impairments, colitis • Side effects include pseudo-membranous colitis, diarrhea • Take with a full glass of water
	Cleocin	*Caps: 75 mg, 150 mg, 300 mg* *Granules: 100 mL*	
Antibiotic Otic Drops with/ without Steroid *These are indicated for patients with acute otitis media with tympanoplasty tubes only!*	**ciprofloxacin 0.3% / dexamethasone 0.1%**	**Adult**: 4 drops twice daily for 7 days **Children > 6 months:** 4 drops twice daily for 7 days	• Ear discomfort and pain is common after instillation of drops
	Ciprodex Otic	*Susp: 7.5 mL*	
	ofloxacin 0.3%	**Adult**: 5 drops in affected ear twice daily for 10 days **Children 1-12 yrs**: 5 drops in affected ear twice daily for 10 days	• Watch for dizziness after instillation, ear ache, taste perversion
	Floxin Otic	*Soln: 5 mL, 10 mL bottles*	
Antipyretics/Pain Relief	**acetaminophen**	**Adult**: 1000 mg every 4-6 hr *Max*: 4 grams/day **Children**: Pounds — Mg dosage 5-8 — 40 mg 9-10 — 60 mg 11-16 — 80 mg 17-21 — 120 mg	• Acetaminophen takes about 45-60 minutes to begin pain relief • Contraindicated in children or adults with hepatitis • **CAUTIOUS USE with any OTC multi-symptom reliever. Do not use if acetaminophen present in multi-symptom product**

continued

OTITIS MEDIA PHARMACOLOGIC MANAGEMENT

American Academy of Pediatrics encourages symptomatic treatment (without antibiotics) initially if the diagnosis of otitis media is uncertain (or there is mild disease) and the child is > 6 months old. If antibiotics are used, the initial antibacterial agent for most children is amoxicillin (for children who are not penicillin allergic). The starting dosage of amoxicillin is recommended at 80-90 mg/kg/day in divided doses. This exceeds the FDA approved dosage for otitis media. There are no antibiotics with specific approval for use in adults for otitis media. It seems reasonable to use the same antibiotics for adults that are used for children. These have been incorporated into this table.

Class	Drug Generic name (Trade name®)	Dosage How supplied	Comments
		Pounds / Mg dosage 22-26: 160 mg 27-32: 200 mg 33-37: 240 mg 38-42: 280 mg 43-53: 320 mg 54-64: 400 mg 65-75: 480 mg 76-86: 560 mg 87-95: 640 mg > 95: give adult dose *Susp: (160 mg/5 mL) preferred for 24-95 pounds* ***CAUTION - Adult suspension available: 500 mg/15 mL***	• Weight based dosing preferred over age based dosing • Infant drops (80 mg/0.8 mL) preferred for 6-23 pounds
	Tylenol Various generic products available	*Tabs: 325 mg, 500 mg scored* *Pediatric forms: Pediatric drops: 80 mg/0.8 mL* *Liquid: 160 mg/5 mL* *Chew tabs: 80 mg* *Jr. Chew tabs: 160 mg* *Adult susp: 500 mg/15 mL*	
	Feverall Suppositories	*Suppositories: 80 mg, 120 mg, 325 mg*	
	ibuprofen	**Adult**: 200-400 mg every 4-6 hr for pain; *Max*: 2400 mg daily **Children < 6 months:** not recommended Over 6 months: Fever < 102.5°F (39.2°C): 5 mg/kg every 6-8 h Fever > 102.5°F (39.2°C): 10 mg/kg every 6-8 hr *Max*: 40 mg/kg/day - do not exceed adult dose	• Ibuprofen takes about 30 minutes to provide pain relief • Contraindicated in children or adults with gastritis or gastric ulcers • Caution with aspirin allergy • Avoid aspirin, anticoagulants; may increase risk of bleeding • Caution advised with hepatic or renal impairment

continued

ENT Disorders

OTITIS MEDIA PHARMACOLOGIC MANAGEMENT

American Academy of Pediatrics encourages symptomatic treatment (without antibiotics) initially if the diagnosis of otitis media is uncertain (or there is mild disease) and the child is > 6 months old. If antibiotics are used, the initial antibacterial agent for most children is amoxicillin (for children who are not penicillin allergic). The starting dosage of amoxicillin is recommended at 80-90 mg/kg/day in divided doses. This exceeds the FDA approved dosage for otitis media. There are no antibiotics with specific approval for use in adults for otitis media. It seems reasonable to use the same antibiotics for adults that are used for children. These have been incorporated into this table.

Class	Drug Generic name (Trade name®)	Dosage How supplied	Comments
	Advil	Ibuprofen dose by: Weight (pounds) – Dose 9-10 – 25 mg 11-16 – 50 mg 17-21 – 75 mg 22-26 – 100 mg 27-32 – 125 mg 33-37 – 150 mg 38-42 – 175 mg 43-53 – 200 mg 54-64 – 250 mg 65-75 – 300 mg 76-86 – 350 mg 87-95 – 400 mg > 95 – give adult dose	• **Never exceed adult dose in children**

ENT Disorders

CONSULTATION/REFERRAL

- ENT referral for recurrent (3 occurrences in 6 months or 4 in one year)
- ENT consultation for headache (may signal meningitis, epidural abscess)
- ENT referral for mastoiditis
- Refer if language delay detected
- Refer/consult for neonates

FOLLOW-UP

- Recheck ears in 4 weeks and follow until resolution or referral
- Re-evaluate sooner if symptoms persist

EXPECTED COURSE

- Improvement in 48-72 hours
- At 4 weeks approximately 50% will still have middle ear effusion (MEE)
- At 3 months about 10% will still have MEE

POSSIBLE COMPLICATIONS

- Tympanic membrane perforation
- Conductive and/or sensorineural hearing loss
- Acute mastoiditis
- Meningitis
- Epidural abscess
- Language delay from hearing loss

VERTIGO
(Dizziness)

DESCRIPTION

The sensation or impression that an individual is moving, or that objects around him are moving, when actually no movement is occurring.

ETIOLOGY

- A disturbance in the equilibratory apparatus with either peripheral or central causes

Peripheral Etiologies:

- Otogenic
  - ◊ Ménière's disease
  - ◊ Myringitis
  - ◊ Infections of inner ear
  - ◊ Otitis media
  - ◊ Acute labyrinthitis
  - ◊ Obstructed eustachian tubes
  - ◊ Benign positional vertigo
- Toxic
  - ◊ Excessive alcohol ingestion
  - ◊ Salicylates
  - ◊ Potent diuretics
  - ◊ Ototoxic drugs (especially aminoglycosides)
- Environmental
- Motion sickness
- Neurological
- 8th cranial nerve tumors (acoustic neuroma)

Central Etiologies:

- Circulatory
  - ◊ Transient ischemic attacks (TIA)
  - ◊ Postural hypotension
- Neurologic
  - ◊ Multiple sclerosis
  - ◊ Temporal lobe seizures
  - ◊ Cervical vertebra disorders
  - ◊ Syphilis
- Other
  - ◊ Hypothyroidism
  - ◊ Psychiatric illness

More than 90% of patients with vertigo have peripheral causes. Elderly patients are more likely to have central etiologies.

INCIDENCE

- Unknown
- Usually in 20-60 year olds

RISK FACTORS

- History of migraines
- Risk factors for cardiovascular disease
- Anxiety/depression/stress

Assess risk factors for migraines, cardiovascular disease, exposure to toxins.

ASSESSMENT FINDINGS

All findings listed below are possible depending on the etiology:

- Asymptomatic except vertigo
- Nystagmus when extraocular movements are tested (peripheral or central)
- Tinnitus (peripheral or central)
- Hearing loss, (peripheral) ear pain
- Paroxysmal, episodic attacks of vertigo (peripheral)
- Carotid bruit (central)
- Persistent vertigo (central)
- Headache, diplopia, slurred speech (central)
- Hypotension (central)

ASSESSMENT FINDINGS IN MOST COMMON CAUSES OF VERTIGO

Benign positional vertigo:

- Vertigo
- Nystagmus with shifts in head position
- No hearing loss or tinnitus
- Nausea, vomiting

Vestibulopathy:

- Vertigo with position changes
- No hearing loss
- No tinnitus
- Nausea, vomiting
- Often follows gastrointestinal or upper respiratory infections

Ménière's Disease:

- Sudden vertigo
- Tinnitus
- Hearing loss
- Ear fullness
- Nausea
- Vomiting

DIFFERENTIAL DIAGNOSIS

- Vestibular disease
- Acoustic neuroma, other tumors
- Cardiac and vascular pathologies; cerebral ischemia
- Sensory deficits
- Psychiatric illnesses
- Metabolic disorders: diabetes mellitus
- Syphilis

DIAGNOSTIC STUDIES

- Neuro exam: test cerebellar function, assess cranial nerves (especially CN VIII), presence of nystagmus
- Hearing: Audiometry to discern hearing loss, Rinne and Weber tests
- Labs: hematocrit/hemoglobin to rule out anemia, TSH, syphilis serology
- Consider fasting blood sugar levels to rule out diabetes and hypoglycemia
- CV: Blood pressure checks in 3 positions to rule out hypotension
- Auditory Brainstem Response to rule out acoustic neuroma
- Consider CT/MRI to rule out central lesions
- Consider in selected patients the Nylen-Barany maneuver or Hallpike maneuver
- Electronystagmography (ENG) to help differentiate central and peripheral lesions

PREVENTION

- Teach safety measures to patients who have vertigo

NONPHARMACOLOGIC MANAGEMENT

- Depends on etiology
- Rest in bed with eyes closed during acute attack
- Handrails at home for chronic multisensory deficits
- Good lighting
- Use of a cane or walker

PHARMACOLOGIC MANAGEMENT

- Depends on etiology
- Antihistamines: meclizine (Antivert®), promethazine (Phenergan®), dimenhydrinate (Dramamine®), transdermal scopolamine

VERTIGO PHARMACOLOGIC MANAGEMENT

Class	Drug Generic name (Trade name®)	Dosage How supplied	Comments
Antihistamines *Mechanism of action not known but possibly has depressant action on hyperstimulated labyrinthine action*	**dimenhydrinate**	**Adults and > 12 years:** Take 1 or 2 tabs every 4-6 hours *Max*: 8 tabs/24 hours **Children 6-12 years**: Give ½ to 1 tab every 6-8 hours *Max*: 3 tablets/24 hours **Children 2 to < 6 years**: Give ½ tab every 6-8 hours *Max*: 1.5 tablets/24 hours	• Pregnancy Category B • May cause drowsiness. Caution against using during activities requiring mental alertness • Avoid CNS depressants while taking • Cautious use in patients with asthma, glaucoma, or BPH
	Dramamine	*Tabs: 50 mg* *Chewtabs: 50 mg* *Capsules: 50 mg* *Liquid: 12.5 mg/4 mL; 12.5 mg/5 mL*	
	meclizine	**Adults and > 12 years:** 25-100 mg daily in divided dosage	• Pregnancy Category B • May cause drowsiness. Caution against using during activities requiring mental alertness • Avoid CNS depressants while taking • Cautious use in patients with asthma, glaucoma, or BPH • Classified as "possibly effective"
	Antivert	*Tabs: 12.5 mg, 25 mg, 50 mg*	

ENT Disorders

CONSULTATION/REFERRAL

- Refer if any neurological symptoms exist
- Refer any problems that are disabling and/or progressive
- Refer to ENT for other or unknown etiologies

FOLLOW-UP

- Dependent on etiology

EXPECTED COURSE

- Dependent on etiology, but generally, peripheral causes have better prognosis than central causes

ALLERGIC RHINITIS

DESCRIPTION

Inflammation of the mucous membranes of the nasal tract with subsequent mucosal edema, clear discharge, sneezing, and nasal stuffiness

ETIOLOGY

- Any substance or condition which causes an IgE mediated response characterized by rupture of mast cells and release of histamines, leukotrienes, prostaglandins, and other substances
- Most common seasonal allergens are pollens from grass, trees, and weeds
- Most common perennial allergens are mold, animal dander, dust mites

INCIDENCE

- Up to 20% of children
- Up to 30% of adolescents
- Usually diminishes with age
- Most common age of onset is 10-20 years

RISK FACTORS

- Family history
- Other atopic diseases (e.g., asthma, atopic dermatitis, allergic conjunctivitis, food allergy)
- Repeated exposure to the allergic substance
- Noncompliance with treatment

ASSESSMENT FINDINGS

- "*Allergic shiners*": dark discolored areas beneath the lower eyelids as a result of impeded lymphatic and venous drainage
- Conjunctival injection
- Pale, boggy turbinates with clear nasal secretions
- "*Allergic salute*": transverse crease on tip of nose due to long-term wiping of nose in an upward direction
- Mouth breathing
- Palpable lymph nodes
- Enlarged tonsils and adenoids

DIFFERENTIAL DIAGNOSIS

- Vasomotor rhinitis
- Rhinitis medicamentosa
- Infection
- Tumors
- Nasal foreign body

DIAGNOSTIC STUDIES

- CBC: eosinophilia if acute reaction
- Consider cultures if infection is suspected
- Allergy testing: antihistamines will suppress reaction to skin allergy testing
- Sinus films if indicated; CT scan
- Diagnostic allergen prick tests
- RAST (Radioallergosorbent test): used in patients in whom a severe reaction is possible

PREVENTION

- Minimize continuous exposure to commonly known allergens
- Remove offending allergens/avoid exposure
- Adherence to pharmacological regimen
- **Avoidance of allergen is first line of treatment**

NONPHARMACOLOGIC MANAGEMENT

- Avoidance/elimination of offending allergen (e.g., frequent vacuuming, dusting, remove feather pillows from bedroom, change air conditioner filter frequently, removal of house plants, pet control, removal carpentry, stuffed animals)
- Surgical removal of polyps
- Surgical reduction of turbinates to relieve obstruction

PHARMACOLOGIC MANAGEMENT

- Saline nasal spray helps to "wash" offending particles which are trapped in airways
- Antihistamines (nonsedating and sedating available)
- Nasal steroids (preferred agent for most cases)
- Systemic steroids (avoid if possible & use only short-term)
- Topical cromolyn (mast cell stabilizer)
- Decongestants, oral or topical

ALLERGIC RHINITIS PHARMACOLOGIC MANAGEMENT

Class	Drug Generic name (Trade name®)	Dosage How supplied	Comments
Antihistamines - First Generation **General comments** Avoid simultaneous use of CNS depressants Care when driving or engaging in activities that require attention Most available over the counter This product has not been reviewed and approved by the FDA	**diphenhydramine**	**Adult**: 25-50 mg every 4-6 hr; *Max*: 300 mg/day **Children < 6 yrs:** individualize **6-12 yrs:** 12.5-25 mg every 4-6 hr *Max*: 150 mg/day	• Pregnancy Category B • Cautious use in patients with glaucoma, difficulty urinating due to an enlarged prostate gland, COPD • Avoid alcohol within 6 hours of taking • May cause profound drowsiness in some patients
	Benadryl	*Chew tabs: 12.5 mg* *Tabs: 25 mg* *Liquid: 12.5 mg/5 mL* *Injection: 50 mg/mL*	
	hydroxyzine	**Adults**: 25 mg 3-4 times a day **Children < 6 yrs:** 50 mg daily in divided doses **> 6 yrs:** 50-100 mg daily in divided doses	• Pregnancy Category C • Unable to establish safety during pregnancy • May produce drowsiness in any dose. Appropriate care advised • If used in geriatric patients, should administer a low dose and monitor carefully
	Atarax Vistaril	*Caps: 25 mg, 50 mg* *Suspension: 25 mg/5 mL; available in 4 oz.; 1 pt.*	
Antihistamine Second Generation **General comments** Does not typically produce drowsiness (except cetirizine) and usually dosed once daily	**cetirizine**	**Adults and Children ≥ 12 years:** 5-10 mg daily **Children 6-11 years**: 5-10 mg based on symptom relief 2-5 yrs: 2.5 mg daily or twice daily	• Pregnancy Category B • Caution regarding activities requiring mental alertness, produces drowsiness because of its affinity for H1 receptors • Dosage adjustment needed for ages 77 and older, renal and hepatic impairment • Take without regard to food • Consider taking in the evening
	Zyrtec	*Tabs: 10 mg;* *Chew tabs: 5 mg; 10 mg* *Syrup: 1 mg/mL; 4 oz. bottle*	
	levocetirizine	**Adult and children ≥ 12 years:** 5 mg once daily in the evening **Children 6-11 yrs:** 2.5 mg once daily in the evening **Children 6 months - 5 yrs:** 1.25 mg once daily in the evening	• Pregnancy Category B • Adjust dose for renal impairment; contraindicated in children 6 months to 11 years with renal impairment • Avoid engaging in activities requiring mental alertness • Avoid concurrent use alcohol or CNS depressants
	Xyzal	*Tabs: 5 mg scored;* *Oral solution: 0.5 mg/mL*	

continued

ALLERGIC RHINITIS PHARMACOLOGIC MANAGEMENT

Class	Drug Generic name (Trade name®)	Dosage How supplied	Comments
	fexofenadine	**Adult and Children ≥ 12 years**: 180 mg daily or 60 mg twice daily **Children 2-11 years**: 30 mg twice daily	• Pregnancy Category C • Shake bottle well before use • Reduce dose for renal impairment • Allegra ODT contains phenylalanine (other Allegra products do not) • Avoid aluminum and magnesium containing antacids • Less effective if taken with fruit juices; therefore, take with water • Do not expect sedation
	Allegra	*Tabs: 30 mg, 60 mg, 180 mg* *ODT tab: 30 mg* *Susp: 6 mg/mL*	
	loratadine	**Adult and Children** ≥ 6 yrs: 10 mg daily **Children 2-5 yrs**: 5 mg once daily	• Pregnancy Category B • Children use chew tabs or syrup • Adjustment needed for renal or hepatic impairment • Do not expect sedation
	Claritin	*Chew Tabs: 5 mg* *Redi Tabs: 10 mg* *Syrup: 1 mg/mL*	
	desloratadine	**Adults**: 5 mg daily **Children 6 mo-11 mo:** 1 mg (2 mL) daily 1-5 yr: 1.25 mg (2.5 mL) daily 6-11 yr: 2.5 mg (5 mL) daily	• Pregnancy Category C • Children use RediTabs or syrup • Do not expect sedation
	Clarinex	*Tabs: 5 mg* *Redi Tabs: 2.5 mg* *Syrup: 0.5 mg/mL*	
Topical nasal steroids *Exert glucocorticoid activity on the nasal mucosa and thus have local anti-inflammatory effects* General comments Indicated for perennial, seasonal allergic rhinitis Improvement of symptoms usually attended by 2 weeks but most derive benefit after a few days.	**budesonide** Rhinocort AQ	**Adult**: *Starting dose*: 1 spray (32 mcg) per nostril daily *Usual*: 2-4 sprays per nostril daily *Max*: 4 sprays per nostril daily **Children 6-12 years:** Initial: 1 spray per nostril daily Usual: 1-2 sprays per nostril daily Max: 2 sprays per nostril daily *8.6 grams (120 metered sprays)*	• Pregnancy Category C • Gently shake container and pump prior to use • Individualize dosage for symptoms • Even though there is minimal systemic absorption of intranasal steroids, possible growth retardation when used in pediatric patients • Rare risk of glaucoma, increased intraocular pressure, cataracts can occur • Avoid exposure to chicken pox or measles

continued

ALLERGIC RHINITIS PHARMACOLOGIC MANAGEMENT

Class	Drug Generic name (Trade name®)	Dosage How supplied	Comments
Discontinue if no improvement in symptoms after 3 weeks Use lowest dose possible, especially in children since there is risk of systemic effects Epistaxis may occur with any if mucous membranes become dried or injured from use	**fluticasone** Flonase	**Adult**: 2 sprays (50 mcg/ spray) each nostril daily or 1 spray per nostril 2 times daily **Children > 4 years:** *Initial*: 1 spray each nostril daily *Max*: 2 sprays each nostril daily *16 gram container, 120 sprays*	• Pregnancy Category C • Individualize dosage for symptoms • Even though there is minimal systemic absorption of intranasal steroids, possible growth retardation when used in pediatric patients • Rare risk of glaucoma, increased intraocular pressure, cataracts can occur • Avoid exposure to chicken pox or measles • Improvement in symptoms may occur as soon as 12 hours but may not be achieved for several days
	mometasone Nasonex	**Adult and ≥ 12 years**: 2 sprays (50 mcg/spray) each nostril daily **Children**: **2-11 yr**: 1 spray per nostril daily *17 gram, 120 sprays*	• Pregnancy Category C • Individualize dosage for symptoms • Even though there is minimal systemic absorption of intranasal steroids, possible growth retardation when used in pediatric patients • Rare risk of glaucoma, increased intraocular pressure, cataracts can occur • Avoid exposure to chicken pox or measles • No change in dosage required for geriatric patient
	triamcinolone Nasacort	**Adult**: 2 sprays (55 mcg/ spray) per nostril daily **Children**: **6-12 yr**: *Initial*:1 spray each nostril/day *Max*: 2 sprays each nostril once daily *16.5 gram, 120 sprays*	• Pregnancy Category C • Individualize dosage for symptoms • Even though there is minimal systemic absorption of intranasal steroids, possible growth retardation when used in pediatric patients • Rare risk of glaucoma, increased intraocular pressure, cataracts can occur • Avoid exposure to chicken pox or measles • Shake well before each use • Improvement in symptoms may occur as soon as 12 hours but may not be achieved for several days

CONSULTATION/REFERRAL

- Allergist for testing when persistent symptoms occur despite treatment
- ENT for sinus related etiologies
- Emergency department for severe allergic response to allergens

FOLLOW-UP

- 2-4 weeks after initial evaluation and then every 3-6 months depending on patient and severity of symptoms

EXPECTED COURSE

- Allergies tend to diminish in severity as individuals age
- Allergic response is heightened each time allergen is contacted

POSSIBLE COMPLICATIONS

- Otitis media
- Secondary infections of sinuses, tonsils, pharynx
- Sinusitis
- Epistaxis
- Facial changes (e.g., allergic salute, allergic shiners)

COMMON COLD

(Rhinosinusitis, Nasopharyngitis, Upper Respiratory Illness)

DESCRIPTION

An infection of the upper respiratory tract caused by a virus. The symptoms may last for 3-10 days and are usually self-limiting.

ETIOLOGY

- Rhinoviruses are the most common cause
- Influenza viruses
- Parainfluenza viruses
- Adenoviruses
- Coronaviruses

INCIDENCE

- Adolescents/Adults: 2-4 annually
- School Children: 7 annually
- Kindergarten: 12 annually

RISK FACTORS

- Exposure to infected individuals
- Psychological stress
- Touching of contaminated surfaces and subsequent touching of nose or conjunctiva (portal of entry)

ASSESSMENT FINDINGS

- Most common symptoms reported: Nasal stuffiness, sneezing, scratchy, irritated throat/hoarseness
- Red/irritated nasal mucosa with mucus discharge
- Malaise, headache
- Cough
- Occasionally fever

DIFFERENTIAL DIAGNOSIS

- Allergic rhinitis
- Influenza
- Sinusitis
- Mumps
- Rubeola

DIAGNOSTIC STUDIES

- Usually none indicated
- CBC if symptoms persist: elevated WBC indicates bacterial infection
- Culture of nasal washings (usually not helpful)

If CBC indicates bacterial infection, consider differential diagnoses.

PREVENTION

- Good hand washing
- Avoid exposure to infected individuals
- Adequate rest
- Stress management
- Zinc lozenges (thought to prevent viral replication) and vitamin C have failed to demonstrate clinical efficacy in preventing common cold

Use of intra-nasal zinc products may produce loss of smell transiently or permanently.

NONPHARMACOLOGIC MANAGEMENT

- Increased rest
- Fluids
- Humidify inspired air
- Discontinue tobacco products
- Hard candy or lozenges for scratchy throat
- Saline nose drops and bulb syringe for infants
- Avoid tobacco products and alcohol
- Teach patients that hand washing is the single most effective preventive measure

PHARMACOLOGIC MANAGEMENT

All products are used for symptom relief.
Antihistamines are used to dry nasal secretions.
Topical decongestants (sympathomimetics) reduce edema in nasal passages, promote drainage, and are available over the counter.
Examples: Oxymetazoline (Afrin®, Duration®) and Phenylephrine (Neosynephrine®)

COMMON COLD PHARMACOLOGIC MANAGEMENT

Many over the counter products are available as single agents and combinations of antihistamines and decongestants. None speed resolution of infection but may help alleviate symptoms.

Class	Drug Generic name (Trade name®)	Dosage How supplied	Comments
Antihistamines - First Generation General comments Avoid simultaneous use of CNS depressants Care when driving or engaging in activities that require attention Most available over the counter	**diphenhydramine** Benadryl Various generics	**Adult**: 25-50 mg every 4-6 hr; *Max*: 300 mg/day **Children < 6 yrs**: individualize **6-12 yrs**: 12.5-25 mg every 4-6 hr *Max*: 150 mg/day *Chew tabs: 12.5 mg* *Tabs: 25 mg* *Liquid: 12.5 mg/5 mL* *Injection: 50 mg/mL*	• Pregnancy Category B • Cautious use in patients with glaucoma, difficulty urinating due to an enlarged prostate gland, COPD • Avoid alcohol within 6 hours of taking • May cause profound drowsiness in some patients

continued

COMMON COLD PHARMACOLOGIC MANAGEMENT

Many over the counter products are available as single agents and combinations of antihistamines and decongestants. None speed resolution of infection but may help alleviate symptoms.

Class	Drug Generic name (Trade name®)	Dosage How supplied	Comments
Antihistamine Second Generation General comments Does not typically produce drowsiness (except cetirizine) and usually dosed once daily	**fexofenadine** Allegra	**Adult and Children ≥ 12 years**: 180 mg daily or 60 mg twice daily **Children 2-11 years**: 30 mg twice daily *Tabs: 30 mg, 60 mg, 180 mg; ODT tab: 30 mg* *Suspension: 6 mg/mL in 300 mL*	• Pregnancy Category C • Shake bottle well before use • Reduce dose for renal • impairment • Allegra ODT contains phenylalanine (other Allegra • products do not) • Avoid aluminum and magnesium containing antacids • Less effective if taken with fruit juices; therefore, take with water • Do not expect sedation
Oral decongestants *Act on adrenergic receptors affecting sympathetic tone of the blood vessels and causing vasoconstriction* *This results in mucous membrane shrinkage and improved ventilation*	**pseudoephedrine tabs** Sudafed Various generics	**Adults and children > 12 years**: *Usual*: two 30 mg tablet every 4-6 hours *Max*: 8 tabs in 24 hours *Alternative*: one 120 mg tablet every 12 hours *Alternative*: one 240 mg ext rel tab once/24 hours **Children 6-12 years:** *Usual*: one 30 mg tab every 4-6 hours *Max*: 4 tabs in 24 hours **Children 6-11 years:** *Alternative*: two teaspoons every 4-6 hours *Max*: 8 teaspoons in 24 hours **Children 4-5 years:** *Usual*: One teaspoon every 4-6 hours *Max*: 4 teaspoons in 24 hours *Tabs: 240 mg, 120 mg, 60 mg, 30 mg* *Liquid: 15 mg/5 mL*	• Pregnancy Category C • Do not use in patients with • hypertension. Cautious use in patients with thyroid disease, CAD, PAD, arrhythmias, prostate disease, and glaucoma • Do not crush, divide, or dissolve tablets

Antihistamines have NOT been shown to alleviate symptoms; however, over the counters are widely used.

In 2007, FDA issued a warning discouraging use of OTC cough and cold products in children ≤ 2 years of age.

PREGNANCY/LACTATION CONSIDERATIONS

- Medications usually avoided if possible
- Most oral decongestants considered safe for short term use, though Pregnancy Category C

FOLLOW-UP

- None usually needed

EXPECTED COURSE

- Complete resolution by 10 days

POSSIBLE COMPLICATIONS

- Sinusitis
- Pneumonia
- Otitis media
- Asthma in individuals who have asthma triggered by viral infections

Avoid aspirin in children to reduce the risk of Reye's Syndrome.

EPISTAXIS
(Nosebleed)

DESCRIPTION

Severe bleeding which occurs from the nose, nasal cavity, or part of the nasopharynx.

This is a symptom, not a disease.

ETIOLOGY

- Idiopathic (most common)
- Epistaxis digitorum (nose picking)
- Bleeding tendency (associated with aplastic anemias, leukemias, hereditary coagulopathies, decreased platelet and clotting functions)
- Infection of the sinuses or upper respiratory tract
- Hypertension
- Liver disease
- Trauma

Kiesselbach's plexus is part of the anterior portion of the septum and is particularly subject to injury and, thus, is a frequent site of anterior hemorrhages.

INCIDENCE

- Most common in children < 15 years and adults > 50 years

RISK FACTORS

- Idiopathic (most common)
- Epistaxis digitorum (nose picking)
- Blood dyscrasias/coagulopathy
- Chronic/acute sinus infections
- Uncontrolled hypertension
- Hepatitis or other liver diseases
- Alcohol abuse
- Blunt nose trauma
- Cocaine use

ASSESSMENT FINDINGS

- Nostril hemorrhage
- Dried blood in nares from prior bleeds
- Hemoptysis
- Nausea from swallowing blood
- Hematemesis

DIFFERENTIAL DIAGNOSIS

- Because epistaxis is a symptom, not a disease, the underlying cause must be identified (see Etiology)

DIAGNOSTIC STUDIES

- Usually none
- CBC if bleeding severe
- Hemoglobin to evaluate for anemia, platelet count
- Clotting studies as indicated

- Liver function tests (may be elevated)

PREVENTION

- Avoid placing objects in nose
- Keep fingernails short
- Management of hypertension, upper respiratory infections
- Lubricate nares during upper respiratory infections if tendency to have nosebleeds
- Humidification at night to prevent drying of mucous membranes
- General measures to stop nosebleeds if they occur

NONPHARMACOLOGIC MANAGEMENT

- Ice packs over nose helps hemostasis
- Upright posture and head tilted forward to prevent blood from reaching posterior pharynx
- Teach patient proper technique to apply pressure to nose by pinching nostrils during times of bleeding
- Nasal endoscopy for cauterization
- Multiple brands of nasal packing available for anterior bleeds
- Surgical cauterization/arterial ligation for intractable bleeds

PHARMACOLOGIC MANAGEMENT

- Analgesics if needed
- Phenylephrine spray (Neo-Synephrine®)
- Vasoconstrictor-impregnated cotton pledget (0.25% phenylephrine or 1:1000 epinephrine)
- Silver nitrate cautery with silver nitrate stick for anterior bleed if area is visible

CONSULTATION/REFERRAL

- ENT referrral for severe anterior bleeds, posterior nasal bleeds, recurrent bleeds
- Consider referral in the elderly (can be severe)

FOLLOW-UP

- Depends on etiology and severity of hemorrhage

EXPECTED COURSE

- Prognosis depends on underlying cause
- For idiopathic epistaxis, prognosis is excellent with proper treatment

POSSIBLE COMPLICATIONS

- Hemorrhage
- Sinusitis
- Abscess
- Tachycardia, hypertension, arrhythmias from systemic effects of topical vasoconstrictors

INFLUENZA
(Grip, Grippe, Flu)

DESCRIPTION

A highly contagious, acute viral illness of the respiratory tract which involves the nasal mucosa, pharynx, respiratory tract and the conjunctiva. Most frequent time of occurrence is during winter months.

ETIOLOGY

- Influenza virus types A and B
- H1N1 ("Swine flu") is a variant of influenza A

INCIDENCE

- Occurs world-wide
- Virus undergoes phenomenon of *antigenic variation* (minor genetic alterations which account for human inability to develop lasting immunity and thus an unending need for vaccination)
- Prevalence is highest in school age population
- Severe disease occurs more frequently in the elderly, pregnant women in the 3rd trimester, infants, and patients with chronic diseases

RISK FACTORS

- Closed or crowded conditions (e.g., schools, prisons, nursing homes)
- Poor hand hygiene
- Presence of chronic disease, especially respiratory ailments

ASSESSMENT FINDINGS

- High fever of sudden onset
- Cough
- Rhinorrhea
- Pharyngitis
- Headache
- Malaise, myalgias, and arthralgias
- Irritated mucous membranes
- Cervical lymphadenopathy
- GI complaints in children

DIFFERENTIAL DIAGNOSIS

- Common cold
- RSV and other viral illnesses
- Pneumonia
- Tonsillitis

DIAGNOSTIC STUDIES

- Usually none are needed to make diagnosis during an epidemic
- Nasal swab for typing (A or B)
- CBC: leukocytosis
- Chest x-ray if pneumonia is suspected

Immunize Annually
Persons at high risk for complications - Especially cardiac and pulmonary patients, and others with chronic diseases ***6-23 month old*** ***Groups at high risk to transmit disease -*** Health care workers

- Immunization is > 70% effective against preventing the disease
- Must immunize *annually* with new vaccine

Do NOT administer if patient has had an anaphylactic reaction to eggs.

NONPHARMACOLOGIC MANAGEMENT

- Minimize contact with others (i.e., home from work or school)
- Saline nose drops/spray for nasal congestion
- Increased fluids
- Rest
- Good hand washing
- Cessation of tobacco products and alcohol
- Humidify air to prevent drying of respiratory secretions
- Patient education regarding disease, treatment, comfort measures, etc.

PHARMACOLOGIC MANAGEMENT

Oral Antiviral Agents	
Influenza Type A	Influenza Type B
Zanamivir Oseltamivir	Zanamivir Oseltamivir

Amantadine and rimantadine are no longer used as lone agents for treatment of influenza A and B because of resistance.

INFLUENZA PHARMACOLOGIC MANAGEMENT

Class	Drug Generic name (Trade name®)	Dosage How supplied	Comments
Oral Antiviral Agents *inhibit virus neuraminidase with the possibility of alteration of viral particle aggregation and particle release*	**oseltamivir** Tamiflu	**Adult and > 13 years:** 75 mg twice daily for 5 days **Renal impairment (CrCL 10-30 mL/min):** 75 mg daily **Children < 15 kg:** 30 mg twice daily **> 15-23 kg:** 45 mg twice daily **> 23-40 kg:** 60 mg twice daily **> 40 kg:** 75 mg twice daily **Adult**: 75 mg twice daily for 5 days Cr CL 10-30 mL/min: 75 mg daily **Children < 1 yr:** not recommended < 15 kg: 30 mg twice daily 16-23 kg: 45 mg twice daily 24-40 kg: 60 mg twice daily > 40 kg: 75 mg twice daily	• Pregnancy Category C • Children less than 1 year not recommended • Treatment should begin within 2 days of onset of symptoms of influenza • Oral capsules may be opened and mixed with sweetened liquids • Monitor for neurologic and behavioral symptoms like hallucinations, delerium, abnormal behaviors • Most common adverse reactions are nausea and vomiting • Potential for interference between live influenza vaccines and oseltamivir is possible • Do not administer within 2 weeks before or 48 hours after administration of oseltamivir • Inactivated influenza vaccine can be administered at any time relative to use of oseltamivir
		PROPHYLAXIS	
		Adult and > 13 years: 75 mg once daily for 10 days **< 15 kg:** 30 mg once daily for 10 days **> 15-23 kg:** 45 mg once daily for 10 days **> 23-40 kg:** 60 mg once daily for 10 days **> 40 kg:** 75 mg once daily for 10 days *Tabs: 30 mg, 45 mg, 75 mg* *Oral suspension: 12 mg/ 1 mL in 25 mL bottles*	• Prophylaxis recommended following close contact with an infected individual • Safety and efficacy of prophylaxis demonstrated for up to 6 weeks in immunocompetent patients • Safety demonstrated up to 12 weeks in immunocompromised patients • Duration of protection lasts as long as dosing is continued • No dosage adjustment necessary for mild to moderate renal dysfunction or geriatric patients • Follow manufacturer's instructions for mixing powder form

continued

INFLUENZA PHARMACOLOGIC MANAGEMENT

Class	Drug Generic name (Trade name®)	Dosage How supplied	Comments
	zanamivir	**Adults and > 7 years:** 10 mg twice daily for 5 days. 2 doses should be taken on the first day provided 2 hours separates doses	• Pregnancy Category C • Not recommended for treatment or prophylaxis of influenza in individuals with underlying airway disease (asthma, COPD). Bronchospasm can occur • Patients who take inhaled bronchodilators should take them PRIOR to taking zanamivir • NO clinically significant drug interactions are known to occur • Elderly patients may need assistance in using the device
	Relenza	**PROPHYLAXIS** **Adults and > 7 years:** 10 mg once daily for 10 days *Blister for oral inhalation: 5 mg blisters of powder on a ROTADISK for oral inhalation via DISKHALER, 5 ROTADISKS and 1 DISKHALER device*	• Pregnancy Category C • Not recommended for treatment or prophylaxis of influenza in individuals with underlying airway disease (asthma, COPD). Bronchospasm can occur • Patients who take inhaled bronchodilators should take them PRIOR to taking zanamivir • NO clinically significant drug interactions are known to occur • Elderly patients may need assistance in using the device

PREGNANCY/LACTATION CONSIDERATIONS

- Safe to immunize during pregnancy

FOLLOW-UP

- None needed if disease is uneventful and no symptoms linger
- Follow-up for complications is dependent on severity of disease and medical status of patient
- Follow-up needed if symptoms persist longer than 10 days or if gradual improvement does not occur over 3-5 days

EXPECTED COURSE

- Favorable outcome

POSSIBLE COMPLICATIONS

- Pneumonia
- Otitis media
- Acute sinusitis
- Croup
- Bronchitis
- Death

Influenza can cause significant morbidity in patients at age extremes and those with existing co-morbidities.

SINUSITIS
(Acute Rhinosinusitis, Acute Bacterial Rhinosinusitis)

DESCRIPTION

Inflammation of the paranasal sinuses due to bacterial, viral, or fungal infection; or allergic reaction.

ETIOLOGY

Acute sinusitis	**Bacterial** *Streptococcus* sp. (most common) *Haemophilus influenza* (common in smokers) *Staphylococcus* sp.
	Viral Rhinovirus Coronavirus Influenza A & B Parainfluenza virus Respiratory syncytial virus
Chronic sinusitis	Gram negative more likely Anaerobic organisms

Vast majority of cases of rhinosinusitis are due to viruses NOT bacteria.

INCIDENCE

- Common in all ages
- Males = Females
- Common in early Fall and early Spring

RISK FACTORS

- Allergies, asthma
- Tooth abscess (25% of chronic sinusitis is due to tooth abscess)
- Cigarette smoking
- Swimming in contaminated water
- Any condition which results in swollen nasal mucous membranes
- Anatomical abnormalities which prevent normal mucosal drainage

ASSESSMENT FINDINGS

- Fever
- Nasal congestion and/or discharge (may be purulent and/or bloody)
- Headache
- Sore throat from persistent postnasal discharge
- Pain over cheeks and upper teeth (maxillary sinuses)
- Pain and tenderness over eyebrows (frontal sinuses)
- Pain and tenderness behind and between eyes (ethmoid sinuses)
- Cough
- Postnasal discharge
- Periorbital edema

Bacterial infection more likely if: symptoms > 10 days, worsening of symptoms after initial improvement, persistent purulent nasal discharge, fever, unilateral face or tooth pain.

DIFFERENTIAL DIAGNOSIS

- Viral, bacterial, or allergic rhinitis
- Dental abscess
- Headaches
- Wegener's granulomatosis

DIAGNOSTIC STUDIES

- CBC: elevated WBC count if bacterial infection
- Sinus x-rays: opaque areas seen on radiographs; air-fluid levels seen
- CT scan: most useful tool to evaluate recurrent sinusitis but unable to differentiate viral from bacterial infection
- Transillumination: opacification with air-fluid levels if sinus cavity is infected

PREVENTION

- Promote drainage by avoiding irritants which increase swelling in mucous membranes and cause retention of sinus exudate
- Good hand washing to prevent upper respiratory infections
- Management of allergic rhinitis

NONPHARMACOLOGIC MANAGEMENT

- Avoid environmental irritants (cigarette smoke)
- Manage allergic rhinitis appropriately

- Humidified air can improve mucus clearance
- Irrigation of sinuses with normal saline nose drops or spray
- Increase fluid intake
- Patient education regarding disease, treatment options, etc.
- May switch to antibiotic with β-lactamase coverage if first course of antibiotics ineffective
- Decongestants: oral route preferred over topical
- Analgesics for headache
- Consider antihistamines/topical nasal steroids if allergy is pre-disposing factor

PHARMACOLOGIC MANAGEMENT

- Antibiotics: for acute infections and patients with moderate to severe infection

ACUTE SINUSITIS PHARMACOLOGIC MANAGEMENT

Reserve antibiotics for patients who have been given decongestants/analgesics for 10 days who have (1) maxillary/facial pain and (2) purulent nasal discharge; if severe illness, treat sooner. For patients with IgE mediated reaction to penicillin or cephalosporins, must use another medication class.

Class	Drug Generic name (Trade name®)	Dosage How supplied	Comments
Antibiotics - Penicillin *inhibits cell wall synthesis of Gram positive bacteria (Staph, Strep) and are most effective against organisms with rapidly dividing cell walls* **General comments** Indicated for infections caused by penicillinase-sensitive microorganisms Generally well tolerated; watch for hypersensitivity reactions	**amoxicillin**	**Adult:** **Mild to moderate sinusitis:** *Usual*: 500 mg every 12 hours for 7-10 days *Alternate*: 250 mg every 8 hours for 7-10 days **Severe sinusitis:** *Usual*: 875 mg every 12 hr for 7-10 days; *Alternate*: 1000 mg three times daily for 10 days usually **Children > 3 months and < 40 kg:** **Mild to moderate sinusitis:** *Usual*: 20 mg/kg/day in divided doses every 8 hours *Alternate*: 25 mg/kg/day every 12 hours for 7-10 days **Severe sinusitis:** *Usual*: 40 mg/kg/day in divided doses every 8 hours *Alternate*: 45 mg/kg/day every 12 hours for 7 -10 days *Alternate*: 90 mg/kg/day in divided doses every 8 or 12 hours - do not exceed max adult dose	• Pregnancy Category B • **DO NOT USE IN PATIENTS WHO HAD HIVES OR ANAPHYLAXIS TO PENICILLIN** • Amoxicillin contains a beta lactam ring in its chemical structure. Therefore, penicillin is rendered ineffective if the organism produces the enzyme, beta lactamase • Decrease dose for renal impairment • Children > 40 kg should be dosed as an adult • Children's dose of amoxicillin should never exceed maximum adult dose • Consider high dose amoxicillin for severe sinusitis or likelihood of drug resistant *Streptococcus pneumoniae*
	Amoxil	*Capsules: 250 mg, 500 mg* *Tabs: 500 mg, 875 mg* *Suspension: 250 mg/5 mL; 400 mg/5 mL* *Pediatric drops: 50 mg/mL*	

continued

ACUTE SINUSITIS PHARMACOLOGIC MANAGEMENT

Reserve antibiotics for patients who have been given decongestants/analgesics for 10 days who have (1) maxillary/facial pain and (2) purulent nasal discharge; if severe illness, treat sooner. For patients with IgE mediated reaction to penicillin or cephalosporins, must use another medication class.

Class	Drug Generic name (Trade name®)	Dosage How supplied	Comments
Extended Spectrum Penicillin *inhibits cell wall synthesis of Gram positive bacteria (Staph, Strep) and are most effective against organisms with rapidly dividing cell walls* **General comments** Addition of clavulanic acid (as potassium) extends antimicrobial spectrum (covers many Gram negative organisms too) and protects PCN molecule if the organism produces beta lactamase Clavulanic acid associated with diarrhea Monitor for PCN hypersensitivity	**amoxicillin/clavulanic acid (as potassium)**	**Adult**: **Mild to moderate sinusitis:** *Usual*: One 250 mg tablet every 8 hours for 10 days *Alternate*: One 500 mg tablet every 12 hours for 10 days **Severe sinusitis:** *Usual*: One 875 mg tablet every 12 hours for 10 days *Alternate*: Two 1000 mg tablets every 12 hours for 10 days **Children > 3 months:** **Mild to moderate sinusitis:** *Usual*: 25 mg/kg/d in two divided doses every 12 hours for 10 days; (Must use 200 mg/5 mL susp or 400 mg/5 mL susp for this regimen).- do not exceed adult dose *Alternate*: 20 mg/kg/day in three divided doses every 8 hours for 10 days (Must use 125 mg/5 mL susp or 250 mg/5 mL susp for this regimen) - do not exceed adult dose **Severe sinusitis:** *Usual*: 45 mg/kg/d in 2 divided doses every 12 hours for 10 days (Must use 200 mg/5 mL susp or 400 mg/5 mL susp for this regimen) - do not exceed adult dose *Alternate*: 40 mg/kg/day in three divided doses given every 8 hours for 10 days (Must use 125 mg/5 mL susp or 250 mg/5 mL susp for this regimen) - do not exceed adult dose	• Pregnancy Category B • **DO NOT USE IN PATIENTS WHO HAD HIVES OR ANAPHYLAXIS TO PENICILLIN** • Two 500 mg amoxicillin/clavulanic acid tablets are NOT equivalent to one 1000 mg amoxicillin/clavulanic acid tablet • Do not substitute Augmentin 200mg/5 mL and 400 mg/5 mL suspensions for Augmentin ES-600. These are NOT interchangeable • Children: Base dose on amoxicillin component • Children > 40 kg should be dosed as an adult • Alternate dose for severe sinusitis based on severity of infection or likelihood of drug resistant drug resistant *Streptococcus pneumoniae* • Take with meals to minimize gastrointestinal side effects • Contraindicated in severe renal impairment (CrCl < 30 mL/min), dialysis, or history of Augmentin associated cholestatic jaundice/hepatic dysfunction • Chewtabs contain phenylalanine

continued

ACUTE SINUSITIS PHARMACOLOGIC MANAGEMENT

Reserve antibiotics for patients who have been given decongestants/analgesics for 10 days who have (1) maxillary/facial pain and (2) purulent nasal discharge; if severe illness, treat sooner. For patients with IgE mediated reaction to penicillin or cephalosporins, must use another medication class.

Class	Drug Generic name (Trade name®)	Dosage *How supplied*	Comments
		Alternate: 90 mg/kg/day in two divided doses every 12 hours for 10 days (Must use 600 mg/5 mL susp for this regimen) - do not exceed adult dose	
	Augmentin XR	*Tabs: XR 1000 mg amoxicillin (62.5 mg clavulanic acid)*	
	Various	*250 mg (62.5 mg clavulanic acid), 500 mg (125 mg clavulanic acid), 875 mg (125 mg clavulanic acid)* *Chew tabs: amoxicillin 125 mg (clavulanate 31.25 mg), 200 mg (28.5 mg clavulanic acid), 250 mg (62.5 mg clavulanic acid), 400 mg (57 mg clavulanic acid)* *Suspension: 125 mg/5 mL (31.25 mg clavulanic acid), 200 mg/5 mL (28.5 mg clavulanic acid), 250 mg/5 mL (62.5 mg clavulanic acid), 400 mg/5 mL (57 mg clavulanic acid), 600mg/5 mL (42.9 mg clavulanic acid)*	

continued

ACUTE SINUSITIS PHARMACOLOGIC MANAGEMENT

Reserve antibiotics for patients who have been given decongestants/analgesics for 10 days who have (1) maxillary/facial pain and (2) purulent nasal discharge; if severe illness, treat sooner. For patients with IgE mediated reaction to penicillin or cephalosporins, must use another medication class.

Class	Drug Generic name (Trade name®)	Dosage How supplied	Comments
	cefprozil	**Adult:** **Mild sinusitis:** *Usual*: 250-500 mg every 12 hours for 10 days **Moderate to severe sinusitis:** *Usual*: 500 mg every 12 hours for 10 days **Children 2- 12 years:** **Mild sinusitis:** *Usual*: 7.5 mg/kg every 12 hours for 10 days *Max:* 500 mg/dose **Moderate to severe sinusitis:** *Usual*: 15 mg/kg every 12 hours *Max:* 500 mg/dose	• Pregnancy Category B • **DO NOT USE IN PATIENTS WHO HAD HIVES OR ANAPHYLAXIS TO PENICILLIN** • Decrease dose for renal impairment • Well tolerated • Children's dose should not exceed adult dose
Cephalosporins ***Second generation*** *Inhibit cell wall synthesis of bacteria* *Contains beta lactam ring like Penicillin* **General comments** For patients who had skin rash to penicillin, OK to use cephalosporin Provides coverage of many Gram positive and Gram negative bacteria but NOT those organisms that produce beta lactamase Well tolerated	**cefprozil**	**Adult:** **Mild sinusitis:** *Usual*: 250-500 mg every 12 hours for 10 days *Max*: 500 mg/day **Moderate to severe sinusitis:** *Usual*: 500 mg every 12 hours for 10 days *Max*: 1000 mg/day **Children 2- 12 years:** **Mild sinusitis:** *Usual*: 7.5 mg/kg every 12 hours for 10 days *Max:* 500 mg/dose **Moderate to severe sinusitis:** *Usual*: 15 mg/kg every 12 hours *Max:* 500 mg/dose	• Pregnancy Category B • **DO NOT USE IN PATIENTS WHO HAD HIVES OR ANAPHYLAXIS TO PENICILLIN** • Decrease dose for renal impairment • Well tolerated
	Cefzil	*Tab: 250 mg, 500 mg* *Suspension: 125 mg/5 mL, 250 mg/5 mL*	

continued

ACUTE SINUSITIS PHARMACOLOGIC MANAGEMENT

Reserve antibiotics for patients who have been given decongestants/analgesics for 10 days who have (1) maxillary/facial pain and (2) purulent nasal discharge; if severe illness, treat sooner. For patients with IgE mediated reaction to penicillin or cephalosporins, must use another medication class.

Class	Drug Generic name (Trade name®)	Dosage How supplied	Comments
	cefuroxime	**Adult > 13 years old:** **Sinusitis:** *Usual*: 250 mg every 12 hours for 10 days **Children 3 months-12 years:** **Sinusitis:** *Usual*: 30 mg/kg/day in 2 divided doses for 10 days *Max*: 1 gram/day	
	Ceftin	*Tab: 250 mg Suspension: 125 mg/5 mL, 250 mg/5 mL*	
Cephalosporins Third generation *Exactly as for second generation cephalosporins but provides broader coverage of Gram negative organisms; beta-lactamase producing organisms* **General comments** For patients who had skin rash to penicillin, OK to use cephalosporin Generally well tolerated	**cefpodoxime**	**Adult ≥ 12 years:** **Sinusitis**: *Usual*: 200 mg every 12 hr for 10 days **Children (2 months to 12 years):** *Usual*: 5 mg/kg every 12 hours for 10 days *Max*: 200 mg/dose	• Pregnancy Category: B • **DO NOT USE IN PATIENTS WHO HAD HIVES OR ANAPHYLAXIS TO PENICILLIN** • Decrease dose for renal impairment • Children's dose should not exceed adult dose • Cefpodoxime: Take tabs with food; suspension may be given without regard to food
	Vantin Various generics	*Tabs: 100 mg and 200 mg* *Suspension: 50 mg/5 mL, 100 mg/5 mL*	
	cefdinir	**Adult > 13 years:** *Usual*: 300 mg every 12h (or 600 mg every 24 hours) for 10 days **Children 6 months-12 yr:** *Usual*: 7 mg/kg every 12 hr or 14 mg/kg daily for 10 days *Max*: 300 mg per dose	• Separate medication by at least 2 hours when giving with iron supplements (except iron fortified cereals)
	Omnicef Various generics	*Tabs: 300 mg* *Suspension: 125 mg/5 mL, 250 mg/5 mL*	

continued

ACUTE SINUSITIS PHARMACOLOGIC MANAGEMENT

Reserve antibiotics for patients who have been given decongestants/analgesics for 10 days who have (1) maxillary/facial pain and (2) purulent nasal discharge; if severe illness, treat sooner. For patients with IgE mediated reaction to penicillin or cephalosporins, must use another medication class.

Class	Drug Generic name (Trade name®)	Dosage How supplied	Comments
	ceftibuten	**Adult > 12 years:** *Usual*: 400 mg/day for 10 days **Children 6 months to 11 years:** *Usual*: 9 mg/kg/day for 10 days *Max*: 400 mg/day	• Ceftibuten suspension must be administered at least 2 hours before or 1 hour after a meal
	Cedax Various generics	*Tabs: 400 mg* *Susp: 90 mg/5 mL, 180 mg/5 mL*	
Macrolides *Inhibit protein synthesis by binding to the 50S ribosomal subunit* **General comments** Good choice for patients with an allergic reaction to penicillin or cephalosporins Avoid concomitant aluminum or magnesium containing antacids	**azithromycin**	**Adults:** *Usual*: 500 mg daily for 3 days *Alternative*: 2 grams as a single dose **Children > 6 months old:** *Usual*: 10 mg/kg once daily for three days *Max*: 500 mg daily	• Pregnancy Category B • Azithromycin 2 gram single dose MUST be taken on an empty stomach; multiday doses may be taken without regard to food • Cautious use in patients with either renal or hepatic dysfunction
	Zithromax® Various generics	*Tabs: 500 mg, 250 mg* *Powder: 2 grams/bottle* *Susp: 100 mg/5 mL, 200 mg/5 mL*	
	clarithromycin	**Adults:** *Usual*: One gram once daily for 14 days *Alternative*: 500 mg twice daily for 14 days **Children:** *Usual*: 7.5 mg/kg every 12 hours for 10 days *Max*: 1 g daily	• Pregnancy Category C • Cautious use in patients with either renal or hepatic dysfunction • Clarithromycin may be involved in drug reactions involving CYP 450 system; special care when prescribing concurrently with 3A4 substrate medications • Common side effect is an abnormal taste in mouth while taking tablet or suspension
	Biaxin XL, Biaxin Various generics	*Tabs: 500 mg* *Ext Rel Tabs: 500 mg* *Susp: 125 mg/5 mL, 250 mg/5 mL*	

continued

ACUTE SINUSITIS PHARMACOLOGIC MANAGEMENT

Reserve antibiotics for patients who have been given decongestants/analgesics for 10 days who have (1) maxillary/facial pain and (2) purulent nasal discharge; if severe illness, treat sooner. For patients with IgE mediated reaction to penicillin or cephalosporins, must use another medication class.

Class	Drug Generic name (Trade name®)	Dosage How supplied	Comments
Quinolones *Antibiotic inhibits the action of DNA gyrase which is essential for the organism to be able to replicate itself* **General comments** Broad spectrum antimicrobial agents Monitor for QT prolongation and photosensitivity Avoid in ages < 18 years, pregnant women due to potential impairment in bone and cartilage formation Monitor for hypoglycemic reactions	**levofloxacin** Levaquin	**Adults > 18 years:** *Usual*: 500 mg once daily for 10-14 days *Alternative*: 750 mg daily for 5 days **Children**: not recommended *Tabs: 250 mg, 500 mg, 750 mg* *Oral soln: 480 mL*	• Pregnancy Category C • Reduce dose for impaired renal function • Avoid drugs that prolong QT interval • Absorption significantly decreased by dairy products, multivitamins, and calcium containing products • Possible increased risk of tendinitis or tendon rupture • Causes photosensitivity
	moxifloxacin Avelox	**Adults** *Usual*: One tablet once daily for 10 days **Children**: not indicated *Tabs: 400 mg*	
Oral decongestants Act on adrenergic receptors affecting sympathetic tone of the blood vessels and causing vasoconstriction This results in mucous membrane shrinkage and improved ventilation	**pseudoephedrine tabs**	**Adults and children > 12 years:** *Usual*: Two 30 mg tablet every 4-6 hours *Max*: 8 tabs in 24 hours *Alternative*: One 120 mg tablet every 12 hours *Alternative*: One 240 mg ext rel tab once/24 hours **Children 6 to 12 years:** *Usual*: One 30 mg tab every 4-6 hours *Max*: 4 tabs in 24 hours **Children 6-11 years:** *Alternative*: Two teaspoons every 4-6 hours *Max*: 8 teaspoons in 24 hours **Children 4-5 years:** *Usual*: One teaspoon every 4-6 hours *Max*: 4 teaspoons in 24 hours	• Pregnancy Category C • Do not use in patients with hypertension. Cautious use in patients with thyroid disease, CAD, PAD, arrhythmias, prostate disease, and glaucoma • Do not crush, divide, or dissolve tablets

continued

ACUTE SINUSITIS PHARMACOLOGIC MANAGEMENT

Reserve antibiotics for patients who have been given decongestants/analgesics for 10 days who have (1) maxillary/facial pain and (2) purulent nasal discharge; if severe illness, treat sooner. For patients with IgE mediated reaction to penicillin or cephalosporins, must use another medication class.

Class	Drug Generic name (Trade name®)	Dosage How supplied	Comments
	Sudafed brand Various generics	*Ext Rel Tabs: 240 mg* *Tabs: 30, 60, 120 mg,* *Liquid: 15 mg/5 mL*	
	phenylephrine	**Adults and children > 12 years**: *Usual*: One 10 mg tab every 4-6 hours *Max*: 4 tabs in 24 hours **Children 6-11 years**: *Usual*: Two teaspoons every 4-6 hours *Max*: 8 teaspoons in 24 hours **Children 4-5 years:** *Usual*: One teaspoon every 4-6 hours *Max*: 4 teaspoons in 24 hours	
	Sudafed PE brand Various generics	*Tabs: 10 mg* *Liquid: 2.5 mg/5 mL*	

PREGNANCY/LACTATION CONSIDERATIONS

- Sinusitis may be aggravated by physiologic nasal congestion due to pregnancy
- Mild decongestant use considered safe for short-term use
- Avoid antibiotics unless absolutely necessary
- Avoid tetracyclines, quinolones, sulfa during pregnancy or lactation

CONSULTATION/REFERRAL

- Refer to ENT for recurrent infections or infection that will not clear
- Consider immediate referral for periorbital cellulitis
- Stiff neck may indicate meningitis

FOLLOW-UP

- Indicated until clinically free of infection

EXPECTED COURSE

- Good prognosis for acute sinusitis
- Chronic sinusitis frequently recurs unless causative factor is treated (e.g. allergic rhinitis, drainage problems) or eliminated (e.g., mechanical obstruction)

POSSIBLE COMPLICATIONS

- Abscess
- Meningitis
- Periorbital cellulitis

EPIGLOTTITIS
(Supraglottitis)

DESCRIPTION

A life-threatening infection of the epiglottis and surrounding tissues that can cause sudden and critical narrowing of the airway.

This is a medical emergency and requires immediate hospitalization for airway management and antimicrobial treatment.

ETIOLOGY

- *Haemophilus influenza* type B (incidence has decreased since Hib vaccine in use)
- *Streptococcus* sp.
- *Staphylococcus*
- Viral pathogens

INCIDENCE

- Uncommon in children < 2 years
- Most common age > 7 years old
- May occur at any age including adults

RISK FACTORS

- Foreign body aspiration

ASSESSMENT FINDINGS

- Fever is usually the first symptom
- Adults have sore throat and odynophagia as predominant symptoms
- Abrupt onset of high fever and sore throat
- Anterior neck with tender adenopathy
- Beefy red pharynx
- Drooling or spitting out of saliva because too painful to swallow
- Muffled voice
- Dyspnea, tachypnea, and inspiratory stridor if respiratory compromise occurs
- "Sniffing posture" (child leans forward and hyperextends neck to maintain patent airway)

Do not attempt to visualize the pharynx if epiglottitis is suspected!

DIFFERENTIAL DIAGNOSIS

- Croup: has characteristic brassy cough not usually found in epiglottitis
- Bacterial tracheitis
- Foreign body aspiration
- Peritonsillar abscess

DIAGNOSTIC STUDIES

- Diagnosis made usually with history and appearance of child/adult
- Do NOT use tongue depressor in examination until airway is secured
- Lateral neck x-ray: characteristic finding is enlarged edematous epiglottitis ("thumbprint" sign); contraindicated unless airway secured
- CBC: elevated WBC

PREVENTION

- Hib immunization for toddlers & young children

Treatment of Acute Epiglottitis:
Airway management (priority intervention) and administration of appropriate antimicrobials!

NONPHARMACOLOGIC MANAGEMENT

- **Maintain patent airway!**
- Arrange for transfer to quickest medical facility which can intubate/manage airway
- Keep patient calm, quiet
- Have supplemental oxygen available until transfer

PHARMACOLOGIC MANAGEMENT

- Intravenous antibiotics to cover gram positive organisms, β-lactamase- producing organisms, and *H. influenza* type B

CONSULTATION/REFERRAL

- Refer to nearest medical facility which can provide intubation/airway management

FOLLOW-UP

- Dependent on patient's condition

EXPECTED COURSE

- Approximately 8% mortality
- Good prognosis if airway management and appropriate antibiotic therapy are initiated in a timely manner

POSSIBLE COMPLICATIONS

- Sudden closure of airway resulting in hypoxia, arrest, and death
- Pneumonia

INFECTIOUS MONONUCLEOSIS

(Mono, Kissing Disease)

ENT Disorders

DESCRIPTION

Viral illness characterized by malaise and fatigue.

ETIOLOGY

- Epstein-Barr virus (EBV) of the herpes family of viruses (almost entirely)

Incubation period is 4-8 weeks.

INCIDENCE

- About 50/100,000 people; up to 5% in susceptible college students
- By young adulthood, about 90% people are seropositive
- 30 times more common in whites than blacks
- Most common age is teens and early twenties

RISK FACTORS

- Contact with oral secretions of an infected person

ASSESSMENT FINDINGS

- Malaise and fatigue
- Tetrad:
  - ◊ Fatigue can last days to weeks
  - ◊ Fever
  - ◊ Pharyngitis can be painful, severe, and exudative
  - ◊ Lymphadenopathy: anterior and posterior cervical nodes; but posterior nodes more common
- Splenomegaly (found in 50% of patients)
- Headache
- Tonsillitis
- Mild hepatomegaly
- Palatal petechiae

DIFFERENTIAL DIAGNOSIS

- Group A β-hemolytic streptococcal infection (detection does not rule out IM and IM does not rule out co-infection with *Streptococcus*)
- Cytomegalovirus (CMV)
- Adenovirus
- Herpes simplex
- Lymphoma/Leukemia
- Rubella
- Viral hepatitis
- Viral tonsillitis

DIAGNOSTIC STUDIES

- CBC: lymphocytosis, atypical lymphs 20% of time
- Monospot used for screening of heterophil antibodies: usually positive by 2nd or 3rd week of illness. 90% of adolescents have positive monospot by third week of illness
- EBV titers (for unusual presentation or prolonged symptoms-more expensive than monospot)
- Atypical monocytes
- Liver enzymes: often elevated
- Ultrasound to diagnose or follow splenomegaly

PREVENTION

- Avoid contact with secretions of infected persons
- Good handwashing
- Isolation NOT necessary
- No blood donation for at least 6 months

NONPHARMACOLOGIC MANAGEMENT

- Rest
- No vigorous exercise, contact sports, or heavy lifting for about 2 months because of potential for splenic rupture (may resume activities sooner if spleen returns to prior non-enlarged state)
- Warm, salt water gargles
- Teach that convalescence may take weeks
- Avoid stress
- Eat well balanced diet with extra fluids

PHARMACOLOGIC MANAGEMENT

- Acetaminophen for fever, aches, pain /other analgesics (aspirin should be avoided because of risk of Reye's syndrome)
- Antiviral medications have not been shown to decrease length or severity of infection

Avoid ampicillin or amoxicillin in patients with infectious mononucleosis due to increased susceptibility to reactions (i.e., characteristic "Ampicillin Rash").

- Avoid steroids unless severe pharyngeal erythema (use may prolong illness)

CONSULTATION/REFERRAL

- For marked pharyngeal swelling that may threaten airway (consider steroids)
- Symptoms persisting longer than 2 weeks
- Immunocompromised individuals

FOLLOW-UP

- In 1-2 weeks and more often if patient's condition dictates

EXPECTED COURSE

- Duration is variable
- Acute phase lasts about 2 weeks
- Complete resolution may take several weeks

POSSIBLE COMPLICATIONS

- Chronic EBV infection (chronic fatigue syndrome)
- Splenic rupture (rare)
- Encephalitis
- Airway obstruction
- Blood dyscrasias
- Other complications effecting nearly every body system

PERITONSILLAR ABSCESS
(Quinsy)

DESCRIPTION

Complication of pharyngitis or tonsillitis that manifests itself initially as a cellulitis and develops into an infection between the anterior and posterior tonsillar pillars.

ETIOLOGY

- Polymicrobial is usual
- *Streptococcus sp.* most common
- *Staphylococcus aureus*
- *Haemophilus influenzae*
- Anaerobic bacteria

INCIDENCE

- Rare in young children, though they are more susceptible
- More common in adolescents/young adults (15-30 years of age)

RISK FACTORS

- Concurrent or previous pharyngitis/tonsillitis/ supraglottitis
- Penetrating trauma in the nasopharyngeal area

ASSESSMENT FINDINGS

- Fever
- Severe sore throat
- Dysphagia
- Trismus: pain on opening of mouth
- Erythematous, swollen, soft palate
- Displaced uvula
- Medially displaced tonsil
- Unilateral neck and/or ear pain
- Torticollis toward side of abscess
- Cervical adenopathy

CRITERIA FOR HOSPITAL ADMISSION

- Inability to swallow
- Trismus
- Incision and drainage

DIFFERENTIAL DIAGNOSIS

- Epiglottitis
- Severe tonsillitis/pharyngitis
- Peritonsillar cellulitis
- Retropharyngeal abscess

DIAGNOSTIC STUDIES

- Ultrasound or CT with contrast will show abscess
- Throat culture
- CBC: leukocytosis
- Lateral neck X-rays if retropharyngeal abscess or epiglottitis is part of differential
- Diagnosis can be made after physical exam usually

PREVENTION

- Early, appropriate treatment of pharyngitis/tonsillitis
- Tonsillectomy after severe or recurrent peritonsillar abscess

NONPHARMACOLOGIC MANAGEMENT

- Inpatient admission
- Maintain patent airway until referral to emergency department or ENT

PHARMACOLOGIC MANAGEMENT

- Intravenous penicillin for *Streptococcus* infections
- Intravenous cephalosporins for *Staphylococcus* infections
- IV steroids are adjunctive (use is controversial)

Penicillin is drug of choice if no contraindications.

CONSULTATION/REFERRAL

- Referral to ENT for likely incision and drainage

FOLLOW-UP

- Peritonsillar abscesses tend to recur; teach patients early signs and symptoms

- Oral course of antibiotics for 10-14 days after incision and drainage
- Tonsillectomy may be indicated 6 weeks after acute event

EXPECTED COURSE

- Complete recovery

POSSIBLE COMPLICATIONS

- Airway obstruction
- Recurrence if abscess is not incised and drained

PHARYNGITIS/TONSILLITIS

DESCRIPTION

An acute inflammation of the pharynx/tonsils.

ETIOLOGY

Causes	
Viral*	**Bacterial**
Rhinovirus **Adenovirus** **Parainfluenza** **Epstein-Barr virus (mononucleosis)**	Group A **β**-hemolytic *Streptococcus*** Haemophilus influenzae *Mycoplasma pneumonia* *Chlamydia pneumoniae* *Neisseria gonorrhoeae* No pathogen can be isolated in many cases

** Most common pathogen*
*** Common depending on time of year*

INCIDENCE

- Prevalent in school age population, but occurs in all age groups (5-18 years most common age group)
- More common during winter months

RISK FACTORS

- Age
- Exposure during Group A **β**-hemolytic *Streptococcus* (GABHS) infection outbreaks
- Family history of rheumatic fever places higher risk if GABHS is untreated
- Crowded conditions
- Daycare attendance
- Chronic illness (e.g., diabetes mellitus)
- Oral sex

ASSESSMENT FINDINGS

- Sore throat and pharyngeal edema
- Tonsillar exudate and/or enlarged tonsils
- Malaise
- Clinical findings are not specific for diagnosis of bacterial or viral illness

- Suggestive of *streptococcal* infection:
  - ◊ Cervical adenopathy
  - ◊ Fever > 102°F (38.8°C)
  - ◊ Absence of other upper respiratory findings (cough, nasal congestion, etc.)
  - ◊ Petechiae on soft palate
- Suggestive of viral infection:
  - ◊ Conjunctivitis, nasal congestion, hoarseness, cough, diarrhea or viral rash

Modified Center Clinical Prediction Rule for Group A *Streptococcus* infection	
Tonsillar exudates	+1 point
Tender anterior chain cervical adenopathy	+1 point
Fever by history	+1 point
Age < 15 years	+1 point
Age 15-45	0 points
Age > 45	-1 point
Cough (almost always excludes *Streptococcus*)	-1 point
3-4 points: Treat empirically for strep 2 points: Rapid *Streptococcus* test, treat if positive 1 point: Unlikely *Streptococcus* 0 or -1 points: Do not test or treat	

DIFFERENTIAL DIAGNOSIS

- Upper respiratory illness
- Tonsillitis

- Mononucleosis
- Peritonsillar abscess
- Epiglottitis

DIAGNOSTIC STUDIES

- Rapid streptococcal test (5-10% false negatives)
- CBC: WBC shift to the left
- Monospot if infectious mononucleosis suspected

PREVENTION

- Avoid contact with infected persons during outbreaks
- Good hand washing, especially during cold weather months
- Teach patients not to share drinking glasses, eating utensils, etc.
- Prompt treatment of individuals with family history of rheumatic fever

NONPHARMACOLOGIC MANAGEMENT

- Gargling with warm salt water
- Increase amount of fluids consumed
- Patient education regarding disease, course and treatment

PHARMACOLOGIC MANAGEMENT

Antipyretics/analgesics (acetaminophen, ibuprofen) for fever and throat pain.

Medication (based on patient's age or weight)	Treatment
Penicillin G	One IM injection
Penicillin V Amoxicillin Erythromycin	Requires 10 days of treatment
First generation cephalosporins	Requires 10 days of treatment
Second generation cephalosporins	5 days of treatment
Azithromycin	Requires 5 days of treatment

ENT Disorders

PHARYNGITIS/TONSILLITIS PHARMACOLOGIC MANAGEMENT

Class	Drug Generic name (Trade name®)	Dosage How supplied	Comments
Antipyretics	**acetaminophen**	**Adult**: *Usual*: 650 mg every 4-6 hr **Infants/Children**: *Usual*: 10-15 mg/kg/dose every 4-6 hours *Max*: 5 doses/24 hours Max Dose 1.625 g/day	*Tylenol Dose by weight:* Pounds — Mg per dose 24-35 — 160 mg 36-47 — 240 mg 48-59 — 320 mg 60-71 — 400 mg 72-95 — 480 mg
	Tylenol	*Tabs: 325 mg scored* *Pediatric Forms:* *Pediatric drops 80 mg/0.8 mL* *Liquid: 160 mg/5 mL* *Chew tabs: 80 mg* *Jr. Chew tabs: 160 mg*	
	acetaminophen	**Children < 3 months:** not recommended 3-11 mo: 80 mg every 6 hr prn 1-3 yr: 80 mg every 4 hr 3-6 yr: 120 mg every 4-6 hr 6-12 yr: 650 mg every 4-6 hr	
	Feverall Supp	*Suppositories: 80 mg, 125 mg, 325 mg*	
	ibuprofen	**Adult**: 200-400 mg every 4-6 hr prn **Children < 6 months:** not recommended **> 6 months:** *Fever <102.5°*: 5 mg/kg every 6-8 hr *Fever >102.5°*: 10 mg/kg every 6-8 hr Max *dose:* 40 mg/kg/day	*Ibuprofen Dose by weight:* Pounds — Mg per dose 12-17 — 50 mg 18-23 — 100 mg 24-35 — 150 mg 36-47 — 200 mg 48-59 — 250 mg 60-71 — 300 mg 72-95 — 400 mg
	Advil Motrin	*Tabs: 200 mg gelcap, tab, liquigels* *Chew tabs: 50 mg, 100 mg scored* *Suspension: 100 mg/5 mL* *Oral Drops: 40 mg/mL*	

continued

ENT Disorders

PHARYNGITIS/TONSILLITIS PHARMACOLOGIC MANAGEMENT

Class	Drug Generic name (Trade name®)	Dosage How supplied	Comments
Penicillin *inhibits cell wall synthesis of Gram positive bacteria (Staph, Strep) and are most effective against organisms with rapidly dividing cell walls* <u>General comments</u> Most common reaction to oral penicillins are gastric: nausea, vomiting, diarrhea Reactions to penicillin are more likely to occur in patients who have had allergies to other medications and/or asthma 10 day minimum treatment required to eradicate *Streptococcus*	**penicillin G**	**Adults**: 1.2 million units IM as a single dose **Older pediatric patients:** 900,000 units IM as a single injection **Infants and pediatric patients < 60 lbs**: 300,000-600,000 units IM as a single injection	• Pregnancy Category B • Give deep IM • Use with caution in patients with significant allergies or asthma • Avoid concurrent use of tetracyclines as they may antagonize the action of penicillin • Inactivated by gastric acid, must be given IM
	Various generics		
	penicillin V potassium	**Adults and children ≥ 12 years:** 125-250 mg every 6-8 hours for 10 days	• Pregnancy Category B • Penicillin V is an analog of penicillin G • For use with mild to moderate infections • Higher blood levels are obtained when taken on an empty stomach
	Pen V K	*Tabs: 250 mg, 500 mg*	
	amoxicillin	**Adults**: *Usual:* 500 mg every 12 hr for 10 days *Alternate:* 875 mg every 12 hr for 10 days **Children 2 months - 12 years:** *Usual*: 25 mg/kg/day in 2 divided doses *Max*: do not exceed adult dose	• Pregnancy Category B • Amoxicillin is not stable in the presence of beta lactamase producing organisms • Considered first line agent in most cases unless patient has had antibiotic exposure in the last 90 days
	Various generics	*Capsules: 250 mg, 500 mg* *Tabs: 500 mg, 875 mg* *Suspension: 250 mg/5 mL; 400 mg/5 mL* *Pediatric drops: 50 mg/mL*	

continued

PHARYNGITIS/TONSILLITIS PHARMACOLOGIC MANAGEMENT

Class	Drug Generic name (Trade name®)	Dosage How supplied	Comments
First Generation Cephalosporins *inhibit cell wall synthesis by bacteria* General comments More effective against rapidly reproducing organisms with cell walls Monitor for hypersensitivity reactions: rash, urticaria, angioedema and pruritis	**cephalexin** Keflex	**Adults**: 1-4 g daily in divided doses PO every 6-12 hours *Max*: 4 g/24 hours *Alternate*: 500 mg PO every 12 hours **Children > 1 year of age:** 25-50 mg/kg/day PO divided every 6-12 hours *Max*: 4 g/24 hours *Alternate*: 25-50 mg/kg/day PO divided every 12 hours *Max*: 4 g/24 hours *Caps: 250 mg, 500 mg, 750 mg* *Susp: 125 mg/5 mL, 250 mg/5 mL*	• Pregnancy Category B • **DO NOT USE IN PATIENTS WHO HAD HIVES OR ANAPHYLAXIS TO PENICILLIN** • Dosage reduction needed for renal impairment • Give without regard to meals • PT should be monitored in patients at risk: renal or hepatic impairment, poor nutritional state • After mixing suspension, store in refrigerator for up to 14 days
	cefadroxil Duricef	**Adults**: 1 g daily in single or divided doses twice daily for 10 days **Children**: 30 mg/kg/day in a single or 2 divided doses for 10 days *Max*: 1 g/day *Caps: 500 mg, 1000 mg,* *Tablets: 1000 mg* *Susp: 250 mg/5 mL, 500 mg/5 mL*	• Pregnancy Category B • **DO NOT USE IN PATIENTS WHO HAD HIVES OR ANAPHYLAXIS TO PENICILLIN** • Dosage reduction needed for renal impairment • No dosage reduction needed for geriatric patients
Second Generation Cephalosporin *Not stable in the presence of beta lactamase producing organisms*	**cefuroxime** Ceftin	**Adults**: 250-500 mg twice daily **Children**: *Usual*: 20 mg/kg/day in 2 divided doses for 10 days *Max*: 1 gram/day *Tabs: 250 mg, 500 mg* *Suspension: 125 mg/5 mL; 250 mg/5 mL*	• Pregnancy Category B • **DO NOT USE IN PATIENTS WHO HAD HIVES OR ANAPHYLAXIS TO PENICILLIN** • Decrease dose for renal impairment • Well tolerated • Children's dose should not exceed adult dose
	cefprozil	**Adult**: 500 mg daily for 10 days **Children**: 7.5 mg/kg every 12 hours for 10 days *Max*: 500 mg daily	

continued

PHARYNGITIS/TONSILLITIS PHARMACOLOGIC MANAGEMENT

Class	Drug Generic name (Trade name®)	Dosage How supplied	Comments
	Cefzil	*Tabs: 250 mg, 500 mg* *Susp: 125 mg/5 mL;* *250 mg/5 mL*	
Macrolides *Inhibit protein synthesis by binding to the 50S ribosomal subunit* **General comments** Not considered first line for treatment of pharyngitis Good choice for patients with an allergic reaction to penicillin or cephalosporins Avoid concomitant aluminum or magnesium containing antacids	**azithromycin** Zithromax Various generics	**Adults**: 500 mg day 1, then 250 mg days 2-5 **Children**: 10 mg/kg on day 1 followed by 4 days of 5 mg/kg *Max*: Day 1: 500 mg *Max*: Days 2-5: 250 mg *Tabs: 250 mg, 500 mg* *Susp: 100 mg/5 mL,* *200 mg/5 mL*	• Pregnancy Category B • Cautious use in patients with either renal or hepatic dysfunction • Avoid concomitant use of aluminum or magnesium containing antacids • Cautious use if renal or hepatic impairment • Hypersensitivity reactions may recur after initial successful symptomatic treatment

CONSULTATION/REFERRAL

- Evidence of acute renal failure and reddish, tea-colored urine (2-3 weeks post infection) may indicate acute poststreptococcal glomerulonephritis
- Tonsillar edema and upper airway obstruction

FOLLOW-UP

- None usually needed
- Patient no longer considered contagious after 24 hours on antibiotic
- Follow up culture not recommended

EXPECTED COURSE

- Peak fever and pain on days 2 and 3
- Lasts 4-10 days

POSSIBLE COMPLICATIONS

- Upper airway obstruction
- Acute poststreptococcal glomerulonephritis after streptococcal infection
- Splenic rupture in infectious mononucleosis infection (rare)
- Rheumatic fever after streptococcal infections
- Peritonsillar abscess

Do not use tetracyclines or sulfonamides for *Streptococcus* eradication because of resistance.

References

Arroll, B., & Kenealy, T. (2005). Antibiotics for the common cold and acute purulent rhinitis. Cochrane Database of Systematic Reviews(3), CD000247. doi: 10.1002/14651858.CD000247.pub2

Balfour, H. H., Jr., Holman, C. J., Hokanson, K. M., Lelonek, M. M., Giesbrecht, J. E., White, D. R., . . . Brundage, R. C. (2005). A prospective clinical study of Epstein-Barr virus and host interactions during acute infectious mononucleosis. Journal of Infectious Diseases, 192(9), 1505-1512. doi: 10.1086/491740

Bickley, L. S., & Szilagyi, P. G. (2008). Bates' guide to physical examination and history taking (10th ed.). Philadelphia: Lippincott Williams & Wilkins.

Block, S. L. (2005). Otitis externa: providing relief while avoiding complications. Journal of Family Practice, 54(8), 669-676. doi: jfp_0805_5408c [pii]

Bousquet, J., Khaltaev, N., Cruz, A. A., Denburg, J., Fokkens, W. J., Togias, A., . . . Williams, D. (2008). Allergic Rhinitis and its Impact on Asthma (ARIA) 2008 update (in collaboration with the World Health Organization, GA(2)LEN and AllerGen). Allergy, 63 Suppl 86, 8-160. doi: 10.1111/j.1398-9995.2007.01620.x

Burton, M. J., & Doree, C. J. (2004). Interventions for recurrent idiopathic epistaxis (nosebleeds) in children. Cochrane Database of Systematic Reviews(1), CD004461. doi: 10.1002/14651858.CD004461.pub2

Carrat, F., Vergu, E., Ferguson, N. M., Lemaitre, M., Cauchemez, S., Leach, S., & Valleron, A. J. (2008). Time lines of infection and disease in human influenza: a review of volunteer challenge studies. American Journal of Epidemiology, 167(7), 775-785. doi: 10.1093/aje/kwm375

Choby, B. A. (2009). Diagnosis and treatment of streptococcal pharyngitis. American Family Physician, 79(5), 383-390.

Chonmaitree, T., Revai, K., Grady, J. J., Clos, A., Patel, J. A., Nair, S., . . . Henrickson, K. J. (2008). Viral upper respiratory tract infection and otitis media complication in young children. Clinical Infectious Diseases, 46(6), 815-823. doi: 10.1086/528685

Devlin, B., Golchin, K., & Adair, R. (2007). Paediatric airway emergencies in Northern Ireland, 1990-2003. Journal of Laryngology and Otology, 121(7), 659-663. doi: 10.1017/S0022215107000588

Dickens, K. P., Nye, A. M., Gilchrist, V., Rickett, K., & Neher, J. O. (2008). Clinical inquiries. Should you use steroids to treat infectious mononucleosis? Journal of Family Practice, 57(11), 754-755. doi: jfp_5710i [pii]

Douglas, R., & Wormald, P. J. (2007). Update on epistaxis. Current Opinion in Otolaryngology & Head and Neck Surgery, 15(3), 180-183. doi: 10.1097/MOO.0b013e32814b06ed

Drug facts and comparisons 2010. (2010). St. Louis: Wolters Kluwer Health.

Ebell, M. H. (2004). Epstein-Barr virus infectious mononucleosis. American Family Physician, 70(7), 1279-1287.

Eichner, E. R. (2007). Sports medicine pearls and pitfalls--defending the spleen: return to play after infectious mononucleosis. Current Sports Medicine Reports, 6(2), 68-69.

Ernst, D., & Lee, A. (2010). Nurse practitioners prescribing reference. New York: Haymarket Media Publication.

Fiore, A. E., Shay, D. K., Broder, K., Iskander, J. K., Uyeki, T. M., Mootrey, G., . . . Cox, N. J. (2009). Prevention and control of seasonal influenza with vaccines: recommendations of the Advisory Committee on Immunization Practices (ACIP), 2009. MMWR Recomm Rep, 58(RR-8), 1-52. doi: rr5808a1 [pii]

Gerber, M. A., Baltimore, R. S., Eaton, C. B., Gewitz, M., Rowley, A. H., Shulman, S. T., & Taubert, K. A. (2009). Prevention of rheumatic fever and diagnosis and treatment of acute Streptococcal pharyngitis: a scientific statement from the American Heart Association Rheumatic Fever, Endocarditis, and Kawasaki Disease Committee of the Council on Cardiovascular Disease in the Young, the Interdisciplinary Council on Functional Genomics and Translational Biology, and the Interdisciplinary Council on Quality of Care and Outcomes Research: endorsed by the American Academy of Pediatrics. Circulation, 119(11), 1541-1551. doi: 10.1161/CIRCULATIONAHA.109.191959

Geva, A., Oestreicher-Kedem, Y., Fishman, G., Landsberg, R., & DeRowe, A. (2008). Conservative management of acute mastoiditis in children. International Journal of Pediatric Otorhinolaryngology, 72(5), 629-634. doi: 10.1016/j.ijporl.2008.01.013

Gilber, D. N., Moellering, R. C., Eliopoulos, G. M., & Sande, M. A. (2010). The sanford guide to antimicrobial therapy (40th ed.). Sperryville, VA: Antimicrobial Therapy;.

Glynn, F., & Fenton, J. E. (2008). Diagnosis and management of supraglottitis (epiglottitis). Current Infectious Disease Reports, 10(3), 200-204.

Guldfred, L. A., Lyhne, D., & Becker, B. C. (2008). Acute epiglottitis: epidemiology, clinical presentation, management and outcome. Journal of Laryngology and Otology, 122(8), 818-823. doi: 10.1017/S0022215107000473

Hahn, R. G., Knox, L. M., & Forman, T. A. (2005). Evaluation of poststreptococcal illness. American Family Physician, 71(10), 1949-1954.

Hanif, J., Tasca, R. A., Frosh, A., Ghufoor, K., & Stirling, R. (2003). Silver nitrate: histological effects of cautery on epithelial surfaces with varying contact times. Clinical Otolaryngology and Allied Sciences, 28(4), 368-370. doi: 727 [pii]

Harper, S. A., Bradley, J. S., Englund, J. A., File, T. M., Gravenstein, S., Hayden, F. G., . . . Zimmerman, R. K. (2009). Seasonal influenza in adults and children--diagnosis, treatment, chemoprophylaxis, and institutional outbreak management: clinical practice guidelines of the Infectious Diseases Society of America. Clinical Infectious Diseases, 48(8), 1003-1032. doi: 10.1086/598513

Harvey, R. J., Debnath, N., Srubiski, A., Bleier, B., & Schlosser, R. J. (2009). Fluid residuals and drug exposure in nasal irrigation. Otolaryngology - Head and Neck Surgery, 141(6), 757-761. doi: 10.1016/j.otohns.2009.09.006

Higgins, C. D., Swerdlow, A. J., Macsween, K. F., Harrison, N., Williams, H., McAulay, K., . . . Crawford, D. H. (2007). A study of risk factors for acquisition of Epstein-Barr virus and its subtypes. Journal of Infectious Diseases, 195(4), 474-482. doi: 10.1086/510854

Infant deaths associated with cough and cold medications--two states, 2005. (2007). MMWR. Morbidity and Mortality Weekly Report, 56(1), 1-4.

Institute for Clinical Systems Improvement. (2008). Diagnosis and treatment of respiratory illness in children and adults. Retrieved from http://www.guideline.gov/content.aspx?id=12294

Johnson, R. F., Stewart, M. G., & Wright, C. C. (2003). An evidence-based review of the treatment of peritonsillar abscess. Otolaryngology - Head and Neck Surgery, 128(3), 332-343. doi: 10.1067/mhn.2003.93

Mackay, I. M. (2008). Human rhinoviruses: the cold wars resume. Journal of Clinical Virology, 42(4), 297-320. doi: 10.1016/j.jcv.2008.04.002

Mak, T. K., Mangtani, P., Leese, J., Watson, J. M., & Pfeifer, D. (2008). Influenza vaccination in pregnancy: current evidence and selected national policies. Lancet Infectious Diseases, 8(1), 44-52. doi: 10.1016/S1473-3099(07)70311-0

Marshall, I. (2006). WITHDRAWN: Zinc for the common cold. Cochrane Database of Systematic Reviews(3), CD001364. doi: 10.1002/14651858.CD001364.pub2

Morris, P. S. (2009). Upper respiratory tract infections (including otitis media). Pediatric Clinics of North America, 56(1), 101-117, x. doi: 10.1016/j.pcl.2008.10.009

Neuhauser, H. K., Radtke, A., von Brevern, M., Lezius, F., Feldmann, M., & Lempert, T. (2008). Burden of dizziness and vertigo in the community. Archives of Internal Medicine, 168(19), 2118-2124. doi: 10.1001/archinte.168.19.2118

Pfoh, E., Wessels, M. R., Goldmann, D., & Lee, G. M. (2008). Burden and economic cost of group A streptococcal pharyngitis. Pediatrics, 121(2), 229-234. doi: 10.1542/peds.2007-0484

Rosenfeld, R. M. (2007). Clinical practice guideline on adult sinusitis. Otolaryngology - Head and Neck Surgery, 137(3), 365-377. doi: 10.1016/j.otohns.2007.07.021

Rosenfeld, R. M., Andes, D., Bhattacharyya, N., Cheung, D., Eisenberg, S., Ganiats, T. G., . . . Witsell, D. L. (2007). Clinical practice guideline: adult sinusitis. Otolaryngology - Head and Neck Surgery, 137(3 Suppl), S1-31. doi: 10.1016/j.otohns.2007.06.726

Rosenfeld, R. M., Brown, L., Cannon, C. R., Dolor, R. J., Ganiats, T. G., Hannley, M., . . . Witsell, D. L. (2006). Clinical practice guideline: acute otitis externa. Otolaryngology - Head and Neck Surgery, 134(4 Suppl), S4-23. doi: 10.1016/j.otohns.2006.02.014

Schlosser, R. J. (2009). Clinical practice. Epistaxis. New England Journal of Medicine, 360(8), 784-789. doi: 10.1056/NEJMcp0807078

Steyer, T. E. (2002). Peritonsillar abscess: diagnosis and treatment. American Family Physician, 65(1), 93-96.

Tasman, W., & Jaeger, E. A. (2005). Duane's clinical ophthalmology on CD-ROM. Philadelphia: J.B. Lippincott Co.

Viehweg, T. L., Roberson, J. B., & Hudson, J. W. (2006). Epistaxis: diagnosis and treatment. Journal of Oral and Maxillofacial Surgery, 64(3), 511-518. doi: 10.1016/j.joms.2005.11.031

Wallace, D. V., Dykewicz, M. S., Bernstein, D. I., Blessing-Moore, J., Cox, L., Khan, D. A., . . . Tilles, S. A. (2008). The diagnosis and management of rhinitis: an updated practice parameter. Journal of Allergy and Clinical Immunology, 122(2 Suppl), S1-84. doi: 10.1016/j.jaci.2008.06.003

Young, J., De Sutter, A., Merenstein, D., van Essen, G. A., Kaiser, L., Varonen, H., . . . Bucher, H. C. (2008). Antibiotics for adults with clinically diagnosed acute rhinosinusitis: a meta-analysis of individual patient data. Lancet, 371(9616), 908-914. doi: 10.1016/S0140-6736(08)60416-X

Yueh, B., Collins, M. P., Souza, P. E., Boyko, E. J., Loovis, C. F., Heagerty, P. J., . . . Hedrick, S. C. (2010). Long-term effectiveness of screening for hearing loss: the screening for auditory impairment--which hearing assessment test (SAI-WHAT) randomized trial. Journal of the American Geriatrics Society, 58(3), 427-434. doi: 10.1111/j.1532-5415.2010.02738.x

Zalmanovici, A., & Yaphe, J. (2007). Steroids for acute sinusitis. Cochrane Database of Systematic Reviews(2), CD005149. doi: 10.1002/14651858.CD005149.pub2

4

ENDOCRINE DISORDERS

Endocrine Disorders

Diabetes Mellitus Type 1 229

Diabetes Mellitus Type 2 231

Hypoglycemia 239

Hyperthyroidism 240

Hypothyroidism 242

Thyroid Nodule 244

Cushing's Syndrome 245

Addison's Disease 246

Gynecomastia 248

*Precocious Puberty 249

References *251*

**Denotes pediatric diagnosis*

Endocrine Disorders

DIABETES MELLITUS
Type 1

DESCRIPTION

A leading serious chronic illness of children and young adults characterized by insulin deficiency, hyperglycemia, and glucosuria.

ETIOLOGY

- Insulin deficiency and hyperglycemia result from destruction of **β**-cells of the pancreas
- **β**-cell destruction may be a result of genetic predisposition in combination with environmental triggers

INCIDENCE

- Mean age at onset is 8 to 12 years; peaking in adolescence
- Approximately 10% of all diabetics
- Highest incidence is in Caucasian-Americans
- Males = Females

Type 1 diabetes mellitus may occur in patients as old as the 3rd or 4th decade.

RISK FACTORS

- Diabetes mellitus Type 1 or 2 in a first-degree relative
- Presence of HLA DR3, DR4, B8, B15 genes on Chromosome 6

ASSESSMENT FINDINGS

- Acute onset of polydipsia, polyphagia, polyuria ("the 3 Ps"), weight loss, fatigue
- Dehydration
- Decreased energy level
- Confusion
- Fruity odor to breath if diagnosed during diabetic ketoacidosis
- Failure to grow and gain weight in small children and infants

DIFFERENTIAL DIAGNOSIS

- Diabetes mellitus Type 2
- Pancreatic disease
- Salicylate poisoning
- Acute poisonings

DIAGNOSTIC STUDIES

- Fasting plasma glucose ≥ 126 mg/dL (on 2 occasions) OR Random glucose level ≥ 200 mg/dL
- Oral glucose tolerance test if diagnosis is questionable
- Glucosuria
- Ketonuria
- Glycosylated hemoglobin > 6.5%
- Electrolytes
- C-peptide insulin level
- Urinalysis for presence of glucose or ketones
- HLA typing

PREVENTION OF COMPLICATIONS

- Normoglycemia by "tight control": maintenance of HgbA1C based on age
- Children < 6 years: 7.5-8.5%
- Children 6-12 years: < 8%
- Adolescents: 13-19: < 7.5% (would rather < 7% if no recurrent episodes of hypoglycemia)
- Smoking avoidance or cessation
- Exercise daily
- Maintenance of ideal body weight
- Education about insensate foot care
- Limit dietary fat intake

MANAGEMENT

- Multidisciplinary treatment: integration of insulin therapy (cornerstone of therapy), nutrition management, exercise
- *Assessments*:
  - ◊ Physical examinations every three months focused on growth, development and sexual development (poor glucose control affects growth)
  - ◊ Blood pressure at each visit; cardiac examination
  - ◊ Funduscopic and vision examination at time of diagnosis, then, annual dilated eye exam and anytime having visual problems
  - ◊ Oral examination

- ◊ Palpation of thyroid
- ◊ Abdominal examination
- ◊ Skin examination
- ◊ Neurological examination
- ◊ Examine feet for pulses, cleanliness, odor, swelling, mobility, nail thickness, bruises, pressure points; include sensory evaluation

- *Insulin therapy*:

Summary of Insulin Therapy	
Rapid acting	Lispro/Aspart - works almost immediately with injection (may be used in lieu of regular insulin)
Short acting	Humalog, NovoLog insulin before meals and snacks
Peakless (mimics basal insulin)	Glargine insulin: Lantus, Levemir
Insulin Pump	Use only Humalog or NovoLog
Calculation of Daily Insulin Requirements	
Adults	0.8 to 1 u/kg/day
Children	0.25 u/kg/day
Adolescents	1.25-1.5 u/kg/day due to accelerated growth and metabolic rate
Insulin pump delivers individualized basal metabolic rate with bolus at meal times	

Type 1 Diabetes Mellitus by Injection
Glargine Insulin: subcutaneous daily based on calculated requirements and then adjusted according to blood sugar values
Humalog or Novolog insulin: before meals and snacks (can initiate dose at 1 unit insulin/10 grams carbohydrate; adjust according to blood sugar values)
***Correction Factor for elevated blood sugar > 150*: Subtract 100 from the blood sugar and divide by 50. Administer this number of units of insulin**
Example: Blood sugar is 200 mg/dL. 200-100=100. Divide 100/50=2 units insulin to correct elevated blood sugar

- *Nutrition therapy*:
  - ◊ Goal is a well balanced diet providing consistency in timing and intake
  - ◊ American Diabetic Association diet recommended: based on food exchanges

- *Exercise*:
  - ◊ Regular aerobic exercise is preferred
  - ◊ Recommended daily to increase the number of insulin receptors and insulin secretion; allows more efficient glucose utilization

- *General*:
  - ◊ Formulate sick day plan
  - ◊ Develop contingency plan for management of hypoglycemia
  - ◊ Medic alert bracelet
  - ◊ School personnel/co-workers should be aware

After initial diagnosis and insulin therapy initiated, *honeymoon phase* characterized by decreased insulin needs. This usually lasts 3-6 months. Then, insulin needs accelerate.

PREGNANCY/LACTATION CONSIDERATIONS

- Goal is maintenance of fasting plasma glucose (FPG) from 60-105 mg/dL and postprandial level < 120 mg/dL
- Dietary management:
  - ◊ Well-balanced meals with a limited intake of concentrated sweets
  - ◊ Refer to registered dietitian and diabetes educator
- Self-monitoring of glucose 4 or more times a day
- Breastfeeding is encouraged because of its positive effect on HDLs
- 28 weeks: maternal assessment of fetal activity should begin, with daily kick counts
- 32 weeks: twice weekly nonstress testing
- Increased risk of maternal and fetal complications:
  - ◊ Accelerates development of retinopathy and pregnancy-induced hypertension
  - ◊ Spontaneous abortion and congenital anomalies
  - ◊ Macrosomia, shoulder dystocia, hypoglycemia, hypokalemia, stillbirth

CONSULTATION/REFERRAL

- Endocrinologist
- Diabetic educator
- Registered dietitian
- Obstetrician during pregnancy

FOLLOW-UP

- Frequency of visits dependent on course of illness
- Hemoglobin A_1C every 3 months
- Screen for microalbuminuria annually
- Annual total urinary protein once positive for microalbuminuria

- Annual serum creatinine in adults and in children if proteinuria is present
- Lipid profile, if > 2 years of age, at diagnosis, then annually once control is established
- Annual ECG in adults
- Thyroid function tests every 2-3 years
- Ophthalmology exam after 3-5 years of diagnosis; annually, thereafter
- Annual influenza immunization

EXPECTED COURSE

- Lifetime illness with course dependent on glucose control
- Use of insulin pump shown to decrease complications, but requires intensive management and training

POSSIBLE COMPLICATIONS

- Ketoacidosis
- Hypoglycemia
- Chronic microvascular disease: retinopathy, renal failure, peripheral neuropathy
- Skin ulcerations, gangrene of lower extremities
- Macrovascular disease, premature atherosclerosis

DIABETES MELLITUS
Type 2

DESCRIPTION

Abnormal insulin secretion, resistance to insulin in target tissues, and/or decrease in insulin receptors.

ETIOLOGY

- Influenced by genetics as well as environmental factors
- High body mass with central obesity is strongest environmental factor
- Inactivity

INCIDENCE

- 300/100,000
- Incidence is rising in all age groups; especially if born after year 2000
- Increased in African-Americans, American Indians, Latino-Americans, Pacific Islanders, Mexican-Americans

RISK FACTORS

- Obesity
- History of gestational diabetes
- History of delivery of macrosomic infant
- Family history of Type 2 diabetes

ASSESSMENT FINDINGS

- Usually discovered on routine examination
- Chemisty panel and urinalysis: glucosuria, proteinuria and hyperglycemia
- Obesity
- Polydipsia, polyuria, polyphagia
- Fatigue
- Blurred vision
- Chronic skin infections
- Balanitis sometimes seen in elderly males
- Chronic candidal vulvovaginitis in women
- May present with hyperosmolar state or coma

Long Term Effects of Hyperglycemia
Hypertension
Nephropathy
Coronary artery disease, myocardial infarction
Peripheral neuropathy
Cerebrovascular accident
Severe peripheral vascular insufficiency

DIFFERENTIAL DIAGNOSIS

- Diabetes mellitus Type 1
- Gestational diabetes
- Cushings's syndrome
- Pheochromocytoma
- Corticosteroid use

DIAGNOSTIC STUDIES

American Diabetes Association Diagnostic Criteria	
Fasting Plasma Glucose	≥ 126 mg/dL and confirmed on a different day
Random Plasma Glucose	≥ 200 mg/dL with symptoms OR 2 hour plasma glucose ≥ 200 mg/dL during an oral GTT with 75 g glucose load OR ≥ 200 mg/dL and confirmed on a different day
Pre-diabetes (Impaired fasting glucose)	Fasting glucose between 100 mg/dL and 125 mg/dL, and confirmed on a different day
Hgb A1C	≥ 6.5%

- Screening: ADA recommends adults over age 45 years be screened every 3 years, more often with fasting plasma glucose close to 126 mg/dL
- To differentiate Type 1 from Type 2 diabetes mellitus: C peptide levels will be below normal in Type 1 diabetes mellitus; and normal or above normal in Type 2 diabetes mellitus

PREVENTION

- Weight loss to attain a normal BMI, exercise 150 minutes/week
- Focus on education regarding: obesity, low fat/calorie diet, exercise, sequelae, treatments

NONPHARMACOLOGIC MANAGEMENT

- Weight loss: primary goal of obese patient; even modest weight loss of 5-10 pounds is helpful in increasing insulin sensitivity
- Nutrition plan:
  - ◊ 3 visits with registered dietitian at diagnosis and ongoing follow-up visits semi-annually to annually
  - ◊ ≈ 50% carbohydrates
  - ◊ ≈ 30% protein
  - ◊ ≈ 20% fat (limit cholesterol to 300 mg/day)
- Avoid alcohol
- Avoid smoking
- Exercise
  - ◊ To increase insulin secretion, glucose utilization and HDL levels
  - ◊ Endurance exercise is optimal (e.g., walking)
  - ◊ Perform stress test first if older than age 35 years and diabetic
- Periodic physical examinations:
  - ◊ Blood pressure and cardiac examination
  - ◊ Funduscopic and vision examination at time of diagnosis, then if diabetic for 5 years or more or if having visual problems
  - ◊ Oral examination
  - ◊ Thyroid palpation
  - ◊ Skin examination
  - ◊ Neurological examination
  - ◊ Abdominal examination
  - ◊ Examine feet for pulses, cleanliness, odor, swelling, mobility, nail thickness, bruises, pressure points; include sensory evaluation

PHARMACOLOGIC MANAGEMENT

- Initiate metformin at diagnosis unless contraindicated
- Classes considered first line: biguanides (metformin), sulfonylureas, alpha-glucosidase inhibitors, deipeptidyl peptidase-4 (DDP-4), and insulin
- Classes considered second line: GLP-1, meglitinides and thiazolidinediones

DIABETES MELLITUS TYPE 2 PHARMACOLOGIC MANAGEMENT

Class	Drug Generic name (Trade name®)	Dosage How supplied	Comments
Biguanides *decrease production of glucose in the liver; decrease absorption of glucose in the intestine, and improve insulin sensitivity by increasing peripheral glucose uptake and utilization* **General comments** Lactic acidosis is a rare but serious metabolic complication Does not produce hypoglycemia unless caloric intake is deficient, there is strenuous exercise without caloric compensation, or in elderly, debilitated or malnourished patients May produce weight loss, improvement of lipid profiles May be used as monotherapy or in combination with TZD, insulin, sulfonylureas Metformin should be temporarily discontinued in patients undergoing radiologic studies involving intravascular administration of iodinated contrast materials because use of such products may result in acute alteration of renal function	**metformin**	**Immediate Release** **Adult:** Metformin 500 mg twice a day. Increase in increments of 500 mg weekly *Max:* 2000 mg daily in 2 divided doses *Alternate*: 850 mg once daily with meals. Increase in increments of 850 mg every 2 weeks *Max*: 2550 mg per day in divided doses **Children 10-16 years:** 500 mg twice a day, given with meals. Increase in increments of 500 mg weekly *Max*: 2000 mg daily in divided doses **DO NOT USE XR in children**	• Pregnancy Category B • Give twice daily with food • Avoid in binge drinkers • Careful use in patients with CHF, renal and hepatic dysfunction • Diarrhea, flatulence are common initial side effects. Usually resolves by 2 weeks • Goal is to decrease fasting plasma glucose and Hgb A1C levels to norm or near norm • Monitor blood glucose to determine lowest effective dose
		Extended Release **Adult:** 500 mg once daily with evening meal. Increase by 500 mg increments not sooner than once weekly *Max*: XR 2000 mg/day	• In elderly patients, do not use extended release tabs unless creatinine clearance is not reduced • Give once daily with the evening meal • Swallow whole, never crush or chew • Do not use in children
	Glucophage Various generics	*Tabs: 500 mg, 850 mg, 1000 mg*	
	Glucophage XL Various generics	*Ext. Rel. Tabs: 500 mg, 750 mg*	
Thiazolidinediones (TZD) *inhibit gluconeogenesis in the liver, improve insulin liver sensitivity in the skeletal muscle and adipose tissue, (and consequently reduce circulating insulin levels in hyperinsulinemic patients)*	**pioglitazone**	**Adult > 18 yrs**: *Initial*: 15 mg or 30 mg once daily *Usual*: individualized *Max*: 45 mg/day **Children**: not established	• Pregnancy Category C • Monitor ALT prior to initiation, then periodically per the clinical judgment of the health care provider

continued

DIABETES MELLITUS TYPE 2 PHARMACOLOGIC MANAGEMENT

Class	Drug Generic name (Trade name®)	Dosage How supplied	Comments
<u>**General comments**</u> Can exacerbate or cause congestive heart failure Not recommended in patients with symptomatic heart failure. Contraindicated in patients with Class III or IV heart failure Depends on the presence of insulin for its action May be used as monotherapy or in combination with metformin, insulin, sulfonylureas	Actos	*Tabs: 15 mg, 30 mg, 45 mg*	• Do not initiate in patients with hepatic dysfunction. If ALT increases > 3 times the upper limits of normal and remains elevated, pioglitazone should be discontinued • Monitor for fluid retention which may exacerbate CHF • No adjustment necessary for renal dysfunction • May increase risk of fractures in post menopausal women • Can be taken without regard to meals
Meglitinides *potentiate insulin secretion from pancreas (short-acting secretagogue)* <u>**General comments**</u> Do not use with insulin May be used as monotherapy or with metformin	**repaglinide**	**Adult**: 0.5 mg within 30 minutes of meal or at meal time 2-4 times daily for patients not previously treated or with Hgb A1C < 8%. Titrate by doubling dose at intervals of at least 1 week *Max*: 16 mg/day *Alternate*: In patients previously treated with antidiabetic agents and Hbg A1C > 8%, initially 1-2 mg with 2-4 meals daily. Titrate by doubling dose at intervals of at least 1 week. *Max*: 16 mg/day	• Pregnancy Category C • Pre-prandial dosing only • If a meal is skipped (or added), skip (or add) a repaglinide dose • Should not be used with sulfonylureas • Use with caution in hepatic, elderly, or debilitated patients. They may be very sensitive to hypoglycemic effects of repaglinide • Dose adjustment recommended for renal dysfunction • Do not take with gemfibrozil
	Prandin	*Tabs: 0.5 mg, 1 mg, 2 mg*	
Alpha glucosidase inhibitors *delay absorption of carbohydrates following a meal resulting in a smaller rise in glucose elevation* <u>**General comments**</u> Contraindicated in patients with inflammatory bowel disorders May be used as monotherapy, with a sulfonylurea, or with insulin	**miglitol**	**Adult**: give one tablet 30 minutes before meals *Initial*: 25 mg three times daily, may start at 25 mg daily and gradually increase to three times daily. Increase to 50 mg three times daily after 4-8 weeks. *Usual*: 50 mg three times daily *Max*: 100 mg three times a day **Children**: not recommended	• Pregnancy Category B • These agents do NOT enhance action of insulin • Dosage adjustment needed for renal dysfunction. No adjustment needed for hepatic dysfunction • If hypoglycemia results, do not administer sucrose (absorption will be delayed) instead, administer dextrose • Flatulence and diarrhea are common side effects

continued

DIABETES MELLITUS TYPE 2 PHARMACOLOGIC MANAGEMENT

Class	Drug Generic name (Trade name®)	Dosage How supplied	Comments
	Glyset	*Tabs: 25 mg, 50 mg, 100 mg*	
	acarbose	**Adult:** 25 mg three times daily. Take with first bite of main meal. Increase at 4-8 week intervals *Max*: 100 mg three times a day *Max < 60 kg*: 50 mg three times daily *Max > 60 kg*: 100 mg three times daily	• Pregnancy Category B • Patients with low body weight may be at increased risk for elevated serum transaminases • Contraindicated in inflammatory bowel disease • Cautious use in renal dysfunction • Monitor blood glucose 1 hour post prandially initially during titration, then glycosylated hemoglobin • Monitor serum transaminases every 3 months during 1st year and periodically thereafter
	Precose	*Tabs: 25 mg, 50 mg, 100 mg*	
DDP IV Inhibitors *Dipeptidyl-peptidase-4 (DDP-IV) inhibitors enhance biologically active GLP-1 to increase insulin secretion and suppress glucagon secretion. Preserves beta cell potential. Weight neutral* **General comments** May be used in combination with metformin, TZD, sulfonylurea, insulin	**sitagliptin**	**Adult:** *Initial*: 100 mg daily *Usual*: 100 mg once daily *Max*: 100 mg daily **Children < 18:** not recommended	• Pregnancy Category B • Dosage adjustment needed for moderate or severe renal dysfunction • Take with or without food • Monitor renal function prior and periodically • May need to lower dose of sulfonylurea initially • Caution with digoxin, monitor pulse rate • Monitor for pancreatitis
	Januvia	*Tabs: 25 mg 50 mg, 100 mg*	
	saxagliptin	**Adult**: May use 2.5-5 mg once daily *Initial*: 2.5 mg or 5 mg once daily taken regardless of meals *Usual*: 5 mg *Max*: 5 mg daily	• Pregnancy Category B • May need to lower dose of sulfonylurea initially • Dosage adjustment needed for moderate or severe renal dysfunction. No adjustment needed for hepatic dysfunction • Take with or without food • Monitor for drug interactions with 3A4/5 inhibitors
	Onglyza	*Tabs: 2.5 mg, 5 mg*	

continued

DIABETES MELLITUS TYPE 2 PHARMACOLOGIC MANAGEMENT

Class	Drug Generic name (Trade name®)	Dosage How supplied	Comments
Glucagon-like Peptide (GLP-1) *promotes release of insulin from pancreatic beta cells in the presence of elevated glucose concentrations* **General comments** May be used with metformin, sulfonylurea, or a TZD Weight loss is desired side effect	**exenatide** Byetta	**Adults:** *Initial*: 5 mcg two times daily subcutaneously within 60 minutes before morning and evening meals (at least 6 hours apart); After one month, may increase to 10 mcg *Usual*: 10 mcg twice daily *Max*: 10 mcg twice daily *Forms: 5 mcg /1.2 mL prefilled pen (60 doses); 10 mcg/2.4 mL prefilled pen (60 doses)*	• Pregnancy Category C • Cautious use in patients with end stage renal disease • NO dosage adjustment needed for hepatic dysfunction • Must be refrigerated prior to first dose, then kept at room temperature • Administer SC injection in thigh, abdomen, or upper arm within 60 minute period before morning and evening meals. Do not administer after a meal • If dose missed, resume as prescribed with the next dose • Common side effect is nausea and anorexia • May decrease the effectiveness of oral contraceptives
Sulfonylurea Agents *stimulates release of insulin from functioning pancreatic beta cells* *Secondary failure may occur with extended therapy* **General comments** Sulfonylureas may be potentiated by many drugs: NSAIDs, quinolones, highly protein bound drugs, beta blocking agents, thiazides, others	**glimepiride** Amaryl	**Adults:** Initially 1-2 mg once daily with breakfast or first main meal. After reaching a dose of 2 mg, increase by up to 2 mg at 1-2 mg intervals if needed. *Usual*: 1-4 mg once daily *Max*: 8 mg/day *Tabs: 1 mg, 2 mg, 4 mg*	• Pregnancy Category C • Cautious use with renal or hepatic dysfunction, elderly or debilitated • Once 8 mg has been reached and fasting glucose is in the range of > 150 mg/dL, insulin may be recommended • Monitor blood glucose for 1-2 weeks when transferring patient from a longer acting sulfonylurea to glimepiride
Administration of oral hypoglycemic drugs is associated with increased cardiovascular mortality compared to treatment with diet alone or insulin Contraindicated in diabetic ketoacidosis. This is treated with insulin	**glipizide**	**Adults:** *Initial*: 5 mg before breakfast. Increase by 2.5–5 mg every few days *Max*: 15 mg once daily dose *Max*: 40 mg daily in divided doses 30 minutes before meals **Elderly, debilitated, hepatic impairment** *Initial*: 2.5 mg daily	• Pregnancy Category C • Cautious use in renal or hepatic dysfunction
	Glucotrol	**Adults**: *Initial*: 5 mg with breakfast *Usual*: 5-10 mg once daily *Max*: 20 mg once daily *Tabs: 5 mg, 10 mg*	• Pregnancy Category C • Do not crush, chew or divide

continued

DIABETES MELLITUS TYPE 2 PHARMACOLOGIC MANAGEMENT

Class	Drug Generic name (Trade name®)	Dosage How supplied	Comments
	Glucotrol XL	*Ext Rel Tabs: 5 mg, 10 mg*	

COMBINATION DRUGS FOR DIABETICS

Combination Type	Fixed-Dose Combination, mg	Trade Name®
DPP IV and biguanide	Sitagliptin-metformin (50/500, 50/1000)	Janumet
Meglitinide and biguanide	Repaglinide and metformin (1/500, 2/500)	PrandiMet
Sulfonylurea and biguanide	Glipizide and metformin (2.5/250, 2.5/500, 5/500)	Metaglip
	Glyburide and metformin (1.25/250, 2.5/500, 5/500	Glucovance
TZD and biguanide	Pioglitazone and metformin (15/500, 15/850)	Actoplus Met
	Rosiglitazone and metformin (2/500, 4/500, 2/1000, 4/1000)	Avandamet
TZD and sulfonylurea	Rosiglitazone and glimepiride (4/1, 4/2, 4/4)	Avandaryl

Drug abbreviations: DPP IV, Dipeptidyl peptidase-4 inhibitor; TZD, thiazolidinediones

Some drug combinations are available in multiple fixed doses. Each drug is reported in milligrams

INSULINS			
Insulin Preparation	Onset in hours	Peak in hours	Duration hours
Novolog®	< 0.25	1-3	3-5
Levemir®	1	0	24
Lantus®	1.1	0	> 24
Apidra®	0.25	1	2-4
Humulog®	< 0.25	1	3.5-4.5
Humulog® mix 75/25	< 0.25	0.5-1.5	24
Humulog® mix 50/50	< 0.25	1	16
Novolin® R	0.5	2.5-5	8
Humulin® 70/30	0.5	2-12	24
Humulin® 50/50	0.5	3-5	24
Novolin® 70/30	0.5	2-12	24
Humulin® N	1-2	6-12	18-24
Novolin® N	1-5	4-12	24

Adapted from Ernst, D. & Lee, A. (Eds.) (2010). Nurse practitioner prescribing reference. NY: Haymarket Media Publications

- *Insulin*
  - ◊ Recommended early in course of oral therapy, though often used when oral agents have been exhausted
  - ◊ 0.2 u/kg or 10 units of peakless insulin recommended as initial insulin therapy
  - ◊ If unable to achieve glycemic goals, administer mealtime insulin
- Other Pharmacologic Therapy
  - ◊ Antihypertensive treatment for blood pressure > 130/80 mm Hg, preferably with ACE inhibitors
  - ◊ HMG-CoA reductase inhibitors ("statins") preferred for hyperlipidemia

PREGNANCY/LACTATION CONSIDERATIONS

- Oral agents are generally avoided; however, metformin has been used to treat pregnant women with "pre-gestational diabetes"
- Sulfonylureas are avoided because they cross the placenta and can cause fetal hyperinsulinemia
- Universal screening at 24 to 28 weeks gestation for detection of gestational diabetes. If glucose > 140 mg/dL one hour after 50 grams oral glucose load, 3-hour GTT is recommended
- Refer to registered dietitian and diabetes educator
- Addition of insulin if glucose > 90 mg/dL fasting or ≥ 120 mg/dL on 2 or more occasions in a two week period
- Self-monitoring of glucose four times a day or more
- Women with gestational diabetes have an increased risk of developing Type 2 diabetes mellitus later, thus follow-up is warranted
- Increased risk of maternal and fetal complications:
  - ◊ Pregnancy accelerates development of retinopathy and pregnancy-induced hypertension
  - ◊ Increased risk of spontaneous abortion, stillbirth, and congenital anomalies
  - ◊ Increased risk of macrosomia resulting in shoulder dystocia

Screen women with gestational diabetes 6-12 weeks postpartum and continue surveillance throughout lifetime.

CONSULTATION/REFERRAL

- Endocrinologist
- Registered dietitian
- Diabetic educator
- Ophthalmologist
- Early referral to foot specialist when needed

FOLLOW-UP

- Success is measured by glycemic control and avoidance of tissue organ damage
- Annual total urinary protein once microalbuminuria present; then total urinary protein
- Annual lipid profile
- Annual serum creatinine
- Annual ECG
- Thyroid function tests if indicated
- If treated with diet, fasting glucose ≤ 126 mg/dL
- If treated with medication, hemoglobin A_1C every 3 months; goal is < 7%
- Annual dilated eye and visual examination at time of diagnosis, then annually, or if complaints of visual problems
- Foot inspection at each visit
- Education at each visit

EXPECTED COURSE

- Dependent on glucose control; poor control results in increased risk of vascular complications
- Usually complications develop 10-15 years after onset but can present earlier, if DM undetected for years before diagnosis

POSSIBLE COMPLICATIONS

- Nephropathy, renal failure
- Peripheral neuropathy
- Retinopathy
- Cardiovascular and peripheral vascular disease
- Glaucoma, cataracts, blindness
- Skin ulcerations, gangrene of lower extremities; limb amputations
- Charcot foot

HYPOGLYCEMIA

DESCRIPTION

Excessive secretion of epinephrine along with dysfunction of the central nervous system as a reaction to insufficient plasma glucose.

ETIOLOGY

- Reactive
  - ◊ Alimentary hyperinsulinism due to gastrectomy, gastrojejunostomy, pyloroplasty, or vagotomy
  - ◊ Ingestion of fructose or galactose by a child with fructose intolerance or galactosemia
  - ◊ Leucine sensitivity in infants
- Idiopathic
- Insulinoma
- Imbalance between production of glucose by the liver and its utilization in peripheral tissue
- Post-GI surgery associated with dumping syndrome

INCIDENCE

- Most prevalent in older adults

RISK FACTORS

- Hormone deficiencies
- Enzyme defects
- Severe malnutrition with muscle wasting and fat depletion
- Third trimester of pregnancy
- Liver disease
- Alcoholism
- Salicylates
- Insulinoma (Islet cell tumor)
- Exogenous insulin, sulfonylureas, quinine, disopyramide, pentamidine
- Endotoxic shock

ASSESSMENT FINDINGS

CNS dysfunction (if glucose dropping gradually):

- Headache
- Visual disturbance
- Confusion, elderly with recurrent hypoglycemia may have dementia-like presentation
- Hunger
- Clumsiness
- Convulsions
- Loss of consciousness

Excessive epinephrine secretion (if sudden decrease in glucose):

- Diaphoresis
- Tremor
- Nervousness
- Dizziness
- Anxiety

Symptoms of hypoglycemia correlate with low blood glucose and are reversed with increases in blood glucose.

DIFFERENTIAL DIAGNOSIS

- CNS disorders
- Emotional disorders
- Factitious disease: self-induction by injection of insulin or ingestion of oral hypoglycemic agents

DIAGNOSTIC STUDIES

- Best to perform when patient is symptomatic: simultaneous plasma glucose, plasma insulin, and C peptide levels
- Diagnostic is:
  - ◊ Plasma insulin level: elevated (values vary in laboratories)
  - ◊ C peptide level: increased
  - ◊ Plasma glucose: decreased
  - ◊ Reversal of symptoms with ingestion of glucose
- Cortisol level
- Drug assay, including sulfonylureas and alcohol
- Liver function studies
- CT scan or abdominal ultrasound to assess for tumors
- If postprandial hypoglycemia suspected, 3-hour oral glucose tolerance test

NONPHARMACOLOGIC MANAGEMENT

- Avoidance of fasting is all that is usually required
- Oral carbohydrate for alert patient (oral fruit juice)
- Surgery is treatment of choice for insulinoma
- High protein diet with restricted carbohydrates,

frequent small meals

- Avoid causative agents
- Counseling if hypoglycemia is self-induced

PHARMACOLOGIC MANAGEMENT

- If there is confusion or coma: initially, intravenous bolus of 25-50 gram glucose as 50% concentrate, followed by constant glucose infusion, until able to eat a meal
- Glucagon intramuscular, subcutaneous
- Hormone replacement in pituitary or adrenal insufficiency

Must identify and treat underlying cause.

CONSULTATION/REFERRAL

- Hormone deficiencies: endocrinologist
- Insulinoma: endocrinologist to confirm diagnosis, then surgeon

FOLLOW-UP

- Variable, dependent on etiology and treatment

EXPECTED COURSE

- With recognition of cause and appropriate treatment, prognosis is favorable

POSSIBLE COMPLICATIONS

- Risk associated with surgery for insulinoma
- Tissue damage or death if glucose deficit is prolonged

HYPERTHYROIDISM

(Thyrotoxicosis)

DESCRIPTION

Clinical state that results when the body's tissues are exposed to an increased level of circulating thyroid hormone. Manifestations are related to excessive metabolic activities in body tissues.

ETIOLOGY

- Most common cause is Graves' disease, an autoimmune disorder with a genetic component
- Other causes include thyroid nodules, ingestion of thyroid hormones, pituitary gland dysfunction, and thyroiditis (Hashimoto's)

INCIDENCE

- Common, affects 0.1% of women and 0.3% of men
- Typical patient is mid-20-40 years old at diagnosis

RISK FACTORS

- Family history of thyroid disease
- Thyroid replacement hormone ingestion
- Other autoimmune disorders

ASSESSMENT FINDINGS

- Weight loss incongruent with daily dietary intake and exercise level
- Most common symptoms are nervousness, dyspnea, intolerance to heat and perspiring, palpitations and tachycardia
- Thyroid enlargement (2 to 6 times) may be accompanied by vascular thrill or bruit
- Atrial fibrillation, systolic murmur, cardiac failure
- Fatigue, weakness, diminished quadriceps strength
- Bowel movements frequent and soft
- Skin changes, warm, moist, hyperpigmented, smooth, flushes easily
- Hair and nails soft and thin
- Labile emotions
- Tremors, rapid deep tendon reflexes
- Oligomenorrhea
- Vision changes, blurred, double, photophobia, tearing
- Exophthalmos, eyelid retraction and lag
- Accelerated growth in children

Most common presentation in patients > 60 years is atrial fibrillation.

DIFFERENTIAL DIAGNOSIS

- Anxiety
- Arrhythmias
- Diabetes mellitus, Types 1 and 2
- Malignancy
- Menopause
- Normal aging
- Pheochromocytoma
- Pregnancy

DIAGNOSTIC STUDIES

- TSH: low or not detectable
- T_4 - increased most commonly
- T_3 - increased occasionally
- Free thyroxine index - increased
- CBC and liver function tests prior to and during treatment on antithyroid drugs

95% of patients with hyperthyroidism have suppressed TSH and elevated T_4.

PREVENTION

- Periodically monitor TSH of patient on thyroid replacement therapy

NONPHARMACOLOGIC MANAGEMENT

- Surgery: thyroidectomy, although not the preferred method of treatment, may be offered if remission does not occur after use of antithyroid drugs; hypothyroidism is frequent long-term outcome

PHARMACOLOGIC MANAGEMENT

- Treatment consists of reducing symptoms and decreasing thyroid hormone synthesis
  - ◊ Symptom management: beta-blockers (atenolol, propanolol, metoprolol)
  - ◊ Decreasing hormone synthesis: antithyroid drugs (methimazole, propylthiouracil), radiocontrast agents, other agents
- Goal is to attain euthyroid state within 3-8 weeks

PREGNANCY/LACTATION CONSIDERATIONS

- PTU is used at lowest dose that keeps serum T_4 at upper limit of normal
- PTU does not cross the placenta
- Pregnancy is an absolute contraindication to the use of radioactive iodine (RAI)

CONSULTATION/REFERRAL

- Surgeon if thyroidectomy is chosen as form of management
- Emergency department for thyroid storm, an extreme form of hyperthyroidism
- Endocrinologist for management during pregnancy and in children
- Ophthalmologist for patient with Grave's ophthalmopathy

FOLLOW-UP

- Long term evaluation for recurrence of hyperthyroidism or development of hypothyroidism is necessary, regardless of treatment choice
- TSH and T_4 every 4 weeks until euthyroid, then every 3 to 6 months while on antithyroid drugs
- TSH at 6 weeks, 12 weeks, 6 months, and annually if RAI therapy used
- Baseline CBC to be repeated if agranulocytosis is suspected
- Liver function tests (LFT): rare hepatic abnormality effect of antithyroid drugs

EXPECTED COURSE

- With antithyroid drug therapy there is a 25-90% chance of permanent remission
- With RAI or surgery, great majority of patients eventually become hypothyroid

Graves's Disease has a high rate of relapse after medications are stopped.

POSSIBLE COMPLICATIONS

- An episode of major depression commonly follows treatment of hyperthyroidism, possibly due to unmasking of depression, or damaged relationships due to behavior changes or illness' effect on neurotransmitters
- Thyroid storm: an extreme form of hyperthyroidism characterized by severe anxiety, fever, nausea, vomiting, abdominal pain and cardiac failure
- Visual disturbance due to ophthalmopathy
- Myxedema
- Cardiac failure in patients with underlying heart disease

HYPOTHYROIDISM

DESCRIPTION

Clinical state that results from either a reduction in the amount of circulating free thyroid hormone, or from resistance to the action of thyroid hormone.

ETIOLOGY

- Majority of cases are due to primary thyroid gland failure from autoimmune destruction (Hashimoto's thyroiditis)
- Ablative therapy for hyperthyroidism
- Other causes are congenital, and secondary or tertiary, due to pituitary or hypothalamic disease

INCIDENCE

- Predominant age is > 40 years
- Females > Males

RISK FACTORS

- Increasing age
- Family history
- Postpartum
- Pituitary disease
- Hypothalamic disease
- Autoimmune diseases
- History of head or neck irradiation
- Treatment of hyperthyroidism

ASSESSMENT FINDINGS

- Severity of clinical symptoms range from asymptomatic to myxedema coma
- Lethargy, delayed deep tendon reflexes
- Mild weight gain, swelling of hands and feet, macroglossia, periorbital edema
- Intolerance to cold
- Constipation
- Menstrual irregularities, decreased libido, infertility
- Memory loss, dull facial expression, depression
- Muscle cramps, arthralgias, paresthesias
- Coarse dry skin, hair loss from body and scalp, brittle nails
- Bradycardia, enlarged heart
- Reduced systolic and increased diastolic blood pressure
- Anemia
- Hyponatremia
- Atrophic or enlarged thyroid

Expect lipid levels to be elevated in patients with hypothryoidism. Treat lipids if still elevated after TSH < 10.

DIFFERENTIAL DIAGNOSIS

- Depression
- Dementia
- Chronic heart failure
- Kidney failure
- Many others because presenting symptoms are usually vague

DIAGNOSTIC STUDIES

- Serum TSH is increased in thyroprivic and goitrous hypothyroidism (often > 20 μu/ml); normal or undetectable in pituitary or hypothalamic hypothyroidism
- T_4 decreased most commonly; occasionally T_3 decreased
- Free T_4 index ↓ = T_3 resin uptake x total serum T_4

Endocrine Disorders

Subclinical hypothyroidism: slightly elevated TSH and nonspecific symptoms; monitor TSH every 3 months. Treatment increases risk of osteopenia/porosis.

PREVENTION

- Periodic monitoring of thyroid hormone levels for those patients being treated for hyperthyroidism
- Newborn screening with T_4 at 2-6 days of age

Congenital hypothyroidism: Educate parents about etiology, importance of treatment with L-thyroxine to prevent mental retardation and need for follow-up care.

NONPHARMACOLOGIC MANAGEMENT

- Educate parents that children may manifest behavioral problems at the beginning of treatment
- Assess growth and development in children
- High fiber diet to prevent constipation
- Diet for weight loss/fat reduction if obese
- Educate regarding need for lifelong compliance with thyroid replacement medication and need to report signs of toxicity, infection, or cardiac symptoms
- Annual lipid level assessment

PHARMACOLOGIC MANAGEMENT

- L-thyroxine daily, beginning at lower dose in elderly or in presence of cardiac disease
- In young, healthy patients, 1.6 mcg/kg/daily is full anticipated dose
- Older patients should be started at 25-50 mcg/kg/day and increased to 1.0 mcg/kg/daily as symptoms and side effects are monitored
- Adult: maintenance: 100-200 mcg/day
- Children: < 6 months: 8-10 mcg/kg/day
  6 mo-1 yr: 6-8 mcg/kg/day
  1-5 yr: 5-6 mcg/kg/day
  6-12 yr: 4-5 mcg/kg/day
- Tabs: 25 mcg; 50 mcg; 88 mcg; 100 mcg; 112 mcg; 137 mcg; 150 mcg; 175 mcg; 200 mcg; 300 mcg

Start low and go slow when initiating replacement in older patients.

L-thyroxine should be given on an empty stomach. In children, may crush tabs and mix in 5-10 mL of water.

PREGNANCY/LACTATION CONSIDERATIONS

- L-thyroxine dose requirements rise by 25-50% beginning in first trimester starting at 8 weeks
- TSH should be assessed at 8 weeks gestation and at 20 to 24 weeks gestation
- Reduce L-thyroxine to prepregnancy dose immediately after delivery
- Breastfeeding is not a contraindication to L-thyroxine therapy

CONSULTATION/REFERRAL

- Refer to pediatric endocrinologist: congenital hypothyroidism
- Refer to ER and endocrinologist for myxedema coma
- Endocrinologist for secondary or tertiary hypothyroidism

FOLLOW-UP

- Measure TSH after patient has been on L-thyroxine for 6 weeks, and every 6-8 weeks until within normal limits, then annually, unless symptomatic
- Examine periodically for signs of thyrotoxicity (e.g., tremor or tachycardia)
- Congenital hypothyroidism: monitor T4 and TSH periodically
- Acquired hypothyroidism: monitor initial response to medication at 4 to 6 weeks with TSH and by symptoms, then monitor TSH annually

EXPECTED COURSE

- Improvement is expected 2 weeks after initiation of medication
- Signs and symptoms should resolve in 3 to 6 months
- Lifelong therapy is needed

POSSIBLE COMPLICATIONS

- Myxedema coma: life-threatening, severe hypothyroidism; may require intravenous L-thyroxine and cardiorespiratory assistance
- Thyrotoxicity
- Treatment induced CHF in elderly or patient with CAD
- Bone demineralization due to over-treatment over a long period
- Mental retardation associated with congenital hypothyroidism if not treated
- Growth and development delays in children

THYROID NODULE

DESCRIPTION

Thyroid mass that is discrete and may function without influence from the pituitary gland (autonomously).

ETIOLOGY

- Unknown

INCIDENCE

- Most common in elderly and women
- Uncommon in children, but if present, >60% are malignant
- < 5% are malignant in adults
- Common in iodine deficient areas

RISK FACTORS

- Iodine deficiency
- Exposure to ionizing radiation: history of irradiation to head, neck, or chest
- Family history

ASSESSMENT FINDINGS

- Both benign and malignant nodules often asymptomatic
- May have symptoms of either hypothyroidism or hyperthyroidism
- Fixed, firm, nontender, large nodules not accompanied by symptoms of thyroid dysfunction more likely to be malignant
- Multiple nodules occur in Hashimoto's thyroiditis
- Hoarseness, dysphagia
- Cervical lymphadenopathy

DIFFERENTIAL DIAGNOSIS

- Benign nodules
- Malignant nodules
- Cysts

DIAGNOSTIC STUDIES

- Thyroid function tests: serum thyroid stimulating hormone (TSH) and free-thyroxine index (FTI) often normal
- High resolution ultrasound helpful in distinguishing cysts from solid lesions
- Fine needle aspiration biopsy: best method to determine malignancy if TSH is normal or increased
- If TSH is decreased, scintigraphy is best method to evaluate malignancy

Initial evaluation starts with assessing thyroid function. Order a thyroid stimulating hormone (TSH) first!

NONPHARMACOLOGIC MANAGEMENT

- Adequate iodine intake
- Surgery if needle biopsy indicates thyroid cancer

PHARMACOLOGIC MANAGEMENT

- Follow guidelines for hypothyroidism or hyperthyroidism if thyroid function affected

PREGNANCY/LACTATION CONSIDERATIONS

- Avoid radionuclide scan

CONSULTATION/REFERRAL

- Endocrinologist if unresponsive to treatment
- Surgeon for malignant or disfiguring nodules

FOLLOW-UP

- Annual evaluation of benign nodules for size and thyroid function if euthyroid
- Follow guidelines for hypothyroid and hyperthyroid if thyroid function is abnormal
- Malignant nodules will require thyroid replacement postoperatively to suppress serum TSH level; thyroid scan and chest x-ray at 6 months, then annually thereafter

EXPECTED COURSE

- Malignant nodules: good survival rate, require annual evaluation
- Benign nodules require long-term management of thyroid dysfunction

POSSIBLE COMPLICATIONS

- Recurrence of tumor
- Complications of hyperthyroidism or hypothyroidism or pharmacologic therapy

CUSHING'S SYNDROME

DESCRIPTION

Cushing's syndrome is an overexposure of the tissues to corticosteroids from exogenous (medications) or endogenous sources (pituitary, adrenal, tumor, etc.). Cushing's Disease, the most common cause of Cushing's syndrome, is glucocorticoid excess related to excessive production of adrenocorticotropic hormone (ACTH) by the pituitary gland.

ETIOLOGY

- The most common cause is adrenocorticotropic hormone-dependent etiologies: pituitary adenoma, non pituitary adrenocorticotropic hormone-producing tumors
- ACTH-independent etiology: autonomous cortisol production from adrenal tissue
- Exposure to exogenous sources of corticosteroids

INCIDENCE

- Females > Males 3:1
- Rare in infancy and childhood

RISK FACTORS

- Long term use of corticosteroids
- Adrenal tumor
- Pituitary tumor

ASSESSMENT FINDINGS

- Truncal obesity, dorsal cervical fat pad ("buffalo hump")
- Amenorrhea, clitoral hypertrophy
- Central weight gain
- Edema, moon face
- Abdominal striae, thin skin with poor wound healing, ecchymosis
- Hirsutism
- Hypertension
- Weakness and fatigue
- Glucosuria, polyuria, polydipsia
- Osteoporosis
- Personality changes, mood changes
- Slow growth in children
- Hyperpigmentation

DIFFERENTIAL DIAGNOSIS

- Obesity
- Diabetes Mellitus, Types 1 and 2
- Syndrome X
- Alcoholism
- Depression

DIAGNOSTIC STUDIES

- Preferred test is late night salivary cortisol or 24 hour urinary free cortisol (elevated is positive)
- 24 hour urinary free cortisol; must obtain 3 or more samples and concurrent 24 hour urinary creatinine clearance
- Persistently elevated serum cortisol is typical of Cushing's syndrome
- CT abdomen to visualize adrenals and detect adrenal source
- Pituitary MRI with gadolinium contrast to detect pituitary source
- X-ray of lumbar spine: osteoporosis common

PREVENTION

- Limit corticosteroid use

NONPHARMACOLOGIC MANAGEMENT

- Surgery is treatment of choice if tumor is present
- High protein diet, potassium supplements
- Educate: early treatment of infection, daily weights, emotional lability
- Reduce pituitary ACTH production:
    - Transphenoidal resection
    - Radiation
- Reduce adrenocortical cortisol secretion:
    - Bilateral adrenalectomy

PHARMACOLOGIC MANAGEMENT

- Medical therapy alone is not usually appropriate
- Medication should be prescribed and managed by an endocrinologist

CONSULTATION/REFERRAL

- Endocrinologist
- Surgeon

FOLLOW-UP

- Replacement glucocorticoid therapy may be needed for up to 1 year after surgery (lifelong if bilateral adrenalectomy is performed)
- Stress need for gradual glucocorticoid withdrawal
- Patient should wear identification bracelet stating need for glucocorticoid replacement
- Patients exhibiting signs of recurrence should undergo measurement of urine free cortisol

EXPECTED COURSE

- Normal hypothalamic-pituitary-adrenal activity is expected within 3 to 24 months of surgery if at least one adrenal gland remains
- Recurrence occurs in a minority of patients
- If surgery is not feasible, lifelong medical therapy is required
- Pregnancy can cause exacerbation

POSSIBLE COMPLICATIONS

- Osteoporosis
- Metastasis of malignant tumors

ADDISON'S DISEASE
(Hypoadrenocorticism)

DESCRIPTION

Hypofunction of the adrenal gland which results in inadequate release of glucocorticoids and mineralocorticoids, also called hypoadrenocorticism.

ETIOLOGY

- 80% of cases due to autoimmune process which causes adrenal destruction
- Acute withdrawal after long-term corticosteroid therapy

INCIDENCE

- All ages affected; predominantly 30-50 year olds
- Females > Males

RISK FACTORS

- Family history of adrenal insufficiency
- Autoimmune adrenal insufficiency
- Cytomegalovirus (CMV)
- Autoimmune deficiency syndrome (AIDS)
- Prolonged use of steroids followed by a stressor such as infection, trauma, or surgery
- Medications that potentiate adrenal failure:
  - ◊ Rifampin
  - ◊ Phenytoin (Dilantin®)
  - ◊ Ketoconazole (Nizoral®)
  - ◊ Opiates
- Other immune disorders

ASSESSMENT FINDINGS

- Slowly progressive symptomology
- Fatigue, weakness, anorexia, nausea and vomiting, weight loss, amenorrhea
- Hypotension
- Depression
- Salt craving
- Cutaneous and mucosal pigmentation (e.g., tanning, freckles, blue-black areolas and mucous membranes)
- Cold intolerance

DIAGNOSTIC STUDIES

- Early stages of disease:
  - ◊ Subnormal rise in cortisol levels after adrenal stimulation with ACTH
- Later stages:
  - ◊ Serum sodium, chloride, and bicarbonate: decreased
  - ◊ Serum potassium: increased
  - ◊ ECG: nonspecific ST segment changes
  - ◊ EEG: generalized slowing
  - ◊ Serum calcium: increased
  - ◊ BUN, creatinine: increased
  - ◊ CBC: normocytic anemia, lymphocytosis, eosinophilia
  - ◊ Low cortisol levels 8-9 AM
- Abdominal CT scan: small adrenals if due to autoimmune; enlarged adrenals due to non-autoimmune etiologies
- Chest x-ray: decreased heart size

DIFFERENTIAL DIAGNOSIS

- Hyperparathyroidism
- Secondary or tertiary adrenocortical insufficiency
- Depression
- Myopathies
- Heavy metal poisoning
- Anemia

NONPHARMACOLOGIC MANAGEMENT

- Correct precipitating factors
- Diet with adequate sodium, chloride, and potassium replacement

PHARMACOLOGIC MANAGEMENT

- Synthetic hydrocortisone 15-20 mg every morning and 10 mg at 4-5 PM
- Intravenous NaCl to treat dehydration

The 5 Ss of Addison disease management: Salt, Sugar, Steroids, Support, Search for precipitating illness.

CONSULTATION/REFERRAL

- Endocrinologist

FOLLOW-UP

- Periodic assessment of:
  - ◊ Blood pressure
  - ◊ Electrolytes/blood sugar
  - ◊ Strength
  - ◊ Appetite
  - ◊ Plasma renin
  - ◊ Heart size

EXPECTED COURSE

- Excellent prognosis
- Requires lifelong replacement therapy with monitoring for adequacy and avoidance of overdose
- 100% lethal without treatment

POSSIBLE COMPLICATIONS

- Acute adrenal crisis (more likely in elderly)
- Psychosis
- Hyperkalemia
- Hyperpyrexia
- Osteoporosis
- Complications of steroid therapy

GYNECOMASTIA

DESCRIPTION

Occurrence of mammary tissue hypertrophy in males causing enlargement of one or both breasts.

Type 1: Benign adolescent hypertrophy
Type 2: Physiologic gynecomastia
Type 3: Stimulated by obesity
Type 4: Pectoral muscle hypertrophy

ETIOLOGY

- Estrogen-androgen imbalance related to effects of puberty, aging, or drugs
- In newborns, from stimulation by maternal hormones
- Estrogen secreting tumor

INCIDENCE

- Occurs in 2/3 of normal males during early puberty
- Occurs in 40-60% of men over age 50 years (medications are usual cause)

RISK FACTORS

- Obesity
- Adrenal hyperplasia
- Klinefelter's syndrome
- Bronchogenic carcinoma
- Drugs:
  - ◊ Tricyclic antidepressants, phenothiazine, diazepam
  - ◊ Ketoconazole (Nizoral®)
  - ◊ Nonsteroidal agents
  - ◊ Spironolactone, methyldopa, digitalis
  - ◊ Phenytoin (Dilantin®)
  - ◊ Cimetidine (Tagamet®)
- Heavy marijuana smoking
- Alcoholism
- Carcinoma of the liver
- Family history
- Thyroid disease: hypo/hyperthyroidism

ASSESSMENT FINDINGS

- Firm, solitary irregular lumps of fat may be attached to underlying skin
- May be unilateral, usually bilateral
- Often tender
- No nipple retraction, increase in pigmentation, ulceration, or nipple discharge
- Testicular size and mass normal considering Tanner staging/Sexual maturity rating
- No thyromegaly, tachycardia, or diaphoresis
- No axillary lymphadenopathy
- No abdominal organomegaly or masses

Gynecomastia may take 1-3 years to regress in adolescent males or may never regress.

DIFFERENTIAL DIAGNOSIS

- Pseudogynecomastia: fatty tissue around breast, no glandular tissue
- Breast cancer
- Obesity
- Cyst
- Neurofibroma

DIAGNOSTIC STUDIES

- None needed for pubertal gynecomastia unless accompanied by abnormalities which demand further evaluation (i.e., breast size > 5 cm, tender mass, recent onset, progressive or unknown duration, signs of malignancy, feminization, signs and symptoms of hyperthyroidism)
- Mammography and/or sonography helpful in differentiating physiological from pathological
- Initial workup: Serum hCG, PSA, LH, testosterone, estradiol levels
- Chest x-ray

PREVENTION

- Education about avoidance of precipitating drugs

MANAGEMENT

- Reassure adolescents of transient nature (< 2 years duration)
- Reassure postpubertal males of negative evaluation and lack of pathology

- Seek exogenous source of estrogen if there is increased nipple pigmentation
- Include breast examination for adolescent males; discuss in matter of fact manner; boys may not raise questions independently

CONSULTATION/REFERRAL

- Endocrinologist if accompanied by abnormal exam findings: TSH, testosterone, estradiol levels
- Surgeon for abnormal breast findings or for subcutaneous mastectomy

FOLLOW-UP

- Evaluate pubertal boys every 3-6 months until resolved

EXPECTED COURSE

- Type 1: should normalize in 2 years or less, but may take up to 3 years
- Type 2: Resolves without treatment
- Type 3: Weight loss can improve gynecomastia
- Drug induced: withdrawal of drug usually results in improvement or resolution

POSSIBLE COMPLICATIONS

- Negative impact on self-image or lifestyle may justify surgical removal

PRECOCIOUS PUBERTY

DESCRIPTION

Premature physical maturation resulting in the appearance of secondary sexual characteristics, accelerated growth, and onset of puberty (before age 7 years in Caucasian girls, 6 years in African-American girls, and before age 9 years in boys). Normal mean age of sexual development in girls is 10 to 13 years, and in boys 11 to 16 years.

ETIOLOGY

- 90% of girls have no underlying pathology
- Boys are often found to have central nervous system disorders (e.g., hamartomas, astrocytomas, or gliomas)
- 50% of male cases are idiopathic
- Exogenous source of estrogen (e.g., child's ingestion of mother's oral contraceptives)

INCIDENCE

- Females > Males
- Some cases are familial
- 1 in 5,000 children in U.S. affected

RISK FACTORS

- Familial precocious puberty
- CNS trauma or inflammation
- CNS tumors and space-occupying lesions
- Congenital adrenal hyperplasia
- Gonadal tumors
- Hypothyroidism

ASSESSMENT FINDINGS

- Progression of sexual development is normal but early development of:
  - ◊ Pubic hair
  - ◊ Axillary hair
  - ◊ Breasts
  - ◊ Testicular enlargement
  - ◊ Rapid onset acne
  - ◊ Body odor
- Sperm and ova are mature resulting in fertility
- Advanced bone age
- Advanced linear growth: child is initially tall for age, then epiphyses close, resulting in eventual short stature
- Increased appetite
- Emotional lability
- Genital maturation
- Leukorrhea

- Vaginal bleeding, menarche

DIFFERENTIAL DIAGNOSIS

- CNS tumors
- CNS trauma
- Exposure to exogenous estrogens
- Acquired hypothyroidism
- Adrenal hyperplasia
- Obesity

- **Adrenarche: presence of pubic hair, typically in girls aged 5-8 years of age**
- **Premature thelarche: isolated precocious development of breast tissue**
- **Pseudoprecocious puberty: due to testicular or ovarian tumor**
- **Premature pubarche: isolated appearance of pubic hair**

DIAGNOSTIC STUDIES

- Tanner staging/Sexual maturity rating
- Chart height, weight and note percentile
- Luteinizing hormone (LH) and follicle stimulating hormone (FSH): present (detectable) in precocious puberty
- Blood testosterone level (boys): elevated
- Blood estradiol level (girls): may be low in early stages, then elevated
- Dehydroepiandrosterone sulfate (DHEA-S): elevated
- TSH to rule out hypothyroidism as etiology
- X-ray of hand and wrist to determine bone age (advanced bone age requires further study because not associated with precocious puberty)
- Skeletal age: advanced osseous maturation
- MRI, CT, pelvic ultrasound, testicular ultrasound to rule out tumors or cysts of ovaries, testicles, or adrenals: enlarged ovaries and uterus and enlarged pituitary gland in precocious puberty

NONPHARMACOLOGIC MANAGEMENT

- Educate:
    - ◊ Greater risk for sexual abuse
    - ◊ Safe storage of oral contraceptives
    - ◊ Effect on peer relationships, body image and sexuality

PHARMACOLOGIC MANAGEMENT

- Administration of gonadotropin-releasing hormone by pediatric endocrinologist
    - ◊ Leuprolide acetate for depot suspension (Lupron Depot-PED®) (intramuscular)

CONSULTATION/REFERRAL

- Referral to pediatric endocrinologist for elimination of cause, or if idiopathic, for administration of gonadotropin-releasing hormone
- Early referral is important to avoid early epiphyseal closure and short stature
- Early referral is also important, especially for boys, because they are more likely to have CNS or other tumors

FOLLOW-UP

- Evaluate every 3 to 6 months
- Drug therapy is discontinued once adequate height is achieved
- Mother's menstrual history is considered when deciding when to let menstruation commence

EXPECTED COURSE

- Sex hormone levels remain suppressed as long as therapy is continued
- Once therapy is discontinued, puberty resumes. Menarche and ovulation appear within a few months
- Drug therapy does not reverse changes that have already occurred:
    - ◊ Breast size will not be reduced
    - ◊ Height will not diminish

POSSIBLE COMPLICATIONS

- Sexual abuse, pregnancy
- Social and psychological ramifications
- Short stature

References

Baskin, H. J., Cobin, R. H., Duick, D. S., Gharib, H., Guttler, R. B., Kaplan, M. M., et al. (2002). American association of clinical endocrinologists medical guidelines for clinical practice for the evaluation and treatment of hyperthyroidism and hypothyroidism. Endocrine Practice, 8(6), 457-469.

Boelaert, K., Torlinska, B., Holder, R. L., & Franklyn, J. A. (2010). Older subjects with hyperthyroidism present with a paucity of symptoms and signs: A large cross-sectional study. Journal of Clinical Endocrinology and Metabolism, 95(6), 2715-2726.

Bolen, S., Feldman, L., Vassy, J., Wilson, L., Yeh, H. C., Marinopoulos, S., et al. (2007). Systematic review: Comparative effectiveness and safety of oral medications for type 2 diabetes mellitus. Annals of Internal Medicine, 147(6), 386-399.

Burke, C. W. (1985). Adrenocortical insufficiency. Clinics in Endocrinology and Metabolism, 14(4), 947-976.

Burns, C. E., Brady, M. A., Blosser, C., Starr, N. B., & Dunn, A. M. (2009). Pediatric primary care (4th ed.). Philadelphia: W.B. Saunders

Buse, J. B., Ginsberg, H. N., Bakris, G. L., Clark, N. G., Costa, F., Eckel, R., et al. (2007). Primary prevention of cardiovascular diseases in people with diabetes mellitus: A scientific statement from the american heart association and the american diabetes association. Circulation, 115(1), 114-126.

Castro, M. R., & Gharib, H. (2005). Continuing controversies in the management of thyroid nodules. Annals of Internal Medicine, 142(11), 926-931.

Cooper, D. S., Doherty, G. M., Haugen, B. R., Kloos, R. T., Lee, S. L., Mandel, S. J., et al. (2009). Revised american thyroid association management guidelines for patients with thyroid nodules and differentiated thyroid cancer. Thyroid, 19(11), 1167-1214.

Cronin, C. C., Callaghan, N., Kearney, P. J., Murnaghan, D. J., & Shanahan, F. (1997). Addison disease in patients treated with glucocorticoid therapy. Archives of Internal Medicine, 157(4), 456-458.

Cryer, P. E., Axelrod, L., Grossman, A. B., Heller, S. R., Montori, V. M., Seaquist, E. R., et al. (2009). Evaluation and management of adult hypoglycemic disorders: An endocrine society clinical practice guideline. Journal of Clinical Endocrinology and Metabolism, 94(3), 709-728.

De Berardis, G., Sacco, M., Evangelista, V., Filippi, A., Giorda, C. B., Tognoni, G., et al. (2007). Aspirin and simvastatin combination for cardiovascular events prevention trial in diabetes (accept-d): Design of a randomized study of the efficacy of low-dose aspirin in the prevention of cardiovascular events in subjects with diabetes mellitus treated with statins. Trials, 8, 21.

Domino, F., Baldor, R., Golding, J., Grimes, J., & Taylor, J. (2011). The 5-minute clinical consult 2011. Philadelphia: Lippincott Williams & Wilkins.

Elamin, M. B., Murad, M. H., Mullan, R., Erickson, D., Harris, K., Nadeem, S., et al. (2008). Accuracy of diagnostic tests for cushing's syndrome: A systematic review and metaanalyses. Journal of Clinical Endocrinology and Metabolism, 93(5), 1553-1562.

Ernst, D., & Lee, A. (2010). Nurse practitioners prescribing reference. New York: Haymarket Media Publication.

Ferri, F. (2010). Ferri's 2010 clinical advisor. Philadelphia: Mosby Elsevier.

Gaede, P., Lund-Andersen, H., Parving, H. H., & Pedersen, O. (2008). Effect of a multifactorial intervention on mortality in type 2 diabetes. New England Journal of Medicine, 358(6), 580-591.

Geffner, D. L., & Hershman, J. M. (1992). Beta-adrenergic blockade for the treatment of hyperthyroidism. American Journal of Medicine, 93(1), 61-68.

Gharib, H., Tuttle, R. M., Baskin, H. J., Fish, L. H., Singer, P. A., & McDermott, M. T. (2005). Subclinical thyroid dysfunction: A joint statement on management from the american association of clinical endocrinologists, the american thyroid association, and the endocrine society. Journal of Clinical Endocrinology and Metabolism, 90(1), 581-585; discussion 586-587.

Haller, M. J., Atkinson, M. A., & Schatz, D. (2005). Type 1 diabetes mellitus: Etiology, presentation, and management. Pediatric Clinics of North America, 52(6), 1553-1578.

Hegedus, L. (2004). Clinical practice. The thyroid nodule. New England Journal of Medicine, 351(17), 1764-1771.

Helfand, M. (2004). Screening for subclinical thyroid dysfunction in nonpregnant adults: A summary of the evidence for the U.S. Preventive services task force. Annals of Internal Medicine, 140(2), 128-141.

Kahn, S. E., Haffner, S. M., Heise, M. A., Herman, W. H., Holman, R. R., Jones, N. P., et al. (2006). Glycemic durability of rosiglitazone, metformin, or glyburide monotherapy. New England Journal of Medicine, 355(23), 2427-2443.

Lania, A., Persani, L., & Beck-Peccoz, P. (2008). Central hypothyroidism. Pituitary, 11(2), 181-186.

Midyett, L. K., Moore, W. V., & Jacobson, J. D. (2003). Are pubertal changes in girls before age 8 benign? Pediatrics, 111(1), 47-51.

Nathan, D. M. (2006). Thiazolidinediones for initial treatment of type 2 diabetes? New England Journal of Medicine, 355(23), 2477-2480.

Nathan, D. M., Buse, J. B., Davidson, M. B., Ferrannini, E., Holman, R. R., Sherwin, R., et al. (2008). Management of hyperglycaemia in type 2 diabetes mellitus: A consensus algorithm for the initiation and adjustment of therapy. Update regarding the thiazolidinediones. Diab tologia, 51(1), 8-11.

Nathan, D. M., Buse, J. B., Davidson, M. B., Ferrannini, E., Holman, R. R., Sherwin, R., et al. (2009). Medical management of hyperglycemia in type 2 diabetes: A consensus algorithm for the initiation and adjustment of therapy: A consensus statement of the american diabetes association and the european association for the study of diabetes. Diabetes Care, 32(1), 193-203.

Nicolucci, A. (2008). Aspirin for primary prevention of cardiovascular events in diabetes: Still an open question. JAMA, 300(18), 2180-2181.

Nieman, L. K., Biller, B. M., Findling, J. W., Newell-Price, J., Savage, M. O., Stewart, P. M., et al. (2008). The diagnosis of cushing's syndrome: An endocrine society clinical practice guideline. Journal of Clinical Endocrinology and Metabolism, 93(5), 1526-1540.

Ogawa, H., Nakayama, M., Morimoto, T., Uemura, S., Kanauchi, M., Doi, N., et al. (2008). Low-dose aspirin for primary prevention of atherosclerotic events in patients with type 2 diabetes: A randomized controlled trial. JAMA, 300(18), 2134-2141.

Paris, C. A., Imperatore, G., Klingensmith, G., Petitti, D., Rodriguez, B., Anderson, A. M., et al. (2009). Predictors of insulin regimens and impact on outcomes in youth with type 1 diabetes: The search for diabetes in youth study. Journal of Pediatrics, 155(2), 183-189 e181.

Phillip, M., Battelino, T., Rodriguez, H., Danne, T., & Kaufman, F. (2007). Use of insulin pump therapy in the pediatric age-group: Consensus statement from the european society for paediatric endocrinology, the lawson wilkins pediatric endocrine society, and the international society for pediatric and adolescent diabetes, endorsed by the american diabetes association and the european association for the study of diabetes. Diabetes Care, 30(6), 1653-1662.

Pignone, M., Alberts, M. J., Colwell, J. A., Cushman, M., Inzucchi, S. E., Mukherjee, D., et al. (2010). Aspirin for primary prevention of cardiovascular events in people with diabetes: A position statement of the american diabetes association, a scientific statement of the american heart association, and an expert consensus document of the american college of cardiology foundation. Diabetes Care, 33(6), 1395-1402.

Rosenstock, J., Ahmann, A. J., Colon, G., Scism-Bacon, J., Jiang, H., & Martin, S. (2008). Advancing insulin therapy in type 2 diabetes previously treated with glargine plus oral agents: Prandial premixed (insulin lispro protamine suspension/lispro) versus basal/bolus (glargine/lispro) therapy. Diabetes Care, 31(1), 20-25.

Samuels, M. H. (2000). Effects of variations in physiological cortisol levels on thyrotropin secretion in subjects with adrenal insufficiency: A clinical research center study. Journal of Clinical Endocrinology and Metabolism, 85(4), 1388-1393.

Screening for thyroid disease: Recommendation statement. (2004). Annals of Internal Medicine, 140(2), 125-127.

Silverstein, J., Klingensmith, G., Copeland, K., Plotnick, L., Kaufman, F., Laffel, L., et al. (2005). Care of children and adolescents with type 1 diabetes: A statement of the american diabetes association. Diabetes Care, 28(1), 186-212.

Singh, S. R., Ahmad, F., Lal, A., Yu, C., Bai, Z., & Bennett, H. (2009). Efficacy and safety of insulin analogues for the management of diabetes mellitus: A meta-analysis. Canadian Medical Association Journal, 180(4), 385-397.

Standards of medical care in diabetes--2010. (2010). Diabetes Care, 33 Suppl 1, S11-61.

Summary of revisions for the 2010 clinical practice recommendations. (2010). Diabetes Care, 33 Suppl 1, S3.

Sun, S. S., Schubert, C. M., Chumlea, W. C., Roche, A. F., Kulin, H. E., Lee, P. A., et al. (2002). National estimates of the timing of sexual maturation and racial differences among us children. Pediatrics, 110(5), 911-919.

Surks, M. I., & Hollowell, J. G. (2007). Age-specific distribution of serum thyrotropin and antithyroid antibodies in the us population: Implications for the prevalence of subclinical hypothyroidism. Journal of Clinical Endocrinology and Metabolism, 92(12), 4575-4582.

Tabak, A. G., Jokela, M., Akbaraly, T. N., Brunner, E. J., Kivimaki, M., & Witte, D. R. (2009). Trajectories of glycaemia, insulin sensitivity, and insulin secretion before diagnosis of type 2 diabetes: An analysis from the whitehall II study. Lancet, 373(9682), 2215-2221.

Tamborlane, W. V., Beck, R. W., Bode, B. W., Buckingham, B., Chase, H. P., Clemons, R., et al. (2008). Continuous glucose monitoring and intensive treatment of type 1 diabetes. New England Journal of Medicine, 359(14), 1464-1476.

Teilmann, G., Pedersen, C. B., Jensen, T. K., Skakkebaek, N. E., & Juul, A. (2005). Prevalence and incidence of precocious pubertal development in denmark: An epidemiologic study based on national registries. Pediatrics, 116(6), 1323-1328.

Trivalle, C., Doucet, J., Chassagne, P., Landrin, I., Kadri, N., Menard, J. F., et al. (1996). Differences in the signs and symptoms of hyperthyroidism in older and younger patients. Journal of the American Geriatrics Society, 44(1), 50-53.

Trzepacz, P. T., Klein, I., Roberts, M., Greenhouse, J., & Levey, G. S. (1989). Graves' disease: An analysis of thyroid hormone levels and hyperthyroid signs and symptoms. American Journal of Medicine, 87(5), 558-561.

Endocrine Disorders

[illegible]

[illegible]

[illegible]

[illegible]

[illegible]

[illegible]

[illegible]

[illegible]

[illegible]

5

GASTROINTESTINAL DISORDERS

Gastrointestinal Disorders

Gastroesophageal Reflux Disease (GERD) 259

Peptic Ulcer Disease (PUD) 263

Acute Gastroenteritis 267

Cholecystitis 270

Viral Hepatitis 274

Diverticulitis 277

Appendicitis 280

Irritable Bowel Syndrome 281

Inflammatory Bowel Disease 285

Crohn's Disease 285

Ulcerative Colitis 287

Constipation 288

Hemorrhoids 293

* Pyloric Stenosis 294

* Hirschsprung's Disease 295

* Intussusception 296

* Colic 297

Pinworms 298

* Encopresis 300

* Recurrent Abdominal Pain 301

References.. *303*

* Denotes pediatric diagnosis

Gastrointestinal Disorders

GASTROINTESTINAL REFLUX DISEASE
(GERD)

DESCRIPTION

Movement of gastrointestinal contents up the esophagus or larynx facilitated by decreased lower esophageal sphincter (LES) tone. Some reflux is physiologic.

INCIDENCE

- Affects up to 1/3 of Americans at some time in their lives
- Affects 81% of patients 60 years of age or older
- Common in pregnant women

RISK FACTORS

- Factors which may reduce LES tone:
  - ◊ Alcohol
  - ◊ Anticholinergic medications
  - ◊ Calcium channel blockers
  - ◊ Chocolate, peppermint
  - ◊ Fatty foods
  - ◊ Hormones: estrogen, progesterone, glucagon, secretin
  - ◊ Pregnancy
  - ◊ Meperidine
  - ◊ Nicotine
  - ◊ Theophylline
- Aging
- Zenker's diverticulum
- Irritation of esophageal mucosa by:
  - ◊ NSAIDs
  - ◊ Tetracycline
  - ◊ Quinidine
  - ◊ Caffeine
- Increased gastric acid secretion: acidic foods
- Delay in gastric emptying: fatty foods
- Zollinger-Ellison syndrome
- Obesity
- Diabetes mellitus, diabetic gastroparesis

ASSESSMENT FINDINGS

- Pyrosis (heartburn) is cardinal symptom, burning beneath sternum, typically postprandial and nocturnal
- Regurgitation, ("sour, hot"): 60%
- Chest pain: 33%
- Dysphagia (present in long standing heartburn): 15-20%
- Esophageal pain referred to neck, mid-back, and upper abdomen
- Chronic cough
- Chronic sore throat/hoarseness
- Erosion of teeth by acid
- Ulceration: hematemesis, fatigue, anemia
- Barrett's esophagitis (small number of patients): replacement of the squamous epithelium of the esophagus by columnar epithelium, which may be further complicated by adenocarcinoma in 2-5% of cases

DIFFERENTIAL DIAGNOSIS

- Cardiac disease
- Esophageal spasm or infection
- Cholelithiasis
- Peptic ulcer disease
- Lower respiratory infection: bronchitis, pneumonia
- Asthma
- Pulmonary edema

DIAGNOSTIC STUDIES

- Patient with one episode of heartburn that responds well to nonpharmacologic and acid suppressant therapy may require no further investigation
- Endoscopy necessary for patients with GERD symptoms who have not responded to empirical trial of PPI therapy
- Endoscopy with biopsy necessary at presentation for patients with esophageal GERD syndrome with troublesome dysphagia
- Manometry: motility test to determine LES and esophageal function
- Ambulatory esophageal pH testing to detect pathologic reflux
- Endoscopy to observe effects of esophagitis and obtain biopsy for histology
- 50% of symptomatic patients have NERD (nonerosive reflux disease)

NONPHARMACOLOGIC MANAGEMENT

- Education: physical causes of GERD, common aggravating and ameliorating factors, and lifestyle changes to control GERD:
  - ◊ Avoid recumbence until 2 hours after meals
  - ◊ Elevate head of bed, including entire chest
  - ◊ Reduce size of meals and amount of fat, acid, spices, caffeine, and sweets
  - ◊ Smoking cessation
  - ◊ Reduce alcohol consumption
  - ◊ Lose weight if indicated
  - ◊ Avoid stooping, bending after meals and tight fitting garments
- Surgical interventions, crural tightening or fundoplication, reserved for patient with stricture, hemorrhage, Barrett's esophagitis, chronic aspiration or intractable symptoms

GASTROESOPHAGEAL REFLUX DISEASE PHARMACOLOGIC MANAGEMENT

Class	Drug Generic name (Trade name®)	Dosage How supplied	Comments
Antacids *Neutralizes hydrochloric acid in the stomach to rapidly cause pH to rise* **General comments** Blocks absorption of many drugs: digoxin, tetracyclines, benzodiazepines, iron and others	**calcium carbonate** *Tums* *Various generics*	**Adults**: chew 2-4 tabs as symptoms occur *Max*: 15 tablets in 24 hours **Children**: not recommended *Tabs: 200 mg* *Packs of 12, 36, 75, 150 tablets*	• Pregnancy Category C • Do not use maximum dosage for more than 2 weeks • FDA has not evaluated and approved this OTC product for reflux • Produces rapid relief of heartburn symptoms • Use with caution in patients with CHF, renal failure, edema, cirrhosis
H2 antagonists *Inhibit gastric acid secredtion by inhibiting H2 receptors of the gastric parietal cells* **General comments** Symptomatic response to therapy does not preclude gastric malignancy Onset of antisecretory action is about 1 hour with inhibition of secretion for 10-12 hours	**cimetidine** Tagamet	**Adult and children > 16 years:** *Initial*: 800 mg two times daily for 12 weeks *Alternative*: 400 mg 4 times daily for 12 weeks *Max*: 12 weeks **Children < 16 yr:** not recommended *Tabs: 300 mg, 400 mg*	• Pregnancy Category B • Cimetidine associated with many 3A4 drug interactions • Long term therapy may be associated with B_{12} deficiency • May take several days for relief to occur • Allow one hour between H_2 blocker and antacid consumption • Dose adjustment needed for renal and hepatic impairment
	ranitidine	**Adult**: 150 mg twice daily *Max*: 6 grams in hypersecretory conditions **Children ≥ 1 mo-16 yr:** 5-10 mg/kg/day in 2 divided doses *Max*: 300 mg/day	• Pregnancy Category B • Efferdose is 25 mg. Dissolve in (no less than) 5 mL water. Do not chew, swallow whole or dissolve on the tongue • Contains phenylalanine • Potential drug interactions with procainamide, warfarin, glipizide and others • Dose adjustment needed for renal and hepatic impairment • No dosage adjustment needed for geriatric patients

continued

GASTROESOPHAGEAL REFLUX DISEASE PHARMACOLOGIC MANAGEMENT

Class	Drug Generic name (Trade name®)	Dosage How supplied	Comments
	Zantac	*Tabs: 150 mg, 300 mg* *Efferdose: 25 mg effervescent tabs* *Syrup: 15 mg/mL*	
	famotidine	**Adults**: *With symptoms of GERD*: 20 mg twice daily for up to 6 weeks *Treatment of esophagitis due to GERD*: 20 or 40 mg twice daily for up to 12 weeks **Children 1-6 yr:** *Initial*: 1 mg/kg/day divided in 2 doses *Max*: 40 mg daily	• Pregnancy Category B • 20 mg twice daily was superior to 40 mg at bedtime for improvement of symptoms • No drug interactions have been identified • No dosage adjustment needed for geriatric patients • Dose adjustment needed for renal and hepatic impairment
	Pepcid	*Tabs: 20 mg, 40 mg* *Susp: 40 mg/5 mL*	
Proton Pump Inhibitors *Potently suppress gastric acid secretion by inhibiting the hydrogen/potassium pump in gastric parietal cells*	**dexlansoprazole**	**Adult ≥ 18 years**: GERD 30 mg daily for 4 weeks	• Pregnancy Category B • Take without regard to food • NO dosage adjustment is necessary for geriatric patients or renal impairment • Dosage adjustment needed for hepatic impairment
	Dexilant	*Tabs: 30 mg, 60 mg*	
<u>**General comments**</u> Therapy > 3 years may lead to B12 malabsorption Take at same time each day Usually best if taken before a meal when hydrogen/potassium pumps are most active Symptomatic response does not preclude the presence of gastric malignancy May interfere with drugs for which gastric pH affects bioavailability PPI may be associated with an increased risk of osteoporosis related fractures of the hip, wrist or spine. Use lowest dose and shortest duration of PPI appropriate for the patient's condition	**esomeprazole**	**Adult**: 20-40 mg once daily for 4-8 weeks **Children 1-11 years**: 10-20 mg once daily for up to 8 weeks **12-17 years**: 20 mg or 40 mg once daily for up to 8 weeks	• Pregnancy Category B • May affect plasma levels of antiretroviral drugs • No dosage adjustment needed for renal or hepatic insufficiency
	Nexium	*Caps: 20 mg, 40 mg e-c delayed release* *Susp: 20 mg, 40 mg per packet*	
	lansoprazole	*Short term treatment of symptomatic GERD:* > 30 kg: 30 mg once daily for up to 12 weeks	
	Prevacid	*Caps: 15 mg, 30 mg* *Solutabs: 15 mg, 30 mg* *Oral Susp packets: 15 mg, 30 mg*	

continued

GASTROESOPHAGEAL REFLUX DISEASE PHARMACOLOGIC MANAGEMENT

Class	Drug Generic name (Trade name®)	Dosage How supplied	Comments
Daily treatment longer than 3 years may lead to malabsorption of Vitamin B12. Consider this diagnosis if clinical symptoms occur	**omeprazole**	**Adults**: 20 mg up to 4 weeks *If esophagitis accompanies GERD:* 20 mg daily for 4-8 weeks **Children**: > 20 kg: 20 mg once daily 10-20 kg: 10 mg once daily 5-10 kg: 5 mg once daily	• Pregnancy Category C • Possible drug interactions with antiretroviral therapy, diazepam, warfarin, phenytoin and others • No dosage adjustment necessary in the elderly or with renal impairment • Dosage adjustment needed for hepatic impairment
	Prilosec	*Caps: 10 mg, 20 mg, 40 mg* *Oral susp packets: 2.5 mg, 10 mg*	
	pantoprazole	For short-term treatment of erosive esophagitis associated with GERD: **Adults**: 40 mg once daily for up to 8 weeks **Children 5 years and older:** > 15 to < 40 kg: 20 mg once daily for up to 8 weeks **5 years and older:** > 40 kg: 40 mg once daily for up to 8 weeks	• Pregnancy Category B • Possible drug interactions with antiretroviral therapy, diazepam, warfarin, phenytoin and others • No dosage adjustment necessary in the elderly
	Protonix	*Del. Rel. Tabs: 20 mg, 40 mg* *Susp: 40 mg/packet*	

CONSULTATION/REFERRAL

- Cardiologist: severe chest pain, radiating pain
- Gastroenterologist:
  - ◊ Dysphagia
  - ◊ Unexplained weight loss
  - ◊ Vomiting
  - ◊ GI bleeding
  - ◊ Anemia
  - ◊ Palpable abdominal mass
  - ◊ Recurrent or refractory symptoms
  - ◊ Long history of alcohol and/or nicotine abuse
  - ◊ Regular NSAID use

FOLLOW-UP

- CBC
- Screen for B12 deficiency after long-term PPI use
- Barrett's esophagitis: endoscopy and biopsy every 1 to 2 years

EXPECTED COURSE

- Most patients respond well to combined nonpharmacologic and pharmacologic therapies, but symptoms return once medication is withdrawn

POSSIBLE COMPLICATIONS

- Ulceration
- Stricture
- Barrett's esophagitis
- High-grade dysplasia
- Esophageal adenocarcinoma
- Aspiration pneumonia

PEPTIC ULCER DISEASE
(PUD)

DESCRIPTION

An ulceration involving the stomach or the duodenum. This is a common problem.

ETIOLOGY

- *Helicobacter pylori* infection: bacteria attach to gastric epithelial cells and secrete enzymes which break down the mucous layer
- NSAID-related ulcers: NSAID use results in the inhibition of prostaglandin synthesis
- Zollinger-Ellison syndrome: tumors in the walls of the pancreas or intestines secrete high levels of gastrin

INCIDENCE

- Uncommon before puberty; incidence increases with age
- 1-2% of U.S. population
- Duodenal ulcer 4 times more common than gastric ulcer

RISK FACTORS

- NSAID use, especially multiple NSAIDs at high doses
- Concomitant use of NSAIDs and systemic corticosteroids
- Cigarette smoking
- Excess alcohol
- Stress
- Previous ulcer disease
- *H. pylori* infection
- Age > 60 years

ASSESSMENT FINDINGS

- Duodenal ulcer:
  - ◊ Burning epigastric pain awakens patient early morning and is relieved by food and antacids
- Gastric ulcer:
  - ◊ Nausea and vomiting
  - ◊ Pain exacerbated by eating
  - ◊ Early satiety
- Acute GI hemorrhage:
  - ◊ Coffee ground emesis
  - ◊ Tarry, black, or bloody stools
- Iron deficiency anemia due to occult blood loss
- Epigastric tenderness
- Perforation: board-like abdomen with rebound tenderness

DIFFERENTIAL DIAGNOSIS

- Gastroesophageal reflux disease (GERD)
- Gastric carcinoma
- Drug induced dyspepsia (coffee, theophylline, digitalis)
- Myocardial infarction, cardiac disease
- Esophageal spasm
- Cholelithiasis
- Lower respiratory infection
- Pancreatitis

DIAGNOSTIC STUDIES

- CBC, metabolic panel (to help identify patients with "alarm" symptoms (e.g., anemia, elevated liver enzymes)
- *H. pylori* serologic antibody measurement
- Endoscopy for direct visualization
- Double contrast barium radiography of the upper gastrointestinal system: ulcer appears as discrete crater
- Urea breath test, biopsy for H. pylori
- Serum gastrin: elevated in Zollinger-Ellison syndrome

PREVENTION

- Eradicate *H. pylori*
- Attempt alternative therapeutics to avoid long-term NSAID use
- Use lowest dose of NSAID that is effective
- Concomitant use of NSAID and misoprostol (Cytotec®) or proton pump inhibitor

NONPHARMACOLOGIC MANAGEMENT

- Avoid cigarette smoking, caffeine, and any foods that exacerbate symptoms
- Lifestyle modifications
- Surgery (vagotomy or gastroduodenal anastomosis) reserved for ulcers resistant to medical treatment

PHARMACOLOGIC MANAGEMENT

- Based on etiology

NSAID-related ulcers:
- Misoprostol (Cytotec®) or proton pump inhibitor (PPI) use along with NSAID: preventive for both duodenal and gastric NSAID-related ulcer complications (e.g., perforation)
- Treat NSAID-related duodenal ulcers for 4-12 weeks with PPI
- Discontinue NSAID if possible
- Consider COX-2 inhibitor

H. pylori-related ulcer:
- Quadruple therapy for 2 weeks
    - 98% eradication rate
    - PPI plus 2 antibiotics; clarithromycin and amoxicillin (alternatives are tetracycline, metronidazole, rifampin)
- Single antibiotic regimens discouraged

Zollinger-Ellison syndrome:
- Proton pump inhibitors
- Surgical correction if pharmacologic therapy fails
    - Definitive therapy is removal of gastrinoma
    - Vagotomy to reduce acid secretion
    - Parathyroidectomy if Zollinger-Ellison syndrome is associated with multiple endocrine neoplasia type 1 (MEN1)

PEPTIC ULCER DISEASE PHARMACOLOGIC MANAGEMENT

Class	Drug Generic name (Trade name®)	Dosage How supplied	Comments
Prostaglandins *Have antisecretory and mucosal protective properties. Increases bicarbonate and mucus production in the stomach*	**misoprostol** Cytotec	**Adults**: 200 mcg 4 times daily with food *Alternate*: 100 mcg 4 times daily with food *Tabs: 100 mcg, 200 mcg*	• Pregnancy Category X • When using in women of childbearing age, misoprostol may be prescribed if she has had a negative pregnancy test 2 weeks prior to beginning therapy, has contraceptive measures in place, and has received oral and written warnings about misoprostol. Begin on the second or third day of the next menses. • No dosage adjustment needed for elderly patients or renal impairment

continued

PEPTIC ULCER DISEASE PHARMACOLOGIC MANAGEMENT

Class	Drug Generic name (Trade name®)	Dosage How supplied	Comments
Proton Pump Inhibitors *Potently suppress gastric acid secretion by inhibiting the hydrogen/potassium pump in gastric parietal cells* General comments Therapy > 3 years may lead to B12 malabsorption Take at same time each day Usually best if taken before a meal when hydrogen/potassium pumps are most active Symptomatic response does not preclude the presence of gastric malignancy May interfere with drugs for which gastric pH affects bioavailability PPI may be associated with an increased risk of osteoporosis related fractures of the hip, wrist, or spine. Use lowest dose and shortest duration of PPI appropriate for the patient's condition Daily treatment longer than 3 years may lead to malabsorption of Vitamin B12 Consider this diagnosis if clinical symptoms occur	**dexlansoprazole**	**Adult ≥ 18 years**: 30 mg daily for 4 weeks	• Pregnancy Category B • Take without regard to food • No dosage adjustment is necessary for geriatric patients or renal impairment • Dosage adjustment needed for hepatic impairment
	Dexilant	*Tabs: 30 mg, 60 mg*	
	esomeprazole	**Adult**: 20-40 mg once daily for 4-8 weeks **Children 1-11 years**: 10-20 mg once daily for up to 8 weeks **12-17 years**: 20 mg or 40 mg once daily for up to 8 weeks	• Pregnancy Category B • May affect plasma levels of antiretroviral drugs • No dosage adjustment needed for renal or hepatic insufficiency
	Nexium	*Caps: 20 mg, 40 mg e-c delayed release* *Susp: 20 mg, 40 mg per packet*	
	omeprazole	**Adults**: 20 mg up to 4 weeks **Children**: > 20 kg: 20 mg once daily 10-20 kg: 10 mg 5-10 kg: 5 mg	• Pregnancy Category B • Possible drug interactions with antiretroviral therapy, diazepam, warfarin, phenytoin and others • No dosage adjustment needed in the elderly or with renal impairment • Dosage adjustment needed for hepatic impairment
	Prilosec	*Caps: 10 mg, 20 mg, 40 mg* *Oral Susp: 2.5 mg, 10 mg*	
	pantoprazole	**Adults**: 40 mg once daily for up to 8 weeks **Children 5 years and older:** > 15 to < 40 kg: 20 mg once daily for up to 8 weeks 5 years and older: > 40 kg: 40 mg once daily for up to 8 weeks	• Pregnancy Category B • Possible drug interactions with antiretroviral therapy, diazepam, warfarin, phenytoin and others • No dosage adjustment needed in the elderly or with renal impairment
	Protonix	*Delayed release tabs: 20 mg, 40 mg* *Susp: 40 mg/packet*	

H. pylori Regimens (examples)	
PPI Based Treatments	Nexium® triple therapy (esomeprazole 40 mg daily, amoxicillin 1000 mg twice daily and clarithromycin 500 mg twice daily) for 10 days Prevacid® triple therapy (lansoprazole 30 mg twice daily, amoxicillin 1000 mg twice daily and clarithromycin 500 mg daily) for 10-14 days Prilosec® triple therapy (omeprazole 20 mg twice daily, amoxicillin 1000 mg twice daily and clarithromycin 500 mg daily) for 10 days

H. pylori Regimens (examples)	
H2 Receptor Based Treatments	Axid® triple therapy (nizatidine 300 mg at bedtime with any antibiotic combination) for 14 days Pepcid® triple therapy (famotidine 40 mg at bedtime with any antibiotic combination) for 14 days Tagamet® triple therapy (cimetidine 800 mg at bedtime with any antibiotic combination) x 14 days

CONSULTATION/REFERRAL

- Refer patients with Zollinger-Ellison syndrome to gastroenterologist
- Refer patients who have failed treatment to gastroenterologist

FOLLOW-UP

- Monitor clinical response of duodenal ulcer
- Confirmation of eradication of *H. pylori* is by *H. pylori* stool antigen test, CLO test biopsy, or urea breath test (serology is limited in usefulness due to the persistence of antibodies for years after successful treatment)
- Gastric ulcer: endoscopy with cytology and biopsy to confirm healing at 6 to 12 weeks
- Symptom improvement does not imply absence of malignancy

EXPECTED COURSE

- Recurrence of *H. pylori* infection is rare (< 1%), but possible with a positive response to *H. pylori* therapy
- NSAID-related gastric ulcers may require months of therapy
- Zollinger-Ellison syndrome: complete surgical removal of gastrinoma cures 25% of patients

POSSIBLE COMPLICATIONS

- Hemorrhage
- Perforation
- Gastric outlet obstruction

ACUTE GASTROENTERITIS
(AGE)

DESCRIPTION

Acute infection causing inflammation of the stomach and intestinal lining resulting in vomiting, diarrhea, and fever.

ETIOLOGY

- Infection is by the fecal-oral route, and possibly by the respiratory route
- Pathogens invade the intestinal mucosa, resulting in a decreased area available for fluid absorption
- Viruses (most common), bacteria, and parasites are responsible
- Most infections in healthy hosts in the U.S. are viral
    - ◊ Rotavirus is most common pathogen in age < 1 year, but found in adults too
    - ◊ The other 3 most common pathogens in adults are: norovirus, enteric adenovirus and astrovirus
- Bacterial infections are less common, but usually more severe
    - ◊ *Campylobacter jejuni* most common bacterial pathogen in children
    - ◊ *Salmonella* most common cause of food-borne illness in the U.S.
    - ◊ Other common pathogens: *Shigella, Escherichia coli, Yersinia enterocolitica, Clostridium difficile*
- Parasitic
    - ◊ *Giardia lamblia* most common parasitic agent in U.S.

INCIDENCE

- Common in all ages
- Incidence is decreasing in U.S.

RISK FACTORS

- Improper handwashing and food preparation
- Day care center attendance
- Recent use of antibiotics (*C. difficile* common)
- Lack of sanitation
- Immunocompromised status
- Recent travel to developing countries

ASSESSMENT FINDINGS

- Hyperactive bowel sounds
- Diarrhea (3 or more loose stools in 24 hours)
- Blood in stool
- White cells in the stool (common with *Salmonella, Shigella, Campylobacter)*
- Nausea and vomiting usually precede diarrhea
- Anorexia
- Fever
- Tenesmus (a strong urge to defecate caused by an anal sphincter spasm)
- Abdominal cramps
- Dehydration
    - ◊ Poor skin turgor
    - ◊ Dry mucous membranes
    - ◊ Flattened or sunken fontanels
    - ◊ Tachycardia, tachypnea
    - ◊ Oliguria
- Lethargy
- Pale skin color

Assessment Findings in Volume Depleted Infants and Children			
Finding	**Mild**	**Moderate**	**Severe**
Anterior Fontanelle	Normal	Sunken	Markedly sunken
Eyes	Normal	Sunken	Markedly sunken
Skin Appearance	Normal	Cool	Cool, mottled
Turgor	Normal	Reduced	Tenting present
Urine Output	Mildly reduced	Markedly reduced	Little to no urine output
Pulse	Normal	Increased	Increased and weak
Physical Signs	Thirsty	Listless	Lethargic

DIFFERENTIAL DIAGNOSIS

- Viral, bacterial, or parasitic infection
- Inflammatory bowel disease
- Medication/food intolerances
- Appendicitis
- Irritable bowel syndrome
- Fecal impaction

CHARACTERISTICS OF COMMON GI INFECTIONS			
AGENT	**ONSET**	**SIGNS/SYMPTOMS**	**COMMENTS**
S. aureus	30 min to 6 hrs	Nausea, vomiting, cramps, soft stool	Creamy food is common source (egg salad, cream filled pastries), undercooked poultry
Salmonella	6-72 hrs	Nausea, vomiting, cramps, bloody stool, WBCs in stool	Undercooked poultry, red meats, Contaminated pets, turtles, reportable
Shigella	Usually 2-4 days	Abdominal pain, fever, watery diarrhea, WBCs in stool	Fecal-oral route; homosexual transmission, reportable
E. coli	10 hrs to 6 days	Cramps, no fever, watery diarrhea	Causative agent of Traveler's diarrhea, contaminated water/food are common sources
Campylobacter	1-7 days	Nausea, vomiting, fever, abdominal pain, watery, bloody diarrhea, WBCs in stool	Causative agent is undercooked poultry, unpasteurized milk, contaminated H_2O
Giardia (Protozoan)	1-4 weeks	Foul smelling stools, abdominal pain, flatulence	Spread by fecal-oral route, contaminated H_2O is a common source
C. difficile	Observed after antibiotic usage, commonly fluoroquinolones and clindamycin	Fever, leukocytosis, bloody, watery diarrhea, cramps, WBCs in stool	Discontinue antibiotics if possible, rehydrate aggressively; tissue culture most sensitive for diagnosis

DIAGNOSTIC STUDIES

- Usually none necessary unless symptoms are severe and last > 48 hours
- Stool for WBC: rare scattered leukocytes are normal; may suggest Crohn's disease, ulcerative colitis, ischemic colitis, *Shigella, Salmonella, Campylobacter*
- Stool cultures: *Shigella, Salmonella, Campylobacter, E. coli* commonly identified
- Blood or mucus present in stool
- Stool for ova and parasites
- Urinalysis, culture, and sensitivity
- In infants and elderly consider assessment for dehydration: BUN, specific gravity, electrolytes

PREVENTION

- Hygiene
- Avoidance of risk factors
- *Shigella*: culture all symptomatic contacts and treat those with positive stool cultures; report to local health department

NONPHARMACOLOGIC MANAGEMENT

- Correct dehydration, orally if possible
- Mild dehydration (3-5% volume loss): 50 mL/kg or 5 teaspoons per pound over 4 hours
- Moderate dehydration (6-9% volume loss): 100 mL/kg or 10 teaspoons/pound over 4 hours
- Rehydrating with soft drinks, gelatin, and apple juice is not advisable due to the high carbohydrate, low electrolyte composition; commercially prepared rehydration products help avoid this problem: Pedialyte®, CeraLyte®, Infalyte®
- Age appropriate diet as soon as possible
- Reintroduce solid foods within 24 hours of onset of diarrhea
- BRAT diet no longer recommended because it provides inadequate protein, fat, and calories
- May develop temporary lactose intolerance
- Monitor oral intake, urine output, and bowel movements; count wet diapers

GASTROENTERITIS PHARMACOLOGIC MANAGEMENT

Class	Drug Generic name (Trade name®)	Dosage How supplied	Comments
Antiemetic *Mechanism of action is unknown but thought to work in the medulla oblongata through which emetic impulses are conveyed to the vomiting center*	**promethazine**	**Adults**: 12.5-25 mg every 4-6 hours as needed **Children ≥ 2 years:** 0.5 mg/kg at 4-6 hour intervals *Max*: 25 mg	• **May cause fatal respiratory depression in children. Do not use under 2 years of age** • Pregnancy Category C • Cautious use in a dehydrated patient
	Phenergan	*Tabs: 12.5 mg, 25 mg, 50 mg* *Suppositories: 12.5 mg, 25 mg, 50 mg*	• Cautious use in sleep apnea asthma, lower respiratory disorders, seizure disorders, glaucoma, GI or urinary obstruction • Potentiates CNS depression • If given IM, must be a deep IM injection
	trimethobenzamide	**Adult**: 300 mg 3-4 times daily **Children**: not recommended	• Safety in pregnancy not established • Cautious use in a dehydrated patient
	Tigan	*Caps: 300 mg* *Injectable: 100 mg/mL*	• Cautious use in sleep apnea, asthma, lower respiratory disorders, seizure disorders, glaucoma, GI or urinary obstruction • Potentiates CNS depression • Consider reducing dose in renal impairment and geriatric patients

PHARMACOLOGIC MANAGEMENT

Use of antidiarrheal agents is discouraged; the offending agent must be excreted.

Organism	Treatment
S. aureus	Antibiotics not recommended
Salmonella	Antibiotics not recommended because it prolongs carrier state by slowing excretion of organisms. Treatment recommended (Bactrim® or ciprofloxacin) for patients with valvular heart disease, immunocompromised states
Shigella	Bactrim® bid for 3-5 days; If acquired outside U.S., ciprofloxacin for 10 days
E. coli	Bactrim® bid for 3 days; may use ciprofloxacin (Cipro®) in adults
Campylobacter	Erythromycin qid for 5 days or Cipro® bid for 7 days
Giardia (Protozoan)	Metronidazole tid for 5 days
C. difficile	Metronidazole 3-4 daily for 10-14 days, Questran® for diarrhea

PREGNANCY/LACTATION CONSIDERATIONS

- Antibiotics indicated when there is a bacterial pathogen identified
- Refer if there is dehydration, intractable symptoms, or bloody diarrhea

CONSULTATION/REFERRAL

- Parenteral rehydration for intractable symptoms, extremes in age, or shock
- Neurologic symptoms
- Severe abdominal pain

FOLLOW-UP

- Telephone contact within 24 hours, 3 days

EXPECTED COURSE

- Both viral and bacterial gastroenteritis is usually self-limiting and resolves without medication in 5 days unless patient is at age extremes or immunocompromised
- Salmonella infection: diarrhea may continue for up to 2 weeks

POSSIBLE COMPLICATIONS

- Cardiovascular collapse from dehydration and acidosis
- Colonic perforation/septicemia
- Carrier state

CHOLECYSTITIS

DESCRIPTION

Inflammation of the gallbladder usually associated with gallstone disease; can be acute or chronic.

ETIOLOGY

- Gallstone obstruction of the gallbladder-cystic duct junction results in inflammation (90-95%) and acute pain
- In a small number of cases, gallbladder inflammation occurs without stone formation
- Obstruction of common bile duct can cause jaundice, light colored stools, and biliary colic
- Obstruction of pancreatic duct can produce pancreatitis, pain over the upper abdomen, nausea and vomiting
- Gallbladder sludge

Test	Classic	with Bile Duct Obstruction	with Pancreatitis
CBC	Mild leukocytosis	Leukocytosis	Leukocytosis
Bilirubin	Normal or Mild elevation	Elevated	Elevated
Amylase	Normal	Usually Elevated	Elevated
LFTs	Slightly elevated	Normal	Elevated
ALP	Normal	Elevated	Normal
GGT	Normal	Elevated	Normal

INCIDENCE

- Increases with age and BMI; most common in ages 50 to 70 years
- Females > Males (2:1)
- Very common in Native Americans

RISK FACTORS

- Pregnancy
- Rapid weight loss
- Obesity
- Gallstones
- Surgery or trauma
- Sickle cell anemia
- Parenteral alimentation over prolonged period

ASSESSMENT FINDINGS

- Patients are usually ill-appearing, febrile and tachycardic
- Murphy's sign: inspiratory arrest with deep palpation of right upper quadrant (RUQ) (classic sign)
- RUQ pain, may be unremitting, with or without rebound pain, may radiate to right shoulder or subscapular area
- Nausea and vomiting/anorexia
- Attack follows meal (especially high in fat) by 1-6 hours
- Low grade fever
- Palpable RUQ mass

A patient with acute cholecystitis usually lies very still because peritoneal inflammation is present and worsens with movement.

DIFFERENTIAL DIAGNOSIS

- Peptic ulcer disease
- Cardiac disease
- Pancreatitis
- Hepatitis
- Bowel obstruction
- Appendicitis

Fatty food intolerance that produces pain, belching, or pain a few minutes after eating is NOT typical of gallbladder disease.

DIAGNOSTIC STUDIES

- Ultrasound is most sensitive and specific test to diagnose cholecystitis
- Ultrasound demonstrates presence of gallstones, thickening of wall of gallbladder (4-5 mm), fluid, and enlargement
- HIDA scan helpful if ultrasound is negative but patient is suspected of having cholecystitis (Positive scan demonstrates gallbladder disease if the gallbladder is unable to be visualized due to cystic duct obstruction)
- Endoscopic retrograde cholangiopancreatography (ERCP) used to see biliary and pancreatic ducts to detect common bile duct stones

A HIDA scan (cholescintigraphy) is indicated if the diagnosis of gallbladder disease is still considered and the ultrasound is negative.

PREVENTION

- Avoid risk factors
- During parenteral feeding, administer cholestyramine (Questran®) daily

NONPHARMACOLOGIC MANAGEMENT

- Severe attacks: nothing by mouth
- Mild attacks: avoid fatty meals
- Nasogastric tube for persistent nausea or abdominal distention
- Laparoscopic or open cholecystectomy within 72 hours of diagnosis

CHOLECYSTITIS PHARMACOLOGIC MANAGEMENT

Class	Drug Generic name (Trade name®)	Dosage How supplied	Comments
Endogenous bile acids *Dissolution of radiolucent, noncalcified gallstones < 20 mm in diameter for patient who refuse cholecystectomy or who are at risk during cholecystectomy*	**bile acid** Actigall	8-10 mg/kg per day in 2-3 divided doses Prevention: 300 mg twice daily *Caps: 300 mg*	• Pregnancy Category B • Not for calcified, radio-opaque or radiolucent bile pigment stones • Obtain sonogram at 6 and 12 months • After complete dissolution repeat sonogram in 1-3 months, then discontinue • Used to prevent gallstone formation in patients undergoing rapid weight loss • Measure liver enzymes at 1 and 3 months then every 6 months while taking
	bile acid Urso forte	**Adults**: 13-15 mg/kg per day in 2-4 divided doses *Tabs: 250 mg, 500 mg scored*	• Pregnancy Category B • Take with food • Reduced absorption with bile acid sequestrants and aluminum containing antacids • Not for calcified, radio-opaque or radiolucent bile pigment stones • Obtain sonogram at 6 and 12 months • After complete dissolution repeat sonogram in 1-3 months, then discontinue • Used to prevent gallstone formation in patients undergoing rapid weight loss • Measure liver enzymes at 1 and 3 months then every 6 months while taking
Antiemetic *Mechanism of action is unknown but thought to work in the medulla oblongata through which emetic impulses are conveyed to the vomiting center*	**promethazine** Phenergan	**Adults**: 12.5-25 mg every 4-6 hours as needed **Children ≥ 2 years:** 0.5 mg/kg at 4-6 hour intervals *Max*: 25 mg *Tabs: 12.5 mg, 25 mg, 50 mg* *Suppositories: 12.5 mg, 25 mg, 50 mg*	• **May cause fatal respiratory depression in children. Do not use under 2 years of age** • Pregnancy Category C • Cautious use in a dehydrated patient • Cautious use in sleep apnea, asthma, lower respiratory disorders, seizure disorders, glaucoma, GI or urinary obstruction • Potentiates CNS depression • If given IM, must be a deep IM injection

continued

CHOLECYSTITIS PHARMACOLOGIC MANAGEMENT

Class	Drug Generic name (Trade name®)	Dosage How supplied	Comments
	trimethobenzamide Tigan	**Adult**: 300 mg 3-4 times daily **Children**: not recommended *Caps: 300 mg* *Injectable: 100 mg/mL*	• Safety in pregnancy not established • Cautious use in a dehydrated patient • Cautious use in sleep apnea, asthma, lower respiratory disorders, seizure disorders, glaucoma, GI or urinary obstruction • Potentiates CNS depression • Consider reducing dose in renal impairment and geriatric patients

CONSULTATION/REFERRAL

- Outpatient if symptoms mild
- Surgeon if biliary colic > 6 hours, toxic appearing, or intractable pain

FOLLOW-UP

- Throughout postoperative period

EXPECTED COURSE

- Stones may recur in bile ducts after cholecystectomy

POSSIBLE COMPLICATIONS

- Empyema of the gallbladder: bacterial invasion of the gallbladder
- Emphysematous cholecystitis: infection with a gas-forming bacteria
- Perforation: requires aggressive fluid replacement, antibiotics and emergency surgical exploration
- Cholecystenteric fistula: gallbladder perforates into duodenum or colon; should be treated as a bowel obstruction with fluid replacement, nasogastric suction, and surgical exploration

VIRAL HEPATITIS

DESCRIPTION

Viral infection affecting the liver. Five viral agents with different antigenic properties are known to be responsible, all causing illnesses that are clinically similar, with various degrees of severity. Hepatitis B, C, and D can cause chronic infections.

ETIOLOGY

Hepatitis Type	Mode of Transmission
Hepatitis A (HAV)	Contaminated food - H_2O, fecal-oral route
Hepatitis B (HBV)	Blood borne/body fluids
Hepatitis C (HCV)	Blood borne
Hepatitis D (HDV)	Blood borne/body fluids
Hepatitis E (HEV)	Fecal-oral

Hepatitis D virus (HDV) is transmitted only after infection with HBV.

Hepatitis Type	Incubation Period
A	2-7 weeks
B	6-23 weeks
C	2-26 weeks
D	2-8 weeks
E	2-9 weeks

INCIDENCE

HAV:
- Occurrence increases with age; rare in infants due to maternal antibodies
- More common in temperate climates; occurs most often in late fall and early winter
- 33% of Americans have antibodies

HBV:
- Endemic areas are Alaska, Southeast Asia, Pacific Islands, Africa
- Perinatal transmission to newborns is 80%

HCV:
- Most common cause of both acute and chronic viral hepatitis
- Accounts for 43% of cases of new hepatitis in the U.S.

HDV:
- 5% of those infected with HBV are also infected with HDV

HEV:
- Sporadic incidence in Asia, Africa, and Central America

RISK FACTORS

HAV and HEV:
- Travel to endemic areas
- Ingestion of contaminated food, water, milk, or shellfish
- Men who have sex with men
- Crowded living conditions
- Lower socioeconomic status

HBV:
- Injecting drug use
- Men who have sex with men
- Engaging in sexual activity with multiple partners
- Health care workers
- Renal dialysis patients
- Body piercing, tattoo recipients (not likely but possible)
- All adolescents are considered high risk

HCV:
- Low socioeconomic status, homelessness
- Sharing toothbrushes, razors
- Men who have sex with men
- HIV positive status increases risk of HCV if exposed
- Injecting drug use
- Tattoos and body piercing
- Transfusions, renal dialysis

HDV:
- Infection with HBV

ASSESSMENT FINDINGS

- Children often asymptomatic
- Vast majority of adults are asymptomatic or minimally symptomatic
- Illness is often more severe in the elderly
- Malaise, fever, jaundice, dark urine are most common symptoms
- Nausea, vomiting, anorexia, abdominal pain (RUQ), liver enlargement
- Clay-colored stools
- Markedly elevated serum alanine aminotransferase (ALT), aspartate aminotransferase (AST)
- Bilirubin, alkaline phosphatase may be elevated
- Transient neutropenia and lymphopenia followed by lymphocytosis
- Measure PT, PTT, albumin, glucose, electrolytes (for severe hepatitis)

In all types of hepatitis, ALT levels are higher than AST.

DIFFERENTIAL DIAGNOSIS

Children and adolescents:
- Hemolytic-uremic syndrome
- Reye's syndrome
- Chronic hemolytic diseases
- Wilson's disease
- Cystic fibrosis
- Infectious mononucleosis
- CMV
- Coxsackievirus
- Toxoplasmosis
- Acute cholangitis (infection of the bile duct)
- Drug toxicity and poisonings

Adults:
- All differential diagnoses for adolescents and children
- Hepatic malignancy
- Autoimmune, alcoholic, or ischemic hepatitis
- Acute cholecystitis
- Disseminated sepsis

DIAGNOSTIC STUDIES

Consider testing for co-infection with HDV in men who have sex with men who are infected with HBV.

Hepatitis Marker Nomenclature	
IgM = Immunoglobulin M Anti-HAV = Hepatitis A antibody Anti-HBs = Hepatitis B surface antibody HBeAg = Hepatitis B e antigen HCV RNA = Hepatitis C ribonucleic acid Anti-HDV = Hepatitis D antibody	IgG = Immunoglobulin G Anti-HBc = Hepatitis B core antigen HBsAg = Hepatitis B surface antigen PCR = Polymerase chain reaction Anti-HCV = Hepatitis C antibody Anti-HEV = Hepatitis E antibody

Hepatitis Type	Markers of Acute Disease	Markers of Chronic Disease/Infectivity	Markers of Recovery
A	IgM anti-HAV	None	IgG anti-HAV
B	IgM anti-HBc (the core) HBsAg *(can also indicate chronic infection)*	HBsAg HBeAg *(high infectivity)*	Anti-HBs *(surface antibody)*
C	PCR HCV-RNA *(sensitive within 10 days of exposure)* Anti-HCV *(may be negative early)*	Anti-HCV	Undetectable HCV-RNA
D	Anti-HDV	Total anti-HDV	None
E	IgM anti-HEV	None	None

Gastrointestinal Disorders

Hepatitis B Lab Interpretation		
Markers	**Results**	**Interpretation**
HBsAg Anti-HBc Anti-HBs	Negative Negative Negative	No infection No immunity
HBsAg Anti-HBc Anti-HBs	Negative Positive Positive	Immune due to natural infection
HBsAg Anti-HBc Anti-HBs	Negative Negative Positive	Immune due to immunization
HBsAg Anti-HBc IgM anti-HBc Anti-HBs	Positive Positive Positive Negative	Acutely infected
HBsAg Anti-HBc IgM anti-HBc Anti-HBs	Positive Positive Negative Negative	Chronically infected

Source: Guidelines for Viral Hepatitis Surveillance and Case Management. (July 14, 2005). Atlanta, GA: Center for Disease Control.

PREVENTION

Hepatitis A

- Sanitation and hygiene
- Hepatitis A vaccine: two-dose vaccine schedule for use in persons over 12 months who are at risk of contracting hepatitis A
- Exposure: Passive immunization with human gamma globulin (IG) for persons who are immunodeficient, nonimmunized or under immunized
- Combination Hepatitis A/B vaccine: Twinrix (three dose vaccine)

Hepatitis B

- Avoidance of risk behaviors and universal precautions
- Hepatitis B vaccine for all newborns and those at risk
- Exposure: Hepatitis B immunoglobulin (HBIG) along with Hepatitis B vaccine to unimmunized or anti-HBs-negative persons
- Infants born to HBsAg-positive women should receive Hepatitis B vaccine within 12 hours of birth along with HBIG
- Screen all pregnant women for Hepatitis B
- Combination Hepatitis A/B vaccine: Twinrix (three dose vaccine)

Hepatitis C

- Universal precautions
- No immunization available

Hepatitis D

- Universal precautions
- Prevention of HBV with immunization (since HDV cannot be transmitted in the absence of HBV)

Hepatitis E

- Sanitation and hygiene

NONPHARMACOLOGIC MANAGEMENT

- Measurement of PT, PTT, albumin, electrolytes, glucose, and CBC
- Education regarding illness, transmission, and cost and side effects of treatment
- Liver biopsy is done to determine extent of liver involvement (especially HBV, HCV)
- High calorie diet, best tolerated in morning
- Abstain from alcohol
- Avoid large doses of acetaminophen, iron and drugs metabolized by the liver
- Blood precautions for patients with Hepatitis B and C
- Maintain fluid balance

PHARMACOLOGIC MANAGEMENT

General:

- Cholestyramine (Questran®) alleviates pruritus
  Adult: 1 packet/scoop (5 g) mixed with food or fluids 1-2 times daily
  Children: not recommended
- Avoid steroids, glucocorticoids

No treatment is recommended for acute hepatitis B.

Hepatitis B (chronic):

- Interferon-alpha (IFN-a®)
- Emtricitabine
- Lamivudine (Epivir®)
  Adult: 300 mg daily or 150 mg twice daily
  Children: < 3 months not recommended
  3 months - 16 years: 4 mg/kg twice daily
  Max: 300 mg daily
  Tabs: 150 mg, 300 mg
  Oral Solution: 10 mg/mL
  Epivir HBV Solution: 5 mg/mL

Hepatitis C:

- Pegylated interferon + ribavirin
- Interferon alfa (for acute episode)
- Pegylated Interferon alfa 2a
- Pegylated Interferon alfa 2b

CONSULTATION/REFERRAL

- Gastroenterologist for Hepatitis B, C, D
- For liver biopsy if disease persists

FOLLOW-UP

- 6 to 12 months after acute illness, measure ALT, AST, bilirubin and globulin levels
- 6 months after acute illness measure HBsAg or HBeAg to determine whether there is chronic infection
- Surveillance for hepatocellular carcinoma

EXPECTED COURSE

HAV:
- Excellent prognosis; once acute infection resolves, expect liver functions to return to normal

HBV:
- Chronic hepatitis develops in 2% of immunocompetent adults
- Chronic hepatitis develops in >90% of infants infected perinatally
- 40% of chronic hepatitis cases result in cirrhosis
- Hepatocellular carcinoma may occur, although this usually happens several decades after primary infection

HCV:
- 85% of acute infections become chronic, some will progress to cirrhosis and hepatocellular carcinoma
- 15% of acute infections will have spontaneous resolution

POSSIBLE COMPLICATIONS

- Chronic active infection
- Hepatocellular carcinoma
- Cirrhosis
- Glomerulonephritis
- Fulminant hepatitis and hepatic necrosis
- Pancreatitis

DIVERTICULITIS

DESCRIPTION

Diverticula, outpouchings that can occur along the wall of the large intestine, become infected, with resultant inflammation.

ETIOLOGY

- Aerobic and anaerobic bacteria invade diverticula

INCIDENCE

- Diverticulosis, the presence of diverticula, is common; especially in Western cultures where low fiber diets predominate
- Diverticulitis is uncommon, increases with age
- 2200-3000/100,000 in U.S.

RISK FACTORS

- Low fiber, low residue diet
- Diverticulosis
- Age > 50 years

ASSESSMENT FINDINGS

- Abdominal pain (due to tension in the wall of the colon), typically left lower quadrant, with or without palpable mass
- Rebound tenderness, board like rigidity
- Anorexia
- Nausea and vomiting
- Diarrhea, constipation
- Abdominal distention
- Fever

DIFFERENTIAL DIAGNOSIS

- Gynecologic disorders
- Urologic disorders
- Appendicitis
- Ulcerative colitis
- Lactose intolerance
- Crohn's disease
- Irritable bowel syndrome
- Colon cancer
- Infective colitis
- Ischemic colitis

DIAGNOSTIC STUDIES

- Abdominal computed tomography (CT) scan, with or without contrast, is least invasive and provides the most information about presence, location, and extent of inflammation but cannot detect presence of bleeding
- Barium enema used to diagnose diverticulosis
- CBC: leukocytosis
- SED rate elevated
- Colonoscopy/flexible sigmoidoscopy to rule out malignancy, ulcerative colitis, or ischemic colitis

Colonoscopy and flexible sigmoidoscopy are usually contraindicated during acute diverticular episode. Generally, a colonoscopy is performed about 6 weeks after the acute episode to allow the colon to heal before insufflating the colon.

PREVENTION

- High fiber diet

Many patients have been advised to avoid seeds, nuts, corn because they could become lodged in a diverticula and produce diverticulitis. Most colorectal surgeons do not believe that these should be avoided.

NONPHARMACOLOGIC MANAGEMENT

- Rest
- NPO during acute episode; advance to clear liquids in small volume at frequent intervals, advance to high fiber diet
- Surgery may be indicated if patient experiences frequent recurrences
- Recommend high fiber diet

Gastrointestinal Disorders

DIVERTICULITIS PHARMACOLOGIC MANAGEMENT

First line treatment for diverticulosis is a high fiber diet (20-30 grams daily). This should not be initiated during an acute episode of diverticulitis. Oral antibiotics are recommended for treatment of mild diverticulitis. Coverage must include gram-negative rods with a quinolone PLUS metronidazole; OR a sulfa drug PLUS metronidazole.

Class	Drug Generic name (Trade name®)	Dosage How supplied	Comments
Anti-Infectives *Intravenous antibiotics for severe cases: triple therapy; ampicillin, gentamicin (Garamycin®) and metronidazole (Flagyl®)* **General Comment** Antibiotics are usually continued for 7-10 days	**ciprofloxacin** Cipro	**Adult**: 500 mg twice daily for 7-14 days *Tabs: 250 mg, 500 mg*	• Pregnancy Category C • **Quinolones are associated with increased risk of tendon rupture in all ages** • Cipro XR is only indicated for urinary tract infections. Use ciprofloxacin for diverticulitis • Dosage adjustment needed for renal impairment • Quinolones should not be used for pediatric patients • Drug interactions with theophylline, methylxanthines, glyburide, NSAIDs and others
	metronidazole Flagyl	**Adult**: 500 mg every 6-8 hours for 7-14 days *Max*: 4 grams/24 hours 750 mg three times a day for 7-10 days *Tabs: 250 mg, 500 mg* *Caps: 375 mg*	• Pregnancy Category B • Alcohol should be avoided while taking metronidazole and for at least 3 days after last dose • Potentiates the anticoagulant effect of warfarin and other anticoagulants • Dosage adjustment needed for hepatic impairment
	sulfamethoxazole-trimethoprim Bactrim Bactrim DS	**Adult**: 2 regular tabs or one DS twice daily for 7-10 days *Tabs: 80/400 mg* *Tabs: 160/800 mg*	• Pregnancy Category C • Use in conjunction with a quinolone or metronidazole • **CONTRAINDICATED in patients with sulfa allergies** • Increased risk of thrombocytopenia in patients receiving thiazide diuretics • Monitor serum digoxin levels • Potentiates oral hypoglycemics • Discontinue at first sign of rash or sign of adverse reaction: fatalities associated with sulfonamides have occurred secondary to Stevens Johnson syndrome, toxic epidermal necrolysis, aplastic anemia, and agranulocytosis

CONSULTATION/REFERRAL

- Gastroenterologist if moderate or severe symptoms exist
- Indications for surgical consult:
  - ◊ Severe, repeated, or extensive disease
  - ◊ Carcinoma suspected
  - ◊ Abdominal drainage, colostomy, or colon resection indicated

EXPECTED COURSE

- Symptoms completely resolve in 1 to 2 weeks
- Greater than 2/3 of patients fully recover without recurrence
- Colon resection is almost always curative

POSSIBLE COMPLICATIONS

- Perforation
- Abscess formation
- Sepsis
- Enteroenteric or enterovesical fistula
- Peritonitis

APPENDICITIS

DESCRIPTION

Inflammation of the vermiform appendix, which is a projection from the apex of the cecum.

ETIOLOGY

Obstruction of the appendix secondary to stool, inflammation, stricture, foreign body, or neoplasm. The obstructed lumen prevents drainage. The resultant increased pressure decreases mucosal blood flow, and the appendix becomes hypoxic

INCIDENCE

- Most common between ages 5 and 50 years
- Males > Females

RISK FACTORS

- Family history
- Abdominal neoplasm

ASSESSMENT FINDINGS

- Abdominal pain, usually severe and initially throughout the abdomen, or periumbilical area, later becomes localized to the right lower quadrant (RLQ)
- Anorexia, abdominal pain, nausea and vomiting are most common symptoms (in this order)
- Constipation and diarrhea occur after the pain
- Maximum abdominal tenderness and rigidity occurs over the right rectus muscle (McBurney's point)
- Psoas sign: pain with right thigh extension
- Obturator sign: pain with internal rotation of flexed right thigh
- Fever, usually 99-101° F (37.2-38.3°C)
- Patients frequently flex the right lower extremity when supine to relieve muscle tension
- May have urinary frequency, urgency, and dysuria
- Decreased bowel sounds
- Elderly may present with weakness, anorexia, tachycardia, and abdominal distention

A rectal exam should be performed on all patients with suspected appendicitis. Retrocecal appendix presents with tenderness on rectal exam.

A pelvic exam on all females with lower abdominal pain to rule out pelvic inflammatory disease, adnexal mass, ectopic pregnancy, or uterine pathology.

DIFFERENTIAL DIAGNOSIS

- Mittelschmerz
- Ruptured ectopic pregnancy
- Pelvic inflammatory disease

- Gastroenteritis
- Gastric ulcer, duodenal ulcer
- Cholecystitis
- Urinary tract infection
- Inflammatory bowel disease
- Recurrent abdominal pain
- Renal calculi

Diverticulitis, ileitis, inflammatory bowel disease, and some GYN disorders can present with right sided abdominal pain.

DIAGNOSTIC STUDIES

- Urinalysis: may be positive for red blood cells and leukocytes
- Urine pregnancy test: negative
- KUB: may show gas filled appendix
- CT scan: diagnostic test of choice

NONPHARMACOLOGIC MANAGEMENT

- Keep NPO
- Instruct to refrain from using laxatives, enemas, or from applying heat to the abdomen
- Prompt surgery is the treatment of choice: appendectomy

PHARMACOLOGIC MANAGEMENT

- Preoperative antibiotics may be prescribed by surgeon (e.g., cefoxitin)

CONSULTATION/REFERRAL

- Prompt surgical referral

FOLLOW-UP

- Routine postoperative assessment is at 2 weeks and 6 weeks
- May require postoperative antibiotics if perforation has occurred

EXPECTED COURSE

- Quick recovery usually follows surgery
- Activity should be restricted for 2-6 weeks

POSSIBLE COMPLICATIONS

- Ruptured appendix, often manifested by cessation of pain
- Abscess
- Peritonitis

IRRITABLE BOWEL SYNDROME
(IBS)

DESCRIPTION

Common intestinal disorder manifested by cramping, abdominal pain, bloating, and changes in bowel habits (e.g., constipation and/or diarrhea). This syndrome is further divided into other classifications depending on the patient's predominant symptoms: IBS-D (diarrhea predominant), IBS-C (constipation predominant), IBS-M (mixed diarrhea and constipation), and IBS-A (constipation alternating with diarrhea).

ETIOLOGY

- Unknown
- Stress is believed to be a factor

INCIDENCE

- Common: affects 15% of population of U.S.
- Rare in children and adolescents
- Predominant age: late 20's
- Female > Male

RISK FACTORS

- Family history

ASSESSMENT FINDINGS

- Crampy abdominal pain in lower quadrant
- Constipation and/or diarrhea
- Mucus in stools
- Abdominal distention
- No significant weight loss
- No bleeding, persistent severe pain, or fever

"Alarm symptoms" or atypical symptoms of IBS are rectal bleeding, nocturnal pain, and weight loss.

DIFFERENTIAL DIAGNOSIS

- Inflammatory bowel disorders
- Gastroenteritis
- Ingestion of antacids containing magnesium
- Lactose intolerance
- Celiac sprue
- Thyroid disorders

DIAGNOSTIC STUDIES

- CBC, chemistries: normal
- Serum IgA antibody to tissue transglutaminase (positive if celiac disease)
- Sedimentation rate: normal
- Stool for ova, parasites, occult blood: negative
- Colonoscopy to rule out other disorders: may show spasm or increased mucosal folds (has a low diagnostic yield and not cost-effective)

If Crohn's disease is suspected, colonoscopy will be performed to intubate the terminal ileum for a biopsy.

NONPHARMACOLOGIC MANAGEMENT

- Consider a trial of lactose free diet
- Exclusion of gas-producing foods
- Stress management
- Heat to abdomen
- Education about illness
- Avoid stimulants known to cause difficulty

IRRITABLE BOWEL SYNDROME PHARMACOLOGIC MANAGEMENT

Class	Drug Generic name (Trade name®)	Dosage How supplied	Comments
Bulk Producing Agents *Hold water in the stool to increase bulk, stimulating peristalsis* **General comments** Onset of action is 12-72 hours Site of action is small and large intestines	**psyllium** Various generics	**Adults ≥ 12 years**: 3.4 g in 8 oz. liquid 1-3 times daily	• New users should start with one dose/day and gradually increase to 3 doses/day • Take at first sign of irregularity • Separate bulk from other medications by at least 2 hours before and after bulk • Do not use if rectal bleeding is present or if constipation lasts > 7 days • Drink with at least 8 ounces of fluid/dose. Inadequate amounts of fluid can cause choking if psyllium swells

continued

IRRITABLE BOWEL SYNDROME PHARMACOLOGIC MANAGEMENT

Class	Drug Generic name (Trade name®)	Dosage How supplied	Comments
Stool Softeners/ Surfactants *Facilitate admixture of fat, water to soften stool* **General comments** Onset of action is 12-72 hours Site of action is small and large intestines Beneficial in anorectal conditions where passage of firm stool is painful	**docusate** Colace Doxidan Surfak	**Adult**: 50-300 mg daily **Children 2-11 yr**: 50-150 mg Colace Glycerin supp for children/infants: 1.2 g, one daily for children > 2 yr *Caps: 50 mg, 100 mg* *Liquid: 10 mg/mL* *Syrup: 60 mg/15 mL*	• Pregnancy Category C • Individualize treatment • Discontinue if rectal bleeding occurs • Discontinue if no bowel movement occurs • Use daily until bowel movements are normal
Stimulants/Irritants *Work by having a direct action on the intestinal mucosa, alters secretion of water and electrolytes* **General comments** Onset of action is 6-10 hours Site of action is the colon If more thorough evacuation is desired, castor oil is a consideration	**bisacodyl** Dulcolax Various generics	**Adults and > 12 years**: 5-15 mg in a single dose once daily **Children 6-11 years**: 5 mg once daily Suppositories: same as oral dosage *Tabs: 5 mg* *Suppository: 10 mg*	• Pregnancy Category C • Swallow whole, do not chew • Do not take within 1 hour of antacids or milk • Discontinue if rectal bleeding occurs • Discontinue if no bowel movement occurs • Suppository produces bowel movement in 15-60 minutes • Do not use castor oil during pregnancy. It may induce premature labor
	senna Senokot Ex-Lax	**Adults and Children > 12 years**: 2 tabs once daily *Max*: 4 tabs twice daily **Children 2-6 years**: ½ tab once a day *Max*: 1 tablet twice daily **Children 6-11 years**: 1 tab once daily *Max*: 2 tabs twice daily *Tabs: 8.6 mg*	• Pregnancy Category C • Do not use longer than one week • Discontinue if rectal bleeding occurs • Discontinue if no bowel movement occurs • Should produce a bowel movement in 6-12 hours
Antidiarrheal Agents *Slow intestinal motility and affects movement of water and electrolytes in bowel. Motility is slowed directly by inhibiting peristalsis in the circular and longitudinal muscles in the intestine*	**loperamide** Various generics	**Adult**: *Initial*: 4 mg; then 2 mg after each loose stool *Max*: 16 mg/day for 2 days	• Pregnancy Category C • Clinical improvement usually observed within 48 hours • Contraindicated if bloody diarrhea or temperature > 101°F present

continued

IRRITABLE BOWEL SYNDROME PHARMACOLOGIC MANAGEMENT

Class	Drug Generic name (Trade name®)	Dosage How supplied	Comments
Antispasmodic/ Anticholinergic Agents *GI anticholinergic agents are used to decrease motility of smooth muscle tone. These agents inhibit acetylcholine which reduces muscle tone and decreases secretions. Antispasmodics decrease GI motility by acting on the smooth muscles of the intestines*	**dicyclomine** (antispasmodic) Bentyl	**Adult**: initial 20 mg four times a day, increase to 40 mg four times a day if tolerated *Caps: 10 mg* *Tabs: 20 mg*	• Pregnancy Category B • Contraindicated in glaucoma, GI or GU obstruction, paralytic ileus, severe ulcerative colitis, myasthenia gravis • The only oral dose shown to be effective is 160 mg/day. Start at 80 mg/day because of side effects • May increase heart rate. Cautious use in cardiac patients • May cause drowsiness, blurred vision
	hyoscyamine sulfate (antispasmodic) Levsin	**Adult**: 1-2 tabs every 4 hours as needed, maximum 12 tabs/24 hours *Tabs: 0.125 mg*	• Pregnancy Category C • Contraindicated in glaucoma, GI or GU obstruction, paralytic ileus, severe ulcerative colitis, myasthenia gravis • May increase heart rate. Cautious use in cardiac patients. • May cause drowsiness, blurred vision
	phenobarbital 48.6 mg/ hyoscyamine sulfate 0.3111 mg/ atropine sulfate 0.0582 mg/ scopolamine hydrobromide 0.0195 mg/ (anticholinergic/ antispasmodic) Donnatal Extentabs	**Adult**: One tablet twice daily *Max*: 2 tabs daily	• Pregnancy Category C • Contraindicated in glaucoma, GI, GU obstruction, paralytic ileus, severe ulcerative colitis, myasthenia gravis • May increase heart rate. Cautious use in cardiac patients • May cause drowsiness, blurred vision • Phenobarbital may decrease the effect of anticoagulants • Phenobarbital is habit forming • Dosing adjustment needed for patients with hepatic impairment
	phenobarbital 16.2 mg/ hycosamine 0.1037 mg/ atropine sulfate .0194 mg/ scopolamine .0065 mg (anticholinergic/ antispasmodic) Donnatal tabs	**Adult**: 1-2 tabs 3-4 times a day *Max*: 8 tabs daily	• Pregnancy Category C • Contraindicated in glaucoma, GI, GU obstruction, paralytic ileus, severe ulcerative colitis, myasthenia gravis • May increase heart rate. Cautious use in cardiac patients. • May cause drowsiness, blurred vision

CONSULTATION/REFERRAL

- Gastroenterologist for treatment failure

FOLLOW-UP

- Variable, dependent on symptoms

EXPECTED COURSE

- Recurrence with stress to be expected
- Does not increase risk of inflammatory bowel disease or colon cancer

INFLAMMATORY BOWEL DISEASE
(IBD)

DESCRIPTION

Inflammatory bowel diseases (IBD) are chronic disorders of the GI tract distinguished by the recurrent inflammatory involvement of intestinal segments. Two main types are Crohn's disease and ulcerative colitis.

CROHN'S DISEASE

DESCRIPTION

Chronic, slowly progressive transmural inflammation of the small intestine (most common), and/or large intestine, often involving the terminal ileum; disease ranges from mild to refractory in severity. Typically several locations of the intestines with sections in between are unaffected.

ETIOLOGY

- Idiopathic

INCIDENCE

- Females > Males
- 15% have family history
- Caucasians > African-Americans or Asians
- Peak age at onset is 15 to 25 years, then smaller peak at 55 to 65 years
- Three- to sixfold increased incidence in Jewish population

RISK FACTORS

- Family history
- Cigarette smoking

ASSESSMENT FINDINGS

- Diarrhea, including nocturnal
- Fever
- Abdominal pain and tenderness
- Weight loss
- Abdominal mass
- Fistulas
- Intestinal obstruction (uncommon)
- Hematochezia
- Megacolon
- Extracolonic disease: uveitis, arthritis, dermatitis, sclerosing cholangitis (< 10%)
- Bone age in children usually delayed by 2 years

The hallmarks of Crohn's Disease are fatigue, abdominal pain, prolonged diarrhea with or without bleeding, weight loss, and fever.

DIFFERENTIAL DIAGNOSIS

- Ulcerative colitis, ischemic colitis
- NSAID adverse effects
- Enteritis
- Intestinal pathogenic bacteria
- Malignancy

- Irritable bowel syndrome
- Appendicitis
- Peptic ulcer disease
- Renal colic

DIAGNOSTIC STUDIES

- Colonoscopy with biopsy: submucosal inflammation with pseudopolyps, edema, and strictures; biopsy often reveals granulomatous inflammation
- Antiglycan antibody: elevated in 75% of cases
- Barium X rays
- Sedimentation rate: elevated
- CBC: anemia
- Albumin: below normal if severe disease
- Electrolytes: imbalances
- B_{12}, folate: deficient
- Stool for leukocytes, culture and sensitivity to rule out other causes for symptoms

NONPHARMACOLOGIC MANAGEMENT

- Maintain nutrition and weight:
  - ◊ May be helpful to decrease fat and increase fiber to treat diarrhea
  - ◊ Low lactose diet for small intestine involvement
  - ◊ Low fiber diet if strictures present
- Sitz baths helpful if perirectal disease present
- Drainage of perirectal abscess if present
- Manage extracolonic manifestations
- Refer to Crohn's and Colitis Foundation of America for information and support
- Surgery when indicated:
  - Abscess
  - Intestinal obstruction
  - For ostomy placement

PHARMACOLOGIC MANAGEMENT

- Mesalamine (Asacol®, Pentasa®, Rowasa®) is used for maintenance and is taken daily
- Antibiotics (if perirectal involvement): Metronidazole (Flagyl) reduces bacteria, granuloma formation
- Folate supplement while taking sulfasalazine, which inhibits folate absorption
- Antispasmodics and antidiarrheals may be helpful

PREGNANCY/LACTATION CONSIDERATIONS

- Pregnancy not contraindicated
- Long-term sulfasalazine therapy is associated with reversible sterility in males

CONSULTATION/REFERRAL

- Gastroenterologist

FOLLOW-UP

- Frequency dependent on severity
- Monitor weight, symptoms, CBC, sedimentation rate, Vitamin B_{12}, folate levels
- Changes in weight are helpful in determining need to increase or decrease medications
- Endoscopy indicated if symptoms change
- Annual liver function tests

EXPECTED COURSE

- Chronic illness with recurrences and exacerbations
- Surgery usually needed every 4-7 years for the average patient
- Full activities and normal, but often shortened life can be expected

POSSIBLE COMPLICATIONS

- Fistulae
- Colon perforation
- Toxic megacolon
- Adenocarcinoma
- Malnutrition

ULCERATIVE COLITIS

DESCRIPTION

Chronic inflammation of the colonic mucosa and submucosa; the inflammation is continuous, widespread and superficial, almost always involves the rectum, and may spread throughout the colon.

ETIOLOGY

- Unknown

INCIDENCE

- More common in developed countries
- Peak occurrence ages 15-40 years, and again at 50-70 years
- Increased frequency of occurrence in Jewish population
- Males = Females

RISK FACTORS

- Positive family history

ASSESSMENT FINDINGS

- Fecal incontinence, bloody diarrhea, rectal bleeding
- Tenesmus (cramping pain of the anal or vesical sphincter), abdominal pain
- Weight loss (possibly from malignancy)
- Fever, tachycardia, anemia
- Extracolonic disease features: uveitis, arthritis, dermatitis, sclerosing cholangitis

DIFFERENTIAL DIAGNOSIS

- Infectious colitis
- Ischemic colitis
- Crohn's disease
- Irritable bowel syndrome
- Diarrhea associated with antibiotic use
- Hemorrhoids
- Diverticulitis
- Lactose intolerance
- Arthralgia/arthritis

DIAGNOSTIC STUDIES

- Sigmoidoscopy with biopsy: establishes whether inflammation is present
- Plain abdominal films: identifies toxic megacolon and should be used in UC patients who present with fever, abdominal pain, leukocytosis
- Colonoscopy with biopsy to define extent of involvement
- Air contrast barium enema: often normal in early disease
- CBC to detect anemia and leukocytosis
- Sedimentation rate: elevated
- pANCA (perinuclear antineutrophil cytoplasmic antibody): elevated in 85% of patients
- Serum electrolytes: hypokalemia

NONPHARMACOLOGIC MANAGEMENT

- Complete bowel rest indicated in acute fulminant disease only
- Surgery is curative and should be considered in cases of disease that is unresponsive to 2-3 weeks of medical therapy
- Referral to Crohn's and Colitis Foundation of America

PHARMACOLOGIC MANAGEMENT

- Sulfasalazine is the treatment of choice for mild exacerbations and for chronic treatment
- Steroid enemas or suppositories are used for proctitis or proctosigmoiditis
- Oral and parenteral steroids are used to manage more severe exacerbations
- In patients unresponsive to steroids, immune modulators are used
- Antidiarrheal should be used cautiously

PREGNANCY/LACTATION CONSIDERATIONS

- Sulfasalazine, topical and oral 5-ASA, and corticosteroids have not been associated with birth defects and can be used in pregnancy and lactation
- Congenital abnormalities have been associated with the use of azathioprine

CONSULTATION/REFERRAL

- Gastroenterologist
- Severe colitis requires prompt hospitalization

FOLLOW-UP

- Regular, close practitioner/patient relationship is important for the detection of exacerbations, complications, and for emotional support
- Patients with extensive or long-standing disease require surveillance for colorectal cancer (every 1-2 years after disease present for 7-8 years) with annual colonoscopy with biopsies

EXPECTED COURSE

- Variable, dependent on extent of disease
- Chronic illness with remissions and exacerbations

POSSIBLE COMPLICATIONS

- Toxic megacolon
- Perforation
- Colon cancer
- Fluid and electrolyte imbalances
- Liver disease
- Stricture formation

CONSTIPATION

DESCRIPTION

Painful, difficult passage of small amounts of hard, dry stool, usually fewer than three times a week.

ETIOLOGY

- Slow, sluggish colonic contractions cause excessive absorption of water by the colon; hard, dry stools move through the colon slowly

INCIDENCE

- Reported most often at age extremes
- The most common GI complaint in the U.S.

RISK FACTORS

- Age extremes
- Inadequate intake of dietary fiber
- Inadequate fluid intake
- Sedentary lifestyle
- Ignoring the urge to defecate
- Change in daily routine
- Medications
  - ◊ Antidepressants
  - ◊ Anticholinergics
  - ◊ Antihypertensives
  - ◊ Antihistamines
  - ◊ Calcium supplements
  - ◊ Iron supplements
  - ◊ Narcotics
  - ◊ Antacids containing aluminum
  - ◊ Diuretics
  - ◊ Anticonvulsants
- Irritable bowel syndrome
- Laxative abuse
- Neurologic, metabolic, and endocrine disorders
- Diverticulosis
- Hirschsprung's disease
- Intestinal obstruction

ASSESSMENT FINDINGS

- Decrease in number of bowel movements compared to patient's "usual" ("usual" is 3-5 times weekly)
- Hard, dry stools
- Pain and difficulty with defecation
- Abdominal distention

DIFFERENTIAL DIAGNOSIS

- Encopresis secondary to constipation
- Irritable bowel syndrome
- Colorectal cancer
- Obstipation (fecal impaction)
- Hirschsprung's disease
- Anorectal stenosis
- Anal fissure
- Hemorrhoids
- Hypothyroidism
- Depression

DIAGNOSTIC STUDIES

- Abdominal x-ray if structural abnormalities: suspected accumulation of stool in the sigmoid colon
- Barium enema if obstruction or Hirschsprung's disease is suspected
- Sigmoidoscopy or colonoscopy for visualization and biopsy
- Colorectal transit study (Sitz marker study) used for chronic constipation; demonstrates how quickly food moves through the colon
- Anorectal manometry to evaluate anal sphincter muscle function
- Stool for occult blood: negative
  - ◊ Should be repeated on at least 3 different stool specimens on different days before being considered negative
- Thyroid studies: normal

PREVENTION

- Establish regular toileting routine; respond to the urge to have a bowel movement
- High fiber diet (20 to 35 grams/day): beans, whole grains, bran, fruit, vegetables
- Adequate intake of water and juice (1.5 to 2 liters/day) and elimination of caffeine, which has a dehydrating effect
- Adequate exercise
- Avoidance of medications that contribute to constipation
- Limit use of laxatives, enemas, and stool softeners

NONPHARMACOLOGIC MANAGEMENT

- Dietary and lifestyle changes (see Prevention)

CONSTIPATION PHARMACOLOGIC MANAGEMENT

Class	Drug Generic name (Trade name®)	Dosage How supplied	Comments
Bulk Producing Agents *Hold water in the stool to increase bulk, stimulating peristalsis* **General comments** Onset of action is 12-72 hours Site of action is small and large intestines All may inhibit the action of tetracyclines, salicylates, digitalis, oral anticoagulants, nitrofurantoins and others	**psyllium**	**Adults ≥ 12 years**: 3.4 g in 8 oz. liquid 1-3 times daily **Children < 6 yr:** not recommended **6-11 yr:** 1.7 g powder in 8 oz. liquid	• New users should start with one dose/day and gradually increase to 3 doses/day • Take at first sign of irregularity • Separate bulk from other medications by at least 2 hours before and after bulk • Do not use if rectal bleeding is present or if constipation lasts > 7 days • Drink with at least 8 ounces of fluid/dose. Inadequate amounts of fluid can cause choking if psyllium swells
	Various generics	*Powder: 3.4 g per rounded tablespoon* *Wafers: 3.4 g per 2 wafers* *Capsules: 0.52 g/cap*	
	methylcellulose	**Adult**: 1 heaping tablespoon in 8 oz. water 1-3 times daily **Children > 6 yr**: 1/2 adult dose	• Do not use if rectal bleeding is present or if constipation lasts > 7 days • Drink with at least 8 ounces of fluid/dose
	Citrucel	*Powder: 2 g per 19 g powder*	

continued

CONSTIPATION PHARMACOLOGIC MANAGEMENT

Class	Drug Generic name (Trade name®)	Dosage How supplied	Comments
	polycarbophil	**Adult**: 2 tabs 1-4 times daily with water **Children 6-12 yr**: 1 tab 1-4 times daily	• Do not use if rectal bleeding is present or if constipation lasts > 7 days • Drink with at least 8 ounces of fluid/dose
	Fibercon	*Caps: 625 mg*	
Stool Softeners/ Surfactants *Facilitate admixture of fat, water to soften stool* **General comments** Onset of action is 12-72 hours Site of action is small and large intestines Beneficial in anorectal conditions where passage of firm stool is painful	**docusate**	**Adult**: 50-300 mg daily **Children 2-11 yr**: 50-150 mg Colace Glycerin supp for children/infants: 1.2 g, one daily for children > 2 yr	• Pregnancy Category C • Individualize treatment • Discontinue if rectal bleeding occurs • Discontinue if no bowel movement occurs • Use daily until bowel movements are normal
	Colace Doxidan Surfak	*Caps: 50 mg, 100 mg* *Liquid: 10 mg/mL* *Syrup: 60 mg/15 mL* *Supp: 1.2 g*	
Hyperosmotic Agents *Osmotic effect retains fluid in colon, lowers pH and increases peristalsis* **General comments** Onset of action is 1-2 days, but glycerin suppository produces results in 15-60 minutes Site of action is the colon	**lactulose**	**Adult**: 10-20 g in 4 oz. water daily *Max*: 40 g/day **Children**: not recommended	• Pregnancy Category B • 20 g packet equivalent to 30 mL liquid Lactulose • Contains galactose • Can be used long term without monitoring electrolytes • May cause significant distention • with flatulence
	Chronulac Kristalose	*Packet: 10 g, 20 g*	
	polyethylene glycol	**Adult**: 17 g in 8 oz. water daily up to 2 weeks, may need 2-4 days for results **Children**: not recommended	• Pregnancy Category is B • Cautious use in renal disease • Do not use longer than 7 days
	Miralax	*Powder: single dose packets of 17 g*	

continued

CONSTIPATION PHARMACOLOGIC MANAGEMENT

Class	Drug Generic name (Trade name®)	Dosage How supplied	Comments
Stimulants/Irritants *Work by having a direct action on the intestinal mucosa, alters secretion of water and electrolytes* **General comments** Onset of action is 6-10 hours Site of action is the colon If more thorough evacuation is desired, castor oil is a consideration	**bisacodyl** Dulcolax Various generics	**Adults and ≥ 12 years**: 5-15 mg in a single dose once daily **Children 6-11 years**: 5 mg once daily *Suppositories: same as oral dosage* *Tabs: 5 mg* *Suppository: 10 mg*	• Pregnancy Category C • Swallow whole, do not chew • Do not take within 1 hour of antacids or milk • Discontinue if rectal bleeding occurs • Discontinue if no bowel movement occurs • Suppository produces bowel movement in 15-60 minutes • Do not use castor oil during pregnancy. It may induce premature labor
	senna Senokot Ex-Lax	**Adults and Children > 12 years**: 2 tabs once daily *Max*: 4 tabs twice daily **Children 6-11 years**: 1 tab once daily *Max*: 2 tabs twice daily **Children 2-6 years**: ½ tab once a day *Max*: 1 tablet twice daily *Tabs: 8.6 mg*	• Pregnancy Category C • Do not use longer than one week • Discontinue if rectal bleeding occurs • Discontinue if no bowel movement occurs • Should produce a bowel movement in 6-12 hours
Lubricants/Emollients *Work by retarding colonic absorption of water, has secondary effect of softening the stool* **General comments** Onset of action is 6-8 hours Site of action is the colon May decrease absorption of fat soluble vitamins	**mineral oil**	**Adults and children > 12 years**: 15-45 mL taken at bedtime **Children 6-11 years**: 5 to 15 mL taken at bedtime	• No pregnancy rating available • Do not use longer than one week • Do not take with meals; take only at bedtime • Discontinue if rectal bleeding occurs • Discontinue if no bowel movement occurs • Protect product from sunlight
Saline Laxatives *Attract and retain water in the intestinal lumen, increase intraluminal pressure and cholecystokinin release* **General comments** Onset of action is 30 minutes to 3 hours Site of action is small and large intestines	**magnesium sulfate**	**Adults**: 10-15 grams in a glass of water **Children**: 5-10 grams in a glass of water	• Pregnancy Category B • May seriously alter fluid and electrolyte balance. Sulfate salts are the most potent • Use cautiously or avoid in patients on sodium restricted diets, CHF, renal dysfunction or hypertension (up to 20% of magnesium can be absorbed)

continued

CONSTIPATION PHARMACOLOGIC MANAGEMENT

Class	Drug Generic name (Trade name®)	Dosage How supplied	Comments
	magnesium hydroxide Milk of Magnesia	**Adults**: varies by specific product. See package labeling for specific information	

PREGNANCY/LACTATION CONSIDERATIONS

- Stress dietary management
- Bulk-forming agents and occasional stool softeners may be used
- Pregnancy Category B: lactulose, magnesium sulfate

CONSULTATION/REFERRAL

- Gastroenterologist for treatment failure or ongoing constipation
- Surgeon for complications of hemorrhoids, fissures, rectal prolapse

FOLLOW-UP

- Regular follow-up evaluation needed until resumption of regular bowel function
- Monitor electrolytes, BUN, and creatinine of chronic laxative user

EXPECTED COURSE

- Brief, occasional constipation responds well to treatment
- Can become chronic and lifelong

POSSIBLE COMPLICATIONS

- Hemorrhoids
- Anal fissures
- Rectal prolapse
- Laxative abuse syndrome (LAS)
- Fecal impaction
- Fluid and electrolyte imbalances due to laxative use
- Acquired megacolon

Pediatric Pharmacology for Constipation		
Pharmaceutical Agent	**Child Age**	**Dosage Recommended**
Metamucil **mix with 8 oz. juice/water**	2-5 years	3/4 tsp 1-3 times a day
	6-11 years	1/2 tsp 1-3 times a day
	> 12 years	1 Tbsp 1-3 times a day
Mineral Oil	4-11 years	1-4 tsp divided in 1-2 doses daily
	> 12 years	1-3 Tbsp divided in 1-2 doses daily
Milk of Magnesia **dilute with juice or water**	< 2 years	2 mL/kg divided in 1-2 doses daily
	2-5 years	1-3 tsp divided in 1-2 doses daily
	6-11 years	1-2 Tbsp divided in 1-2 doses daily
	> 12 years	2-4 Tbsp divided in 1-2 doses daily
Colace Syrup **20 mg/5 mL**	< 3 years	1/2-1 tsp divided in 1-4 doses
	3-6 years	1-3 tsp divided in 1-4 doses
	> 6 years	1-2 Tbsp divided in 1-4 doses
Maltsupex **mix with 4-8 oz. water/juice**	< 2 years	1-2 tsp divided in 1-2 doses daily
	> 2 years	1-2 Tbsp divided in 1-2 doses daily
Lactulose 10 g/15 mL	> 6 months	1-2 mL/kg divided in 2-3 doses daily

HEMORRHOIDS

DESCRIPTION

Varicose veins of the hemorrhoidal venous plexus.

- *Internal hemorrhoids*: those that occur above the dentate line
- *External hemorrhoids*: folds of perianal skin resulting from prior perianal swelling; symptomatic only when becoming thrombosed

ETIOLOGY

- Veins of the hemorrhoidal plexus become engorged as a result of:
  - ◊ Passage of stool: shearing force, straining
  - ◊ Increased venous pressure (e.g., pregnancy, CHF)

INCIDENCE

- Common in adults
- Males = Females

RISK FACTORS

- Constipation, straining with defecation
- Chronic diarrhea
- Pregnancy: due to constipation and direct effect of gravid uterus
- Hypertension, congestive heart failure
- Prolonged sitting
- Obesity
- Colon malignancy

ASSESSMENT FINDINGS

Internal hemorrhoids:

- Painless bleeding with defecation
- Feeling of incomplete evacuation after bowel movements

External hemorrhoids:

- Anal itching
- Pain with defecation
- Anal protrusion of blue, shiny mass
- Can be acutely painful

DIFFERENTIAL DIAGNOSIS

- Rectal prolapse
- Rectal neoplasm
- Condyloma
- Anal fissure

DIAGNOSTIC STUDIES

- Stool for occult blood: if positive, refer for colonoscopy. Do **not** assume bleeding is due to hemorrhoids. Should be repeated on at least 3 different stool specimens on 3 different days before being considered negative
- Colonoscopy preferred because more of colon able to be visualized during exam
- Anoscopy: visualization of bright red or purple masses
- Sigmoidoscopy

PREVENTION

- Avoid constipation
- Refrain from prolonged sitting and straining with bowel movements

NONPHARMACOLOGIC MANAGEMENT

- Sitz baths alleviate pain
- Education about prevention
- High fiber diet and liberal water intake
- Cold packs
- Rubber band ligation (for internal hemorrhoids only)
- Infrared coagulation (external hemorrhoids)
- Sclerotherapy
- Hemorrhoidectomy for severe cases

PHARMACOLOGIC MANAGEMENT

- See *Constipation*
- Fiber supplements
- Stool softeners
- Analgesic ointment: benzocaine (Hurricaine®), dibucaine (Nupercainal®)
- Corticosteroid preparations (for itching and shrinking swollen hemorrhoids): hydrocortisone

(Anusol-HC®)
Adult: 1 rectally 2-3 times daily
Children: not recommended
Supp: 25mg

PREGNANCY/LACTATION CONSIDERATIONS

- Hemorrhoids that occur with pregnancy usually resolve without treatment after delivery

CONSULTATION/REFERRAL

- Surgeon if conservative management is ineffective

FOLLOW-UP

- None needed unless symptoms persist

EXPECTED COURSE

- May resolve spontaneously or as a result of treatment
- May be recurrent and chronic

POSSIBLE COMPLICATIONS

- Thrombosis
- Rectal prolapse
- Infection
- Incontinence

PLYLORIC STENOSIS

DESCRIPTION

Narrowing of the pyloric sphincter that occurs in infancy; due to hypertrophy of the pyloric muscle and eventual obstruction.

ETIOLOGY

- Probably familial
- More common in first born males

INCIDENCE

- Caucasians
- Males > Females (5:1)
- Usual onset is 3-4 weeks to 5 months of age

RISK FACTORS

- Family history

ASSESSMENT FINDINGS

- Projectile nonbilious vomiting, progressive in severity and frequency
- Usually begins after 2 weeks of age
- Olive-shaped mass palpable in right upper quadrant of abdomen (hypertrophied pylorus)
- Peristaltic waves visible across abdomen after feeding
- Insatiable hunger with weight loss and dehydration

DIFFERENTIAL DIAGNOSIS

- Gastroesophageal reflux
- Inappropriate feeding
- Gastritis
- Congenital adrenal hyperplasia

DIAGNOSTIC STUDIES

- Ultrasound is replacing contrast x-ray: clearly shows hypertrophied pyloric muscles and narrowed pyloric channel
- Upper gastrointestinal series: thin, elongated pyloric canal ("string sign")

MANAGEMENT

- Correction of fluid and electrolyte imbalances
- Surgical correction

CONSULTATION/REFERRAL

- For surgical pyloromyotomy

FOLLOW-UP

- Educate to introduce feedings gradually after surgery
- Routine pediatric care

EXPECTED COURSE

- Surgery remedies disorder

HIRSCHSPRUNG'S DISEASE
(Congenital Aganglionic Megacolon)

DESCRIPTION

Congenital absence of ganglion cells in a section of the wall of the large intestine resulting in lack of motility in that region, accumulation of feces, and dilation of the colon.

ETIOLOGY

- Familial
- Often associated with trisomy 21

INCIDENCE

- Occurs 1 in 2 - 5000 births in the U.S.
- Males > Females

RISK FACTORS

- Family history
- Down syndrome

ASSESSMENT FINDINGS

- Failure to pass meconium within 48 hours of birth
- Constipation, obstipation
- Distended abdomen with palpable mass of feces
- Poor feeding, failure to thrive
- Vomiting
- Explosive diarrhea or flatus after finger rectal exams
- Anemia secondary to chronic blood loss from colon

DIFFERENTIAL DIAGNOSIS

- Acquired megacolon
- Idiopathic constipation, obstipation
- Ileal atresia
- Meconium plug, meconium ileus

DIAGNOSTIC STUDIES

- CBC: anemia, leukocytosis
- Abdominal x-rays: dilated loops of bowel
- Biopsy: absence of ganglion cells

MANAGEMENT

- Removal of accumulated feces
- Correction of fluid and electrolyte imbalances
- Education: diet after surgery, signs of dehydration, colostomy care if needed

CONSULTATION/REFERRAL

- Surgeon for resection of affected bowel and possible colostomy
- Consider referral to pediatric gastroenterologist

FOLLOW-UP

- Throughout recuperative period

EXPECTED COURSE

- Favorable prognosis if corrected before complications occur

POSSIBLE COMPLICATIONS

- Toxic enterocolitis
- Perforated bowel

INTUSSUSCEPTION

DESCRIPTION

An emergent condition in which one bowel segment becomes invaginated into another.

ETIOLOGY

- Idiopathic in infants age 5-9 months (90% of cases)
- Associated with predisposing conditions in neonates, older children, and adults (10% of cases)
- *See* Risk Factors

INCIDENCE

- Peak age is 5-9 months
- Can occur at any age but most common 6-12 months of age
- Up to 4/1000 live births in the U.S.
- Males > Females: 3:2

RISK FACTORS

- Hypertrophy of Peyer's patches (mucous membrane of the small intestine)
- Neoplasm
- Lead paint (in adults)
- Meckel's diverticulum
- Foreign body
- Henoch-Schönlein purpura
- Appendicitis
- Recent viral upper respiratory or gastrointestinal infection (21%)

ASSESSMENT FINDINGS

- Classic triad (frequently late findings):
  - ◊ Abdominal pain, often colicky
  - ◊ Vomiting (almost always occurs)
  - ◊ Bloody stools resembling "currant jelly"
- Lethargy
- Irritability
- May present with right upper quadrant mass
- May present with fever

DIFFERENTIAL DIAGNOSIS

- Intestinal perforation
- Gastroenteritis
- Enterocolitis
- Parasitic infection
- Tumors

DIAGNOSTIC STUDIES

- Stool for occult blood: often positive
- Gold standard for diagnosis is barium enema:
  - ◊ "Coiled spring" appearance
  - ◊ Often therapeutic, may reduce intussusception
- Plain abdominal x-ray to exclude intestinal perforation before barium enema
- Abdominal ultrasound can sometimes identify other etiologies of pain (e.g., appendicitis, ovarian sources, urinary tract source)

MANAGEMENT

- Rehydration
- Emergency nonsurgical or surgical reduction

CONSULTATION/REFERRAL

- Radiologist
- Surgeon

FOLLOW-UP

- Throughout postoperative period

EXPECTED COURSE

- Spontaneous reduction while awaiting surgery is known to occur
- Recurrence rate after barium enema reduction is 10%
- Recurrence rate after surgery is less than 4%

POSSIBLE COMPLICATIONS

- Can be fatal without prompt treatment
- Bowel ischemia
- Bowel perforation
- Sepsis

COLIC

DESCRIPTION

A symptom complex, in an otherwise healthy infant, that is characterized by episodes of inconsolable crying, accompanied by apparent abdominal pain. Tends to occur at predictable times of the day, often in the evening, and may last for several hours.

ETIOLOGY

- Unknown
- Possibly due to immaturity of the gastrointestinal tract

INCIDENCE

- Usually begins at age 3 weeks and resolves by age 3 to 4 months

RISK FACTORS

- Family tension
- First-time parents

ASSESSMENT FINDINGS

- Parent describes infant as:
    - ◊ Rigid
    - ◊ Fists clenched
    - ◊ Legs flexed upon abdomen
    - ◊ Irritable
    - ◊ Frequent flatus
- Normal growth
- Abdomen may be distended due to ingestion of air with crying
- Normal stools
- Normal physical exam

DIFFERENTIAL DIAGNOSIS

- Gastroesophageal reflux
- Infection
- Injury
- Incarcerated hernia
- Food intolerance

NONPHARMACOLOGIC MANAGEMENT

- Educate parents about comfort measures and feeding techniques
    - ◊ Rhythmic rocking in a swing or car
    - ◊ Continuous monotonous noise (e.g., vacuum cleaner, hairdryer, or clothes dryer)
    - ◊ Slow feeding with frequent burping
    - ◊ Pacifier
- Parental reassurance and encouragement with emphasis on infant's healthy status, and normal growth and development
- Formula changes are usually ineffective
- Breastfeeding mothers may be able to identify foods in their diet that contribute

PHARMACOLOGIC MANAGEMENT

- Treatment is controversial
- Simethicone (Mylicon®) 20 mg/0.3 mL
  < 2 yr < 24 pounds: 0.3 mL PRN; max: 3.6 mL/24h
  > 2 yr > 24 pounds: 0.6 mL PRN; max: 7.2 mL/24h

CONSULTATION/REFERRAL

- Breastfeeding consultant as indicated

FOLLOW-UP

- Close telephone contact and more frequent visits for education and support

EXPECTED COURSE

- Usually resolves by itself by age 3 months

PINWORMS
(Enterobiasis)

DESCRIPTION

Intestinal infestation with *Enterobius vermicularis*, a white, thread-like parasite one centimeter in length.

ETIOLOGY

- The eggs of *Enterobius vermicularis* are ingested from contaminated fingers and fomites
- After hatching, become larvae in the intestines and travel to the rectum

INCIDENCE

- The most common parasitic infestation in children in the U.S.
- Predominant age is preschool to 14 years

RISK FACTORS

- Family contact
- Day care center attendance, institutional residence
- Poor hygiene
- Crowded living conditions
- Warm climate

ASSESSMENT FINDINGS

- Perianal itching, vulvovaginitis
- Enuresis
- Abdominal pain
- Irritability, restlessness
- Anorexia
- Parent may directly visualize female worm at night or early in the morning by shining a flashlight on the perianal area

DIFFERENTIAL DIAGNOSIS

- Idiopathic pruritus ani
- Dermatitis
- Lichen planus
- Scabies
- Vaginitis

DIAGNOSTIC STUDIES

- Transparent adhesive tape test ("Scotch" tape test): identification of ova on low power microscopy after touching tape to perianal area

PREVENTION

- Avoidance of risk factors
- Hygiene

NONPHARMACOLOGIC MANAGEMENT

Educate parent and child:
- Careful handwashing, hygiene
- Wash clothing and bedding in hot water at time of treatment
- Ova remain viable for 3 weeks in a moist environment
- Discourage scratching
- Keep hands away from face and mouth

PINWORM PHARMACOLOGIC MANAGEMENT

Class	Drug Generic name (Trade name®)	Dosage How supplied	Comments
Antihelminthics *inhibits the formation of worm's microtubules and causes glucose depletion*	**mebendazole**	**Adults and Children**: 100 mg single dose	• Pregnancy Category C • May cause abdominal pain and diarrhea after administration • Do not use in children < 2 years of age • May repeat after 3 weeks
General comments Cleanliness is important to prevent reinfection	Vermox	*Chew tabs: 100 mg*	
Treat the entire household as well as close contacts May be used to treat other worm infections besides pinworm	**pyrantel pamoate**	**Adults and children:** > 187 pounds: 4 tabs 163-187 pounds: 3.5 tabs 138-162 pounds: 3 tabs 113-137 pounds: 2.5 tabs 88-112 pounds: 2 tabs 63-87 pounds: 1.5 tabs 38-62 pounds: 1 tab 25-37 pounds: 0.5 tab	• No formal pregnancy category has been assigned by the FDA for this medication • Available OTC • Take with food and a full glass of water • Shake suspension well before measuring dose • Do not prescribe for patient taking theophylline
	Antiminth, PinX, Ascarel	*Bottles of 12 tabs*	• May cause dizziness, abdominal pain or diarrhea after taking

PREGNANCY/LACTATION CONSIDERATIONS

- Antihelminthics contraindicated in pregnancy

CONSULTATION/REFERRAL

- Usually none needed
- Pediatric gastroenterology consult may be needed

FOLLOW-UP

- Antihelminthics to be repeated in 2 weeks

EXPECTED COURSE

- Easily resolved, but reinfestation is common

POSSIBLE COMPLICATIONS

- Excoriation and impetigo from scratching
- Urinary tract infection, urethritis
- Endometritis, salpingitis

ENCOPRESIS

DESCRIPTION

Incontinence of stool after age 4 years; at least one event per month for 3 months

- Primary encopresis: child has never been toilet trained successfully
- Secondary encopresis: child previously trained begins to soil

ETIOLOGY

- Unclear
- Appears to be associated with emotional as well as physiologic factors, such as constipation
- Often associated with anger

INCIDENCE

- Males > Females
- Affects >1% of children 4 years and older
- More common in low socioeconomic backgrounds

RISK FACTORS

- Dehydration or inadequate fluid intake
- Inappropriate use of laxatives
- Major life or family stress
- Inappropriate toilet training
- Physical or sexual abuse
- Painful bowel movements
- Changes in diet

ASSESSMENT FINDINGS

- Constipation present > 80% of time
- Painful bowel movements
- Fecal/foul odor surrounds child
- Hiding during play
- Attempting to retain stool
- Large amount of stool noted on abdominal exam
- Stool often of large volume

DIFFERENTIAL DIAGNOSIS

- Developmental delay
- Cerebral palsy
- Hirschsprung's disease
- Anal fissure
- Anorectal stenosis
- Hypothyroidism
- Hypercalcemia

DIAGNOSTIC STUDIES

- If associated with constipation, abdominal x-ray is indicated: may show accumulation of stool

PREVENTION

- Educate parents regarding appropriate toilet training and bowel habits
- Assist with stress management
- Early detection of abuse

NONPHARMACOLOGIC MANAGEMENT

Encopresis without constipation:

- Assist with development of appropriate bowel routine; instruct to use the bathroom at specific times
- Reinforce appropriate bowel habits with rewards

Encopresis with constipation:

- High fiber diet
- Increase fluid intake
- Limit milk intake in child > 1 year of age
- Encourage child to take responsibility for toileting; development of bowel routine
- Sit on toilet 10 minutes twice a day after meals
- Administer enemas to evacuate colon if impacted
- Educate parents not to punish child for soiling
- Biofeedback may be helpful

PHARMACOLOGIC MANAGEMENT

Encopresis without constipation:

- Avoid use of laxatives

Encopresis with constipation:

- Administer stool softeners or laxatives if not impacted
- Mineral oil for children > age 5 years (prevents absorption of fat soluble vitamins; **cautious use!**)

CONSULTATION/REFERRAL

- Psychological counseling may be needed

FOLLOW-UP

- Evaluate in 1 week to determine if colon successfully evacuated
- Repeat enemas if necessary
- Teach parent to use laxatives/enemas if stool is retained for > 48 hours, or if soiling resumes
- Recheck monthly for 6 months
- Continue stool softeners until child has not soiled for 1 month

Use laxatives until child has one soft stool daily. Slowly withdraw laxative and wean off. May take several weeks.

EXPECTED COURSE

- Condition can be managed successfully in 80-90% of cases with aggressive treatment and adequate parental education

POSSIBLE COMPLICATIONS

- High-risk of difficulty with social and family relations
- Psychogenic megacolon
- Recurrent UTI
- Anal fissures

RECURRENT ABDOMINAL PAIN

(Functional Abdominal Pain)

DESCRIPTION

Childhood condition in which there are three or more episodes of functional abdominal pain occurring over a 3 month period.

ETIOLOGY

- Unknown

INCIDENCE

- Affects 10% of school age children
- Peak age is 9 years
- Females > Males

RISK FACTORS

- Emotional stress
- Maternal depression, overprotection, or rigidity
- Defective family coping skills
- Family history

ASSESSMENT FINDINGS

- Abdominal pain
  - ◊ Often periumbilical, may be generalized
  - ◊ May be sharp or dull
  - ◊ Constant, or intermittent
  - ◊ Rarely nocturnal
  - ◊ Accompanied by dramatic response and complicated rituals
- School absenteeism
- May include low grade fever, nausea, and vomiting
- Usually no change in bowel habits, sometimes constipation reported
- Pain medication reported as ineffective

DIFFERENTIAL DIAGNOSIS

- Urinary tract infection
- Gastroenteritis
- Lactose intolerance
- Depression
- Irritable bowel syndrome
- Acute abdomen (e.g., appendicitis)

DIAGNOSTIC STUDIES

- CBC with differential: normal
- Urinalysis: normal
- Urine pregnancy test: negative
- Flat and erect x-ray of abdomen: negative
- Breath hydrogen test: no evidence of lactose intolerance

NONPHARMACOLOGIC MANAGEMENT

- Support patient and family, ensuring that pain is taken seriously
- Introduce the possibility that the pain is functional (inorganic)
- Discuss relationship between stress and pain
- Encourage normal activities, including regular school attendance
- Increase dietary fiber if there is constipation

PHARMACOLOGIC MANAGEMENT

- Pain medication is generally not helpful

CONSULTATION/REFERRAL

- Mental health professional if there is family or behavioral dysfunction

FOLLOW-UP

- Provide ongoing support with emphasis on lack of organic cause and lack of physical danger
- Teach signs and symptoms of emergent pain, acute abdomen

EXPECTED COURSE

- Resolves gradually
- Course variable

References

Allison, J., Herrinton, L., Liu, L., Yu, J., & Lowder, J. (2008). Natural history of severe ulcerative colitis in a community-based health plan. Clinical Gastroenterology and Hepatology, 6(9), 999-1003.

American Academy of Pediatrics Subcommittee on Chronic Abdominal Pain. (2005). Chronic abdominal pain in children. Pediatrics, 115(3), 812-815.

American Academy of Pediatrics Subcommittee on Chronic Abdominal Pain, North American Society for Pediatric Gastroenterology Hepatology, & Nutrition. (2005). Chronic abdominal pain in children. Pediatrics, 115(3), e370-381.

American College of Gastroenterology Chronic Constipation Task Force. (2005). An evidence-based approach to the management of chronic constipation in North America. American Journal of Gastroenterology, 100 Suppl 1, S1-4.

Armstrong, G., Wasley, A., Simard, E., McQuillan, G., Kuhnert, W., & Alter, M. (2006). The prevalence of hepatitis c virus infection in the United States, 1999 through 2002. Annals of Internal Medicine, 144(10), 705-714.

Aro, P., Storskrubb, T., Ronkainen, J., Bolling-Sternevald, E., Engstrand, L., Vieth, M., et al. (2006). Peptic ulcer disease in a general adult population: The kalixanda study: A random population-based study. American Journal of Epidemiology, 163(11), 1025-1034.

Barr, R., Paterson, J., MacMartin, L., Lehtonen, L., & Young, S. (2005). Prolonged and unsoothable crying bouts in infants with and without colic. Journal of Developmental and Behavioral Pediatrics, 26(1), 14-23.

Bethony, J., Brooker, S., Albonico, M., Geiger, S., Loukas, A., Diemert, D., et al. (2006). Soil-transmitted helminth infections: Ascariasis, trichuriasis, and hookworm. Lancet, 367(9521), 1521-1532.

Bickley, L. S., & Szilagyi, P. G. (2003). Bates' guide to physical examination and history taking (8th ed.). Philadelphia: Lippincott Williams & Wilkins.

Bongers, M., Tabbers, M., & Benninga, M. (2007). Functional nonretentive fecal incontinence in children. Journal of Pediatric Gastroenterology and Nutrition, 44(1), 5-13.

Buettcher, M., Baer, G., Bonhoeffer, J., Schaad, U., & Heininger, U. (2007). Three-year surveillance of intussusception in children in Switzerland. Pediatrics, 120(3), 473-480.

Burkhart, C., & Burkhart, C. (2005). Assessment of frequency, transmission, and genitourinary complications of enterobiasis (pinworms). International Journal of Dermatology, 44(10), 837-840.

Burns, C. E., Brady, M. A., Blosser, C., Starr, N. B., & Dunn, A. M. (2009). Pediatric primary care: A handbook for nurse practitioners (4th ed.). Philadelphia: W.B. Saunders.

Burns, C. E., Dunn, A. M., Brady, M. A., Starr, N. B., & Blosser, C. (2008). Pediatric primary care: A handbook for nurse practitioners. Philadelphia: W. B. Saunders.

Campbell, J. (1989). Dietary treatment of infant colic: A double-blind study. Journal of the Royal College of General Practitioners, 39(318), 11-14.

Cataldo, P., Ellis, C., Gregorcyk, S., Hyman, N., Buie, W., Church, J., et al. (2005). Practice parameters for the management of hemorrhoids (revised). Diseases of the Colon and Rectum, 48(2), 189-194.

Ceydeli, A., Lavotshkin, S., Yu, J., & Wise, L. (2006). When should we order a ct scan and when should we rely on the results to diagnose an acute appendicitis? Current Surgery, 63(6), 464-468.

Chen, C., Yang, H., Su, J., Jen, C., You, S., Lu, S., et al. (2006). Risk of hepatocellular carcinoma across a biological gradient of serum hepatitis b virus DNA level. JAMA, 295(1), 65-73.

Chey, W., Wong, B., & and the Pratice Parameters Committee of the American College of Gastronenterology. (2007). American college of gastroenterology guideline on the management of helicobacter pylori infection. American Journal of Gastroenterology, 102(8), 1808-1825.

D'Haens, G., Baert, F., van Assche, G., Caenepeel, P., Vergauwe, P., Tuynman, H., et al. (2008). Early combined immunosuppression or conventional management in patients with newly diagnosed crohn's disease: An open randomised trial. Lancet, 371(9613), 660-667.

Dalrymple, J., & Bullock, I. (2008). Diagnosis and management of irritable bowel syndrome in adults in primary care: Summary of nice guidance. BMJ, 336(7643), 556-558.

Desai, S. P. (2009). Clinician's guide to laboratory medicine (3rd ed.). Houston, TX: Md2b.

Domino, F., Baldor, R., Golding, J., Grimes, J., & Taylor, J. (2011). The 5-minute clinical consult 2011. Philadelphia: Lippincott Williams & Wilkins.

Drugs facts and comparisons. (2010). St. Louis: Wolters Kluwer Health.

Ernst, D., & Lee, A. (2010). Nurse practitioners prescribing reference. New York: Haymarket Media Publication.

Etzioni, D., Mack, T., Beart, R. J., & Kaiser, A. (2009). Diverticulitis in the United States: 1998-2005: Changing patterns of disease and treatment. Annals of Surgery, 249(2), 210-217.

Ford, A., Forman, D., Bailey, A., Axon, A., & Moayyedi, P. (2008). Irritable bowel syndrome: A 10-yr natural history of symptoms and factors that influence consultation behavior. American Journal of Gastroenterology, 103(5), 1229-1239; quiz 1240.

Ghany, M., Strader, D., Thomas, D., Seeff, L., & American Association for the Study of Liver Diseases. (2009). Diagnosis, management, and treatment of hepatitis c: An update. Hepatology, 49(4), 1335-1374.

Gilber, D. N., Moellering, R. C., Eliopoulos, G. M., Chambers, H. F., & Saag, M. S. (2010). Sanford guide to antimicrobial therapy (40th ed.).

Hampel, H., Abraham, N., & El-Serag, H. (2005). Meta-analysis: Obesity and the risk for gastroesophageal reflux disease and its complications. Annals of Internal Medicine, 143(3), 199-211.

Haricharan, R., Seo, J., Kelly, D., Mroczek-Musulman, E., Aprahamian, C., Morgan, T., et al. (2008). Older age at diagnosis of hirschsprung disease decreases risk of postoperative enterocolitis, but resection of additional ganglionated bowel does not. Journal of Pediatric Surgery, 43(6), 1115-1123.

Hirsl-He*f*áej, V., Pustisek, N., Sikani*f*á-Dugi*f*á, N., Domljan, L., & Kani, D. (2006). Prevalence of chlamydial genital infection and associated risk factors in adolescent females at an urban reproductive health care center in croatia. Collegium Antropologicum, 30 Suppl 2, 131-137.

Hyman, P., Milla, P., Benninga, M., Davidson, G., Fleisher, D., & Taminiau, J. (2006). Childhood functional gastrointestinal disorders: Neonate/toddler. Gastroenterology, 130(5), 1519-1526.

Johansson, E., Rydh, A., & Riklund, K. (2007). Ultrasound, computed tomography, and laboratory findings in the diagnosis of appendicitis. Acta Radiologica, 48(3), 267-273.

Kahrilas, P., Shaheen, N., Vaezi, M., Hiltz, S., Black, E., Modlin, I., et al. (2008). American gastroenterological association medical position statement on the management of gastroesophageal reflux disease. Gastroenterology, 135(4), 1383-1391, 1391.e1381-1385.

Kaltenbach, T., Crockett, S., & Gerson, L. (2006). Are lifestyle measures effective in patients with gastroesophageal reflux disease? An evidence-based approach. Archives of Internal Medicine, 166(9), 965-971.

Kaptchuk, T., Kelley, J., Conboy, L., Davis, R., Kerr, C., Jacobson, E., et al. (2008). Components of placebo effect: Randomised controlled trial in patients with irritable bowel syndrome. BMJ, 336(7651), 999-1003.

Keeffe, E., Dieterich, D., Han, S., Jacobson, I., Martin, P., Schiff, E., et al. (2006). A treatment algorithm for the management of chronic hepatitis b virus infection in the United States: An update. Clinical Gastroenterology and Hepatology, 4(8), 936-962.

Kornbluth, A., Sachar, D., & the Practice Parameters Committee of the American College of Gastroenterology. (2010). Ulcerative colitis practice guidelines in adults: American college of gastroenterology, practice parameters committee. American Journal of Gastroenterology, 105(3), 501-523; quiz 524.

Lichtenstein, G., Hanauer, S., Sandborn, W., & the Practice Parameters Committee of American College of Gastroenterology. (2009). Management of crohn's disease in adults. American Journal of Gastroenterology, 104(2), 465-483; quiz 464, 484.

Lim, S., Ng, T., Kung, N., Krastev, Z., Volfova, M., Husa, P., et al. (2006). A double-blind placebo-controlled study of emtricitabine in chronic hepatitis b. Archives of Internal Medicine, 166(1), 49-56.

Liu, J., Wyatt, J., Deeks, J., Clamp, S., Keen, J., Verde, P., et al. (2006). Systematic reviews of clinical decision tools for acute abdominal pain. Health Technology Assessment, 10(47), 1-167, iii-iv.

Loening-Baucke, V. (2007). Prevalence rates for constipation and faecal and urinary incontinence. Archives of Disease in Childhood, 92(6), 486-489.

Lopez, P., Cohn, S., Popkin, C., Jackowski, J., Michalek, J., & Group, A. D. (2007). The use of a computed tomography scan to rule out appendicitis in women of childbearing age is as accurate as clinical examination: A prospective randomized trial. American Surgeon, 73(12), 1232-1236.

M√°ller-Lissner, S., Kamm, M., Scarpignato, C., & Wald, A. (2005). Myths and misconceptions about chronic constipation. American Journal of Gastroenterology, 100(1), 232-242.

Malfertheiner, P., Megraud, F., O'Morain, C., Bazzoli, F., El-Omar, E., Graham, D., et al. (2007). Current concepts in the management of helicobacter pylori infection: The Maastricht III Consensus Report. Gut, 56(6), 772-781.

Mandelblatt, J., Cronin, K., Bailey, S., Berry, D., de Koning, H., Draisma, G., et al. (2009). Effects of mammography screening under different screening schedules: Model estimates of potential benefits and harms. Annals of Internal Medicine, 151(10), 738-747.

Manuel, D., Cutler, A., Goldstein, J., Fennerty, M., & Brown, K. (2007). Decreasing prevalence combined with increasing eradication of helicobacter pylori infection in the United States has not resulted in fewer hospital admissions for peptic ulcer disease-related complications. Alimentary Pharmacology and Therapeutics, 25(12), 1423-1427.

Sandborn, W., Feagan, B., & Lichtenstein, G. (2007). Medical management of mild to moderate crohn's disease: Evidence-based treatment algorithms for induction and maintenance of remission. Alimentary Pharmacology and Therapeutics, 26(7), 987-1003.

Sandborn, W., Regula, J., Feagan, B., Belousova, E., Jojic, N., Lukas, M., et al. (2009). Delayed-release oral mesalamine 4.8 g/day (800-mg tablet) is effective for patients with moderately active ulcerative colitis. Gastroenterology, 137(6), 1934-1943.e1931-1933.

Singh, G., Lingala, V., Wang, H., Vadhavkar, S., Kahler, K., Mithal, A., et al. (2007). Use of health care resources and cost of care for adults with constipation. Clinical Gastroenterology and Hepatology, 5(9), 1053-1058.

Sommerfield, T., Chalmers, J., Youngson, G., Heeley, C., Fleming, M., & Thomson, G. (2008). The changing epidemiology of infantile hypertrophic pyloric stenosis in scotland. Archives of Disease in Childhood, 93(12), 1007-1011.

Sonnenberg, A. (2007). Time trends of ulcer mortality in europe. Gastroenterology, 132(7), 2320-2327.

Suita, S., Taguchi, T., Ieiri, S., & Nakatsuji, T. (2005). Hirschsprung's disease in Japan: Analysis of 3852 patients based on a nationwide survey in 30 years. Journal of Pediatric Surgery, 40(1), 197-201; discussion 201-192.

Sung, J., Kuipers, E., & El-Serag, H. (2009). Systematic review: The global incidence and prevalence of peptic ulcer disease. Alimentary Pharmacology and Therapeutics, 29(9), 938-946.

Tack, J., Talley, N., Camilleri, M., Holtmann, G., Hu, P., Malagelada, J., et al. (2006). Functional gastroduodenal disorders. Gastroenterology, 130(5), 1466-1479.

To, T., Wajja, A., Wales, P., & Langer, J. (2005). Population demographic indicators associated with incidence of pyloric stenosis. Archives of Pediatrics and Adolescent Medicine, 159(6), 520-525.

Turner, D., Walsh, C., Steinhart, A., & Griffiths, A. (2007). Response to corticosteroids in severe ulcerative colitis: A systematic review of the literature and a meta-regression. Clinical Gastroenterology and Hepatology, 5(1), 103-110.

van Marrewijk, C., Mujakovic, S., Fransen, G., Numans, M., de Wit, N., Muris, J., et al. (2009). Effect and cost-effectiveness of step-up versus step-down treatment with antacids, h2-receptor antagonists, and proton pump inhibitors in patients with new onset dyspepsia (diamond study): A primary-care-based randomised controlled trial. Lancet, 373(9659), 215-225.

Vogt, T., Wise, M., Bell, B., & Finelli, L. (2008). Declining hepatitis a mortality in the United States during the era of hepatitis a vaccination. Journal of Infectious Diseases, 197(9), 1282-1288.

Yang, H., McElree, C., Roth, M., Shanahan, F., Targan, S., & Rotter, J. (1993). Familial empirical risks for inflammatory bowel disease: Differences between Jews and non-Jews. Gut, 34(4), 517-524.

6

HEALTH PROMOTION: ADULT

Health Promotion: Adult

Primary, Secondary, Tertiary Prevention 311

Adult Health Promotion and Disease Prevention 311

Screening 311

Education and Counseling 313

Vaccine Schedule for Adults 314

Chemoprophylaxis 316

Special Considerations: Elderly Adults 317

Screening 317

Disease Prevention for the International Traveler 318

Obesity 319

References *321*

PRIMARY, SECONDARY, TERTIARY PREVENTION

Diseases and conditions are better prevented than treated. A focus of delivery of primary care to patients is prevention of disease. Prevention is thought of in terms of primary, secondary, and tertiary prevention.

Primary prevention describes an intervention that prevents a disease or condition from occurring. An example of primary prevention is administration of routine tetanus immunization to a healthy, 42 year old.

Secondary prevention describes an intervention that provides early identification of a disease or condition that has recently developed. Examples of secondary prevention are a screening mammogram in a 50 year old female or screening for elevated cholesterol levels in a 21 year old.

Tertiary prevention describes an intervention that recognizes that a clinical disease is already established. The purpose of the intervention is to minimize complications, treat, and restore the patient to the highest level of function. Examples of tertiary prevention are use of cholesterol lowering medication in a patient with coronary artery disease or use of an oral anti-hyperglycemic medication in a patient with diabetes to achieve normal blood glucose values.

Some recommendations for adults by the U.S. Preventive Services Task Force's (USPSTF) Guide to Clinical Preventive Services 2010

ASPIRIN FOR PRIMARY PREVENTION OF CARDIOVASCULAR EVENTS

- Adults (men age 45-79 and women age 55-79) at risk for coronary heart disease because of age, gender, hypertension, hyperlipidemia, family history, or smoking may benefit from daily dose of aspirin
- Benefit: prevention of myocardial infarction
- Risk: possible gastrointestinal or cerebral bleed (risk may be greater in older adults)
- Optimal dose is not known but 75-325 mg daily is reasonable

SCREENINGS

Abdominal Aortic Aneurysm (AAA)

- Screen all men age 65 to 75 who have ever smoked for AAA, using ultrasound examination
- If negative, do not re-screen

Breast Cancer Screening

- There is insufficient evidence to recommend teaching or performing self-breast exam to help decrease mortality from breast cancer
- Screening with mammography for women aged 50-74 years should be done every 2 years depending on risk for breast cancer
- Women age 40 and older with identified risks may benefit from earlier mammogram screenings
- Current studies demonstrate that women 75 years and older are being screened

Cervical Cancer Screening

- Screening should begin after a woman reaches age 21
- It is unclear as to the optimal age to discontinue screening, but, screening after age 65 yielded low results in previously screened women
- There were no differences in outcomes in patients who were screened annually compared to those screened every 3 years

- Discontinuation of cervical screening after total hysterectomy (for benign reasons) is appropriate

Chlamydia Infection Screening

- Sexually active women ages 24 and younger or 25 and older, even if asymptomatic, are at increased risk for infection and, therefore, should be screened
- There is insufficient evidence to recommend a screening interval but consideration should be given to risk factors for infection, change in partners, pregnancy status
- Risk factors include age, unmarried status, Hispanic and African-American races, history of an STD, having new or multiple sexual partners, inconsistent use of contraceptive barrier products, and cervical ectopy
- Women at increased risk, even if asymptomatic, should be screened
- Benefit is unknown for screening high risk men

Colorectal Cancer Screening

- Beginning at age 50 years, men and women of average risk should be screened using fecal occult blood (FOBT), flexible sigmoidoscopy, colonoscopy, OR double-contrast barium enema (BE)
- Annual FOBT has a high rate of false positives
- Colonoscopy can be performed at 10 year intervals; flexible sigmoidoscopy, BE at 5 year intervals
- Persons at increased risk should consider screening at an earlier age. Examples of increased risk are history of colon cancer in a first degree relative before age 60 years, familial polyposis, ulcerative colitis, personal history of colorectal cancer
- Colonoscopy has the highest degree of sensitivity and specificity of all screening tests available but is more expensive and associated with higher risks

Diabetes Mellitus

- There is insufficient evidence to recommend routine screening for elevated glucose levels in asymptomatic adults
- Screening is recommended for adults who have hypertension, hyperlipidemia, polyuria, or polydipsia
- Screen for type 2 DM in asymptomatic adults with a sustained BP greater than 135/80

Hypertension Screening

- All persons >18 years of age should be periodically screened for hypertension with blood pressure measurement (no recommendation is made as to the intervals between measurements)
- Two abnormal measurements should be made on at least two different visits over a period of one to several weeks before a diagnosis of hypertension should be considered

Lipid Disorders

- Men aged > 35 and women aged > 45 years should be screened for lipid disorders and treated if found to be at high risk for development of coronary artery disease (CAD)
- Men aged 20-35 and women aged 20-45 should be screened if they have other risk factors for coronary artery disease
- Risk factors include: personal history of diabetes, family history of CAD or hyperlipidemia, hypertension or tobacco use
- Screening should include measurement of total cholesterol and HDL only (these can be measured in a non-fasting state). Abnormal results should be confirmed
- Optimal intervals for screening, and age to stop screening, are uncertain

Obesity

- All adult patients should be screened for obesity
- Counseling and behavioral interventions should be offered to promote weight loss in adults who are obese

Screening for Osteoporosis

- Women aged 65 and older should be screened for osteoporosis
- Women at increased risk of fractures should be screened starting at age 60
- Frequency of screening is uncertain

EDUCATION AND COUNSELING

NUTRITION

- Whole grains: at least half of daily consumption should be whole grains
- Vegetables: several daily servings with emphasis on dark green and orange ones
- Fruits: several daily servings of fresh, canned, frozen, or dried
- Milk should be low fat or no fat
- Meat/Beans: lean meats, fish, beans
- Oils: minimize use but avoid solid fats
- Women should consume adequate calcium:
  - ◊ Adults age <25 years: 1200-1500 mg/day
  - ◊ Adults age 25-50 years: 1200 mg/day
  - ◊ Postmenopausal women: 1200-1500 mg/day
  - ◊ Pregnant/nursing women: 1200-1500 mg/day
- Individuals who follow a vegetarian diet should be instructed to consume a wide variety of legumes, grains, nuts, seeds, and vegetables to ensure appropriate protein intake

EXERCISE

- Regular physical activity for all adults (most days of the week) because of its proven efficacy in reducing risk of CHD, hypertension, and obesity, and its positive effect on general well-being
- Progressive activity over several months toward achievement of cardiovascular fitness
- Development and maintenance of muscular strength and joint flexibility
- Inclusion of regular weight-bearing exercise to promote bone density
- Discourage sporadic vigorous exercise in favor of consistently performed, moderate-level activities

SMOKING CESSATION

- On a regular basis, promote smoking cessation for all adults
- Pregnant women should be counseled on the effect of smoking on fetal health
- Parents should be counseled on the effect of smoking on child health
- 87% of cancers of the lung, bronchus, and trachea are associated with smoking
- Smoking significantly increases the risk for many cancers, stroke, CAD, peripheral vascular disease
- Discourage exposure to second hand smoke (environmental tobacco smoke). This increases the risk of lung cancer, heart disease, lower respiratory tract infections in children and infants, increases risk of SIDS, aggravates symptoms of asthma, etc.

SAFETY

- Lap/shoulder belt use
- Bicycle and motorcycle helmets
- Smoke detectors
- Firearm safety
- Avoidance of alcohol/drug use while driving, boating, swimming
- Setting on home hot water tank should not exceed 120° F (48.8° C)
- Poison control contact number: 1-800-222-1222

ALCOHOL ABUSE

- Patients with evidence of alcohol dependence should be offered advice and counseling regarding reduction of consumption, and the role of alcohol in current medical or psychosocial problems
- A decreased risk of coronary artery disease is associated with low to moderate alcohol consumption in adults aged > 65 years (2 drinks/day for men; 1 drink or less/day for women)

DENTAL HEALTH

- Daily flossing and brushing with fluoride toothpaste
- Regular preventive dental care
- Avoidance of tobacco

SEXUALLY TRANSMITTED DISEASES

- Sexual behavior counseling should be based on individual risk factors and local epidemiology
  - ◊ Abstinence
  - ◊ Maintenance of a mutually monogamous sexual relationship
  - ◊ Latex condom use for those with multiple partners, casual partners
  - ◊ Female condom for women whose male partner uses no condom
  - ◊ Diaphragm and spermicide helpful in reducing risk of gonorrhea and chlamydia, but not as effective as male condoms and not proven effective against HIV and other STDs

◊ Pregnant women at risk of STDs should be educated regarding potential fetal risk
◊ Alcohol and drug use is associated with high-risk sexual behavior

CONTRACEPTION

- Contraceptive counseling should be based on information obtained though direct questioning about sexual activity, contraceptive use, and concern about pregnancy

TESTICULAR CANCER

- Patients at high risk for the development of testicular cancer (e.g., those with a history of cryptorchidism or atrophic testes) should be informed of their increased risk and instructed on testicular self-examination and to seek appropriate medical attention if an abnormality is noted

SOLAR DAMAGE

- All adults should receive counseling to avoid excess sun and use protective clothing to prevent solar damage and associated risk of skin cancer
- Basal cell and squamous cell carcinoma are in epidemic proportions in the U.S.

VACCINE SCHEDULE FOR ADULTS

Latest vaccine information: www.cdc.gov/nip

- **Tetanus-diphtheria (Td)**
  ◊ Substitute one time dose of Tdap for Td booster, then boost with Td every 10 years
  ◊ Primary series if not completed is 3 doses: first 2 doses are 4 weeks apart, third dose is 6-12 months after the second dose
  ◊ International travelers should receive a booster every 10 years
  ◊ Pregnancy: if woman received last Td vaccination > 10 years ago, administer Td during second or third trimester; if woman received last Td less than 10 years previously, then Tdap during immediate postpartum period

- **Influenza vaccine**: annual vaccination with current vaccine at or around October
  ◊ Inactivated influenza vaccination is indicated for the following adults:
    * Residents of chronic care facilities
    * Chronic cardiopulmonary disorders
    * Chronic metabolic diseases
    * Hemoglobinopathies
    * Immunosuppression
    * Renal dysfunction
    * Health care providers
    * Pregnancy is not a contraindication to receiving the inactivated influenza vaccine; do not use FluMist®
    * For healthy persons aged 5-49 years who do not have contact with high risk persons, FluMist® may be administered

- **Pneumococcal vaccine**: 1 dose recommended for the following adults:
  ◊ All immunocompetent individuals age 65 years or older
  ◊ High-risk groups:
    * Institutionalized persons age 50 years or older
    * Most chronic diseases
    * Chronic cardiac or pulmonary disease (including asthma)
    * Diabetes mellitus
    * Anatomic asplenia
    * Native American and Alaska Native populations - risk for invasive pneumococcal disease is increased
  ◊ Revaccination recommended after 5 years for individuals at highest risk for morbidity and mortality from pneumococcal infection:
    * Persons > 65 years of age for whom > 5 years has passed and were < 65 years at the

initial vaccination
    * Persons with chronic renal failure or nephrotic syndrome, anatomic asplenia, persons with immunocompromising conditions

- **Measles-mumps-rubella (MMR) vaccine** should be administered to all persons born after 1956 who lack evidence of immunity
  ◊ In adults, administer one dose; a second dose should be administered to young adults in settings where there is risk of infection (schools) or exposure, work in healthcare facilities, plan to travel internationally
  ◊ Not recommended after age 50 years, unless other risk factors are present
  ◊ Contraindicated in pregnancy
  ◊ After immunization, counsel to avoid pregnancy for 4 weeks

- **Hepatitis A vaccine** should be administered in a 2-dose schedule at 0 and 6-12 months
  ◊ High risk groups include:
    * Persons seeking protection for hepatitis A virus infection
    * Men who have sex with men and persons who use injectable drugs
    * Persons with chronic liver disease
    * Persons who receive clotting factor concentrates
    * Persons traveling to or working in countries with high or intermediate endemicity of hepatitis A

- **Hepatitis B vaccine** recommended for all young adults and for susceptible adults in high-risk groups; first 2 doses 1 month apart, then a third dose 6 months later.
  ◊ High risk groups include:
    * Men who have sex with men
    * Injecting drug users and their sex partners
    * History of sexual activity with multiple partners in the last 6 months
    * History of recently acquired sexually transmitted disease
    * International travelers to countries where Hepatitis B vaccine is endemic
    * Recipients of blood products, hemodialysis patients
    * Persons in jobs with frequent exposure to blood products
    * Pregnancy is not a contraindication in a high risk person

- **Meningococcal vaccination**
  ◊ Anatomic or functional asplenia or persistent complement component deficiencies
  ◊ First year college students living in dormitories
  ◊ Military recruits
  ◊ Persons who travel to or live in countries in which meningococcal disease is hyperendemic or epidemic
  ◊ Meningococcal polysaccharide vaccine (MPSV4) is preferred for adults aged $\geq$ 56 years
  ◊ Meningococcal conjugate vaccine (MCV4) is preferred for adults $\leq$ 55 years

- **Human Papillomavirus (HPV)**
  ◊ Recommend 3 doses for females age 19 to 26 years if not previously vaccinated; recommendation begins at age 11 to 12 for females
  ◊ Males age 9 to 26 recommended 3 dose regimen

- **Herpes Zoster**
  ◊ Recommended one dose for immunocompetent persons aged 60 or older who lack evidence of immunity

- **Varicella vaccine, 2 doses given 4-8 weeks apart**
  ◊ Recommended for healthy adults with no history of varicella infection who might be at high risk
  ◊ Do not administer during pregnancy; counsel to avoid pregnancy for 4 weeks after vaccine

Additional information about vaccines and schedules can be obtained at www.cdc.gov/vaccines or 800-CDC-INFO, 24 hours a day, 7 days a week

CHEMOPROPHYLAXIS

NEURAL TUBE DEFECTS

- Daily multivitamins containing 0.4-0.8 mg folic acid are recommended for all fertile women in case of unplanned or planned pregnancy to reduce the risk of neural tube defects
- Daily multivitamin containing folic acid supplementation of 0.4-0.8 mg is recommended for all women planning pregnancy beginning at least 1 month prior to conception and continuing through the first trimester
- Women with a history of a previous pregnancy affected by a neural tube defect who are planning pregnancy are advised to supplement their folic acid intake with 4mg/day beginning 1-3 months prior to conception and continuing through the first trimester of pregnancy

HEPATITIS B EXPOSURE

- Postexposure recommendations: Initiate Hepatitis B immunization and give hepatitis B immune globulin (HBIG) in the following circumstances:
  - ◊ Birth of an infant to a hepatitis B surface antigen (HBsAg)-positive mother
  - ◊ Household exposure of an infant < 1 year of age to a primary caregiver with acute Hepatitis B virus
  - ◊ Percutaneous or permucosal exposure to HBsAg-positive blood
  - ◊ Sexual exposure to a HBsAg-positive person

HEPATITIS A EXPOSURE

- Postexposure recommendations: Initiate Hepatitis A immunization and administer immune globulin as soon as possible within 2 weeks after exposure to:
  - ◊ Sexual contacts
  - ◊ Close household contacts
  - ◊ Staff and children at day care centers where a case is recognized
  - ◊ Staff and patients at custodial institutions where Hepatitis A virus transmission has occurred
  - ◊ Food handlers in establishments where a food handler is diagnosed with Hepatitis A virus

MENINGITIS

- Postexposure prophylaxis rifampin/ciprofloxacin for meningococcal meningitis:
  (Casual contacts do not need prophylaxis)
  - ◊ Household contacts of persons with meningococcal infection
  - ◊ Daycare contacts of persons with meningococcal infection
  - ◊ Individuals with direct exposure to oral secretions of a person with meningococcal infection (e.g., kissing)
  - ◊ The meningococcal vaccine is also recommended for persons age 3 months or older in all outbreaks caused by serogroup A strains, and for persons at least 2 years of age in all outbreaks caused by serogroup C, Y, and W-135 strains

Rifampin is contraindicated during pregnancy.

TETANUS

- Postexposure prophylaxis
  - ◊ Tdap should replace a single dose of Td for adults aged 19-64 years who have not received a dose of Tdap previously
  - ◊ Initiate tetanus toxoid (Td) or Tdap if an individual presents with a minor, clean wound, and > 10 years has elapsed since the last dose
  - ◊ If an individual presents with a serious, contaminated wound, tetanus toxoid or Tdap is recommended if > 5 years has elapsed since the last dose

RABIES

- Individuals at high risk of contact with the rabies virus should receive pre-exposure prophylaxis against rabies:
  - ◊ Animal handlers
  - ◊ Rabies laboratory workers
  - ◊ Persons planning to spend > 1 month in an endemic area
- Persons with frequent exposure should have antibody level checked every 6 months and should receive a booster injection as their titers drop below protective levels
- Indications for postexposure prophylaxis with human rabies immune globulin (HRIG):
  - ◊ Dependent on type of animal and circumstances of attack (consult local health department)

◊ Carnivorous wild animal, bat
◊ Unprovoked attack

SPECIAL CONSIDERATIONS: ELDERLY ADULTS

SCREENING:

CAROTID ARTERY STENOSIS

- Patients > age 60 years at high risk for vascular disease are likely to benefit from screening with auscultation for bruits and follow-up carotid ultrasound
- The most effective intervention to prevent brain attack is still smoking cessation and treatment of hypertension

ABDOMINAL AORTIC ANEURYSM

- Men 65-75 years old with risk factors (e.g., vascular disease, family history of abdominal aortic aneurysm (AAA), hypertension, and smoking) are at highest risk for AAA and would benefit most from abdominal palpation or abdominal ultrasound to screen for AAA

PROSTATE CANCER

- Screening for prostate cancer is controversial and should be limited to individuals with a life expectancy >10 years, using digital rectal exam (DRE) and prostatic specific antigen (PSA), and performed only after the patient has been given information regarding the potential benefit and harm of early detection and treatment
- PSA of 4 ng/mL detects the majority of prostate cancers; however, PSA may not detect early prostate cancer

GLAUCOMA

- African-American patients with diabetes, severe myopia, family history of glaucoma, and/or 65 years of age and older are at greatest risk of developing glaucoma and may benefit from screening for increased intraocular pressure. Effective screening is best performed by an eye specialist with the benefit of proper equipment

HEARING IMPAIRMENT

- Older adults are at risk for hearing impairment, particularly presbycusis (progressive loss of hearing and sound discrimination characterized by inability to hear the consonants "s", "sh", and "f", which are high-frequency sounds)
- Screening for hearing impairment by questioning regarding hearing is recommended
- Audiometric testing is appropriate follow-up if questioning reveals the possibility of hearing difficulty

ACTIVITIES OF DAILY LIVING

- Information regarding ability to perform activities of daily living should be solicited from patients and from family members. Direct questioning may be accompanied by brief standardized questionnaires, but questionnaires are not a reliable substitute for interview. If dementia is suspected, further assessment to exclude primary causes (e.g., depression, physical illness, and medication effect) is important

DEPRESSION

- Clinicians should maintain a high index of suspicion for depressive symptoms in elderly patients who have suffered recent losses, or those with chronic illness

ABUSE

- Elderly dependent adults who present with multiple injuries, or with an unsatisfactory explanation for injuries, should be assessed for abuse and followed accordingly

CERVICAL CANCER

- Women older than 65 years do not appear to benefit from Pap testing if 3 consecutive Pap smears have been normal; however, many women in this age group have not been previously tested on a consistent basis and may still benefit from the screening

POLYPHARMACY

- Older adults tend to be on multiple medications
- "Brown Bag Test": encourage elderly patients to bring all medications for each clinic visit so prescriber may assess medications for drug interactions, contraindications, duplications, etc.

DISEASE PREVENTION FOR THE INTERNATIONAL TRAVELER

For latest information: www.cdc.gov/travel/

MALARIA

- Malaria is transmitted through the bite of an infected female Anopheles mosquito, by blood transfusion, and congenitally
  - ◊ Endemic in Central America, South America, Sub-Saharan Africa, India, Southeast Asia, Middle East, and Oceania
  - ◊ Stay in well screened area, use mosquito nets, clothing to cover body
  - ◊ High-risk hours are between dusk and dawn
  - ◊ Adherence to specific antimalarial drug regimen

TRAVELERS' DIARRHEA

- Risk is associated with travel to developing countries: Latin America, Middle East, Asia, parts of the Caribbean, and southern Europe
- Transmitted through ingestion of fecally contaminated food and fluids
- Educate regarding food and beverage intake
- Avoid raw and undercooked meat and fish, fresh fruit, drinks with ice, local tap water, ground-grown vegetables, foods sold by street venders, and dairy products
- Fluids safest to ingest are bottled carbonated beverages, canned fruit juices, beer, wine, drinks with boiled water (e.g., tea, coffee)
- Cautious use of non antimicrobial medications: bismuth subsalicylate (Pepto-Bismol®), loperamide (Imodium®)
- Antimicrobial agents:
  - ◊ Trimethoprim sulfamethoxazole (Bactrim®, Septra®)
  - ◊ Doxycycline (Vibramycin®)
  - ◊ Norfloxacin (Noroxin®)
  - ◊ Ciprofloxacin (Cipro®)
- Rehydration regimen recommended by World Health Organization (WHO):
  - ◊ Dissolve ½ teaspoon table salt, ½ teaspoon baking soda, ¼ teaspoon KCl, and 2½ tablespoons sucrose in 1 L drinkable water
  - ◊ Drink 2-5 L/day

SCHISTOSOMIASIS

- Avoid swimming in fresh water in endemic areas
- Adequately chlorinated and salt water are safe

HEPATITIS A AND B

- Immunizations are recommended before travel to areas where these diseases may be endemic

TETANUS

- Up to date immunization is recommended before travel outside the U.S.

OBESITY

DESCRIPTION

Condition of increased body weight that leads to increased morbidity and mortality. Defined as weight 20% greater than an individual's ideal body weight. Abdominal (android) obesity carries increased risk for long-term health problems.

ETIOLOGY

- Multifactorial: genetic, social, developmental, psychological, metabolic
- Imbalance between food intake and energy expenditure
- Insulinoma
- Diabetes mellitus
- Glucocorticosteroid drug therapy
- Cushing's syndrome
- Hypothyroidism
- Hypothalamic disorders

INCIDENCE

- On increase in the U.S.
- Prevalence of obesity
  - ◊ 20-30% in adult males
  - ◊ 30-40% in adult females
  - ◊ 11-15% in adolescents

RISK FACTORS

- Decreased socioeconomic status
- High fat diet
- Parental obesity
- Sedentary life-style
- Increased television viewing/computer use, especially among children

ASSESSMENT FINDINGS

- BMI $\geq$ 30 kg/m^2 (BMI 25-29.9 kg/m^2) is considered overweight
- BMI = body weight (kg) / body height (m)^2

A simple way to determine ideal body weight:
  - ◊ Men: 106 lbs + 6 lbs/inch over 5 feet
  - ◊ Women: 100 lbs + 5 lbs/inch over 5 feet

- Abdominal (android) obesity: waist: hip ratio > 0.85 in women and > 0.95 in men. (To obtain, divide waist measurement by hip measurement)
- Use food diaries and self-assessments to determine eating habits

DIAGNOSTIC STUDIES

- Not needed for diagnosis, but can assist with identification of underlying problem and development of treatment plan
- Thyroid function studies
- Lipid profile
- Blood glucose

PREVENTION

- Well-balanced diet following USDA Food Guide Pyramid
- Regular exercise

NONPHARMACOLOGIC MANAGEMENT

- Severely restrictive diets are not recommended
- Counseling regarding life-long behavior changes
- Well-balanced diet following USDA Food Guide Pyramid
- Behavior modification
- Determine caloric requirement for body weight and activity level

PREGNANCY/LACTATION CONSIDERATIONS

- Well-balanced diet should be maintained in pregnancy
- Restrictive caloric intake is not recommended in pregnancy
- Common time of onset or worsening of obesity

CONSULTATION/REFERRAL

- Refer to community organizations for weight loss and maintenance programs (e.g., Weight Watchers)
- Refer for nutritional counseling

FOLLOW-UP

- Long-term frequent follow-up

EXPECTED COURSE

- Chronic condition that is rarely cured
- Long-term maintenance of weight loss difficult
- Dependent on sustained patient motivation

POSSIBLE COMPLICATIONS

- Increased mortality
- Cardiovascular disease
- Diabetes mellitus
- Hypertension
- Hyperlipidemia
- Cholelithiasis especially with rapid weight loss
- Osteoarthritis
- Hypoventilation
- Gout
- Thromboembolism
- Sleep apnea
- Low self-esteem
- Decreased mobility
- Decreased exercise tolerance

References

Centers for Disease Control and Prevention. (2010). Recommended adult immunization schedule — United States, 2010. *MMWR. Morbidity and Mortality Weekly Report, 59*(1), 1-4.

Fiore, A. E., Shay, D. K., Broder, K., Iskander, J. K., Uyeki, T. M., Mootrey, G., et al. (2009). Prevention and control of seasonal influenza with vaccines: Recommendations of the advisory committee on immunization practices (acip), 2009. *MMWR Recomm Rep, 58*(RR-8), 1-52.

Trinite, T., Loveland-Cherr, C., & Marion, L. (2009). The U.S. Preventive services task force: An evidence-based prevention resource for nurse practitioners. *Journal of the American Academy of Nurse Practitioners, 21* (6), 301-306.

U.S. Preventive Services Task Force. (2010). *Guide to clinical preventive services* (3u ed.). Washington, DC: U.S. Government Printing Office.

7

HEALTH PROMOTION: PEDIATRICS

Health Promotion: Pediatrics

Primary, Secondary, Tertiary Prevention 327

Tanner Stages of Physical Development 327

Newborn (Birth to One Month) 328

Two Months (Infant) 331

Four Months (Infant) 332

Six Months (Infant) 333

Nine Months (Infant) 334

Twelve Months (Toddler) 335

Fifteen Months (Toddler) 337

Eighteen Months (Toddler) 338

Two Years (Toddler) 339

Three Years (Toddler) 340

Four Years (Preschool) 341

Five Years (Preschool) 342

Six Years (School Age) 343

Eight Years (School Age) 344

Ten Years (School Age) 345

Early Adolescence (11, 12, 13, and 14 Years) 346

Middle Adolescence (15, 16, and 17 Years) 347

Late Adolescence (18, 19, 20, and 21 Years) 348

Immunizations 349

References *351*

Health Promotion-Pediatrics

PRIMARY, SECONDARY, TERTIARY PREVENTION

Diseases and conditions are better prevented than treated. A focus of delivery of primary care to patients is prevention of disease. Prevention is thought of in terms of primary, secondary, and tertiary prevention.

Primary prevention describes an intervention that prevents a disease or condition from occurring. An example of primary prevention is administration of routine MMR to a healthy, 12 month old.

Secondary prevention describes an intervention that provides early identification of a disease or condition that has recently developed. An example of secondary prevention is PKU screening in a newborn.

Tertiary prevention describes an intervention that recognizes that a clinical disease is already established. The purpose of the intervention is to minimize complications, treat, and restore the patient to the highest level of function. An example of tertiary prevention is treatment of iron deficiency anemia with daily iron supplements in an iron deficient adolescent.

TANNER STAGES OF PHYSICAL DEVELOPMENT

(SEXUAL MATURITY RATING)

FEMALE BREASTS

STAGE 1
- Prepubertal: papilla elevated above chest wall

STAGE 2
- Breast bud stage: breast and papilla form small mound, areola increases in diameter

STAGE 3
- Breast and areola enlarge, no separation in contours

STAGE 4
- Secondary mound formed by areola and papilla about at level of breast

STAGE 5
- Adult breast: nipple projects, areola becomes part of contour of breast

MALE GENITALIA

STAGE 1
- Testes one centimeter, scrotum and penis are size seen in early childhood

STAGE 2
- Slight enlargement of testes (2-3 centimeters), scrotum becomes reddened and textured

STAGE 3
- Further testicular growth (3-4 centimeters), slight enlargement of penis

STAGE 4
- Penis increases in length and diameter, testes enlarge (4-5 centimeters)

STAGE 5
- Adult genitalia, (testes 5 centimeters)

PUBIC HAIR

STAGE 1
- No pubic hair present

STAGE 2
- Sparse, lightly pigmented, straight along border of labia/base of penis

STAGE 3
- Hair becomes more pigmented, coarse, curled, and more abundant

STAGE 4

- Pubic hair is abundant but covers smaller area than found in adult

STAGE 5

- Adult in type and quantity with horizontal distribution

STAGE 6

- Hair grows up linea alba

NEWBORN (NEONATE)

(Birth to One Month)

TERMS

- Preterm: gestational age less than 37 weeks
- AGA (appropriate for gestational age): preterm or term babies whose measurements are between the 10th and 90th percentiles
- SGA (small for gestational age): refers to babies whose measurements fall below the 10th percentile
- LGA (large for gestational age): refers to babies whose lengths and weights are above 90th percentile regardless of age

NEWBORN ASSESSMENT/SCREENING

- Charts for male and female infants and children can be found: www.cdc.gov/growthcharts

Height, weight, and head circumference should always be plotted on growth charts.

NORMAL ASSESSMENT/SCREENING

LENGTH

- Average is 20 inches (50.8 cm)

WEIGHT

- Always compare weight with gestational age
- Average is 7.5 lbs (3.4 kg)
- Weight between 6-9 lbs (2.72 kg-4.1 kg)
- Babies lose 10% of birth weight in first 3 or 4 days of life

HEAD

- Circumference measured at largest circumference above the ears
- Average is 13 to 14 inches (33.0-35.6 cm)

Hydrocephalus: an excess amount of CSF which accumulates in the ventricles.
Microcephalus: a skull that is abnormally small and is usually associated with mental retardation.

- Cranial molding: occurs with vertex delivery due to overriding of cranial bones at the sutures
- Breech delivery: swelling and ecchymosis to presenting part, absence of cranial molding

Caput succedaneum: swelling and/or ecchymosis of the scalp over the presenting part, resolves within a few days.
Cephalhematoma: accumulation of blood which produces swelling that does not cross suture lines, disappears over several weeks to months.

- Fontanels
  - ◊ Posterior (1 cm in diameter) rarely palpable at birth, closes by 2 months of age, slight depression is normal
  - ◊ Anterior (2-3 cm in diameter) remains palpable until 9-18 months, slightly depressed is normal

The anterior fontanel should always be open at birth and about the size of your thumbnail.

EYES

- Red reflex should be present bilaterally
- Absent red reflex may indicate congenital cataracts, retinoblastoma
- PERRL
- Chemical conjunctivitis due to silver nitrate or erythromycin ointment may be seen
- Purulent eye discharge usually associated with gonococcus, chlamydia, or herpes

- Eyes should open symmetrically but may appear puffy (normal)
- Disconjugate gaze is normal in the newborn
- Retinopathy of prematurity (formerly called retrolental fibroplasia): develops in premature infants presumably related to use of high oxygen concentrations, apnea, and sepsis. Resulting blindness is irreversible
- Hypertelorism (wide set eyes): present in Down syndrome

The average visual acuity of a newborns is 20/200 to 20/400.

EARS

- Assess risk factors for hearing problems: NICU admission for > 2 days, congenital CMV, herpes, or rubella infections, bilirubin > 20 mg/dL, family history of hearing problems, abnormalities of the pinna and ear canal
- Inspect ears for positioning
- Low set ears: may indicate renal or genetic abnormality, multisystem syndrome
- Assess gross hearing by observing for startle response to loud noise
- Routine hearing screen performed in newborn nursery: otoacoustic emissions (OAE)
- Auditory evoked response testing for newborns at high risk for neural hearing loss

NARES

- Patency assessed by closing mouth and each naris separately or passing small catheter into nasopharynx

No nasal flaring should be present.

MOUTH

- Palate: intact
- Cleft palate: a fissure in the mid palate usually associated with the cleft lip
- Assess frenulum length

Short frenulum makes tongue movement difficult and impedes speech.

- Epstein's pearls: small, white, cysts on the palate and gums; common
- Natal teeth sometimes present: possible risk of aspiration if very loose

NECK

- Webbing: excessive amounts of skin seen in Turner's and Noonan's syndromes
- Masses: thyroglossal cysts, hematoma in the sternocleidomastoid muscle
- Torticollis: turning of head to one side due to shortening of the sternocleidomastoid muscle

CLAVICLE

- May be fractured in LGA babies delivered vaginally, usually resolves without treatment
- Crepitus sometimes present if clavicle fractured
- Decreased movement of arm on affected side, if clavicle fractured
- Ecchymosis visible from injury

HEART

- Normal rate is 120-160 beats per minute
- Murmurs common (only 10% are significant)
- Marked sinus arrhythmia (normal)
- Femoral pulses equal and strong

Coarctation of the aorta should be suspected when femoral pulses are unequal or weak.

- Dextrocardia, situs inversus: assess PMI location to rule out dextrocardia
- Cardiac murmurs may present with cyanosis or heart failure

SKIN

- No jaundice should be present at birth
- Lanugo: fine, dark, hair over the trunk and shoulders; seen in prematurity
- Vernix: white, greasy, thick material found on infant's skin; seen in prematurity
- Milia: multiple, tiny (1 mm) papules on the forehead, cheeks, and nose; common
- Acrocyanosis: bluish skin changes to feet and hands normal during first few days of life due to heat loss

Observe for peripheral cyanosis which usually indicates cardiac or respiratory problems.

- Meconium staining may occur if first stool is passed in utero. Infant's skin and fingernails may be stained
- "Stork bite" on nape of neck, eyelids; common
- Mongolian spot (hyperpigmented nevi): usually in sacral and gluteal area; common

ABDOMEN

- No masses or distention should be present
- Palpate kidneys to assess for agenesis or

hypoplasia
- Umbilical hernia should be easily reducible if present; common
- Umbilical stump should fall off by the 14th day
- Failure to pass meconium stool within 24 hours of birth is abnormal

GENITALIA (MALE)
- Urethral opening should be at the tip of penis (see Hypospadias in Men's Health Disorders chapter, page 415)

Circumcision is delayed for hypospadias because foreskin may be used during repair.

- Palpate scrotum for presence of testes (see Cryptorchidism in Men's Health Disorders chapter, page 406)
- Testes descended into scrotum or able to be retrieved to scrotum. Must be monitored. If unable to palpate, refer to urologist
- Hydrocele is common (identify by transillumination of scrotum)
- Assess for inguinal hernia

GENITALIA (FEMALE)
- Labia and vagina should be patent
- White discharge may be present (normal), small amount blood tinged discharge may be present (normal for the first few days)

Ambiguous genitalia always abnormal.

PATENT ANUS AND RECTUM
- Both should be patent
- Temperature measurement with rectal thermometer will determine anal patency

HIP DYSPLASIA (see Orthopedic Disorders, page 523)

LOWER EXTREMITY ABNORMALITIES
- Foot curvatures often due to intrauterine molding (in-toeing and out-toeing)
- Tibial curvatures (seldom pathologic)
- Genu varum: bowleg
- Genu valgum: knock-knee
- Club foot (talipes): talipes equinovarus most common, foot is plantar flexed, inverted, and significantly adducted (may require casting/ taping in the nursery)
- Metatarsus adductus: adduction of the forefoot (no treatment needed usually)

NEUROLOGICAL
- Muscle tone: observe tone, symmetry, and movement
- Assess spine for spinal bifida, pilonidal dimple

REFLEXES
- Babinski
- Moro
- Palmar grip
- Rooting
- Sucking
- Stepping/placing response

CRANIAL NERVES (CN)
- CN II (optic): assessed by checking response to bright light (squinting)
- CN III (oculomotor), CN IV (trochlear), CN VI (abducens): tested by observing infant's ability to gaze in all directions
- CN V (trigeminal), CN IX (glossopharyngeal), CN X (vagus), and CN XII (hypoglossal): tested by observing sucking and swallowing
- CN VII (facial): tested by observing symmetrical facial movements during crying
- CN VIII (acoustic): tested by observing startle reaction to loud noise

SCREENING
- Screening varies by state
- Universal screening of phenylketonuria (PKU) and congenital hypothyroidism
- Hemoglobinopathy
- Ideal time for screening of PKU is 24 hours after retained feedings because metabolites may not have been produced before this time

NEWBORN DEVELOPMENT
- Observe interaction of parent(s) with infant for feeding, holding, and caring for baby
- Observe baby's suck reflex and/or attachment
- Observe response to sound, blinking, crying, parents' voice, and face
- Posture should be flexed

ANTICIPATORY GUIDANCE
- Newborn infant will feed every 2-3 hours. Awaken to feed if 4 hours have elapsed without feeding
- Breastfed and formula fed infants usually do not require vitamin D supplementation. Supplementation is needed if the lactating woman's diet is lacking in vitamin D or if formula is not vitamin D fortified and the infant does not have adequate exposure to sunlight

NEVER place infants < 6 months of age in direct sunlight.

- Discuss car seat use (rear facing in the back seat; center placed is safest until 20 pounds (9.1 kg and 1 year of age)
- Place infant on back or side for sleeping

Do not place pillows in infant's crib and always place sides of crib in "up" position.

- Never leave unattended while changing diaper
- Do not use baby powder
- Discuss importance of smoke free environment with caregiver
- Review signs and symptoms of illness and course of action: fever, dehydration, vomiting, jaundice, etc.
- Discuss cord care
- Discuss circumcision if applicable
- Discuss frequency of bowel movements/wet diapers
- Use clothing/blanket to maintain body temperature

TWO MONTHS
(Infant)

NORMAL GROWTH/ASSESSMENT SCREENING
- Length: one inch per month
- Weight: about one ounce per day
- Head circumference: 0.5 inches (1.25 cm) per month
- Plot all on growth chart

EYES
- Red reflex bilaterally
- Dacryostenosis (see Ophthalmic Disorders, page 483)
- Dacryocystitis; common
- Assess for strabismus
- Assess ability to visually track object

EARS
- Assess gross hearing

MOUTH
- Assess suck reflex
- Check for oral candidiasis

HEART
- Evaluate for presence of cardiac murmurs
- Evaluate femoral pulses bilaterally for coarctation of the aorta

SKIN
- Assess for cradle cap
- Assess for diaper rash
- Assess for atopic dermatitis if family history
- Assess for signs of abuse

ABDOMEN
- Assess for abdominal masses
- Assess for umbilical hernia

GENITALIA (MALE)
- Assess for bilaterally descended testes
- Identify hydrocele by transillumination
- Assess for inguinal hernia

GENITALIA (FEMALE)
- Assess for labial adhesions

MUSCULOSKELETAL
- Assess for hip dysplasia
- Assess for torticollis
- Assess for metatarsus adductus

NEUROLOGICAL
- Check palmar grasp
- Check plantar grasp
- Check Moro reflex
- Check stepping response
- Assess rooting reflex
- Check for tonic neck ("fencing" reflex appears at 2-3 months)
- Assess Babinski reflex

SCREENING
- Assess gross hearing
- Assess lead risk
- Developmental screening (e.g., Denver Developmental Screening Tool)

DEVELOPMENT
- Infant should focus on face

- Grasps rattle if placed in hand
- Smiles, coos
- Able to lift head 45° and has some control when torso held upright

ANTICIPATORY GUIDANCE
- Discuss car seat use
- Place infant on back/side for sleeping
- Review signs and symptoms of illness/course of action
- Encourage infant-parent interactions
- Encourage parents to take brief periods of time away from baby
- No solid foods, do not place cereal in bottle
- Do not give plain water to infants < 6 months. This increases the risk of hyponatremia

Honey may expose infant to spores of *Clostridium botulinum*. Avoid until at least 1 year of age.

- Discuss colic, immunizations and possible side effects

FOUR MONTHS
(Infant)

NORMAL GROWTH/ASSESSMENT SCREENING
- Length: one inch (2.5 cm) per month
- Weight: about one ounce (28 g) per day
- Head circumference: 0.5 inches (1.25 cm) per month
- Plot all on growth chart

EYES
- Red reflex should be present bilaterally
- Dacryostenosis (see Ophthalmic Disorders, page 483)
- Dacryocystitis; common
- Assess for strabismus
- Assess ability to visually track object

EARS
- Assess gross hearing

MOUTH
- Assess suck reflex
- Assess for presence of oral candidiasis

HEART
- Evaluate for presence of cardiac murmurs

SKIN
- Assess for cradle cap
- Assess for diaper rash
- Assess for atopic dermatitis, especially if family history
- Assess for signs of abuse

ABDOMEN
- Assess for abdominal masses
- Assess for umbilical hernia

GENITALIA (MALE)
- Assess for bilaterally descended testes (2/3 males have spontaneous descent by 3-4 months)
- Identify hydrocele by transillumination
- Assess for inguinal hernia

GENITALIA (FEMALE)
- Assess for labial adhesions

MUSCULOSKELETAL
- Assess for hip dysplasia
- Assess for metatarsus adductus

NEUROLOGICAL
- Check plantar grasp
- Assess Moro reflex
- Assess stepping response
- Rooting reflex (disappears by 4 months except during sleep)
- Check for tonic neck ("fencing" reflex appears at 2-3 months)
- Assess Babinski reflex

SCREENING
- Gross hearing
- Assess lead risk
- Developmental screening (e.g., Denver Developmental Screening Tool)

DEVELOPMENT
- Infant should focus on face
- Grasps rattle if placed in hand
- Smiles, coos, recognizes caregivers' voice and touch
- Able to hold and control head when held upright
- No head lag when pulled upright
- Raises body on hands

- Rolls prone to supine
- Follows light 180°

ANTICIPATORY GUIDANCE

- Discuss car seat use
- Discuss teething and measures to soothe painful gums
- Avoid bottle propped in bed or held in bed
- No vitamin mineral supplement is needed at this time if formula fed or well-nourished mother who breastfeeds (otherwise, infant may be at risk)
- Discuss childproofing home (small, sharp, or dangerous objects, poisons, medications)
- Discuss introduction of solid foods: cereal first, then pureed fruit and vegetables
- Development of bedtime ritual
- Provide age appropriate toys
- Play peek-a-boo and pat-a-cake
- Have Poison Control Center number in case of accidental ingestion (syrup of ipecac should ONLY be administered when specifically directed by Poison Control Center)

Syrup of ipecac should not be administered:
*** If ingestion of acids, alkalis, hydrocarbons, sharp objects, or seizure-inducing drugs has occurred**
*** To children < 6 months of age**
*** In cases of diminished gag reflexes or coma**

SIX MONTHS
(Infant)

NORMAL GROWTH ASSESSMENT SCREENING

- Length: grows 1/2 inch (1.25 cm) per month
- Weight: gains about 3-4 ounces (90-100 g) per week; doubled birth weight at this age
- Head circumference: 0.25 inches (.8 cm) per month
- Plot all on growth chart

EYES

- Red reflex should be present bilaterally
- Dacryostenosis (see Ophthalmic Disorders, page 483)
- Dacryocystitis; common
- Assess for strabismus
- Assess ability to visually track object

EARS

- Assess gross hearing

MOUTH

- Assess for tooth eruption
- Lower central incisors (6 months)
- Lower lateral incisors (7 months)
- Upper central incisors (7.5 months)

HEART

- Evaluate for presence of cardiac murmurs

SKIN

- Assess for cradle cap
- Assess for diaper rash
- Assess for atopic dermatitis if family history
- Assess for signs of abuse

ABDOMEN

- Assess for abdominal masses
- Assess for umbilical hernia

GENITALIA (Male)

- Assess for bilaterally descended testes (Refer if not palpable bilaterally)
- Identify hydrocele by transillumination
- Assess for inguinal hernia

GENITALIA (FEMALE)

- Assess for labial adhesions

MUSCULOSKELETAL

- Assess for hip dysplasia
- Assess for metatarsus adductus
- Assess for flat feet
- Assess muscle tone

NEUROLOGICAL

- Check plantar grasp
- Moro reflex disappearance at about 6 months
- Stepping response still present
- Tonic neck ("fencing" reflex disappears at about 6 months)
- Assess Babinski reflex

SCREENING

- Gross hearing
- Assess for anemia in the following situations:
  - Low socioeconomic status

- Birthweight < 1500 grams (3.3 lbs)
  - Low iron formula used (not recommended)
  - Whole milk prior to 1 year of age (not recommended)
- Developmental screening (e.g., Denver Developmental Screening Tool)

DEVELOPMENT
- Bears weight and stands when placed
- Sits with support/may be unassisted
- Rolls supine to prone
- No head lag when pulled upright
- Able to place object in opposite hand and in mouth
- Recognizes parents
- Says "dada" or "baba"
- Babbles
- Smiles, squeals, laughs, imitates some sounds

ANTICIPATORY GUIDANCE
- Discuss child proofing home (small, sharp, or dangerous objects, poisons, medications)
- Be aware of hazards at child's level: buckets, electric sockets, etc.
- Discuss introduction of solid foods 2-3 times per day. If solid foods have not been introduced, initiate at this age.
- Needs iron fortified cereal at least twice daily if breast fed
- Needs iron fortified cereal even if infant consumes iron fortified formula
- Discuss foods that are a choking hazard (e.g., nuts, hot dogs, whole grapes, hard candy)
- Introduce a cup for liquids
- Dental care: clean teeth with soft brush and plain water
- Fluoride supplements if not sufficient amounts in drinking water for fluoride supplementation for children over 6 months of age
- Use distraction, schedules, and routines as discipline; be consistent
- Put baby in bed for sleep while still awake

Baby will learn how to console self when awakens at nighttime.

- Play peek-a-boo and pat-a-cake
- Provide opportunities for exploring
- Do not use baby walkers

NINE MONTHS
(Infant)

NORMAL GROWTH/ASSESSMENT SCREENING
- Length: grows 1/2 inch (1.25 cm) per month
- Weight: about 3-4 ounces (90-100 g) per week
- Head circumference: 0.25 inches (.8 cm) per month
- Plot all on growth chart

EYES
- Red reflex should be present bilaterally
- Dacryostenosis (see Ophthalmic Disorders, page 483)
- Dacryocystitis; common
- Assess for strabismus
- Assess ability to visually track object

EARS
- Assess gross hearing

MOUTH
- Assess for tooth eruption
- Upper lateral incisors

HEART
- Evaluate for presence of cardiac murmurs

SKIN
- Assess for cradle cap
- Assess for diaper rash
- Assess for atopic dermatitis if family history
- Assess for signs of abuse

ABDOMEN
- Assess for abdominal masses
- Assess for umbilical hernia

GENITALIA (Male)
- Assess for bilaterally descended testes (Refer if not palpable bilaterally)
- Identify hydrocele by transillumination
- Assess for inguinal hernia

GENITALIA (FEMALE)
- Assess for labial adhesions

MUSCULOSKELETAL

- Assess for hip dysplasia
- Assess for metatarsus adductus
- Assess for flat feet
- Assess muscle tone

NEUROLOGICAL

- Check plantar grasp
- Stepping reflex disappears at 9 months
- Babinski reflex still intact

SCREENING

- Assess gross hearing
- Assess lead risk
- Assess for anemia
- Developmental screening (e.g., Denver Developmental Screening Tool)

DEVELOPMENT

- Crawls, creeps, and scoots
- Sits independently
- Pulls to stand
- Bangs, shakes, drops, and throws objects
- Able to feed self with finger foods
- Responds to own name and understands a few words
- Stranger anxiety develops

ANTICIPATORY GUIDANCE

- Discuss child proofing home (small, sharp, or dangerous objects, poisons, medications, etc.)
- Be aware of hazards at child's level: buckets, electric sockets, bath tub, check hot water thermostat (setting should be $< 120°$)
- Discuss introduction of mashed foods and finger foods, start table foods
- Discuss weaning from bottle
- Discuss nuts, hot dogs, whole grapes, hard candy, tough meat, etc. as choking hazards
- Fluoride supplements if not sufficient amounts in drinking water
- Brush teeth daily and at bedtime
- Use distraction as discipline
- Limit rules, but enforce consistently
- Put baby to bed awake
- Play peek-a-boo and pat-a-cake
- Provide opportunities for exploring
- Do not use baby walkers

TWELVE MONTHS
(Toddler)

NORMAL GROWTH/ASSESSMENT SCREENING

- Length: grows three inches (7.5 cm) annually
- Weight: gains about 4½ to 6½ lbs (2 kg to 3 kg) annually; should have tripled weight by this time
- Head circumference: one inch (2.5 cm) annually
- Plot all on growth chart
- Initial dental screening 12-36 months of age (when cooperative)

EYES

- Red reflex should be present bilaterally
- If dacryostenosis present refer to ophthalmologist
- Dacryocystitis; becoming less common at this age
- Assess for strabismus
- Assess ability to visually track object

EARS

- Assess gross hearing

MOUTH

- Assess teeth for decay and eruption
- Lower first molars (12 months)

HEART

- Evaluate for presence of cardiac murmurs
- Normal heart rate: 80-160 beats per minute

SKIN

- Assess for diaper rash
- Assess for atopic dermatitis if family history
- "Stork bites" usually disappear by this age
- Assess for signs of abuse

ABDOMEN

- Assess for abdominal masses
- Assess for umbilical hernia

GENITALIA (MALE)

- Descended testes
- Identify hydrocele by transillumination (if hydrocele still present at this time, refer to urologist)
- Assess for inguinal hernia

GENITALIA (FEMALE)

- Assess for labial adhesions

MUSCULOSKELETAL

- Assess for hip dysplasia
- Assess for metatarsus adductus
- Assess feet
- Assess gait

NEUROLOGICAL

- Rooting (may be present up to 12 months during sleep)

SCREENING

- Gross hearing
- Assess lead risk
- Assess for anemia if high risk

Consider PPD if:
*** Low socioeconomic status**
*** Prior exposure to tuberculosis**
*** Foreign birth**

- Mantoux skin using purified protein derivative (PPD) test considered most reliable for tuberculosis screening
- Developmental screening (e.g., Denver Developmental Screening Tool)

DEVELOPMENT

- Pulls to stand, may take a few steps
- Bangs blocks together
- Uses pincer grasp and able to point
- Says 2-4 words
- Looks for dropped or hidden objects
- Responds to own name and understands a few words
- Feeds self and drinks from cup
- Waves and says "bye-bye", "dada", and "mama"
- Imitates vocalizations

ANTICIPATORY GUIDANCE

- Child car seat can face forward if child weighs at least 20 pounds (seat must remain in car's rear seat)
- Re-examine home for dangerous objects, poisons
- Home safety around lawnmowers, moving cars in driveway, animals, streets, pool, bathtub, etc.
- Provide healthy food choices and 2-3 nutritious snacks daily (expect decrease in appetite)
- Start on 2% milk, fat is needed for adequate brain development

Begin weaning from bottle.

- Avoid nuts, hot dogs, whole grapes, hard candy, tough meat, etc.
- Allow toddler to feed self (wash hands often; especially before eating)
- Fluoride supplements if not sufficient amounts in drinking water
- Brush teeth daily and at bedtime
- Do not allow child to bite or hit
- Limit rules, but enforce consistently
- Praise, talk, show affection to child
- Provide opportunities for exploring environment
- Expect curiosity about genitals

FIFTEEN MONTHS
(Toddler)

NORMAL GROWTH/ASSESSMENT SCREENING
- Length: three inches (7.5 cm) annually
- Weight: about 4½ to 6½ lbs (2 kg to 3 kg) annually
- Head circumference: one inch (2.5 cm) annually
- Plot all on growth chart

EYES
- Red reflex should be present bilaterally
- Assess for strabismus
- Assess ability to visually track object

EARS
- Assess gross hearing

MOUTH
- Assess teeth for decay and eruption
- Upper first molars (14 months)
- Lower cuspids (16 months)

HEART
- Evaluate for presence of cardiac murmurs

SKIN
- Assess for diaper rash
- Assess for nevi, café au lait spots, and birth marks which have not disappeared
- Assess for signs of abuse

ABDOMEN
- Assess for abdominal masses
- Assess for umbilical hernia

GENITALIA (MALE)
- Assess for bilaterally descended testes
- Assess for inguinal hernia

GENITALIA (FEMALE)
- Assess for labial adhesions

MUSCULOSKELETAL
- Assess for hip dysplasia
- Assess for metatarsus adductus
- Assess feet
- Assess gait

SCREENING
- Assess gross hearing
- Assess lead risk
- Consider PPD if at high risk
- Developmental screening (e.g., Denver Developmental Screening Tool)

DEVELOPMENT
- Walks well and is able to stoop
- Can point to a body part
- Says 3-10 words
- Stacks two blocks
- Follows simple commands
- Feeds self and drinks from cup
- Points, grunts, pulls to show what he wants
- Listens to a story

ANTICIPATORY GUIDANCE
- Use toddler car seat in car's rear seat
- Re-examine home for dangerous objects, poisons
- Recheck home safety
- Supervise around lawnmowers, moving cars in driveway, animals, streets, pools, and bathtubs
- Provide healthy food choices. Do not force to eat
- Discuss nuts, hot dogs, whole grapes, hard candy, tough meat, etc. as choking hazards
- Allow toddler to feed self. Fluoride supplements if not sufficient amounts in drinking water
- Brush teeth daily and at bedtime
- Do not allow child to bite or hit
- Limit rules, but enforce consistently
- Praise, talk, show affection to child. Give individual attention.
- Provide opportunities for exploring environment
- Expect curiosity about genitals

EIGHTEEN MONTHS
(Toddler)

NORMAL GROWTH/ASSESSMENT SCREENING
- Length: grows three inches (7.5 cm) annually
- Weight: about 4½ to 6½ lbs (2 kg to 3 kg) annually
- Head circumference: one inch (2.5 cm) annually
- Plot all on growth chart

EYES
- Red reflex should be present bilaterally
- Assess for strabismus
- Assess ability to visually track object

EARS
- Assess gross hearing

MOUTH
- Assess teeth for decay and eruption
- Upper cuspids (18 months)
- Lower 2nd molars (20 months)

HEART
- Evaluate for presence of cardiac murmurs

SKIN
- Assess for diaper rash
- Assess for nevi, café au lait spots, and birth marks which have not disappeared
- Assess for signs of abuse

ABDOMEN
- Assess for abdominal masses
- Assess for umbilical hernia

GENITALIA (MALE)
- Assess for inguinal hernia

GENITALIA (FEMALE)
- Assess for labial adhesions

MUSCULOSKELETAL
- Assess for hip dysplasia
- Assess for metatarsus adductus
- Assess feet
- Assess gait

SCREENING
- Assess gross hearing
- Assess lead risk
- Consider PPD if at high risk
- Developmental screening (e.g., Denver Developmental Screening Tool)

DEVELOPMENT
- Able to walk backwards
- Can throw a ball
- Says 15-20 words
- Imitates words, uses two word phrases
- Points to multiple body parts
- Shows affection, kisses
- Able to voice 1 or 2 wants
- Listens to a story, points and names objects in book
- Begins to scribble spontaneously
- Stacks 3-4 blocks

ANTICIPATORY GUIDANCE
- Use toddler car seat in car's rear seat
- Do not place child in front seat of car if airbag is present
- Re-examine home for dangerous objects, poisons
- Recheck home safety
- Supervise around lawnmowers, moving cars in driveway, animals, streets, pools, and bathtubs
- Provide healthy food choices. Do not force to eat
- Discuss nuts, hot dogs, whole grapes, hard candy, tough meat, etc. as choking hazards
- Allow toddler to feed self with spoon and hands
- Should no longer use bottles
- Fluoride supplements if not sufficient amounts in drinking water
- Brush teeth daily and at bedtime
- Do not allow child to bite or hit
- Limit rules, but enforce consistently. Reassure child once negative behavior has stopped
- Praise, talk, show affection to child. Give individual attention
- Expect curiosity about genitals
- Assess child's readiness for toilet training

TWO YEARS
(Toddler)

NORMAL GROWTH/ASSESSMENT SCREENING
- Length: grows three inches (7.5 cm) annually
- Weight: about 4½ to 6½ lbs (2 kg to 3 kg) annually
- Head circumference: one inch (2.5 cm) annually
- Plot all on growth chart
- Consider initial dental screening (12-36 months of age)

EYES
- Red reflex should be present bilaterally
- Assess for strabismus
- Assess ability to visually track object

EARS
- Assess gross hearing

MOUTH
- Assess teeth for decay and eruption
- Upper 2nd molars (24 months)

HEART
- Evaluate for presence of cardiac murmurs

SKIN
- Assess for signs of abuse

ABDOMEN
- Assess for abdominal masses
- Assess for umbilical hernia

GENITALIA (MALE)
- Assess for inguinal hernia

GENITALIA (FEMALE)
- Assess for labial adhesions

MUSCULOSKELETAL
- Assess feet
- Assess gait

SCREENING
- Assess lead risk
- Consider PPD if at high risk
- Developmental screening (e.g., Denver Developmental Screening Tool)

DEVELOPMENT
- Able to walk up and down stairs one step at a time
- Can kick a ball
- Says at least 20 words
- Imitates words, uses 2-3 word phrases
- Imitates adults
- Follows two step commands
- Stacks 5 blocks

ANTICIPATORY GUIDANCE
- Use toddler car seat
- Re-examine home for dangerous objects, poisons
- Recheck home safety
- Supervise closely
- Provide healthy food choices. Do not force to eat
- Fluoride supplements if not sufficient amounts in drinking water
- Brush teeth daily and at bedtime
- Begin to encourage self care
- Limit rules, but enforce consistently. Use time-out for behavior: one minute for each year of age
- Assess readiness for toilet training (usually too early for male toddler)
- Expect curiosity about genitals
- Limit television viewing time to one hour per day of age appropriate programming

THREE YEARS
(Toddler)

NORMAL GROWTH/ASSESSMENT SCREENING
- Length: grows three inches (7.5 cm) annually
- Weight: about 4½ to 6½ lbs (2 kg to 3 kg) annually
- Head circumference: one inch (2.5 cm) annually
- Plot all on growth chart
- Initial dental screening if not taken place yet

EYES
- Red reflex should be present bilaterally
- Assess for strabismus
- Assess ability to visually track object
- Normal vision is 20/50
-

EARS
- Assess gross hearing

MOUTH
- Assess teeth for decay and eruption

HEART
- Evaluate for presence of cardiac murmurs
- Normal heart rate is 80-120 beats per minute

SKIN
- Assess for signs of abuse

ABDOMEN
- Assess for abdominal masses
- Assess for umbilical hernia

GENITALIA (MALE)
- Assess for inguinal hernia

GENITALIA (FEMALE)
- Assess for labial adhesions

MUSCULOSKELETAL
- Assess gait

SCREENING
- Vision and hearing if cooperative
- Blood pressure screen; taller and heavier children will have higher blood pressure (consult a pediatric BP table)
- Assess lead risk if not done previously
- Consider PPD if at high risk
- Developmental screening (e.g., Denver Developmental Screening Tool)

DEVELOPMENT
- Able to jump
- Can stand on one foot
- Can kick a ball
- Able to ride a tricycle
- Says name, age, and gender
- Knows gender of others
- Able to copy a circle, cross
- Able to recognize colors

ANTICIPATORY GUIDANCE
- Use toddler car seat in car's rear seat
- Re-examine home for dangerous objects, poisons
- Supervise closely
- Provide healthy food choices. Do not force to eat
- Fluoride supplements if not sufficient amounts in drinking water
- Brush teeth daily and at bedtime
- Encourage self care
- Limit rules, but enforce consistently. Use time-out for unacceptable behavior: 1 minute for each year of age
- Expect curiosity about genitals. Use correct terms when referring to genitals
- Limit television viewing time to one hour daily of age appropriate programming
- Help with fears

FOUR YEARS
(Preschool)

NORMAL GROWTH/ASSESSMENT SCREENING
- Length: grows three inches (7.5 cm) annually
- Weight: about 4½ to 6½ lbs (2 kg to 3 kg) annually
- Head circumference: one inch (2.5 cm) annually
- Plot all on growth chart

EYES
- Red reflex should be present bilaterally
- Assess for strabismus
- Assess ability to visually track object
- Normal vision is 20/40

EARS
- Assess gross hearing

MOUTH
- Assess teeth for decay and eruption

HEART
- Evaluate for presence of cardiac murmurs

SKIN
- Assess for signs of abuse

ABDOMEN
- Assess for abdominal masses
- Assess for umbilical hernia

GENITALIA (MALE)
- Assess for inguinal hernia

GENITALIA (FEMALE)
- Assess for labial adhesions

MUSCULOSKELETAL
- Assess gait

SCREENING
- Vision and hearing (should be cooperative)
- Assess for amblyopia, strabismus, and visual acuity
- Blood pressure screen (consult a pediatric BP table)
- Assess lead risk if not done previously
- Consider PPD if at high risk
- Developmental screening (e.g., Denver Developmental Screening Tool)

DEVELOPMENT
- Able to sing a song
- Can hop on one foot
- Able to throw a ball overhand
- Able to draw a person with three parts
- Able to cut and paste
- Able to build a tower with 10 blocks
- Says first and last name, age, and gender
- Counts to 5
- Able to copy a square
- Able to dress self with supervision

ANTICIPATORY GUIDANCE
- Uses car seat/seat belt depending on size and weight
- Teach about stranger safety, neighborhood safety, and learn to swim if around any type of water activities
- Re-examine home for dangerous objects, poisons
- Continue to supervise closely
- Provide healthy food choices. Do not force to eat
- Fluoride supplements if not sufficient amounts in drinking water
- Educate about preventive and emergency dental care
- Encourage assertiveness, not aggression
- Limit rules, but enforce consistently. Use time-out for unacceptable behavior: 1 minute for each year of age
- Expect curiosity about genitals. Use correct terms
- Limit television viewing to one hour per day of age appropriate screening
- Enroll in school or some specific learning environment

FIVE YEARS
(Preschool)

NORMAL GROWTH/ASSESSMENT SCREENING
- Length: grows three inches (7.5 cm) annually
- Weight: about 4½ to 6½ lbs (2 kg to 3 kg) annually
- Head circumference: negligible growth
- Plot all on growth chart

EYES
- Red reflex should be present bilaterally
- Assess ability to visually track object
- Normal vision is 20/30

EARS
- Assess gross hearing

MOUTH
- Assess teeth for decay and eruption

HEART
- Evaluate for presence of cardiac murmurs

SKIN
- Assess for signs of abuse

ABDOMEN
- Assess for abdominal masses
- Assess for umbilical hernia

GENITALIA (MALE)
- Assess for inguinal hernia

MUSCULOSKELETAL
- Assess gait

SCREENING
- Vision and hearing
- Blood pressure (consult pediatric BP table)
- Assess lead risk if not done previously
- Consider PPD if at high risk
- Developmental screening (e.g., Denver Developmental Screening Tool)

- **DEVELOPMENT**
  - Able to draw a person with body, head, arms, legs
  - Able to recognize most letters and can print some
  - Plays make believe
  - Learns address and phone number
  - Can define at least one word
  - Counts on fingers
  - Able to copy a triangle; knows colors
  - Able to dress self without help
  - Able to skip, tiptoe
  - Begins to understand right and wrong
  - Plays cooperatively and enjoys playmate's company

ANTICIPATORY GUIDANCE
- Uses seatbelt in car's back seat (if weighs 60 pounds or head is higher than back of seat) or booster car seat if doesn't meet weight and height requirements
- Teach about personal hygiene
- Teach about stranger safety, playground safety, pedestrian safety
- Needs after school supervision
- Continue to supervise closely
- Provide healthy food choices
- Fluoride supplements if not sufficient amounts in drinking water
- Educate about preventive and emergency dental care
- Encourage assertiveness, not aggression
- Limit rules, but enforce consistently. Use time-out for unacceptable behavior: 1 minute per year of age
- Encourage self-discipline
- Limit television viewing to one hour per day of age appropriate programming
- Teach how to resolve conflict and deal with anger appropriately
- Household chores

SIX YEARS
(School Age)

NORMAL GROWTH/ASSESSMENT SCREENING
- Length: grows 2½ inches (6.4 cm) annually
- Weight: about 5-7 lbs (2.3 kg to 3.2 kg) annually
- Assess for childhood obesity
- Head circumference: negligible growth
- Plot all on growth chart

EYES
- Red reflex should be present bilaterally
- Assess ability to visually track object
- Normal vision is 20/20

EARS
- Assess gross hearing

MOUTH
- Assess teeth for decay and eruption
- Assess for upper and lower first molars
- Assess for lower central incisors

HEART
- Evaluate for presence of cardiac murmurs
- Normal heart rate is 70-110 beats per minute

SKIN
- Assess for signs of abuse

ABDOMEN
- Assess for abdominal masses
- Assess for umbilical hernia

GENITALIA (MALE)
- Assess for inguinal hernia

MUSCULOSKELETAL
- Assess gait

SCREENING
- Vision and hearing
- Blood pressure (consult pediatric BP table)
- Assess lead risk if not done previously
- Consider PPD if at high risk
- Screen for obesity and offer comprehensive, intensive behavioral interventions to promote improvement in weight loss

SCHOOL PERFORMANCE
- Interview child: Does he/she like school? What subject does he/she like best? Like least? How are grades?
- Interview parent: Any particular concerns? Reading/doing math at grade level?

ANTICIPATORY GUIDANCE
- Review immunization status
- Use seatbelt in back seat of car
- Reinforce personal hygiene
- Teach about stranger safety, playground safety, pedestrian safety
- Needs after school supervision
- Continue to supervise closely
- Provide healthy food choices. Teach about what constitutes healthy choices. Offer comprehensive, intensive behavioral interventions for obesity risk children
- Fluoride supplements if not sufficient amounts in drinking water
- Educate about preventive and emergency dental care
- Enforce rules consistently. Have firm rules for acceptable behavior
- Encourage self-discipline
- Limit TV watching to one hour per day of age appropriate programming
- Teach how to resolve conflict and deal with anger appropriately
- Household chores
- Encourage reading
- Patient should ask questions daily about school and give individual attention
- Answer questions regarding sexuality. Provide age-appropriate books

EIGHT YEARS
(School Age)

NORMAL GROWTH/ASSESSMENT SCREENING
- Use drape for exam
- Length: 2½ inches (6.4 cm) annually
- Weight: about 5-7 lbs (2.3 kg to 3.2 kg) annually
- Assess for childhood obesity
- Head circumference: negligible growth
- Plot height/weight on growth chart

EYES
- Red reflex should be present bilaterally
- Assess ability to visually track object

EARS
- Assess gross hearing

MOUTH
- Assess teeth for decay and eruption
- Assess for upper central incisors (7-8 years)
- Assess for lower lateral incisors (7-8 years)
- Assess for upper lateral incisors (8-9 years)

HEART
- Evaluate for cardiac murmurs

SKIN
- Assess for signs of abuse

ABDOMEN
- Assess for abdominal masses
- Assess for umbilical hernia

GENITALIA (MALE)
- Assess for inguinal hernia
- Assess Tanner stage

GENITALIA (FEMALE)
- Assess for early puberty
- Assess Tanner stage

MUSCULOSKELETAL
- Assess for scoliosis

SCREENING
- Vision and hearing
- Blood pressure (consult pediatric table)
- Assess lead risk
- Consider PPD if at high risk
- Screen for obesity and offer comprehensive, intensive behavioral interventions to promote improvement in weight loss

SCHOOL PERFORMANCE
- Interview child: Does he/she like school? What subject does he/she like best? Like least? How are grades?
- Interview parent: Any particular concerns? Reading/doing math at grade level?

ANTICIPATORY GUIDANCE
- Uses seatbelt
- Reinforce pedestrian, neighborhood, stranger, sports safety
- Reinforce personal hygiene
- Needs after school supervision and supervision with friends
- Provide healthy food choices. Teach about what constitutes healthy choices
- Fluoride supplements if not sufficient amounts in drinking water
- Educate about preventive and emergency dental care
- Enforce rules consistently. Have firm rules for acceptable behavior. Provide consequences
- Encourage self-discipline
- Limit TV watching to one hour per day
- Teach how to resolve conflict and deal with anger appropriately
- Household chores
- Needs personal space
- Encourage reading
- Parent should ask questions daily about school and give individual attention
- Answer questions regarding sexuality. Provide age-appropriate books

TEN YEARS
(School Age)

NORMAL GROWTH/ASSESSMENT SCREENING
- Use drape for exam
- Length: grows 2½ inches (6.4 cm) annually
- Weight: about 5-7 lbs (2.3 kg to 3.2 kg) annually
- Assess for childhood obesity
- Head circumference: negligible growth
- Body mass index

EYES
- Red reflex should be present bilaterally
- Assess ability to visually track object

EARS
- Assess gross hearing

MOUTH
- Assess teeth for decay and eruption
- Assess for lower cuspids (9-10 years)
- Assess for first bicuspids (10-11 years)

HEART
- Evaluate for presence of cardiac murmurs
- Heart rate: 70-110 beats per minute

SKIN
- Assess for signs of abuse

ABDOMEN
- Assess for abdominal masses
- Assess for umbilical hernia

GENITALIA (MALE)
- Assess for inguinal hernia
- Assess for early puberty
- Assess Tanner stage

GENITALIA (FEMALE)
- Assess for early puberty
- Assess Tanner stage

MUSCULOSKELETAL
- Assess for scoliosis

SCREENING
- Vision and hearing
- Blood pressure (consult pediatric table)
- Assess lead risk
- Consider PPD if at high risk
- Screen for obesity and offer comprehensive, intensive behavioral interventions to promote improvement in weight loss

SCHOOL PERFORMANCE
- Interview child: Does he/she like school? What subject does he/she like best? Like least? How are grades?
- Interview parent: Any particular concerns? Reading/doing math at grade level?

ANTICIPATORY GUIDANCE
- Uses seatbelt
- Reinforce sports safety
- Counsel regarding tobacco, alcohol, and drugs
- Reinforce personal hygiene
- Needs after school supervision and supervision with friends
- Provide healthy food choices. Teach about what constitutes healthy choices. Offer comprehensive, intensive behavioral interventions for obesity risk children
- Fluoride supplements if not sufficient amounts in drinking water
- Teach about preventive and emergency dental care
- Enforce rules consistently. Have firm rules for acceptable behavior. Provide consequences
- Encourage self-discipline
- Prepare for sexual development and puberty; encourage abstinence and answer questions
- Teach how to resolve conflict and deal with anger appropriately
- Household chores
- Needs personal space
- Encourage reading; parent should ask questions daily about school; give individual attention
- Encourage child to pursue talents and likes

EARLY ADOLESCENCE
(11, 12, 13, and 14 years)

HISTORY/ASSESSMENT
- Use drape for exam
- Allow adolescent to be primary historian
- Consider interview and examination alone
- Interview parent(s) separately

GROWTH SPURT
- Females: about 11 years of age
- Males: about 13 years of age

EYES
- Red reflex should be present bilaterally
- Assess ability to visually track object

EARS
- Assess gross hearing

MOUTH
- Assess teeth for decay and tooth eruption
- Assess for upper cuspids, lower second bicuspids (11-12 years)
- Assess for lower second molars (11-13 years)
- Assess for upper second molars (12-13 years)

HEART
- Evaluate for presence of cardiac murmurs

SKIN
- Assess for signs of abuse, tattoos, acne

ABDOMEN
- Assess for umbilical hernia

GENITALIA (MALE)
- Assess for inguinal hernia
- Assess Tanner stage
- Ask about whether "wet dreams" are occurring. Educate regarding same
- Discuss/teach testicular self exam, especially if history of undescended testicles or single testicle
- Ask about whether sexually active and about use of birth control, condoms
- Gynecomastia, common

GENITALIA (FEMALE)
- Assess Tanner stage
- Ask about whether menses has started and if regular
- Assess for condyloma or lesions
- Instruct regarding self breast exam
- Ask about whether sexually active and about use of birth control and condoms
- Pregnancy history
- Assess for condyloma or other lesions

MUSCULOSKELETAL
- Assess for scoliosis

SCREENING
- Vision and hearing
- Blood pressure
- Consider screening for major depressive disorder
- Consider PPD if at high risk
- Consider cholesterol screening if family history or risk factors
- If sexually active: test for sexually transmitted diseases; urine for gonorrhea, chlamydia
- Screen for obesity and offer comprehensive, intensive behavioral interventions to promote improvement in weight loss

SCHOOL PERFORMANCE
- How are grades? How much school is missed? For what reasons?
- Does student participate in extracurricular activities?
- Interview parent: Any particular concerns?

ANTICIPATORY GUIDANCE
- Counsel regarding adequate sleep, exercise, healthy habits
- Encourage healthy food choices
- Maintain appropriate weight
- Counsel regarding tobacco, alcohol, and drugs Discuss prevention of substance abuse
- Reinforce personal hygiene
- Counsel regarding body changes during puberty, sexual feelings, sexually transmitted diseases
- Fluoride supplements if not sufficient amounts in drinking water
- Educate about preventive and emergency dental care
- Enforce rules consistently. Have firm rules for acceptable behavior. Provide consequences
- Encourage self-discipline
- Teach how to resolve conflict and deal with

anger appropriately
- Household chores
- Needs personal space
- Parent should ask questions daily about school and after school activities
- Give individual attention
- Encourage child to pursue talents and likes. Discuss college, vocational training, military, and careers
- Take on responsibilities, learn new skills
- Encourage initiation of HPV4 vaccination (3 dose series) for females aged 11 to 12 years and males aged 9 through 26 years to reduce likelihood of HPV infection

MIDDLE ADOLESCENCE
(15, 16, and 17 Years)

HISTORY/ASSESSMENT
- Use drape for exam
- Allow adolescent to be primary historian
- Interview and examination alone
- Interview parent(s) separately

EYES
- Red reflex should be present bilaterally
- Assess ability to visually track object

EARS
- Assess gross hearing

MOUTH
- Assess teeth for decay and tooth eruption
- Assess for upper and lower third molars (17-21 years)

HEART
- Evaluate for presence of cardiac murmurs

SKIN
- Assess for signs of abuse, tattoos, acne, piercing

GENITALIA (MALE)
- Assess for inguinal hernia
- Assess Tanner stage
- Gynecomastia common
- Reinforce importance of testicular self exam, especially if history of undescended testicles and/ or single testicle
- Ask about whether sexually active and about use of birth control and condoms

GENITALIA (FEMALE)
- Assess Tanner stage
- Ask about whether periods are regular and any associated problems
- Pregnancy history
- Reinforce importance of self-breast exam
- Ask about whether sexually active and about use of birth control and condoms
- Assess for condyloma or lesions if sexually active

MUSCULOSKELETAL
- Assess for scoliosis

SCREENING
- Vision and hearing
- Blood pressure
- Height and weight, assess for obesity
- Consider screening for major depressive disorder
- Consider PPD if at high risk
- Consider cholesterol screening if family history or risk factors
- If sexually active: test for sexually transmitted diseases ; urine for gonorrhea/chlamydia
- Screen for obesity and offer comprehensive, intensive behavioral interventions to promote improvement in weight loss

SCHOOL PERFORMANCE
- How are grades? How much school is missed? For what reasons?
- Does student participate in extracurricular activities?
- Interview parent: Any particular concerns?

ANTICIPATORY GUIDANCE
- Counsel regarding adequate sleep, exercise, healthy habits
- Car safety: speed limits, seat belt use, abstinence from alcohol and drugs while driving
- Encourage healthy food choices. Maintain

appropriate weight
- Counsel regarding tobacco, alcohol, and drugs. Discuss prevention of substance abuse
- Reinforce personal hygiene if appropriate
- Counsel regarding sexually transmitted diseases, pregnancy, safe sex
- Fluoride supplements if not sufficient amounts in drinking water (up to age 16 years)
- Educate about preventive and emergency dental care
- Enforce rules consistently. Have firm rules for acceptable behavior. Provide consequences
- Encourage self-discipline
- Teach how to resolve conflict and deal with anger appropriately
- Household chores
- Needs personal space
- Parent should ask questions daily about school and after school activities
- Give individual attention
- Encourage adolescent to pursue talents and interests; discuss college, vocational training, military, careers
- Take on responsibilities, learn new skills

LATE ADOLESCENCE
(18, 19, 20, and 21 Years)

HISTORY/ASSESSMENT
- Use drape for exam
- Adolescent is primary historian
- Interview and examination alone
- Interview parents separately as appropriate

EYES
- Red reflex should be present bilaterally
- Assess ability to visually track object

EARS
- Assess gross hearing

MOUTH
- Assess teeth for decay and eruption
- Assess for upper and lower third molars (17-21 years)

HEART
- Evaluate for presence of cardiac murmurs

SKIN
- Assess for signs of abuse, tattoos, acne

GENITALIA (MALE)
- Assess for inguinal hernia
- Assess Tanner stage
- Gynecomastia (less common than in early adolescence; may be due to drug use)
- Reinforce importance of testicular self exam, especially if history of undescended testicles and/or single testicle
- Ask about whether sexually active and about use of birth control and condoms

GENITALIA (FEMALE)
- Tanner stage
- Ask if regular menses and about any associated problems
- Pregnancy history
- Reinforce importance of self breast exam
- Ask about whether sexually active and about use of birth control and condoms
- First pelvic exam at age 21
- Assess for condyloma or lesions if sexually active

MUSCULOSKELETAL
- Assess for scoliosis

SCREENING
- Vision and hearing
- Blood pressure
- Consider PPD if at high risk
- Consider screening for major depressive disorder
- Consider cholesterol screening if family history or risk factors
- If sexually active: test for gonorrhea, chlamydia, HIV, syphilis, Hepatitis B/C and other sexually transmitted diseases
- Screen for obesity and offer comprehensive, intensive behavioral interventions to promote improvement in weight loss

SCHOOL/JOB PERFORMANCE

- How are grades? How much school is missed? For what reasons?
- Does student participate in extracurricular activities?
- How is job going?

ANTICIPATORY GUIDANCE

- Counsel regarding adequate sleep, exercise, healthy habits
- Car safety: speed limits, seat belt use, abstinence from alcohol, drugs while driving
- Encourage healthy food choices. Maintain appropriate weight
- Counsel regarding tobacco, alcohol, and drugs. Discuss prevention of substance abuse
- Reinforce personal hygiene if appropriate
- Counsel regarding sexually transmitted diseases, pregnancy, safe sex
- Brush teeth and encourage regular dental care
- Enforce rules consistently. Have firm rules for acceptable behavior. Provide consequences
- Encourage self-discipline
- Needs personal space
- Encourage adolescent to pursue talents and interests
- Discuss college, vocational training, military, careers
- Take on responsibilities, learn new skills

IMMUNIZATIONS

The most recent immunization schedules for persons age 0-6 years and 7-18 years can be found at: www.cdc.gov/vaccines/recs/acip

Vaccine	Route	Comments	Contraindications*
Diphtheria, Tetanus, Pertussis (DTaP, DT, Tdap, Td)	IM	Shake vial vigorously to obtain uniform suspension prior to withdrawing each dose. Inspect vaccine visually for particulate matter and/or discoloration prior to administration	Encephalopathy within 7 days of previous dose of DTP or DTaP attributable to vaccine; Age younger than 6 weeks
Haemophilus influenzae type b (Hib)	IM		Age younger than 6 weeks
Hepatitis A (HepA)	IM		Age younger than 12 months
Hepatitis B (HepB)	IM	Consult package insert.	Severe allergic reaction after previous vaccine dose or vaccine component
Human papillomavirus (HPV)	IM		Age younger than 9 years
Influenza, live attenuated (LAIV)	Intranasal spray		Severe allergic reaction to egg protein, pregnancy, known severe immunodeficiency, possible reactive airways disease in child ages 2-4 Age younger than 2 years

continued

Vaccine	Route	Comments	Contraindications*
Measles, mumps, rubella (MMR)	SC	Reconstitute just before using. Use only the diluent supplied with the vaccine. Inject the volume of the diluent shown on the diluent label into the vial of lyophilized vaccine and gently agitate to mix thoroughly. Withdraw the entire contents and administer immediately after reconstitution.	Pregnancy, known severe immunodeficiency; Age younger than 12 months
Meningococcal-conjugate (MCV4)	IM		Age younger than 2 years
Meningococcal-polysaccharide (MPSV4)	SC	Discard single dose MPSV4 if not used after 30 minutes reconstitution	Age younger than 2 years
Pneumococcal conjugate (PCV)	IM		Age younger than 6 weeks
Pneumococcal polysaccharide (PPSV)	IM or SC		Age younger than 2 years
Polio, inactivated (IPV)	IM or SC		Age younger than 6 weeks
Rotavirus	SC		
Varicella (Var)	SC	Discard single dose MPSV if not used after 30 minutes reconstitution	Pregnancy, substantial suppression of cellular immunity; prior to 12 months of age *Severe allergic reaction after previous vaccine dose or vaccine component

Source: www.immunize.org/catf.d/p3084.pdf
Adapted from "Table 5. Contraindications and Precautions to Commonly Used Vaccines" found in CDC, "General Recommendations on Immunization: Recommendations of the Advisory Committee on Immunization Practices (ACIP)." MMWR 2006; 55(No. RR-15), p. 10-14.

IMMUNIZATION DOCUMENTATION MUST INCLUDE:

1. Date of administration
2. Name or common abbreviation of vaccine
3. Vaccine lot number
4. Vaccine manufacturer
5. Administration site
6. Vaccine information statement (VIS) edition date
7. Name and address of vaccine administrator

Vaccine Adverse Event Reporting System (VAERS): 800-822-7967

References

Agency for Healthcare Research and Quality. (2010). Guide to clinical preventive services. Retrieved from http://www.ahrq.gov/clinic/pocketgd.thm.

American Academy of Pediatrics. *Bright futures*. Elk Grove Village, IL: American Academy of Pediatrics.

American Academy of Pediatrics. (2009). *Red book: 2009 report of the committee on infectious diseases* (28th ed.). Elk Grove Village, IL: American Academy of Pediatrics

Burns, C.E., Brady, M.A., Blosser, C., Starr, N.B., & Dunn, A.M. (2009). Pediatric primary care: A handbook for nurse practitioners (4th ed.). Philadelphia: W.B. Saunders.

Centers for Disease Control and Prevention. (2010). Recommended immunization schedules for persons aged 0 through 18 years -- United States, 2010. *MMWR, Morbidity and Mortality Weekly Report, 58*(51 &52), 1-4.

Frankenburg, W. (1992). *Denver II training manual*. Denver, CO: Denver Developmental Materials, Inc.

U.S. Preventtive Services Task Force. (2001). *Guide to clinical preventive services* (3rd ed.). Washington, DC: U.S. Government Printing Office.

8

HEMATOLOGIC DISORDERS

Hematologic Disorders

Iron Deficiency Anemia 357

Anemia of Chronic Disease 361

Glucose-6-Phosphate Dehydrogenase Deficiency 362

Lead Toxicity 364

Sickle Cell Anemia 366

Thalassemia 368

Vitamin B12 Deficiency Anemia 370

Folic Acid Deficiency 372

Leukemia 373

Lymphoma 375

Idiopathic Thrombocytopenia Purpura 376

* Neonatal Hyperbilirubinemia 378

* Rh Incompatibility 379

References 381

**Denotes pediatric diagnosis*

Hematologic Disorders

IRON DEFICIENCY ANEMIA

DESCRIPTION

Microcytic, hypochromic anemia that occurs when iron loss exceeds intake of iron and subsequently, iron stores become depleted. Associated with chronic blood loss.

> **Microcytosis: red blood cell is smaller than average (< 80 fL)**
> **Hypochromia: describes a decreased amount of hemoglobin found in red blood cells**

ETIOLOGY

Common causes:

- Heavy menses
- Gastrointestinal bleeding
- Decreased iron intake, especially vegetarians
- Gastrointestinal neoplasm
- Increased iron requirements
- Pregnancy
- Lactation
- Poor iron absorption

INCIDENCE

- 7-10% of adult population
- Females > Males
- Most common type of anemia in U.S.
- Most common anemia in infancy and childhood, especially at 9-24 months of age (10-20%)

RISK FACTORS

- See Etiology
- Infants and toddlers
- Adolescents
- Pregnancy
- Low birthweight infant
- Low socioeconomic status
- Chronic ASA, NSAID use

ASSESSMENT FINDINGS

- Most are asymptomatic
- Tinnitus
- Headache
- Dyspnea on exertion
- Fatigue
- Tachycardia
- Palpitations
- Inability to concentrate
- Irritability in young children
- Pallor (best seen in conjunctivae)
- Koilonychia (spoon-shaped, brittle nails)
- Cold intolerance
- Frequent infections
- Pica (craving for ice, starch, clay, or other unusual substances)

DIFFERENTIAL DIAGNOSIS

- α- and β- thalassemia trait
- Sideroblastic anemia
- Gastric carcinoma (especially in the elderly)
- Anemia of chronic disease
- Hypothyroidism
- Renal failure
- Lead toxicity

DIAGNOSTIC STUDIES

- Hemoglobin level < 2 standard deviations below the mean for age
- Hemoglobin: < 12 g/dL in adults
- RBC count: decreased
- Mean corpuscular volume (MCV): decreased (<80 fl)
- Red cell distribution width (RDW): increased

> **MCV: describes the size of the average RBC**
> **Anisocytosis: describes the variability of RBC size**
> **RDW: measure of the variability of the RBC size**

- Serum ferritin: decreased (best non-invasive test in adults; earliest lab abnormality)
- Serum iron: decreased
- Total iron-binding capacity (TIBC): increased
- Reticulocyte count: decreased

> **TIBC: ability of the RBC to bind circulating iron**
> **Reticulocyte count: measure of the ability of the bone marrow to produce RBCs**

- Peripheral smear: hypochromic, microcytic red blood cells, anisocytosis, poikilocytosis
- Bone marrow aspiration is gold standard for diagnosis, but rarely needed
- As indicated to diagnose underlying problem

Poikilocytosis: describes different RBC shapes
Anisocytosis: variation in red blood cell size

PREVENTION

- Adequate intake of iron in diet
- Infant diet should include iron-fortified formula and cereal
- Breastfed infants should receive iron supplementation from 4 months of age

NONPHARMACOLOGIC MANAGEMENT

- Diet rich in foods containing protein and iron (e.g., meat, dried beans, dark green, leafy vegetables)
- Increase fiber in diet to counteract constipating effect of iron replacement therapy
- Screening recommended for pregnant women and high-risk infants

Patient Education about Iron Replacement
Teach patients about iron replacement therapy
Take 1-2 hours before meals on empty stomach for greatest absorption
Take with meals if GI upset occurs, but be aware that this decreases iron absorption
Do not take concomitantly with antacids, tetracycline, dairy products
Bowel movements will be very dark in color
Iron is highly toxic, keep out of children's reach
Place iron drops in back of mouth to reduce staining of teeth in infants and young children
Administration of iron with vitamin C enhances absorption

- Transfusion of packed red blood cells indicated if anemia severe and patient symptomatic
- Energy conservation with frequent rest periods
- Attempt to identify hidden source of bleeding

Food may reduce absorption of iron by 50%.

IRON DEFICIENCY ANEMIA PHARMACOLOGIC MANAGEMENT

These products help replenish iron stores within the body. Doses are determined on the elemental iron content of the product. In normal states, the body absorbs ~ 10% of the elemental iron dose; in anemic states, the body absorbs between 20-30% of the elemental iron dose. Practitioners must consider the absorption in relation to not only the product's elemental iron content but also in relation to the Recommended Daily Allowance (RDA)

Class	Drug Generic name (Trade name®)	Dosage How supplied	Comments
Iron *Elemental mineral necessary for several body functions, including red blood cell production and function* **General comments** Therapy/treatment consists of replacing immediate needs as well as replenishing the body's storage of iron	**ferrous fumarate** (33% elemental iron or 330 mg/g)	DOSES ARE DETERMINED BY MG ELEMENTAL IRON **Adult:** **Prophylaxis of Anemia** *Initial*: 60 mg Fe/day *Max*: 60 mg Fe/day **Treatment of anemia** *Initial*: 60-100 mg Fe twice/day *Max:* 60 mg Fe four times/day	• Pregnancy Category Unassigned • Multiple dosage forms of ferrous sulfate tablets exist (e.g., enteric coated, extended release, slow release, timed release); close attention is warranted to the strength and dosage form when ordering or administering • **Black Box Warning regarding accidental overdose in children which can be fatal** • Lower doses may be required in geriatric patients

continued

IRON DEFICIENCY ANEMIA PHARMACOLOGIC MANAGEMENT

These products help replenish iron stores within the body. Doses are determined on the elemental iron content of the product. In normal states, the body absorbs ~ 10% of the elemental iron dose; in anemic states, the body absorbs between 20-30% of the elemental iron dose. Practitioners must consider the absorption in relation to not only the product's elemental iron content but also in relation to the Recommended Daily Allowance (RDA)

Class	Drug Generic name (Trade name®)	Dosage How supplied	Comments
Administration with Vitamin C enhances absorption	Ferro-sequels	Time Rel. Tab: 150 mg (delivers 50 mg elemental iron)	• Do not crush or chew extended release formulation • Do not take with cereal or fiber products
Avoid concomitantly with antacids, tetracycline, dairy products	Fem-iron	Tabs: 63 mg (delivers 20 mg elemental iron)	
May cause dark (black) stools, constipation **Recommended Daily Allowance (RDA)** < 6 m: 0.27 mg/day 7-12 m: 11 mg/day 1-3 yr: 7 mg/day 4-8 yr: 10 mg/day 9-13 yr: 8 mg/day Male: 14-18 yr: 11 mg/day Female: 14-18 yr: 15 mg/day Adult male: 8 mg/day Adult female, premenopausal: 18 mg/day Adult female, post-menopausal: 8 mg/day During Pregnancy: 27 mg/day Lactating: 9-10 mg/day	**ferrous gluconate** (12% elemental iron or 120 mg/g)	**DOSES ARE DETERMINED BY MG ELEMENTAL IRON** **Adults**: **Prophylaxis of Anemia** *Initial*: 60 mg Fe/day *Max*: 60 mg Fe/day **Mild-to-moderate anemia** *Initial*: 60 mg Fe twice/day *Max*: 60 mg Fe four times/day **Children**: **Prophylaxis** *Initial*: 1-2 mg/kg/day *Max*: 15 mg/day **Mild-to-moderate anemia** *Initial*: 3 mg/kg/day of elemental iron in single or divided doses **Elemental Iron: Severe anemia** *Initial*: 4-6 mg/kg/day of elemental iron in single or divided doses	• Pregnancy Category Unassigned • Multiple trade names exist with slight variation, each with slight variation on dosing • Vitamin C enhances absorption • **Black Box Warning regarding accidental overdose in children which can be fatal** • Lower doses may be required in geriatric patients
	Fergon **This product is not recomended for children**	*Tabs: 240 mg (delivers 27 mg iron)*	
	Other trade names	*Tabs: 324 mg (delivers 38 mg elemental iron), 325 mg (delivers 36 mg elemental iron)*	

continued

IRON DEFICIENCY ANEMIA PHARMACOLOGIC MANAGEMENT

These products help replenish iron stores within the body. Doses are determined on the elemental iron content of the product. In normal states, the body absorbs ~ 10% of the elemental iron dose; in anemic states, the body absorbs between 20-30% of the elemental iron dose. Practitioners must consider the absorption in relation to not only the product's elemental iron content but also in relation to the Recommended Daily Allowance (RDA)

Class	Drug Generic name (Trade name®)	Dosage How supplied	Comments
	ferrous sulfate (20% elemental iron or 200 mg/g)	**DOSES ARE DETERMINED BY MG ELEMENTAL IRON** **Adults**: **Prophylaxis of Anemia** *Initial*: 60 mg Fe/day *Max*: 60 mg Fe/day **Mild-to-moderate anemia** *Initial*: 30-65 mg Fe divided into three times/day *Max*: 65 mg/day **Children**: **Prophylaxis** *Initial*: 1-2 mg/kg/day *Max*: 15 mg/day **Mild-to-moderate anemia** *Initial*: 3 mg/kg/day of elemental iron in single or divided dose **Severe anemia** *Initial*: 4-6 mg/kg/day of elemental iron in three divided doses	• Pregnancy Category Unassigned • Multiple concentrations of ferrous oral liquid exist (e.g., 15 mg/mL or 15 mg/0.6 mL); close attention is warranted to the concentration when ordering or administering • Multiple dosage forms of ferrous sulfate tablets exist (e.g., enteric coated, extended release, slow release, timed release); close attention is warranted to the strength and dosage form when ordering or administering • **Black Box Warning regarding accidental overdose in children which can be fatal** • Lower doses may be required in geriatric patients • Do not crush or chew extended release formulation
	Feosol	*Tabs: 200 mg (delivers 65 mg iron)* *Caplet: 50 mg (elemental iron)* *Elixir: 220 mg/5 mL (delivers 44 mg/5 mL elemental iron)*	
	Slow Fe	*Sust. Rel. Tab: 160 mg (delivers 50 mg elemental iron)*	
	Fer-In-Sol Drops	*Elixir: 75 mg/0.6 mL (delivers 15 mg/0.6 mL elemental iron)*	

Adults need about 180 mg of elemental iron daily during anemic states. Children need about 3 mg/kg/d during anemic states.

PREGNANCY/LACTATION CONSIDERATIONS

- Common during pregnancy
- Iron supplementation almost always needed

CONSULTATION/REFERRAL

- If hemoglobin not increased after one month of iron replacement therapy, referral dependent on underlying cause

FOLLOW-UP

- Repeat hemoglobin one month after therapy initiated
- Dependent on underlying cause

EXPECTED COURSE

- Rapid hematological response is typical
- Curable with iron therapy, but recurrence common unless underlying cause successfully managed

Reticulocyte count increases once iron supplementation takes place. This is observable in 3-4 days.

POSSIBLE COMPLICATIONS

- Congestive heart failure
- Tissue hypoxia
- Neurological and intelligence deficits in children

ANEMIA OF CHRONIC DISEASE

DESCRIPTION

Mild to moderate normochromic, normocytic (usually, but can be microcytic) anemia associated with chronic disease. Red blood cell life span is shortened from the normal 120 days to 60-90 days.

Normocytic: describes an average size of RBC
Normochromia: describes the average amount of hemoglobin found in red blood cells

ETIOLOGY

- Unknown

INCIDENCE

- Most common in elderly with chronic illness
- Also seen in children with chronic illness
- Seen in patients with malignancies more than 50% of the time

RISK FACTORS

- Presence of chronic infectious, inflammatory, and/or malignant disease

ASSESSMENT FINDINGS

- Dependent on underlying disease
- Asymptomatic
- Dyspnea on exertion
- Fatigue
- Headache
- Anorexia
- Weight loss
- Lightheadedness after mild exercise

DIFFERENTIAL DIAGNOSIS

- Iron deficiency anemia
- Thalassemia
- Sideroblastic anemia

DIAGNOSTIC STUDIES

- CBC with peripheral smear: normocytic, normochromic red blood cells; leukocytosis common
- Hemoglobin: 7-11 g/dL range
- Serum iron: decreased
- Total iron-binding capacity (TIBC): normal to slightly decreased
- Transferrin saturation: usually decreased
- Serum ferritin: normal or increased
- Red cell distribution width (RDW): normal (11.5-14.5%)
- Mean corpuscular volume (MCV): normal or slightly decreased
- Reticulocyte count: normal or decreased

MANAGEMENT

- Treatment aimed at control of underlying disease process
- Administration of iron is not usually indicated
- Transfusion of packed red blood cells (PRBC) indicated if patient becomes very symptomatic
- Energy conservation with frequent rest periods

CONSULTATION/REFERRAL

- As needed for management of underlying chronic condition

FOLLOW-UP

- As needed for evaluation and management of underlying chronic condition

Anemia of chronic disease is not usually progressive, though hemoglobin/hematocrit may be monitored every 3 months.

EXPECTED COURSE

- Dependent on underlying chronic condition

Iron deficiency anemia can co-exist with anemia of chronic disease. A look at the ferritin level may help differentiate the two anemias.

POSSIBLE COMPLICATIONS

- Worsening of underlying chronic condition

GLUCOSE-6-PHOSPHATE DEHYDROGENASE DEFICIENCY

(G-6-PD Deficiency)

DESCRIPTION

Normocytic anemia caused by absence of glucose-6-phosphate dehydrogenase (G-6-PD). Congenital sex-linked red blood cell enzyme deficiency that leaves the patient susceptible to hemolysis after ingestion of substances with oxidant properties.

ETIOLOGY

- X-linked recessive disorder

INCIDENCE

- Most prevalent in persons of Mediterranean and African descent
- Common in Saudi Arabians, Africans, African Americans
- 16% of African-American males are affected and 1-2% of females
- Affects > 200 million people

RISK FACTORS

- Mediterranean or African descent
- Family history of G-6-PD deficiency

ASSESSMENT FINDINGS

- Symptoms develop 24-48 hours after ingestion of substances that have oxidant properties
- Pallor
- Jaundice
- Dark urine

Most patients with G6PD have no symptoms, but if they ingest specific substances, they will develop an acute hemolytic anemia.

DIFFERENTIAL DIAGNOSIS

- α- and **β**-thalassemia trait
- Sideroblastic anemia
- Anemia of chronic disease
- Hypothyroidism
- Lead toxicity

DIAGNOSTIC STUDIES

- Hemoglobin/hematocrit: decreased during acute episode
- Mean corpuscular volume: normal
- G-6-PD level: decreased, but may be falsely elevated during an acute episode; re-measure level 1-2 weeks after acute episode
- RBC morphology is peculiar and varied
- Peripheral smear: Heinz bodies, schistocytes, bite cells, blister cells

PREVENTION

- Screening of persons with risk factors, family history

MANAGEMENT

- Teach patients to avoid the following substances
  - ◊ Antimalarials (primaquine, chloroquine)
  - ◊ Sulfonamides
  - ◊ Phenacetin
  - ◊ Aspirin
  - ◊ Chloramphenicol
  - ◊ Nitrofurantoin
  - ◊ Furazolidone
  - ◊ Trimethoprim-sulfamethoxazole (Bactrim®)
  - ◊ Fava beans
- Packed red cell transfusion may be necessary

CONSULTATION/REFERRAL

- Consider referral to hematologist to identify variant of type

EXPECTED COURSE

- Excellent prognosis if diagnosed early and person avoids substances that cause hemolysis

After an acute episode, hemoglobin levels can return to normal as soon as 2-6 weeks.

POSSIBLE COMPLICATIONS

- Severe anemia

LEAD TOXICITY
(Plumbism, Lead Poisoning)

DESCRIPTION

Occurs as a result of exposure to lead, characterized by sideroblastic anemia

Sideroblastic anemia occurs when iron is not able to be incorporated into the hemoglobin molecule.

ETIOLOGY

- Exposure to lead either by ingestion or inhalation

INCIDENCE

- Most common in children under 5 years of age
- May occur in adults; Males > Females

RISK FACTORS

- Residing in or frequent visitation to home built before 1960
- Sibling or playmate with lead toxicity
- Child of adult with occupational exposure
- Living near busy highway or hazardous waste dump
- Ingestion of soil containing lead (pica)
- Member of occupation associated with lead over exposure (plumbers, pipe fitters, welders, firing range workers, painters)

ASSESSMENT FINDINGS

Mild:
- Intermittent abdominal pain
- Irritability
- Lethargy
- Mild fatigue
- Myalgias
- Paresthesias
- Learning disorders in children

Moderate:
- Constipation
- Diffuse abdominal pain
- General fatigue
- Headache
- Loss of libido
- Tremor
- Vomiting
- Weight loss

Severe:
- Abdominal colic due to abdominal muscle spasm
- Metallic taste in mouth
- Coma
- Encephalopathy
- Lead lines
- Motor neuropathy (wrist drop)
- Oliguria
- Renal failure
- Seizures

Common symptom of lead toxicity is a gastrointestinal complaint regardless of severity. Adults commonly present with peripheral neuritis in the extensor muscles.

DIFFERENTIAL DIAGNOSIS

- Iron deficiency anemia
- ADD, ADHD, autism
- Mental retardation
- Seizure disorder
- Colic
- Polyneuropathy
- Acute abdominal pain
- Encephalopathy

DIAGNOSTIC STUDIES

- Lead level > 10 mg/dL is considered abnormal (screen is a finger stick)
- Abnormal finger stick screening values should be confirmed by venipuncture test
- Hemoglobin and hematocrit: slightly decreased
- Serum creatinine: elevated
- Erythrocyte protoporphyrin: elevated

There are a lot of false positives on lead levels due to poor specimen collection.

PREVENTION

- Screening of children at risk for lead exposure at 6-11 months of age & then again at 2 years
- Primary prevention in workplace:
    - ◊ Engineering controls: substitution of less hazardous material, isolation via containment structure, appropriate ventilation
    - ◊ Personal protective equipment: respirator
    - ◊ Work practices: removal of lead accumulation, personal hygiene practices, periodic inspection/ maintenance of control equipment

LEAD LEVEL INTERPRETATION

Level Interpretation	
< 9 µg/dL	Unexposed or normal
10-19 µg/dL	Acceptable levels for long-term exposure, retest in 3-6 months
20-44 µg/dL	Close observation and follow-up indicated, retest in 3 months
> 45 µg/dL	Remove from exposure. Recheck 1-3 months. Report to Public Health. Screen all family members
> 60 µg/dL	Removal from exposure, retest within 1 month. Report to Public Health. Screen all family members

NONPHARMACOLOGIC MANAGEMENT

- Increased iron and Vitamin C intake in diet
- Remove source of lead exposure
- Removal of worker from exposure if level > 60 µg/dL
- Reportable to local health department

PHARMACOLOGIC MANAGEMENT

- Lead chelation agent as indicated by lead levels and clinical manifestations (oral or parenteral)
- Oral agent approved for chelation in children: succimer (Chemet®)
  < 12 months: not recommended
  > 12 months: 10 mg/kg every 8 hr for 5 days; then reduce frequency to ever 12 hours for 14 days
- Iron supplementation

CONSULTATION/REFERRAL

- If lead chelation therapy required

EXPECTED COURSE

- If detected early, excellent prognosis

POSSIBLE COMPLICATIONS

- Lead encephalopathy
- CNS toxicity

In children:

- Decreased IQ scores
- Poor muscle coordination
- Shortened attention span
- Increased incidence of behavior problems

SICKLE CELL ANEMIA

DESCRIPTION

A group of genetic disorders characterized by chronic severe hemolytic anemia resulting from destruction of brittle erythrocytes; associated with intermittent episodic events (crises). Sickle cell trait is usually asymptomatic without anemia.

Sickle shaped red blood cells are inflexible, very fragile, and increase the blood's viscosity. Patients should always be well hydrated to help prevent crises.

ETIOLOGY

- Inherited autosomal recessive disorder

INCIDENCE

- Most common of the clinically significant hemoglobinopathies
- Affects more than 80,000 Americans
- 1 in 500 African-Americans have sickle cell disease
- 1 in 1000 Hispanics have sickle cell disease
- 1 in 10 African-Americans carry sickle cell trait
- Also seen to lesser degree in persons from Mediterranean area

RISK FACTORS FOR CRISIS

- Dehydration
- Hypoxemia
- Infection
- Fever

ASSESSMENT FINDINGS

- Asymptomatic in early months of life
- Pallor
- Hand-foot syndrome (symmetric, painful swelling of the hands and feet in infants and young children)
- Failure to thrive
- Acute painful vaso-occlusive episodes, especially of bones, joints, abdomen, and back
- Delayed maturation (physical and sexual); Males > Females
- Increased incidence of streptococcal infections
- Frequency of complications and secondary damage increases with age

The pain associated with sickle cell crises is related to tissue ischemia and necrosis. Repeated crises can lead to organ failure.

DIFFERENTIAL DIAGNOSIS

- Other hemoglobinopathies (e.g., thalassemia)
- Other causes of acute pain in bones, joints, and abdomen (e.g., rheumatic fever, rheumatoid arthritis, osteomyelitis, acute abdomen, leukemia)

DIAGNOSTIC STUDIES

- Sickledex is the screening test; if positive then Hemoglobin electrophoresis
- Sickle cell disease: Hgb S predominates and Hgb A absent
- Sickle cell trait: Hgb S and A are present
- Peripheral smear: few irreversibly sickled RBCs, polynucleated RBCs
- Presence of Howell-Jolly bodies
- Thrombocytosis

PREVENTION

- See *Risk Factors*
- Screening/counseling of couples preconceptually

NONPHARMACOLOGIC MANAGEMENT

- Regular dental care
- Regular developmental assessment
- Keep immunizations up to date
- Good hydration at all times
- Family should have a "sick day plan" (includes early identification of infection and immediate treatment)
  - ◊ Usual childhood activities
  - ◊ Hospitalization for crises
- Maintenance of good nutrition and adequate hydration
- Avoid smoking/alcohol
- Patient/family education about importance of prompt, aggressive treatment of infections
- Teach early recognition of complications
- Screening of all high-risk infants for sickle cell disease

PHARMACOLOGIC MANAGEMENT

- NSAIDs for pain management in milder crises
- Narcotic analgesics may be needed for pain control during severe crises
- Polyvalent pneumococcal vaccine
- Routine childhood immunizations

SICKLE CELL ANEMIA PHARMACOLOGIC MANAGEMENT

Class	Drug Generic name (Trade name®)	Dosage How supplied	Comments
Penicillin General comments Oral solution stable for 14 days if refrigerated	**penicillin V** Penicillin V potassium	**Children**: *Birth-3 yrs*: 125 mg twice/day *3-5 yrs*: 250 mg twice/day *Suspension: 125 mg/5mL, 250 mg/5 mL*	• May stop at 6 years if no pneumococcal infections • If risk factors present, continue penicillin through puberty
Folic acid supplementation	**folic acid** Folvite	**Adult**: *Initial*: 1 mg/day **Children**: *Initial*: 0.5-1 mg/day	
	folacin (folic acid) **cyanocobalamin (Vitamin B12)** **pyridoxine (Vitamin B6)** Foltx	**Adult**: *Initial*: 1-2 tabs daily **Children**: not recommended *Tab: folic acid 2.5 mg, pyridoxine 25 mg, B12 2 mg*	• May cause paresthesias • Contraindicated in patients taking levodopa • May reduce effectiveness of phenytoin

PREGNANCY/LACTATION CONSIDERATIONS

- Highest risk during third trimester and delivery
- Fetal mortality: 35-40%
- Complications during pregnancy: increased number and severity of crises, eclampsia, infections, pulmonary infarction, phlebitis
- Increased risk of prematurity, intrauterine growth restriction, and fetal death
- Best managed by perinatal team in tertiary care center

CONSULTATION/REFERRAL

- Refer to hematologist
- Refer for genetic counseling

FOLLOW-UP

- Dependent on frequency/severity of crises and complications

Patients with fever > 101° F (38.8° C) should be aggressively treated to prevent sickle cell crisis.

EXPECTED COURSE

- Anemia is chronic and lifelong
- Frequent complications occur during adolescence and twenties
- Most common causes of death: infections, embolic events
- Life expectancy of persons with sickle cell trait is not affected

POSSIBLE COMPLICATIONS

- Body image and sexual identity problems
- Low self-esteem
- Priapism
- Aseptic necrosis of femoral head
- Skin ulcerations
- Cardiomegaly
- Abnormal hepatic function
- Infarcts: splenic, cerebral, pulmonary, bone
- Hematuria
- Retinopathy
- Chronic pulmonary disease
- Pneumonia
- Meningitis
- Pyelonephritis
- Sepsis

THALASSEMIA

DESCRIPTION

A group of hereditary disorders that causes an overproduction of specific chains in the hemoglobin molecule. These chains tend to aggregate and precipitate in red blood cells causing premature red blood cell hemolysis. These anemias are characterized by hypochromia and microcytosis.

There are two main types, but multiple variants:

- β-thalassemia: deficient synthesis of **β**-globin chains causing severe anemia, classified by severity and clinical type:
  - ◊ Major (Cooley's anemia, homozygous β-thalassemia): very severe disease; rarely live to adulthood
  - ◊ Intermedia: less severe disease; normal lifespan but delayed puberty
  - ◊ Minor (trait, heterozygous **β**-thalassemia): the least severe disease and most common form; normal lifespan
- α-thalassemia: deficient synthesis of α-globin chains causing mild anemia with variable degrees of clinical disease

ETIOLOGY

- Autosomal recessive

INCIDENCE

- Occurs throughout the U.S.
- Prevalent in the Mediterranean areas, Middle East, India, African, and Southeast Asia
- Thalassemia trait affects 3-5% of above ethnic groups

RISK FACTORS

- Family history of thalassemia

ASSESSMENT FINDINGS

β-thalassemia major:

- Usually becomes symptomatic about 3 months of age
- Pallor
- Failure to thrive
- Increased respiratory rate
- Fatigue
- Splenomegaly/hepatomegaly
- Pathological fractures

α- and β-thalassemia minor (trait):

- Asymptomatic
- Mild pallor
- Mild splenomegaly

DIFFERENTIAL DIAGNOSIS

- Iron deficiency anemia
- Other microcytic, hypochromic anemias

DIAGNOSTIC STUDIES

β-thalassemia major:

- Red blood cells (RBC): decreased
- Hemoglobin: < 5 g/dL
- Hematocrit: may be as low as < 10%
- Peripheral smear: microcytosis, hypochromia, target cells

Hematologic Disorders

Target cell: a red blood cell with a "bull's eye" or "target" in the center of the cell.
Normal red blood cells are biconcave discs.

- Red cell distribution width (RDW): normal or decreased
- Reticulocyte count: increased
- Hemoglobin electrophoresis: used for diagnosis
- Serum ferritin level: normal or increased depending on diet
- Skull and long bone x-rays: cortical thinning and widening of the marrow space

β-thalassemia minor:

- Hemoglobin: slightly decreased or normal
- Hematocrit: 28-40%
- Peripheral smear: microcytosis, hypochromia
- Serum ferritin level: normal or increased
- Hemoglobin electrophoresis: Hgb A2 increased
- Total iron binding capacity (TIBC): normal
- RBC count: normal or increased
- Reticulocyte count: normal or slightly increased

α-thalassemia trait:

- Peripheral smear: microcytosis, hypochromia
- Hematocrit: 28-40%
- Hemoglobin electrophoresis: used for diagnosis
- Hemoglobin electrophoresis: Hgb A2 normal; Hgb F increased

Hemoglobin electrophoresis not required to make diagnosis of *β-thalassemia minor* if patient has a microcytic, hypochromic anemia with normal serum ferritin.

PREVENTION

- Genetic counseling before conception for persons who carry or may be at risk of carrying the gene
- Amniocentesis after 14 weeks gestation

NONPHARMACOLOGIC MANAGEMENT

- Monitor mild cases (alpha and beta thalassemia minor); usually no intervention needed, except, low iron diet
- Regular blood transfusions to maintain hemoglobin > 10 g/dL (thalassemia major)
- Splenectomy if hypersplenism is increasing need for transfusions
- Drinking tea will chelate iron and so may be helpful for patients with high iron in diet
- Evaluation of children of adults with thalassemia
- Regular preventive dental care

PHARMACOLOGIC MANAGEMENT

- Deferoxamine (Desferal®): iron chelation therapy for iron overload
  Adult: initial 1000 mg IM, follow with 500 mg IM every 4 hr for 2 doses, max 6,000 mg daily
- Polyvalent pneumococcal vaccine

PREGNANCY/LACTATION CONSIDERATIONS

- Degree of anemia exacerbated during pregnancy

CONSULTATION/REFERRAL

- Refer for genetic counseling
- Hematologist referral for chelation, beta thalassemia major, or other clinician concerns

FOLLOW-UP

- Frequent lifelong monitoring

EXPECTED COURSE

- Thalassemia major: average lifespan 17 years
- Heart failure and infection are leading causes of death
- *β*-thalassemia minor, α-thalassemia: normal life span

POSSIBLE COMPLICATIONS

β-thalassemia major:

- Chronic hemolysis
- Complications from splenectomy if needed
- Infections, skin ulcerations
- Jaundice
- Enlarged heart
- Cholelithiasis
- Impaired vertical growth
- Delayed onset of puberty
- Hepatomegaly
- Iron overload
- Splenomegaly

There are no dietary restrictions required for patients with thalassemia minor. However, thalassemia major patients should eat an iron poor diet.

VITAMIN B12 DEFICIENCY ANEMIA
(Pernicious Anemia, Cobalamin Deficiency)

DESCRIPTION

Macrocytic anemia due to vitamin B12 deficiency

Macrocytosis: red blood cell is larger than average (> 100 fl)

ETIOLOGY

- Atrophic gastric mucosa
- Gastrointestinal surgery
- Impaired absorption
- Drug induced
- Breastfed infants whose mothers have deficient diets or pernicious anemia

INCIDENCE

- Found mostly in adults > 60 years
- Males = Females
- Most prevalent in Scandinavian and English speaking populations

RISK FACTORS

- Elderly
- Inadequate dietary intake (alcoholics, strict vegetarians)
- GI surgery
- Tapeworm infestation
- Malabsorption syndromes (Sprue, Zollinger-Ellison syndrome)
- Medications (e.g., colchicines, oral chelating agents, biguanides, proton pump inhibitors)
- Chronic disease

ASSESSMENT FINDINGS

- Onset gradual, months to years

A Vitamin B12 deficiency diagnosis starts with an index of suspicion by the health care provider.

Neurological abnormalities:
- Diminished cognition
- Abnormal reflexes
- Ataxia
- Disorientation, memory loss
- Positive Babinski reflex, Romberg's sign
- Dementia
- Weakness/spasticity
- Extremity numbness
- Paresthesias
- Poor finger coordination
- Decreased position and vibratory sense
- Vertigo

Other findings:
- Atrophic glossitis
- Depression
- Dyspnea on exertion
- Hepatomegaly/splenomegaly
- Prematurely graying hair
- Skin becomes waxy
- GI symptoms: diarrhea, constipation, indigestion, anorexia

Deficiency of Vitamin B12 affects the hematologic, neurologic, and skeletal systems.

DIFFERENTIAL DIAGNOSIS

- Alcoholism
- Folic acid deficiency anemia
- Other macrocytic anemias
- Other neurological disorders
- Hepatic dysfunction
- Polypharmacy

DIAGNOSTIC STUDIES

- Mean corpuscular volume (MCV): > 110 fl
- Serum vitamin B12 level: < 200 pg/mL

B12 Levels	
> 300 pg/mL	Normal levels
200-300 pg/mL	B12 deficiency possible
< 200 pg/mL	B12 deficiency very likely

- Peripheral smear: anisocytosis, poikilocytosis

Anisocytosis: variation in red blood cell size
Poikilocytosis: variation in red blood cell shape

- Folate level: 60% of patients with Vitamin B12 deficiency have low folate levels (low folate levels impair B12 absorption)
- Gastric analysis: achlorhydria
- Indirect bilirubin: increased
- LDH: increased
- WBC with differential: hypersegmented neutrophils, decreased WBCs
- Serum ferritin: increased or normal
- Platelets: decreased
- Hemoglobin: normal
- Total iron binding capacity (TIBC): normal

If B12 deficiency is possible, check homocysteine and methylmalonic acid (MMA) levels. These are elevated in patients with B12 deficiency secondary to decreased ability to metabolize B12.

PREVENTION

- Index of suspicion, early detection

NONPHARMACOLOGIC MANAGEMENT

- Increase dietary intake of meats, peas and beans, and other protein rich foods
- Educate about lifelong nature of treatment
- Teach patients to give self-injections of vitamin B12

PHARMACOLOGIC MANAGEMENT

- Vitamin B12 (cyanocobalamin) 1000 mcg/d intramuscularly administered every day for one week, then weekly for one month, then monthly for life
  Children: 100 mcg biweekly for 2-4 weeks, then 30-50 mcg IM monthly for maintenance
- Oral Vitamin B12 supplementation (not as well absorbed as via intramuscular route) but can give 1-2 mg/d for treatment in lieu of injections
- Nasal vitamin B12 delivery:
  Cyancobalamin (Calomist®) 25 mcg/nasal spray
  - ◊ Adult: initial 1 spray each nare daily, may increase to bid dosing if needed
  - ◊ Children: not recommended

  OR

  Cyancobolamin (Nasocabal®) 500 mcg/1 mL spray
  - ◊ Adult: 1 spray in one nostril weekly after B12 levels are stabilized
  - ◊ Children: not recommended

PREGNANCY/LACTATION CONSIDERATIONS

- Deficiency may be seen secondary to increased demand

CONSULTATION/REFERRAL

- Consult hematologist if resistant to B12 therapy

FOLLOW-UP

- Re-evaluate 2 weeks after beginning therapy to determine response
- Monthly vitamin B12 injections
- Endoscopy every 5 years (3 fold increase in gastric carcinoma)

EXPECTED COURSE

- Anemia is reversible, but neurologic deficits may not be reversible with treatment if symptoms > 6 months and severe
- Reticulocyte count rapidly increases and peaks in 7-10 days after treatment initiated
- Hematocrit begins to rise within 1 week after beginning treatment

Vitamin B12 deficiency takes years to develop after dietary intake is insufficient because the daily needs are small compared to the amount stored in the body and liver.

POSSIBLE COMPLICATIONS

- Hypokalemia
- Gastric polyps
- Gastric, colorectal cancer

FOLIC ACID DEFICIENCY ANEMIA

DESCRIPTION

Macrocytic anemia due to folic acid deficiency

ETIOLOGY

- Inadequate folic acid intake, especially in the elderly, chronically ill, alcoholics, infants on goat's milk, kwashiorkor, marasmus
- Malabsorption syndromes (e.g., sprue, short-bowel syndrome, Celiac disease)
- Increased demand for folic acid (e.g., pregnancy, malignancy, severe psoriasis, rapid growth)
- Decreased folic acid utilization with some drugs (e.g., methotrexate, TMPS (Bactrim®), triamterene, phenytoin)

INCIDENCE

- Most common during ages 60-70 years
- Peak incidence in children is at 4-7 months of age

RISK FACTORS

- See *Etiology*
- Low birthweight infant

ASSESSMENT FINDINGS

- Insidious onset
- Similar clinical and hematologic features as vitamin B12 deficiency anemia, but neurological lesions do not occur
- Atrophic glossitis (tongue is red and shiny)
- GI symptoms: indigestion, constipation, diarrhea

Infants:
- Irritability
- Failure to thrive
- Chronic diarrhea

DIFFERENTIAL DIAGNOSIS

- Pernicious anemia

DIAGNOSTIC STUDIES

- Mean corpuscular volume (MCV): > 100 fl
- Hematocrit: decreased
- Hemoglobin: normal
- Red cell distribution width (RDW): elevated
- Reticulocyte count: decreased
- Serum folic acid level: decreased, < 3 ng/mL
- RBC folate level < 150 mg/mL
- Homocysteine levels: elevated because folate needed to convert homocysteine to methionine
- Serum ferritin level: normal
- Total iron binding capacity (TIBC): normal
- Lactic acid dehydrogenase (LDH): elevated
- Vitamin B12 level: normal

It is usual for patients who have a B12 deficiency to have a folate deficiency too. Measure a B12 level in folic acid deficiency anemia.

PREVENTION

- Avoid medications which interfere with folic acid absorption (phenytoin, sulfa drugs)
- Adequate dietary intake of folic acid

NONPHARMACOLOGIC MANAGEMENT

- Increased folic acid intake in diet
- Dietary counseling about foods high in folic acid:
  - ◊ green leafy vegetables
  - ◊ fruits
  - ◊ nuts
  - ◊ liver
  - ◊ foods containing yeast
  - ◊ mushrooms

PHARMACOLOGIC MANAGEMENT

- Folic acid supplementation orally or parenterally; examples:
  Folmor®
  - ◊ (Folic acid 2.5mg + vitamin B12, B6)
  - ◊ Adult: 1-2 tabs daily
  - ◊ Children: not recommended

Foltx® (folic acid 2.5 mg + vitamin B12)
◊ Adult: 1-2 tabs daily
◊ Children: not recommended

PREGNANCY/LACTATION CONSIDERATIONS

- Increased demand for folic acid
- Adequate folic acid intake before and during pregnancy important for prevention of neural tube defects in fetus
- Recommended dosage prepregnancy is 1 mg/day for all women of childbearing age

CONSULTATION/REFERRAL

- Usually not needed

FOLLOW-UP

- Re-evaluate in 2 weeks to determine response to therapy and then every month until stable

EXPECTED COURSE

- Rapid increase in reticulocyte count with peak in 7-10 days after therapy started
- Hematocrit should rise within 1 week of initiation of therapy

POSSIBLE COMPLICATIONS

- Failure to thrive

LEUKEMIA
(ALL, ANLL, CML, CLL)

DESCRIPTION

Hyper/hypo proliferation of blast cells in the bone marrow and other tissues with resultant bone marrow failure. The specific type of leukemia is categorized according to the course of the disease and the type of blast cell which predominates.

- Acute lymphocytic leukemia (ALL): principal type of leukemia in children
- Acute nonlymphoblastic leukemia (ANLL)
- Chronic myelocytic leukemia (CML)
- Chronic lymphocytic leukemia (CLL)

CLL is the most common form of leukemia in adults in the world. It is often discovered incidentally.

ETIOLOGY

- Exact cause unknown
- Some have familial tendency

INCIDENCE

- Account for 33% of pediatric malignancies
- ALL: 75% of all pediatric cases; peaks at 4 years of age
- ANLL: 20% of all cases
- Males > Females
- 70% occurs in adults (CLL and ANLL)

RISK FACTORS

- Family history of leukemia
- Chromosomal abnormalities
- Exposure to teratogens, carcinogens
- Immunocompromised state
- Chemical and drug exposure, especially nitrogen mustard and benzene
- Cigarette smoking

ASSESSMENT FINDINGS

ALL:
- Symptoms appear acutely and progress rapidly
- Fever
- Bleeding tendencies: petechiae, delayed clotting after injury

- Lymphadenitis
- Pallor
- Fatigue
- Hepatosplenomegaly
- Lymphadenopathy
- Gingival swelling

ANLL:
- Pallor
- Fever
- Infection
- Bleeding
- Hepatomegaly
- Gingival hypertrophy

CML:
- Onset usually insidious
- Splenomegaly
- Weight loss
- Fatigue
- Low grade fever
- Anorexia
- Night sweats
- Visual disturbances
- Priapism

CLL:
- Fatigue
- Pallor
- Fever, night sweats, weight loss
- Recurrent infections
- Lymphadenopathy
- Hepatosplenomegaly
- Petechiae

DIFFERENTIAL DIAGNOSIS

- Other diseases of the bone marrow
- Viral or drug induced bone marrow dysfunction

DIAGNOSTIC STUDIES

- CBC: WBC, RBC, and/or platelets decreased
- Differential: increased lymphocytes and blast cells
- Hemoglobin: decreased
- Reticulocyte count: < 0.5%
- Erythrocyte sedimentation rate: usually elevated
- LFTs: may be abnormal
- Coagulation profile: can be abnormal; especially in ANLL
- Bone marrow aspiration used to make actual diagnosis
- Chest X ray: mediastinal mass

Blastocytes identified on CBC are always abnormal. Blastocytes are immature white cells that are normally found in the bone marrow, not serum.

PREVENTION

- Avoidance of known risk factors

NONPHARMACOLOGIC MANAGEMENT

- Radiation
- Keep well hydrated
- Platelet transfusion if count < 20,000 mm3
- RBC transfusion if patient has symptomatic anemia
- Patient/family education
  - ◊ Screen other family members
  - ◊ Avoid aspirin products
  - ◊ Close temperature monitoring if WBC count < 1000
  - ◊ No intense activity or contact sports
  - ◊ Aggressive treatment of infections and potential infections
- Refer patient and family to Leukemia Society of America for educational and supportive resources

PHARMACOLOGIC MANAGEMENT

- Chemotherapy regimens specific for type of leukemia

PREGNANCY/LACTATION CONSIDERATIONS

- Chemotherapy may be used in the second and third trimesters, but plan is specific for type of leukemia

CONSULTATION/REFERRAL

- Refer to oncologist for treatment at diagnosis or suspected diagnosis

FOLLOW-UP

- Close monitoring of WBCs, RBCs, and platelets, other indices as indicated
- Bone marrow studies every week or as appropriate for status
- Follow up bone scans, CT, MRIs as indicated

EXPECTED COURSE

ALL:
- Remission rate is greater than 90% with treatment
- Long-term survival is typical in children

ANLL:
- Remission rate is 60-80% with 20-40% long-term survival

CML:
- Poor long term prognosis

CLL:
- Usually asymptomatic early in course of the disease
- Overall survival is about 9 years after diagnosis

POSSIBLE COMPLICATIONS

- Infection
- Blast crisis

LYMPHOMA

DESCRIPTION

Malignancy of lymphatic system. Two common types:

- Hodgkin's: malignant disease of the lymphatic system characterized by presence of Reed-Sternberg cells
- Non-Hodgkin's: diverse group of lymphomas

Hodgkin's lymphoma, formerly called Hodgkin's disease, is one of the most curable forms of cancer.

ETIOLOGY

- Unknown
- Evidence of links to viral infections

INCIDENCE

Hodgkin's:
- 7900 cases annually
- Males > Females
- Two peak ages: during twenties and again during sixties
- Increased incidence in first-degree relatives and siblings of patients with Hodgkin's

Non-Hodgkin's:
- Twice as common as Hodgkin's
- Peak incidence during sixties

RISK FACTORS

- Immunodeficiency (acquired or inherited)
- Autoimmune disease (lupus, others)
- HIV infection

ASSESSMENT FINDINGS

- Firm, nontender, enlarged lymph nodes in cervical, supraclavicular, axillary, or inguinal areas
- Freely mobile nodes (less common)
- Fever
- Cough
- Night sweats
- Weight loss >10%
- Pruritus
- Fatigue
- Hepatomegaly
- Splenomegaly
- Adenopathy usually asymmetric in Hodgkin's
- Non-Hodgkin often has disseminated adenopathy

DIFFERENTIAL DIAGNOSIS

- Hodgkin's vs. Non-Hodgkin's disease
- Infectious lymphadenopathy (Cat scratch disease)
- Tumor metastasis from other site
- Autoimmune diseases
- Drug reaction

DIAGNOSTIC STUDIES

- Reed-Sternberg cells on biopsy (pathognomonic)
- CBC with differential: anemia
- Peripheral smear
- Chemistry profile
- Erythrocyte sedimentation rate (ESR): elevated
- Liver function tests: elevated
- Renal function tests
- Chest x-ray: mediastinal mass possible

- CT of chest if chest x-ray abnormal
- Bone scan
- Abdominal ultrasound and CT
- Lymph node biopsy
- Bone marrow biopsy

NONPHARMACOLOGIC MANAGEMENT

- Radiation therapy alone or in combination with chemotherapy
- Splenectomy may be done for staging of illness
- Autologous bone marrow transplantation
- Excellent oral hygiene

PHARMACOLOGIC MANAGEMENT

- Chemotherapy
- Interferon
- Polyvalent pneumococcal vaccine
- Influenza immunization annually

PREGNANCY/LACTATION CONSIDERATIONS

- Diagnosis during pregnancy does not have a negative impact on Hodgkin's disease
- Hodgkin's does not have a deleterious affect on fetus

CONSULTATION/REFERRAL

- Referral to oncologist/hematologist

FOLLOW-UP

- Monitor CBC and hydration status
- Periodic examination of involved nodes to monitor response to therapy
- Careful follow-up for early detection of relapse

EXPECTED COURSE

Hodgkin's:
- Dependent on stage
- 83% 5 year survival

Non-Hodgkin's:
- Prognosis dependent on histopathology

POSSIBLE COMPLICATIONS

- Infertility
- Secondary malignancy

IDIOPATHIC THROMBOCYTOPENIA PURPURA
(ITP)

DESCRIPTION

Decrease in the number of platelets in the absence of an identifiable cause; all other causes of thrombocytopenia must be ruled out before a diagnosis of ITP can be made.

Idiopathic thrombocytopenia is always a diagnosis of exclusion.

ETIOLOGY

- Underlying cause unknown
- Defect is due to IgG autoantibodies on platelet surfaces which precipitate autoimmune response

INCIDENCE

- Approximately 22 cases/million in U.S.

Acute ITP:
- Predominant age: 2-9 years old
- Increased incidence in fair-skinned children
- Males=Females

Chronic ITP:
- Predominant age: > 50 years old
- Females > Males (2:1)

RISK FACTORS

- Acute infection
- Cardiopulmonary bypass
- Hypersplenism
- Pre-eclampsia
- Age

ASSESSMENT FINDINGS

- Onset is often acute
- History of viral illness 1-4 weeks prior to onset common in children
- Bleeding can occur with minor accident once platelet count reaches 40,000-60,000 mm^3
- Petechiae, purpura, and/or bruising
- Unusual bleeding in GI and GU tracts
- Epistaxis
- Nonpalpable spleen (if palpable, probably not idiopathic)
- Spontaneous bleeding can occur if platelet count < 20,000 mm^3

DIFFERENTIAL DIAGNOSIS

- Thrombocytopenia secondary to another cause
- Medications: > 150 have been identified
- Hemophilia
- Von Willebrand's disease
- Meningococcemia
- Vitamin K deficiency
- Alcohol ingestion
- Lymphoma
- Systemic lupus erythematosus
- Disseminated intravascular coagulation (DIC)

DIAGNOSTIC STUDIES

- CBC: decreased platelet count < 150,000
- Platelet count: 5,000-75,000/mm^3
- Platelet bound IgG antibody: positive in 80% of patients with ITP
- WBC: normal
- Bleeding time: prolonged
- Hematocrit and hemoglobin: normal unless significant blood loss has occurred
- PT, PTT: normal
- Peripheral smear: megathrombocytes
- Bone marrow aspiration: megakaryocytes

Request a peripheral smear when thrombocytopenia is present. The pathologist will typically identify normal red and white cells; enlarged platelets that are few in number.

PREVENTION

- Avoid unnecessary exposure to medications that inhibit platelet function (e.g., aspirin, heparin), suppress bone marrow

NONPHARMACOLOGIC MANAGEMENT

- Hospitalization for patients with active bleeding
- Consider platelet transfusions
- Splenectomy in patients that fail medical therapy and need prednisone daily to preserve platelets

Pneumococcal vaccine should be administered at least 2 weeks prior to splenectomy.

- Minimal activity to prevent injury or bruising
- No contact sports; especially if spleen is enlarged

PHARMACOLOGIC MANAGEMENT

- Prednisone for 4-6 weeks, then taper off, may need repeat course for chronic ITP

PREGNANCY/LACTATION CONSIDERATIONS

- Prednisone for 10-14 days before delivery
- Thrombocytopenia may be secondary to pre-eclampsia
- Increased fetal mortality

CONSULTATION/REFERRAL

- Surgical referral for splenectomy with medical failure
- Referral to hematologist; especially during pregnancy

FOLLOW-UP

- Frequent platelet counts (daily to weekly depending on severity)

EXPECTED COURSE

Acute ITP:
- 80-85% recover within 4-8 weeks of onset
- 15-20% develop chronic ITP

Chronic ITP:
- Rare spontaneous recovery

POSSIBLE COMPLICATIONS

- 1% mortality due to intracranial bleeding
- Severe blood loss

NEONATAL HYPERBILIRUBINEMIA
(Neonatal Jaundice)

DESCRIPTION

An accumulation of unconjugated bilirubin from destruction of fetal erythrocytes and decreased ability of the liver to excrete this. It is deposited in the skin and sclera and the characteristic yellow color appears.

ETIOLOGY

- Physiologic jaundice
- ABO incompatibility
- Rh incompatibility
- Sepsis
- Breastfeeding
- Dehydration

INCIDENCE

- 60% of term infants and 80% of premature infants exhibit jaundice in the first week of life

RISK FACTORS

- Prematurity
- Rh-positive infant of Rh-negative mother
- ABO incompatibility between mother and fetus
- Family history of hemolytic disease

ASSESSMENT FINDINGS

- Yellow tone to sclera, mucous membranes, skin
- Jaundice appears on the head and face first and then progresses to the trunk and extremities
- It resolves in the opposite direction (extremities, trunk, face)

Diagnosis is aided by applying gentle pressure to the baby's skin. Blanching reveals the normal skin color and the contrast in skin color becomes more evident.

- Bright yellow stools
- Jaundice occurs usually on day 2-3 of life in physiological jaundice
- If jaundice occurs within the first 24 hours of life or after the third day, other causes must be investigated

Always ask how the infant is feeding. Poor feeding is a common predictor of jaundice secondary to breastfeeding.

DIFFERENTIAL DIAGNOSIS

- See *Etiology*

DIAGNOSTIC STUDIES

Findings suggesting nonphysiologic hyperbilirubinemia:
- Serum bilirubin rising at rate greater than 5 mg/dL in 24 hours
- Serum bilirubin > 20 mg/dL in term infant or 10-14 mg/dL in preterm infant
- Conjugated serum bilirubin > 1mg/dL or 10% of total serum bilirubin

Elevated bilirubin levels can be neurotoxic.

Other studies:
- Liver function tests
- Coombs' (direct and indirect) to evaluate for Rh and/or ABO isoimmunization
- CBC to assess for infection

Hematologic Disorders

- G-6-PD levels to assess for G-6-PD deficiency, a cause of kernicterus

PREVENTION

- Early frequent feedings

Increase breastfeedings to 10-12 times/day during the first few days of life.

NONPHARMACOLOGIC MANAGEMENT

- Monitor status closely as long as serum bilirubin levels are < 20 mg/dL
- Good hydration
- Exposure to sunlight
- Phototherapy
- Exchange transfusion
- Treatment of underlying cause if nonphysiologic

Phototherapy may increase risk of dehydration. Monitor hydration status while undergoing phototherapy.

EXPECTED COURSE

- Physiologic jaundice resolves spontaneously without sequelae
- 33% of all infants with untreated hemolytic disease and bilirubin levels >30 mg/dL will develop kernicterus

COMPLICATIONS

- Kernicterus
- Mental retardation
- Deafness
- Quadriplegia
- Complications from phototherapy or exchange transfusion

Kernicterus is rare in the U.S. but occurs due to deposition of bilirubin in brain tissue. This produces a bilirubin encephalopathy. Infants exhibit lethargy and poor feeding.

Rh INCOMPATIBILITY

DESCRIPTION

Anti-Rh antibody production in Rh-negative person after exposure to Rh antigen that results in destruction of red blood cells.

ETIOLOGY

- Most commonly occurs when an Rh-negative woman carries an Rh-positive fetus
- Blood transfusion of Rh-positive blood to Rh-negative recipient

INCIDENCE

- 15% of Caucasian population is Rh negative
- < 5% of all populations is Rh negative

RISK FACTORS

- Rh-negative mother with Rh-positive fetus
- Any maternal fetal hemorrhage
- Ectopic pregnancy
- Placenta abruptio
- Placenta previa
- Spontaneous/induced abortion
- Blood transfusion

ASSESSMENT FINDINGS

- Jaundice in newborn
- Hemolytic transfusion reaction
- Congenital anemia
- Fetal hydrops

DIFFERENTIAL DIAGNOSIS

- ABO incompatibility
- Isoimmunization from another cause

DIAGNOSTIC STUDIES

- Indirect Coombs': positive in mother
- Direct Coombs': positive in infant

PREVENTION

- Rho(D) immune globulin (RhoGAM®) administered to Rh-negative women:
    - ◊ Routinely at 28 weeks gestation
    - ◊ Routinely within 72 hours after delivery of Rh-positive infant
    - ◊ Anytime maternal fetal hemorrhage occurs
    - ◊ After ectopic pregnancy
    - ◊ After spontaneous/induced abortion

RhoGAM® administration does not eliminate the possibility of incompatibility but decreases the likelihood to less than 1%.

NONPHARMACOLOGIC MANAGEMENT

- Phototherapy
- Exchange transfusion
- Early delivery of affected fetus
- Intrauterine transfusion

PHARMACOLOGIC MANAGEMENT

- Diuretics and digoxin for infant that has developed hydrops fetalis

If paternity is uncertain, RhoGAM is given at 28 weeks and routinely within 72 hours after birth.

FOLLOW-UP

- Antibody titer measured frequently during pregnancy in Rh-negative women
- Nonstress testing to determine status of fetus
- Biophysical profile to determine status of fetus

EXPECTED COURSE

- Survival rate of severely affected pregnancies with proper management: 80% - 90%
- Fetuses affected by hydrops fetalis have poor prognosis
- Once a woman is isoimmunized, each subsequent pregnancy more severely affected

POSSIBLE COMPLICATIONS

- Fetal hydrops
- Kernicterus
- Pregnancy loss
- Severe anemia of infant

References

ACOG practice bulletin no. 78: Hemoglobinopathies in pregnancy. (2007). Obstetrics and Gynecology, 109(1), 229-237.

Alleyne, M., Horne, M. K., & Miller, J. L. (2008). Individualized treatment for iron-deficiency anemia in adults. American Journal of Medicine, 121(11), 943-948.

Bartlett, N. L. (2008). Modern treatment of hodgkin lymphoma. Current Opinion in Hematology, 15(4), 408-414.

Beutler, E., & Waalen, J. (2006). The definition of anemia: What is the lower limit of normal of the blood hemoglobin concentration? Blood, 107(5), 1747-1750.

Binns, H. J., Campbell, C., & Brown, M. J. (2007). Interpreting and managing blood lead levels of less than 10 microg/dl in children and reducing childhood exposure to lead: Recommendations of the centers for disease control and prevention advisory committee on childhood lead poisoning prevention. Pediatrics, 120(5), e1285-1298.

Bonds, D. R. (2005). Three decades of innovation in the management of sickle cell disease: The road to understanding the sickle cell disease clinical phenotype. Blood Reviews, 19(2), 99-110.

Burns, C. E., Brady, M. A., Blosser, C., Starr, N. B., & Dunn, A. M. (2009). Pediatric primary care: A handbook for nurse practitioners (4th ed.). Philadelphia: W.B. Saunders.

Chiorazzi, N., Rai, K. R., & Ferrarini, M. (2005). Chronic lymphocytic leukemia. New England Journal of Medicine, 352(8), 804-815.

Cunningham, F. G., Gant, N. F., Leveno, K. J., Gilstrap, L. C., Hauth, J. C., & Wenstrom, K. D. (2005). Williams obstetrics (22nd ed.). New York: McGraw-Hill.

Domino, F., Baldor, R., Golding, J., Grimes, J., & Taylor, J. (2011). The 5-minute clinical consult 2011. Philadelphia: Lippincott Williams & Wilkins.

Ernst, D., & Lee, A. (2010). Nurse practitioners prescribing reference. New York: Haymarket Media Publication.

Eussen, S. J., de Groot, L. C., Clarke, R., Schneede, J., Ueland, P. M., Hoefnagels, W. H., et al. (2005). Oral cyanocobalamin supplementation in older people with vitamin b12 deficiency: A dose-finding trial. Archives of Internal Medicine, 165(10), 1167-1172.

Ferri, F. (2010). Ferri's 2010 clinical advisor. Philadelphia: Mosby Elsevier.

Frank, J. E. (2005). Diagnosis and management of g6pd deficiency. American Family Physician, 72(7), 1277-1282.

George, J. N. (2009). Chronic refractory immune (idiopathic) thrombocytopenic purpura in adults. Up to Date. Retrieved from http://www.uptodate.com/patients/content/topic.do?topicKey=~77D7lgjejgme4R

Godeau, B., Provan, D., & Bussel, J. (2007). Immune thrombocytopenic purpura in adults. Current Opinion in Hematology, 14(5), 535-556.

Harper, J. W., Holleran, S. F., Ramakrishnan, R., Bhagat, G., & Green, P. H. (2007). Anemia in celiac disease is multifactorial in etiology. American Journal of Hematology, 82(11), 996-1000.

Johnson, C. S. (2005). Sickle cell disease. Hematology/Oncology Clinics of North America, 19(5), xi-xiii.

Kumar, V. (2007). Pernicious anemia. MLO: Medical Laboratory Observer, 39(2), 28, 30-21.

Kuppers, R. (2009). The biology of hodgkin's lymphoma. Nat Rev Cancer, 9(1), 15-27.

Larson, R. A. (2006). Management of acute lymphoblastic leukemia in older patients. Seminars in Hematology, 43(2), 126-133.

Lead exposure in children: Prevention, detection, and management. (2005). Pediatrics, 116(4), 1036-1046.

Management of hyperbilirubinemia in the newborn infant 35 or more weeks of gestation. (2004). Pediatrics, 114(1), 297-316.

Manning-Dimmitt, L. L., Dimmitt, S. G., & Wilson, G. R. (2005). Diagnosis of gastrointestinal bleeding in adults. American Family Physician, 71(7), 1339-1346.

Mast, A. E., Blinder, M. A., & Dietzen, D. J. (2008). Reticulocyte hemoglobin content. American Journal of Hematology, 83(4), 307-310.

Moise, K. J., Jr. (2008). Management of rhesus alloimmunization in pregnancy. Obstetrics and Gynecology, 112(1), 164-176.

National Heart Lung and Blood Institute. What is sickle cell anemia. Retrieved from http://www.nhlbi.nih.gov/health/dci/Diseases/Sca/SCA_All.html

Raemaekers, J. M., & van der Maazen, R. W. (2008). Hodgkin's lymphoma: News from an old disease. Netherlands Journal of Medicine, 66(11), 457-466.

Robins, E. B., & Blum, S. (2007). Hematologic reference values for african american children and adolescents. American Journal of Hematology, 82(7), 611-614.

Rund, D., & Rachmilewitz, E. (2005). Beta-thalassemia. New England Journal of Medicine, 353(11), 1135-1146.

Shanafelt, T. D., & Kay, N. E. (2007). Comprehensive management of the cll patient: A holistic approach. Hematology Am Soc Hematol Educ Program, 324-331.

Weiss, G., & Goodnough, L. T. (2005). Anemia of chronic disease. New England Journal of Medicine, 352(10), 1011-1023.

Woolf, A. D., Goldman, R., & Bellinger, D. C. (2007). Update on the clinical management of childhood lead poisoning. Pediatric Clinics of North America, 54(2), 271-294, viii.

9

LACTATION

Lactation

Benefits of Breastfeeding 387

Disadvantages of Breastfeeding 387

Contraindications to Breastfeeding 387

Physiology of Lactation 387

Breastfeeding Technique 388

Maternal Nutrition 388

Vitamin Supplementation of the Breastfed Infant 388

Determination of Adequate Intake 388

Breast Care 389

Storage of Breast Milk 389

Weaning 389

Drugs/Medications 389

Alcohol 389

Smoking 390

Common Problems of Lactation 390
- Plugged Milk Duct 390
- Sore Nipples 390
- Flat or Inverted Nipples 390
- Engorgement 391
- Mastitis 391
- Leaking 391
- Inadequate Let-Down Reflex 392
- Candidal Infection of Nipples 392

Jaundice....................392
References....................*393*

Lactation

BENEFITS OF BREASTFEEDING

MATERNAL

- Economical
- Accelerates uterine involution and decreases postpartal bleeding
- Exerts protective effect against endometrial and breast cancer
- No preparation of milk or bottles needed
- Facilitates maternal weight loss

INFANT

- Decreases rate of respiratory, gastrointestinal, and middle ear infections
- Easy to digest
- Enhances bonding and encourages a close relationship between mother and infant
- May decrease development of allergies
- Decreases constipation
- May help avoid obesity
- Provides protection against sudden infant death syndrome (SIDS)

DISADVANTAGES OF BREASTFEEDING

- Mother may perceive it as an inconvenience
- Time commitment may be perceived as a disadvantage
- Only mother can feed baby

CONTRAINDICATIONS TO BREASTFEEDING

- HIV positive mother
- Active tuberculosis
- Newly diagnosed breast cancer
- Drug abuse by mother
- Infant galactosemia
- Herpes lesion on mother's breasts
- Mother receiving medications that are contraindicated for infant

PHYSIOLOGY OF LACTATION

- Decline of estrogen and progesterone after delivery of placenta initiates increased milk production
- Oxytocin and prolactin are two of the major hormones responsible for lactation
- Oxytocin is responsible for let-down reflex which is necessary for successful breastfeeding
- Prolactin is released as nipple stimulation occurs during sucking. Regulates milk volume and production
- Day 0-2: colostrum is secreted: a thick, sticky, yellow fluid rich in immunoglobulins, vitamin E, and leukocytes. It is higher in protein, fat-soluble vitamins, and minerals than mature milk
- Day 2-4: transitional milk is thinner, more plentiful milk with increased lactose, fat, calories, and water-soluble vitamin content
- Day 4: mature milk: consists of fore milk (first milk expressed from breast at each nursing) and hind milk (milk higher in fat and calories); expressed after the let-down reflex occurs and is essential for adequate infant nutrition

BREASTFEEDING TECHNIQUE

- Infant should be placed facing the mother (belly-to-belly)
- Teach breastfeeding woman different positions for breastfeeding:
  - ◊ Cradle position
  - ◊ Football hold
  - ◊ Side-lying position
- Position should be rotated frequently, especially first few weeks of breastfeeding
- Generally, newborns should breastfeed 8-12 times in 24 hours
- Nursing time: varies widely with each infant; limiting nursing time may increase engorgement. Breast will be emptied usually after 10-20 minutes of nursing
- Removing infant from breast: break suction with finger before removing infant to prevent sore nipples
- Burp infant when changing breasts and after feeding
- Avoid use of pacifiers and bottles which may cause nipple confusion in infant
- Supplemental feedings including water are not usually needed for adequate nutrition

MATERNAL NUTRITION

- Increased fluids are required
- Avoid caffeine (may stimulate infant)
- Increased calorie intake by 500 kcal over prepregnancy requirements
- Continue prenatal vitamins
- Iron supplementation may be needed if diet inadequate
- Calcium supplement if not taking in adequate amounts in diet

VITAMIN SUPPLEMENTATION OF THE BREASTFED INFANT

- Iron supplementation after 6 months of age
- Fluoride started after 6 months of age if living in an area where water is not fluoridated
  Example: Poly-Vi-Flor Drops/Tablets and Drops with Iron
  Base dose on fluoride content of water
  Not recommended for < 4 months of age
  If fluoride content < 0.3 ppm:
  - ◊ 6 months-3 years: 0.25 mg/fluoride/day

  If fluoride content 0.3-0.6 ppm:
  - ◊ 6 months-3 years: not recommended
- Supplementation with vitamin D is recommended for all infants

DETERMINATION OF ADEQUATE INTAKE

- Appropriate weight gain of infant (about one ounce per day for first 6 months)
- Breasts feel full before nursing and soft afterwards
- Infant has 6-8 wet diapers in a 24 hour period
- Infant satisfied
- Infant has at least two soft stools per day
- Audible swallowing while nursing

BREAST CARE

- Wear comfortable, well-fitting bra
- Wash breasts with warm water
- Avoid use of soap due to its drying effect
- Lanolin may be used for soothing and healing
- Fresh air to nipples helpful in drying and healing nipples

STORAGE OF BREAST MILK

- Store in sterilized polypropylene plastic containers
- Write date on container
- Refrigerate or freeze milk immediately after expressing
- Freeze milk that will not be used within 2 days
- Use milk within 3 months if stored in a self-defrosting freezer
- Use milk stored in a traditional freezer within 12 months
- Use oldest milk first
- Thaw under warm running water. Do not heat milk on stove or in microwave
- Do not refreeze breast milk

WEANING

- Breastfeeding alone is adequate until infant is 6 months of age. At this time solid foods may be introduced slowly
- To wean infant, substitute a bottle or cup feeding for a breastfeeding every few days until infant is completely off breast

DRUGS/MEDICATIONS

- Many drugs are excreted in breast milk and have the potential to affect infant
- Health care provider should be consulted before taking any medications
- When a medication must be taken by the lactating woman, take it immediately after breastfeeding so that the infant receives the least amount possible

ALCOHOL

- Occasional alcohol is allowed
- May impair let-down reflex if too high an amount is consumed
- May impair let-down reflex

SMOKING

- Smoking decreases breast milk volume
- Nicotine is excreted in breast milk to infant
- Smoking cessation is recommended
- Never smoke while holding baby

COMMON PROBLEMS OF LACTATION

PLUGGED MILK DUCT

CAUSES

- Infrequent nursing
- Engorgement

ASSESSMENT FINDINGS

- Sore lump in one or both breasts
- No fever

MANAGEMENT

- Moist hot packs to breast lump before and during nursing
- More frequent nursing, especially on affected side
- Do not stop breastfeeding
- Pump or express milk after feeding if infant not emptying breasts
- Breast massage
- Breastfeeding in various nursing positions

SORE NIPPLES

CAUSES

- Improper positioning of infant
- Removing infant from breast without first breaking suction with finger
- Nipple confusion from introduction of bottle nipple or pacifier too early
- Improper latch-on because of short frenulum
- Inappropriate use of breast creams and soaps
- Thrush
- Infant nursing on tip of nipple

ASSESSMENT FINDINGS

- Complaint of pain when infant nurses
- Nipples tender, raw, swollen, or traumatized

MANAGEMENT

- Expose breasts to air or sunlight for short period several times a day. Avoid washing breasts with soap and water
- Avoid use of breast creams
- Breastfeed frequently to avoid vigorous nursing by infant
- Make sure nipple is in the posterior portion of infant's mouth
- Limit nursing time on sore nipple
- Nurse on the least sore side first
- Change bra pads frequently to keep nipples dry
- Wear vented breast shells to protect and dry nipples between feedings
- Avoid use of rubber nipple shield
- Mild analgesics may be required
- Educate regarding positioning and breaking suction with finger when taking infant off breast
- For patients with cracking, blistering, bleeding, or severe pain of nipples, a consultation or referral to a lactation consultant is recommended

FLAT OR INVERTED NIPPLES

CAUSE

- Adhesions of the nipple causing retraction or inversion

ASSESSMENT FINDINGS

- Inverted nipples retract inward when stimulated

MANAGEMENT

- Should be assessed during pregnancy
- Specially designed, vented breast shells with a hole in the center can be worn during the last month of pregnancy. These shells provide slight, constant pressure to draw the nipple out
- Manually pull the nipple out before feeding
- Use a breast pump for a short while before feeding
- Application of ice before nursing to draw out nipple
- Referral to lactation consultant usually necessary

ENGORGEMENT

CAUSES

- Milk stasis in the breast from inadequate emptying
- Skipping or delaying feedings

ASSESSMENT FINDINGS

- Pain in breasts
- Hard, warm, lumpy breasts
- Feeling of fullness in breasts
- Flattened nipples
- Usually occurs in first few weeks of nursing

MANAGEMENT

- Increase frequency of nursing
- Avoid long periods without nursing
- Manual expression of milk
- Hot shower allowing water to flow over breasts
- Apply warm compresses to breasts before nursing
- Apply ice to breasts for relief after nursing
- Hand expression of some milk before feeding to soften breast and facilitate infant attaching to breasts
- Breast massage

MASTITIS

CAUSES

- Plugged milk ducts leading to infection
- Usually caused by staphylococcal or streptococcal organisms
- Predisposing factors
  - ◊ Fatigue, stress
  - ◊ Cracked nipples
  - ◊ Improper-fitting bra
  - ◊ Inadequate emptying of breast
  - ◊ Abrupt weaning

ASSESSMENT FINDINGS

- Breast tenderness and pain
- Lump in one or both breasts
- Fever, chills
- Erythema overlying sore area
- Flu-like symptoms
- Fatigue

MANAGEMENT

- Moist hot packs or warm shower before and during nursing
- More frequent nursing on affected side
- Do not stop breastfeeding
- Rule out other sources of fever
- Acetaminophen for fever
- Analgesics for pain
- Increased rest
- Increased fluids
- If abscess occurs, surgical drainage is required
- Do not wean abruptly
- Antibiotics to cover *Staphylococcus aureus*, the most common causative organism
  Examples: Amoxil 500 mg twice a day for 7-10 days (L1) OR Cephalosporin: cefprozil (Cefzil) 500 mg bid (L2) OR Macrolide: Erythromycin 1.6 g in 2, 3, or 4 divided doses (L2 and L3 early postnatally because associated with pyloric stenosis, so delay at least 6 weeks)

Lactation Risk Categories range from L1 Safest, L2 Safer, L3 Moderately Safe, L4 Possibly Hazardous, and L5 Contraindicated.

LEAKING

CAUSES

- Let-down reflex stimulated by crying infant or even the sight of an infant
- Overly full breasts

MANAGEMENT

- Good supportive bra
- Wearing breast pads without plastic liners; should be changed frequently
- Pressure against nipple with heel of hand when feel let-down sensation
- Increased feeding
- Manual expression of milk if breast overly full

INADEQUATE LET-DOWN REFLEX

CAUSES

- Multifactorial
- Inadequate relaxation
- Fatigued or tense mother
- Infant not nursing long enough

ASSESSMENT FINDINGS

- Breasts not completely emptying

MANAGEMENT

- Allow infant ample time to nurse
- Massage breasts before nursing
- Use relaxation and breathing techniques
- Adequate rest and nutrition
- Oxytocin nasal spray during feeding (limit to 1st week postpartum) Nasal spray 2-3 minutes prior to breast feeding or pumping 100 microliter/spray
- Referral to lactation consultant often necessary

CANDIDAL INFECTION OF NIPPLES

CAUSES

- Infection of either or both breasts with Candida albicans
- May be contracted by infant during delivery and transmitted to mother's breast

ASSESSMENT FINDINGS

- Red, painful itching nipples and areola
- White patches in mouth of infant do not rub off
- Pain, burning, itching, redness of breasts

MANAGEMENT

- Treat infant with oral nystatin (Mycostatin®)
- Treat mother with topical agent, antifungal, to breast
- Apply Nystatin or Clotrimazole cream to breast(s) after breastfeeding
- Keep nipples clean and dry
- Wash antifungal off breast before breastfeeding

JAUNDICE

CAUSE

- Too little colustrum or breastmilk from inadequate feedings

ASSESSMENT FINDINGS

- Yellow skin tone
- Yellow sclera
- Usually occurs after third day of life
- Infant healthy and thriving

MANAGEMENT

- Increase feedings of breastmilk
- Avoid supplementation with milk
- Serum bilirubin measurement
- Rule out pathological causes of jaundice
- Continue breastfeeding
- Usually resolves without harm to infant

References

ACOG Committee Opinion No. 361: Breastfeeding: Maternal and infant aspects. (2007). Obstetrics and Gynecology, 109, 479-480.

American Academy of Pediatrics. (2009a). Breastfeeding. In R. E. Kleinman (Ed.), Peditric nutrition handbook. Elk Grove Village, IL: American Academy of Pediatrics.

American Academy of Pediatrics. (2009b). Red book: 2009 report of the committee on infectious diseases (28th ed.). Elk Grove Village, IL: American Academy of Pediatrics.

Anderson, P. O., & Valdes, V. (2007). A critical review of pharmaceutical galactagogues. Breastfeed Med, 2(4), 229-242. doi: 10.1089/bfm.2007.0013

Bickley, L. S., & Szilagyi, P. G. (2008). Bates' guide to physical examination and history taking (10th ed.). Philadelphia: Lippincott Williams & Wilkins.

Branch, W. T. (2003). Office practice of medicine (4th ed.). Philadelphia: Saunders.

Burns, C. E., Brady, M. A., Blosser, C., Starr, N. B., & Dunn, A. M. (2009). Pediatric primary care: A handbook for nurse practitioners (4th ed.). Philadelphia: W.B. Saunders.

Cunningham, F. G., Gant, N. F., Leveno, K. J., Gilstrap, L. C., Hauth, J. C., & Wenstrom, K. D. (2005). Williams Obstetrics (22nd ed.). New York: McGraw-Hill.

Davidson, M. B., London, M., & Ladewig, P. (2007). Old's Maternal-Newbrn Nursing and Women's Health Across the Lifespan. Upper Saddle River, NJ: Prentice Hall.

Domino, F., Baldor, R., Golding, J., Grimes, J., & Taylor, J. (2011). The 5-minute clinical consult 2011. Philadelphia: Lippincott Williams & Wilkins.

Drug Facts and Comparisons. (2010). St. Louis: Wolters Kluwer Health. Facts & Comparisons.

Ernst, D., & Lee, A. (2010). Nurse practitioners prescribing reference. New York: Haymarket Media Publication.

Ferri, F. (2010). Ferri's 2010 clinical advisor. Philadelphia: Mosby Elsevier.

Hale, T. W. (2008). Medications and mother's milk (10th ed.). Amarillo, TX: Pharmasoft Publishing.

Lawrence, R. A., & Lawrence, R. M. (2005). Breastfeeding: A guide for the medical profession (6th ed.). St. Louis: Mosby.

Uphold, C. R., & Gramham, M. V. (2003). Clinical guidelines in family practice (4th ed.). Gainesville, FL: Barmarrae Books.

Lactation

10

MEN'S HEALTH DISORDERS

Men's Health Disorders

Benign Prostatic Hyperplasia 399

Acute Bacterial Prostatitis 402

Chronic Prostatitis 403

Prostate Cancer 404

Cryptorchidism 406

Epididymitis 407

Testicular Torsion 408

Hydrocele 410

Spermatocele 411

Varicocele 411

Testicular Cancer 412

Inguinal Hernia 414

Hypospadias 415

Phimosis 416

Erectile Dysfunction 417

References *419*

BENIGN PROSTATIC HYPERPLASIA (BPH)

DESCRIPTION

Noncancerous enlargement of the prostate gland associated with LUTS (lower urinary tract symptoms).

ETIOLOGY

- Exact cause unknown
- The presence of androgens is necessary for the development of BPH

INCIDENCE

- Uncommon < 40 years of age
- > 50% of men aged 60 years and 80% of men by age 70 years have some degree of BPH
- High prevalence that progresses with age

RISK FACTORS

- Elevated PSA levels, increased physical activity
- Increasing age

ASSESSMENT FINDINGS

- Weak urinary stream
- Hesitancy and post-void dribbling
- Incomplete emptying of bladder
- Frequency and urgency
- Nocturia
- Incontinence
- Urinary retention
- Hematuria: gross or microscopic
- Firm, smooth, symmetrically enlarged prostate

Size of prostate does not always correlate with symptoms.

DIFFERENTIAL DIAGNOSIS

- Prostatitis
- Prostate cancer
- Urethral stricture
- Neurogenic bladder
- Effect of medications (e.g., sympathomimetics)
- Urinary tract infection
- Bladder cancer

DIAGNOSTIC STUDIES

- Use of American Urological Association Symptom Index (a self-administered tool consisting of seven questions about symptoms of prostatism including incomplete emptying, frequency, intermittency, urgency, a weak stream, hesitancy, and nocturia) for initial evaluation. The index is scored from 0-35 depending on symptoms:
  - ◊ Mild symptoms: score of 0-7
  - ◊ Moderate symptoms: score of 8-19
  - ◊ Severe symptoms: score of 20-35
- Urinalysis: pyuria if residual urine present
- Creatinine for assessment of renal function
- Postvoid residual urine measurement (> 100 mL)
- Prostate specific antigen (PSA): may be elevated, but < 10 ng/mL
- Ultrasound of prostate (not necessary for routine evaluation of the gland)
- Needle biopsy
- IVP, CT or MRI of the prostate

NONPHARMACOLOGIC MANAGEMENT

- Lifestyle modifications may provide relief for patients with mild symptoms (AUA score 0-7)
  - ◊ Limit fluids before bedtime
  - ◊ Frequent voiding
  - ◊ Avoid sympathomimetic or anticholinergic medications (e.g., decongestants) due to increased risk of urinary retention
  - ◊ Avoid caffeine, alcohol, and other beverages that produce diuresis
- Surgical options for patients with moderate to severe symptoms:
  - ◊ Transurethral resection of the prostate (TURP) - gold standard for relief of symptoms related to urinary retention
  - ◊ Transurethral incision of the prostate (TUIP): may be better option for younger men or smaller prostates
  - ◊ Open prostatectomy may be needed for very large prostates (> 100 g). A normal prostate gland in a young man is about 20 grams
- Indications for surgery: severe symptoms, refractory urinary retention, recurrent urinary tract infections, recurrent hematuria, bladder stones, renal insufficiency due to BPH
- Balloon dilation of the prostate in selected patients with smaller prostates

PHARMACOLOGIC MANAGEMENT

- Pharmacologic therapy is indicated in mild to moderate disease (AUA score >8)

BENIGN PROSTATIC HYPERPLASIA PHARMACOLOGICAL MANAGEMENT

Prior to initiating therapy with these products must include appropriate evaluation to identify other conditions such as infection, prostate cancer, stricture disease, hypotonic bladder or other neurogenic disorders that might mimic BPH

Class	Drug Generic name (Trade name®)	Dosage How supplied	Comments
Alpha adrenergic antagonists *Blockade of the alpha adrenergic receptors causes relaxation of smooth muscle in the prostate and neck of the bladder* **General comments** May cause orthostatic hypotension Must be used with caution in patients taking erectile dysfunction medications Seek medical attention for priapism	**doxazosin**	**Adult:** *Initial*: 1 mg/day *Usual*: Titrate for effect *Max*: 8 mg/day **Extended Release** **Adult:** *Initial*: 4 mg/day *Usual*: Titrate for effect *Max*: 8 mg/day	• Drug therapy must be individualized • Increase immediate release dose at 7-14 day intervals; increase extended dose at 3-4 week intervals • Extended release form contraindicated in patients with hepatic dysfunction • Extended release form should be taken daily with breakfast • Do not crush or chew extended release form
	Cardura	*Tabs: 1 mg, 2 mg, 4 mg, 8 mg scored*	
	Cardura XL	*Ext. Rel. Tabs: 4 mg, 8 mg*	
	tamsulosin	**Adult:** *Initial*: 0.4 mg/day *Max*: 0.8 mg/day	• Doses should be taken at a consistent time each day • May increase dose after 2-4 weeks • If higher doses are held for extended periods, resume at lower dose and titrate back
	Flomax	*Caps: 0.4 mg caps*	
	terazosin	**Adult:** *Initial*: 1 mg/day at HS *Usual*: titrate for effect *Max*: 20 mg/day	• Syncope most likely timed with dosage administration • If higher doses are held for extended periods, resume at lower dose and titrate back
	Hytrin	*Tabs: 1 mg, 2 mg, 5 mg, 10 mg* *Caps: 1 mg, 2 mg, 5 mg, 10 mg*	

continued

BENIGN PROSTATIC HYPERPLASIA PHARMACOLOGICAL MANAGEMENT

Prior to initiating therapy with these products must include appropriate evaluation to identify other conditions such as infection, prostate cancer, stricture disease, hypotonic bladder or other neurogenic disorders that might mimic BPH

Class	Drug Generic name (Trade name®)	Dosage How supplied	Comments
Antiandrogenic agents *Inhibit conversion of testosterone to the androgen, DHT. Enlargement of the prostate gland is caused by DHT* **General comments** Pregnant women should not handle product May take 6-12 months to assess benefit of therapy PSA levels will decrease while on this therapy	**dutasteride**	**As Monotherapy** **Adult:** *Initial*: 0.5 mg/day *Max*: 0.5 mg/day **As Combination Therapy** *Initial*: 0.5 mg/day *Max*: 0.5 mg/day in combination with tamsulosin (0.4mg) daily	• Do not crush or chew • If higher doses are held for extended periods, resume at monotherapy dose and titrate back
	Avodart	*Caps: 0.5 mg*	
	finasteride	**As Monotherapy** **Adult:** *Initial*: 5 mg/day *Max*: 5 mg/day **As Combination Therapy** **Adult:** *Initial*: 5 mg/day *Max:* 5 mg/day in combination with doxazosin daily	• Do not crush or chew • May be taken without regard to meals • May decrease amount of ejaculate
	Proscar	*Tabs: 5mg*	

5 alpha-reductase inhibitors will decrease PSA. PSA value must be doubled (to compare with pre-medication result) for purposes of screening for prostate cancer.

CONSULTATION/REFERRAL

- Refer for urological evaluation if refractory to treatment, evidence of renal complications, or if surgery indicated

FOLLOW-UP

- Digital rectal exam annually
- PSA annually

EXPECTED COURSE

- Symptoms improve or stabilize in 70-80% of patients
- 20-30% require treatment due to worsening of symptoms

POSSIBLE COMPLICATIONS

- Acute urinary retention
- Urinary incontinence (nocturnal is common)
- Nocturia
- Urinary tract infection
- Prostatitis
- Hydronephrosis
- Erectile dysfunction from pharmacologic or surgical treatment

ACUTE BACTERIAL PROSTATITIS

DESCRIPTION

Acute inflammatory condition of the prostate that is usually associated with fever, perineal pain and dysuria.

ETIOLOGY

- Translocation of bacteria up the urethra
- Urinary reflux into prostate ducts
- Common organisms: *E. coli, Pseudomonas, Klebsiella, Proteus, Chlamydia trachomatis, Trichomonas vaginalis, N. gonorrhoea*

INCIDENCE

- Most common in ages 30-50 years; especially if sexually active

RISK FACTORS

- Sexual activity, sexual abstinence
- Multiple sexual partners
- Urinary tract infection
- Trauma

ASSESSMENT FINDINGS

- Abrupt onset
- Fever, chills, malaise
- Enlarged, boggy, and tender prostate
- Low back pain
- Perineal pain
- Decreased urinary stream
- Frequency, urgency, dysuria
- Nocturia
- Pain upon defecation and ejaculation

Prostate massage can produce iatrogenic bacteremia. Avoid during acute episodes.

DIFFERENTIAL DIAGNOSIS

- Urinary tract infection
- Chronic prostatitis
- Sexually transmitted disease
- Malignancy
- Acute urinary retention

DIAGNOSTIC STUDIES

- Urinalysis: WBCs, bacteria, hematuria
- Fractional urine examination: third specimen (after prostate massage) has 10-15 or greater WBCs/high-powered field
- Urine culture
- Gram stain, culture and sensitivity of expressed prostatic secretions
- PSA will be increased during acute infection, therefore, do not consider screening for prostate cancer until 4 weeks post treatment

Imaging studies are almost never required unless needed to rule out malignancy.

PREVENTION

- Safe sex practices
- Emptying bladder regularly and frequently

NONPHARMACOLOGIC MANAGEMENT

- Refrain from intercourse and/or use a condom until resolved or treatment completed
- Good hydration
- Sitz bath for pain relief
- Avoid vigorous prostate massage
- Hospitalization may be required if infection severe

PHARMACOLOGIC MANAGEMENT

- Antibiotic treatment for 4 weeks using culture and sensitivity as guide in antibiotic selection
- Consider:
  - ◊ trimethoprim-sulfamethoxazole (Bactrim®)
    Bactrim DS one twice daily for 28 days
  - ◊ ciprofloxacin (Cipro®)
    500 mg daily for 28 days
  - ◊ doxycycline (Vibramycin®)
    100 mg twice daily for one day then daily for 28 days
- NSAIDs may be used for analgesic effect until urine cultures are completed
- Antipyretics
- Stool softeners

CONSULTATION/REFERRAL

- Refer patient with possible abscess or systemic illness to urologist

FOLLOW-UP

- Urinalysis and culture 4-6 weeks after initiating therapy

EXPECTED COURSE

- Variable cure rates

POSSIBLE COMPLICATIONS

- Bacteremia
- Urinary tract infection, epididymitis
- Urinary retention
- Renal parenchymal disease

CHRONIC PROSTATITIS

DESCRIPTION

Chronic inflammatory condition of the prostate that results in recurrent infection, inflammation and difficulty with urination.

ETIOLOGY

- Usually *E. coli, Klebsiella, Proteus, S. aureus, S. faecelis*

INCIDENCE

- Most common > 50 years of age

RISK FACTORS

- Age > 50 years
- Urinary tract infection

ASSESSMENT FINDINGS

- Asymptomatic, but not usually
- Frequency, urgency, dysuria
- Dribbling, hesitancy
- Decreased force of urinary stream
- Pain
  - ◊ With defecation or ejaculation
  - ◊ Perineum
  - ◊ Lower abdomen
  - ◊ Low back
  - ◊ Scrotum
  - ◊ Penis
- Hematuria: gross or microscopic
- Mildly tender prostate gland with enlargement

DIFFERENTIAL DIAGNOSIS

- Acute bacterial prostatitis
- Acute urinary retention
- Benign prostatic hyperplasia
- Prostate cancer
- Urinary tract infection

DIAGNOSTIC STUDIES

- Fractional urine examination: third specimen has 10-15 WBCs/high-powered field
- Urinalysis: WBCs, blood, bacteria
- Urine culture and sensitivity
- Culture of prostatic secretions
- CT and/or ultrasound if indicated to rule out malignancy
- PSA: frequently elevated
- BUN and creatinine
- Cystoscopy (refer to urologist)

Prostate massage can produce iatrogenic bacteremia. Avoid during acute episodes.

NONPHARMACOLOGIC MANAGEMENT

- Sitz bath to relieve pain
- Good hydration
- Avoid coffee, tea, alcohol, and other beverages which can cause diuresis
- Avoid anticholinergics and sympathomimetics which can cause urinary retention
- Surgical resection of prostate for intractable chronic disease in older men

PHARMACOLOGIC MANAGEMENT

Long term antibiotic treatment is usually needed to eradicate infection because the prostate gland has poor absorption of antibiotics.

- Fluoroquinolone daily (e.g., norfloxacin, ciprofloxacin) for 4-12 weeks
  Ofloxacin (Floxin) 300 mg twice daily for 4-12 weeks
  Ciprofloxacin (Cipro) 400 mg twice daily for 4-12 weeks
- Suppression therapy may be needed if a cure is not attainable:
  trimethoprim-sulfamethoxazole (Bactrim DS®): one tablet daily

CONSULTATION/REFERRAL

- Consultation with urologist if unresponsive to antibiotic therapy or cystoscopy needed

FOLLOW-UP

- Urinalysis and urine culture every 30 days until resolved (may be chronic)

EXPECTED COURSE

- May take several months to cure

POSSIBLE COMPLICATIONS

- Bacteremia
- Urinary tract infection, epididymitis
- Urinary retention
- Renal parenchymal disease

PROSTATE CANCER

DESCRIPTION

Malignancy of prostate gland.

ETIOLOGY

- Unknown

INCIDENCE

- Leading cause of cancer in men
- 17% lifetime risk of prostate cancer
- Incidence increases with age, most common after age 60 years

RISK FACTORS

- Family history, especially first degree relative
- Increasing age
- African-American

ASSESSMENT FINDINGS

- Asymptomatic
- Prostate feels hard upon digital examination
- Prostatic nodules may be palpated
- Acute urinary retention possible
- Hematuria possible
- Urinary tract infection
- Anemia
- Back/hip pain radiating into testicular area
- Lymphedema
- Lymphadenopathy

DIFFERENTIAL DIAGNOSIS

- Prostatitis
- Benign prostatic hyperplasia
- Benign prostatic nodules
- Prostate stones

DIAGNOSTIC STUDIES

- Prostatic ultrasound
- Prostate specific antigen (PSA): can be normal but if elevated, usually > 10 ng/mL
- Alkaline phosphatase: elevated with metastasis
- Bone scan: positive if metastasis (always indicted if PSA > 20)
- CT
- MRI not helpful
- Biopsy

Digital rectal exam does NOT significantly increase PSA. Therefore, acceptable to perform DRE and measure PSA on same day.

PSA value > 10 ng/mL should be biopsied. PSA value > 4-9.9 ng/mL is usually biopsied, though only 20% of these men will be diagnosed with prostate cancer. PSA < 4.0 ng/mL does not rule out prostate cancer.

SCREENING

- Annual digital rectal examination beginning at age 40 years
- Annual PSA and digital rectal examination beginning at age 50 years
- Consider screening at age 45 years for those at high risk (first degree relative with prostate cancer, African-American heritage)

NONPHARMACOLOGIC MANAGEMENT

- Surgical intervention: TURP or radical prostatectomy and orchiectomy
- Brachiotherapy (radiation seed therapy)
- Cryotherapy/cryosurgery
- Radiation therapy (electron beam)
- Watchful waiting

PHARMACOLOGIC MANAGEMENT

- Consider
  - ◊ Leuprolide (Lupron®)
    7.5 mg IM monthly
    Also available in every 3 months (22.5 mg IM), or every 4 months (30 mg IM) formulas
  - ◊ Flutamide (Eulexin®) for androgen ablation
- Estrogen therapy
- Chemotherapy

For androgen dependent tumors, decreasing circulating testosterone is helpful. This is done with gonadotropin-releasing hormone (GnRH) agonists such as Lupron®.

CONSULTATION/REFERRAL

- Refer to urologist and oncologist

FOLLOW-UP

- Clinical examination every 3 months for one year; then every 6 months for one year; then annually
- PSA every 3 months for one year; then every 6 months for one year, then annually

EXPECTED COURSE

- Depends on stage at time of diagnosis
- Usually grows slowly
- Cancer confined to prostate: 5-year survival rate is 98%
- Cancer which has spread outside of the prostate: 5-year survival rate is 29%

POSSIBLE COMPLICATIONS

- Urinary retention
- Metastasis
- Pathologic fracture
- Impotence secondary to radical prostatectomy
- Postoperative incontinence

CRYPTORCHIDISM
(Undescended Testicle)

DESCRIPTION

Incomplete descent of one or both testicles into the scrotum.

Testicular descent typically occurs during the 7th or 8th month in utero.

ETIOLOGY

- Not completely understood
- May involve hormonal, mechanical, and/or neural factors

INCIDENCE

- 3% of full term male infants
- 33% of premature male infants

RISK FACTORS

- Family history of cryptorchidism
- Premature birth
- Hypospadias

ASSESSMENT FINDINGS

- Absence of one or both testes upon palpation of scrotum (assess with child or infant in sitting, squatting, or standing positions)
- One or both testicles in a site other than scrotum

This exam is best performed with warm hands with the male sitting, standing or squatting.

A large percentage of males with cryptorchidism will have an inguinal hernia.

DIFFERENTIAL DIAGNOSIS

- Retractile testis (normal testis that ascends into inguinal canal as a result of cremasteric reflex)
- Atrophic testis
- Anorchia: complete absence of testis

DIAGNOSTIC STUDIES

- Ultrasound to identify location of testicle(s)

NONPHARMACOLOGIC MANAGEMENT

- Orchiopexy usually performed by age one year; usually 6-9 months
- Teach self-testicular examination when older
- Educate regarding increased risk of testicular cancer and infertility

PHARMACOLOGIC MANAGEMENT

- Human chorionic gonadotropin (hCG) sometimes recommended for older children (> 6 years) but may be used in much younger children. Caution, may induce precocious puberty

CONSULTATION/REFERRAL

- Refer for urological evaluation if testicle(s) not descended by 4 months of age

FOLLOW-UP

- Follow closely before surgical correction to determine if testicle has descended
- Follow closely after surgical correction to evaluate testicular growth

EXPECTED COURSE

- Spontaneous descent, if it occurs, will usually do so in first 6 months of life (and usually by 3 months of age)
- Usually corrected with surgical therapy
- Lifelong consequence of increased testicular cancer risk (20-46 times higher) even after correction

POSSIBLE COMPLICATIONS

- Testicular cancer
- Decreased fertility rate even with treatment
- Hernia development
- Testicular torsion

EPIDIDYMITIS

DESCRIPTION

Inflammation of the epididymis usually occurring from movement of pathogens from urethra or prostate.

ETIOLOGY

Prepubertal boys:
- Bacterial urinary tract infection
- Underlying congenital defect

Younger than 35 years:
- Usually *Chlamydia trachomatis* or *Neisseria gonorrhoeae* in men <35 years

Older than 35 years:
- Bacterial urinary tract infection
- Prostatitis, urinary instrumentation, or structural lesion

INCIDENCE

- Common, especially in younger, sexually active men or older men with urinary tract infection

The most common cause of acute scrotal pain in prepubertal boys is epididymitis. Testicular torsion is much less common. Both disorders present with scrotal pain, testicular torsion MUST be ruled out first.

RISK FACTORS

- Recent trauma to scrotum
- Multiple sexual partners
- Previous sexually transmitted infection
- Urinary tract infection
- Delaying urination while doing continuous physical labor
- Indwelling urinary catheter
- Urethral instrumentation or surgery
- Increased intra-abdominal pressure as with straining from heavy physical labor

ASSESSMENT FINDINGS

- Gradual development of scrotal pain
- Urethral discharge
- Dysuria, frequency
- Hematuria
- Epididymis very tender, enlarged, and indurated (epididymis is located posterior to testicle)
- Discomfort decreases with elevation of testes
- Scrotal edema and erythema
- Fever, chills
- Cremasteric reflex present and may be painful
- Presentation in children not as dramatic as in older males

If the cremasteric reflex is absent in a male with scrotal pain, suspect testicular torsion.

DIFFERENTIAL DIAGNOSIS

- Testicular torsion
- Orchitis
- Testicular tumor
- Testicular trauma
- Epididymal cyst or tumor
- Spermatocele
- Hydrocele
- Varicocele
- Insect bites to scrotum
- Tuberculous or fungal infection

DIAGNOSTIC STUDIES

- Doppler ultrasound of scrotum
- Urinalysis: pyuria, hematuria
- Urine and urethral Gram stain and culture with sensitivity
- Urethral discharge for chlamydia and gonorrhea testing
- HIV screen
- Syphilis serology

A normal urine analysis and negative culture with epididymitis indicates a sterile epididymitis.

PREVENTION

- Antibiotic prophylaxis before urethral instrumentation or surgery

NONPHARMACOLOGIC MANAGEMENT

- Elevation of scrotum with athletic supporter
- Cool compresses to scrotum or ice packs
- Treat sexual partner if causative agent *N. gonorrhoeae* or *C. trachomatis*
- Refrain from sexual intercourse and/or use condom until resolved/treatment completed

PHARMACOLOGIC MANAGEMENT

- NSAIDs for pain/discomfort

Secondary to UTI:

- Trimethoprim-sulfamethoxazole (Bactrim®)
  8 mg/kg/day trimethoprim and 40 mg/kg/day of sulfamethoxazole twice daily for 10 days
- Do not exceed max adult dose

Secondary to chlamydia/gonorrhea:

- Doxycycline (Vibramycin®) AND ceftriaxone (Rocephin®) intramuscular
  Doxycycline: 100 mg twice daily for 10 days
  Ceftriaxone:
  Adult: 250 mg IM
  Children: 50-75 mg/kg IM (max: adult dose)
- Treat sexual partners

Older men, secondary to UTI:

- Consider
  ◊ Trimethoprim-sulfamethoxazole (Bactrim®)
  Bactrim DS twice daily for 10 days
  ◊ ciprofloxacin (Cipro®) 500 mg po twice daily, lower doses with renal impairment
  ◊ ofloxacin (Floxin®) 200 mg twice daily
  Floxin: 200 mg twice daily

CONSULTATION/REFERRAL

- Immediate referral if testicular torsion cannot be ruled out
- Consult urologist in prepubertal patients, for recurrence, and if unresponsive to therapy

FOLLOW-UP

- Urine cultures posttreatment in prepubertal boys and older men
- Evaluation of prepubertal boys for genitourinary anomaly

EXPECTED COURSE

- Expect improvement within 72 hours if on appropriate antibiotic
- Infection and pain resolve over 2-4 weeks with appropriate treatment

POSSIBLE COMPLICATIONS

- Recurrent epididymitis
- Infertility
- Abscess

TESTICULAR TORSION

DESCRIPTION

An acute ischemic event that occurs when the testis and spermatic cord twist.

ETIOLOGY

- Usually occurs suddenly with no known cause
- History of trauma may be reported; especially a kick to the groin or falling on a hard object
- May be associated with exercise, very cold temperatures, or sexual stimulation

INCIDENCE

- 1/4000 males
- 2/3 of cases occur in adolescents; peak age is 14 years
- Accounts for 40% of cases of acute scrotal pain and swelling

RISK FACTORS

- May be more common in winter
- Paraplegia
- Commonly occurs at puberty
- Bell-clapper deformity

ASSESSMENT FINDINGS

- Sudden, severe, unilateral scrotal pain
- Scrotal edema and erythema
- Firm tender mass which may appear retracted upward; there may be a transverse lie of the testicle
- No relief of pain with testicular elevation
- Lower abdominal pain
- Nausea and vomiting
- Testis is very tender
- Cremasteric reflex absent

Testicular pain associated with testicular torsion is usually abrupt in onset but may occasionally proceed more slowly with increasing severity.

DIFFERENTIAL DIAGNOSIS

- Epididymitis
- Orchitis
- Hydrocele, varicocele, spermatocele
- Testicular tumor
- Incarcerated inguinal hernia
- Trauma

DIAGNOSTIC STUDIES

- Doppler ultrasound of scrotum: demonstrates reduced blood flow
- Urinalysis: normal in 90% of cases

NONPHARMACOLOGIC MANAGEMENT

- Manual relief of torsion; followed by orchidopexy
- Surgical exploration and detorsion or orchiectomy if nonviable testis
- Bilateral orchiopexy

PHARMACOLOGIC MANAGEMENT

- Analgesics

CONSULTATION/REFERRAL

- Emergency-immediate urological referral for correction

FOLLOW-UP

- By urologist at 1-2 weeks post correction
- Annual visits to evaluate for appropriate testicular health until adolescence

EXPECTED COURSE

- Duration of torsion determines if testicle remains viable:
  - ◊ 80-100% salvage if blood flow re-established within 6 hours
  - ◊ < 20% if greater than 24 hours
  - ◊ Decreased spermatogenesis vast majority of time
  - ◊ 66% of salvaged testicles may atrophy in first 2-3 years post-torsion

POSSIBLE COMPLICATIONS

- Infertility, decreased sperm counts
- Testicular atrophy

HYDROCELE

DESCRIPTION

Collection of peritoneal fluid within scrotum.

ETIOLOGY

Infants:
- Usually *communicating*: represents an incomplete closure of processus vaginalis which results in temporary trapping of peritoneal fluid

Adults:
- Usually *non-communicating*: represents closure of the processus vaginalis which traps peritoneal fluid
- Neoplasms
- Infection
- Trauma

Communicating hydroceles have an associated indirect inguinal hernia.

INCIDENCE

- 1% of adult males
- Common in infancy especially in premature infants

RISK FACTORS

- Unknown in many cases
- Exotrophy of bladder
- Peritoneal dialysis

ASSESSMENT FINDINGS

- Painless, swelling in the scrotum
- Fluctuation in size of scrotum in communicating hydrocele
- Scrotum feels heavy and enlarged
- Transillumination of scrotum

DIFFERENTIAL DIAGNOSIS

- Communicating vs. non-communicating hydrocele
- Scrotal trauma; such as falling on a hard object
- Spermatocele
- Varicocele
- Inguinal hernia
- Orchitis, epididymitis
- Scrotal tumor

DIAGNOSTIC STUDIES

- Scrotal ultrasound to differentiate hernia from hydrocele

NONPHARMACOLOGIC MANAGEMENT

Communicating hydrocele:
- Observation and reassurance until one year of age
- Surgical correction if not closed by one to two years of age
- In adults, no treatment required unless symptoms are bothersome. *Tumor must be ruled out prior to monitoring*

Non-communicating hydrocele:
- Surgical drainage of fluid and ligation of processus vaginalis
- Therapy not always required in adults unless causing discomfort or other complication
- *Tumor must be ruled out prior to monitoring*

CONSULTATION/REFERRAL

- Refer for surgical evaluation if hydrocele has not resolved by one year of age or for new hydroceles in adults

FOLLOW-UP

- Follow at 3 month intervals in infants until resolved or referral made

EXPECTED COURSE

- Communicating hydrocele usually resolves within first year of life
- Non-communicating hydroceles rarely resolve spontaneously

POSSIBLE COMPLICATIONS

- Inguinal hernia

SPERMATOCELE

DESCRIPTION

A well circumscribed mass located in the scrotum along the spermatic cord which contains sperm (often found in the head of the epididymis).

ETIOLOGY

- Unknown
- May be due to blockage of the epididymal ducts

ASSESSMENT FINDINGS

- Freely movable, painless, cystic mass
- Maybe tender when palpated
- Located posterior and superior to testicle
- Easily transilluminates
- Circumscribed mass in scrotum

DIFFERENTIAL DIAGNOSIS

- Varicocele
- Hydrocele
- Testicular tumor
- Epididymitis
- Orchitis

DIAGNOSTIC STUDIES

- Scrotal ultrasound
- Aspiration reveals nonviable sperm

MANAGEMENT

- No therapy necessary unless mass becomes bothersome

CONSULTATION/REFERRAL

- Refer to urologist if causing discomfort to patient

EXPECTED COURSE

- Benign

VARICOCELE

DESCRIPTION

Collection of abnormally large dilated veins (usually the internal spermatic vein) in the scrotum, usually situated above the testis.

ETIOLOGY

- Poorly functioning anti-reflux valves of the spermatic veins

INCIDENCE

- Usually found in older adolescents, but may occur at any age
- 80-90% occur on left
- Present in 20% of male population

RISK FACTORS

- Abdominal pathology
- Renal tumor
- Venous obstruction

ASSESSMENT FINDINGS

- Asymptomatic usually
- Presenting complaint is often infertility
- Scrotum resembles "bag of worms"
- Bluish discoloration of scrotum
- Varicocele increases in size when patient standing and with valsalva maneuver
- Testis nontender
- Feeling of heaviness in scrotum

Sudden appearance of a left-sided varicocele in an adult male should prompt evaluation for possible renal tumor.

DIFFERENTIAL DIAGNOSIS

- Hydrocele
- Spermatocele
- Testicular tumor
- Epididymal cyst

DIAGNOSTIC STUDIES

- Doppler ultrasound
- Sperm count: decreased
- Intravenous pyelography to rule out renal tumor or venous obstruction

MANAGEMENT

- If mild, left-sided varicocele present in an adult without infertility, observation is indicated
- Scrotal support
- Surgical correction if infertility present

CONSULTATION/REFERRAL

- Consult urologist in the following situations:
    - ◊ Right-sided varicocele
    - ◊ New onset in adults
    - ◊ Large varicocele
    - ◊ Does not disappear when supine
    - ◊ Pain
    - ◊ Testicular atrophy
    - ◊ Rapidly increasing in size
    - ◊ Infertility
    - ◊ Prepubertal boys
    - ◊ Older males (increased risk of renal tumors)

EXPECTED COURSE

- Surgical intervention will alleviate symptoms, but infertility is rarely reversed

POSSIBLE COMPLICATIONS

- Causes 40% of male infertility
- Testicular atrophy especially post surgery
- Prepubertal boys: failure to develop secondary sex characteristics

TESTICULAR CANCER

DESCRIPTION

Malignant tumor of the testicle. Two types:

- Seminomas account for 40-50% of cases
- Non seminomas: embryonal cell carcinoma, teratoma, choriocarcinoma

CLINICAL STAGING (Skinner/Walter Reed)

- A: tumor limited to testis and cord
- B: tumor of testis and retroperitoneal nodes
- B1: < 6 nodes all < 2 cm
- B2: > 6 nodes all > 2 cm
- B3: positive retroperitoneal nodes > 5 cm
- C: metastases above diaphragm or involving solid abdominal organs

ETIOLOGY

- Unknown

INCIDENCE

- Most common malignancy in males aged 15-35 years
- Peak incidence between ages 20-40 years
- Accounts for 1-2% of all cancers in males

Testicular cancer is one of the most curable solid cancers in the United States. The incidence of cancer has increased in the last 10 years.

RISK FACTORS

- History of cryptorchidism (even if repaired)
- Testicular atrophy
- Caucasian race; rare in African-Americans
- HIV positive status

ASSESSMENT FINDINGS

- Solid, firm, nontender testicular mass
- Sensation of fullness or heaviness in scrotum
- Previous small testicle enlarging to size of normal testicle
- Hydrocele
- Gynecomastia
- Mass does not transilluminate

Both testicles should be examined and compared for size, tenderness, symmetry and presence of nodules.

DIFFERENTIAL DIAGNOSIS

- Hernia
- Hydrocele, spermatocele, varicocele
- Epididymitis
- Benign testicular mass
- Testicular torsion

DIAGNOSTIC STUDIES

- α-fetoprotein: protein (a tumor marker): elevated
- β-human chorionic gonadotropin (β-hCG) (a tumor marker): elevated
- Scrotal ultrasound (gold standard for diagnosis)
- Abdominal and chest CT scan
- Biopsy

PREVENTION

- Monthly self-testicular examination beginning in adolescence

MANAGEMENT

- Dependent on staging
- Radiation therapy
- Chemotherapy
- Surgical intervention: radical orchiectomy

CONSULTATION/REFERRAL

- Refer to urologist for evaluation and treatment

FOLLOW-UP

- Close monitoring of hCG and α-fetoprotein for indication of response to therapy and recurrence
- Periodic chest and abdominal CT for detection of metastasis

EXPECTED COURSE

- Usually complete cure in patients with limited disease
- 70-80% cure in patients with advanced disease
- 5-year survival rate: about 95%

POSSIBLE COMPLICATIONS

- Metastasis
- Complications associated with radiation, chemotherapy, and surgery

INGUINAL HERNIA

DESCRIPTION

- Two types:
  - ◊ Indirect: hernial sac protrudes through the internal inguinal ring into the inguinal canal often descending into the scrotum
  - ◊ Direct: hernial sac protrudes directly through the abdominal wall in the region of Hesselbach's triangle

TERMS

- Incarcerated: one in which the hernia's contents cannot be replaced into the abdomen
- Strangulated: incarcerated hernia in which the blood supply to the entrapped bowel has been diminished; a surgical emergency
- Reducible: the hernia is easily replaced into the abdomen using gentle pressure or may occur spontaneously

ETIOLOGY

- Congenital defect
- Injury

INCIDENCE

- 80% of all hernias are inguinal

Indirect:
- 3.5-5.5% of full term infants; increased incidence in premature infants
- 50% of all hernias in adults are indirect
- Males > Females

Direct:
- More common in middle and later years of life
- Rare in pediatric population

RISK FACTORS

- Male
- Weak abdominal musculature
- Premature
- Twin gestation

ASSESSMENT FINDINGS

- Feeling of heaviness in groin
- Painful or painless swelling or lump in groin or into scrotum which increases when standing or straining
- The bulge is often intermittent and palpable during episodes of increased abdominal pressure (straining)
- In women, bulge may be seen in the labia majora
- Strangulated hernia:
  - ◊ Colicky abdominal pain
  - ◊ Nausea and vomiting
  - ◊ Abdominal distention

Important assessment information to elicit is the location of the bulge and what makes it change in size.

DIFFERENTIAL DIAGNOSIS

- Hydrocele/varicocele/spermatocele
- Epididymitis
- Testicular tumor
- Undescended testicle
- Lymphadenopathy

DIAGNOSTIC STUDIES

- Ultrasound

A presumptive diagnosis can usually be made with history and exam.

NONPHARMACOLOGIC MANAGEMENT

- Educate about signs and symptoms of strangulation
- Do not attempt to reduce a strangulated hernia
- Hernia will not resolve spontaneously, surgical correction (herniorrhaphy) is required

CONSULTATION/REFERRAL

- Refer to surgeon for evaluation
- Refer immediately if strangulated

EXPECTED COURSE

- Complete recovery without sequelae if treated promptly and appropriately

POSSIBLE COMPLICATIONS

- Strangulation of hernia

HYPOSPADIAS

DESCRIPTION

Congenital abnormality in which the urethral opening is on the underside of the penis (ventral surface).

ETIOLOGY

- Multifactorial

INCIDENCE

- Occurs in 1/300 male infants

RISK FACTORS

- Family history
- Increased incidence in whites
- Exogenous progesterone intake by mother during pregnancy
- Presence of undescended testicles, inguinal hernia, or hydrocele

ASSESSMENT FINDINGS

- Urethra located on ventral surface of penis
- Urinary stream aims downward
- Foreskin may not be present
- Chordee (bowing of the penis due to fibrous band of tissue pulling on penis)

DIFFERENTIAL DIAGNOSIS

- Ambiguous genitalia

DIAGNOSTIC STUDIES

- None usually needed

MANAGEMENT

- Circumcision must NOT be done, foreskin may be needed for surgical repair
- Surgical repair usually at age 6-18 months

CONSULTATION/REFERRAL

- Refer to urologist for surgical repair

EXPECTED COURSE

- Usually excellent prognosis

POSSIBLE COMPLICATIONS

- Erectile dysfunction if chordee present

PHIMOSIS

DESCRIPTION

Foreskin which is too tight, preventing retraction over the glans penis.

ETIOLOGY

- Physiologic: present at birth and resolves spontaneously by 3 years of age
- Congenital: unresolved physiologic phimosis
- Acquired: recurrent infection or irritation

INCIDENCE

- 1% of adolescent males

RISK FACTORS

- Poor hygiene
- Diabetes mellitus
- Presence of an STD

ASSESSMENT FINDINGS

- Unretractable foreskin
- Pain with erection
- Balanitis may be present

DIFFERENTIAL DIAGNOSIS

- Allergic reaction

DIAGNOSTIC STUDIES

- None usually needed

PREVENTION

- Good hygiene
- Parental education about care of uncircumcised infant
- Circumcision at birth (controversial)

NONPHARMACOLOGIC MANAGEMENT

- Normal cleansing and gentle stretching of foreskin
- Often nocturnal erections will stretch ring and problem resolves without other intervention
- Circumcision if there is urinary obstruction

CONSULTATION/REFERRAL

- Refer for surgical evaluation for circumcision

EXPECTED COURSE

- Complete resolution if treated appropriately

POSSIBLE COMPLICATIONS

- Urinary tract infection
- Stricture
- Inflammation of the prepuce
- Balanitis

ERECTILE DYSFUNCTION

DESCRIPTION

Inability to achieve or maintain an erection satisfactorily to effect penetration and ejaculation. Transient or occasional impotence is common and not necessarily evidence of pathology. A pattern of repeated (> 25%) episodes over more than a month should be investigated, however.

Always consider concurrent medical disorders when men present with erectile dysfunction. Aging is not a cause.

ETIOLOGY

- 50% organic in nature
  - ◊ Spinal cord injury
  - ◊ Surgical procedures
  - ◊ Diabetes mellitus: reported in up to 50% of men with diabetes
  - ◊ Heavy metal toxicity
  - ◊ Medications (e.g., phenothiazines, tricyclic antidepressants, selective serotonin-reuptake inhibitors, exogenous estrogen, many antihypertensives)
  - ◊ Drug abuse (e.g., heroin, morphine, methadone, barbiturates)
  - ◊ Chronic alcoholism
  - ◊ Heavy smoking
  - ◊ Hypo/hyperthyroidism
  - ◊ Addison's disease
  - ◊ Cushing's syndrome
  - ◊ Acromegaly
  - ◊ Hyperprolactinemia
  - ◊ Prostatic cancer
  - ◊ Arterial insufficiency
- Psychogenic

INCIDENCE

- Affects up to 10% of men at any given point in time, but much higher incidence in treatment of hypertension

RISK FACTORS

- See Etiology

ASSESSMENT FINDINGS

- Dependent on underlying etiology
- Inability to achieve or maintain an erection
- Absence of nocturnal erection may indicate organic cause

DIAGNOSTIC STUDIES

- Determined by suspected underlying etiology
- CBC and complete metabolic panel
- Hormone levels: free testosterone, prolactin level
- Fasting blood sugar
- Thyroid stimulating hormone
- Consider testosterone level (low levels may be cause of erectile dysfunction
- Digital rectal exam to rule out prostate causes
- Testing of nocturnal erection at home with use of a "snap gauge" or a formal tumescence study in a sleep laboratory (tends to be intact with physiologic causes)
- Doppler estimation of penile blood flow if vascular cause suspected

PREVENTION

- Good glucose control in diabetes mellitus
- Avoid (if possible) medications that may cause erectile dysfunction as well as marijuana and alcohol

NONPHARMACOLOGIC MANAGEMENT

- Psychologic support
- Education regarding causes
- Change in medications which may cause impotence
- Penile implants for patients with refractory impotence
- Vacuum suction device
- Vascular surgery for those with vascular insufficiency

CONSULTATION/REFERRAL

- Referral to urologist, vascular surgeon, neurologist depending on underlying pathology

ERECTILE DYSFUNCTION PHARMACOLOGIC MANAGEMENT

Class	Drug Generic name (Trade name®)	Dosage How supplied	Comments
PDE-5 Inhibitors General comments Patients should be healthy enough for sexual activity Patients should receive counseling to report sudden changes in vision Priapism lasting greater than 4 hours should be evaluated Transient hypotension may be noted	**sildenafil** Viagra	**Adult**: *Initial:* 50 mg 1/2 to 4 hours before sexual activity *Max:* 100 mg *Tabs: 25 mg, 50 mg, 100 mg*	• Avoid concomitant use of nitrates or alpha-blockers • Use with caution in patients with recent MI, CVA • May use lower starting dose in elderly or patients with diminished renal or hepatic function
	tadalafil Cialis	**As Needed Use** **Adult:** *Initial:* 10 mg before sexual activity *Max*: 20 mg daily **Daily Use** **Adult:** *Initial:* 2.5 mg/day *Max:* 5 mg/day *Tabs: 2.5 mg, 5 mg, 10 mg, 20 mg*	• Avoid concomitant use of nitrates • Use caution if patient on alpha-blocker • May be taken without regard to meals • Use with caution in patients with recent MI, CVA • May use lower starting dose in elderly or patients with diminished renal or hepatic function
	vardenafil Levitra	**Adult:** *Initial:* 10 mg 1 hour before sexual activity *Max:* 20 mg/day *Tabs: 2.5 mg, 5 mg, 10 mg, 20 mg*	• Avoid concomitant use of nitrates • Use caution if patient on alpha-blocker • Avoid in renal dialysis patients • May use lower starting dose in elderly or patients with diminished renal or hepatic function

FOLLOW-UP

- Frequent follow-up is indicated

EXPECTED COURSE

- Dependent on underlying cause

POSSIBLE COMPLICATIONS

- Complications from treatments (e.g., priapism)
- Low self-esteem
- Disruption in sexual relationships

References

Akre, O., Pettersson, A., & Richiardi, L. (2009). Risk of contralateral testicular cancer among men with unilaterally undescended testis: a meta analysis. International Journal of Cancer, 124(3), 687-689. doi: 10.1002/ijc.23936

Allen, N. E., Key, T. J., Appleby, P. N., Travis, R. C., Roddam, A. W., Tjonneland, A., . . . Riboli, E. (2008). Animal foods, protein, calcium and prostate cancer risk: the European Prospective Investigation into Cancer and Nutrition. British Journal of Cancer, 98(9), 1574-1581. doi: 10.1038/sj.bjc.6604331

Atkins, J. M., Taylor, J. C., & Kane, S. F. (2010). Acute and overuse injuries of the abdomen and groin in athletes. Curr Sports Med Rep, 9(2), 115-120. doi: 10.1249/JSR.0b013e3181d40080

Baldisserotto, M. (2009). Scrotal emergencies. Pediatric Radiology, 39(5), 516-521. doi: 10.1007/s00247-008-1134-0

Baskin, L. S., & Ebbers, M. B. (2006). Hypospadias: anatomy, etiology, and technique. Journal of Pediatric Surgery, 41(3), 463-472. doi: 10.1016/j.jpedsurg.2005.11.059

Bent, S., Kane, C., Shinohara, K., Neuhaus, J., Hudes, E. S., Goldberg, H., & Avins, A. L. (2006). Saw palmetto for benign prostatic hyperplasia. New England Journal of Medicine, 354(6), 557-566. doi: 10.1056/NEJMoa053085

Bray, F., Richiardi, L., Ekbom, A., Pukkala, E., Cuninkova, M., & Moller, H. (2006). Trends in testicular cancer incidence and mortality in 22 European countries: continuing increases in incidence and declines in mortality. International Journal of Cancer, 118(12), 3099-3111. doi: 10.1002/ijc.21747

Brown, C. T., Yap, T., Cromwell, D. A., Rixon, L., Steed, L., Mulligan, K., . . . Emberton, M. (2007). Self management for men with lower urinary tract symptoms: randomised controlled trial. BMJ, 334(7583), 25. doi: 10.1136/bmj.39010.551319.AE

Burnett, A. L., & Wein, A. J. (2006). Benign prostatic hyperplasia in primary care: what you need to know. Journal of Urology, 175(3 Pt 2), S19-24. doi: 10.1016/S0022-5347(05)00310-1

Burns, C. E., Brady, M. A., Blosser, C., Starr, N. B., & Dunn, A. M. (2009). Pediatric primary care: A handbook for nurse practitioners (4th ed.). Philadelphia: W.B. Saunders.

Carlson, W. H., Kisely, S. R., & MacLellan, D. L. (2009). Maternal and fetal risk factors associated with severity of hypospadias: a comparison of mild and severe cases. J Pediatr Urol, 5(4), 283-286. doi: 10.1016/j.jpurol.2008.12.005

Centers for Disease Control and Prevention. (2007). Updated recommended treatment regimens for gonococcal infections and associated conditions — United States, April 2007. Retrieved from www.cdc.gov/std/treatment/2006/GonUpdateApril2007.pdf

Domino, F., Baldor, R., Golding, J., Grimes, J., & Taylor, J. (2011). The 5-minute clinical consult 2011. Philadelphia: Lippincott Williams & Wilkins.

Drug Facts and Comparisons. (2010). St. Louis: Wolters Kluwer Health. Facts & Comparisons.

Ernst, D., & Lee, A. (2010). Nurse practitioners prescribing reference. New York: Haymarket Media Publication.

Grubb, R. L., 3rd, Pinsky, P. F., Greenlee, R. T., Izmirlian, G., Miller, A. B., Hickey, T. P., . . . Andriole, G. L. (2008). Prostate cancer screening in the Prostate, Lung, Colorectal and Ovarian cancer screening trial: update on findings from the initial four rounds of screening in a randomized trial. BJU International, 102(11), 1524-1530. doi: 10.1111/j.1464-410X.2008.08214.x

Jemal, A., Siegel, R., Ward, E., Hao, Y., Xu, J., & Thun, M. J. (2009). Cancer statistics, 2009. CA: A Cancer Journal for Clinicians, 59(4), 225-249. doi: 10.3322/caac.20006

Karmazyn, B., Steinberg, R., Kornreich, L., Freud, E., Grozovski, S., Schwarz, M., . . . Livne, P. (2005). Clinical and sonographic criteria of acute scrotum in children: a retrospective study of 172 boys. Pediatric Radiology, 35(3), 302-310. doi: 10.1007/s00247-004-1347-9

Mena, L. A., Mroczkowski, T. F., Nsuami, M., & Martin, D. H. (2009). A randomized comparison of azithromycin and doxycycline for the treatment of Mycoplasma genitalium-positive urethritis in men. Clinical Infectious Diseases, 48(12), 1649-1654. doi: 10.1086/599033

Peate, I. (2007). Men's health: The practice nurses' handbook. Hoboken, NJ: Wiley-Interscience.

Pettersson, A., Richiardi, L., Nordenskjold, A., Kaijser, M., & Akre, O. (2007). Age at surgery for undescended testis and risk of testicular cancer. New England Journal of Medicine, 356(18), 1835-1841. doi: 10.1056/NEJMoa067588

Pontari, M. A., Joyce, G. F., Wise, M., & McNaughton-Collins, M. (2007). Prostatitis. Journal of Urology, 177(6), 2050-2057. doi: 10.1016/j.juro.2007.01.128

Powell, T. M., & Tarter, T. H. (2006). Management of nonpalpable incidental testicular masses. Journal of Urology, 176(1), 96-98; discussion 99. doi: 10.1016/S0022-5347(06)00496-4

Qaseem, A., Snow, V., Denberg, T. D., Casey, D. E., Jr., Forciea, M. A., Owens, D. K., & Shekelle, P. (2009). Hormonal testing and pharmacologic treatment of erectile dysfunction: a clinical practice guideline from the American College of Physicians. Annals of Internal Medicine, 151(9), 639-649. doi: 10.1059/0003-4819-151-9-200911030-00151

Rundle, A., & Neugut, A. I. (2008). Obesity and screening PSA levels among men undergoing an annual physical exam. Prostate, 68(4), 373-380. doi: 10.1002/pros.20704

Saigal, C. S., Movassaghi, M., Pace, J., & Joyce, G. (2007). Economic evaluation of treatment strategies for benign prostatic hyperplasia--is medical therapy more costly in the long run? Journal of Urology, 177(4), 1463-1467; discussion 1467. doi: 10.1016/j.juro.2006.11.083

Sandlow, J. (2004). Pathogenesis and treatment of varicoceles. BMJ, 328(7446), 967-968. doi: 10.1136/bmj.328.7446.967

Schroder, F. H., Hugosson, J., Roobol, M. J., Tammela, T. L., Ciatto, S., Nelen, V., . . . Auvinen, A. (2009). Screening and prostate-cancer mortality in a randomized European study. New England Journal of Medicine, 360(13), 1320-1328. doi: 10.1056/NEJMoa0810084

Suzuki, S., Furui, S., Okinaga, K., Sakamoto, T., Murata, J., Furukawa, A., & Ohnaka, Y. (2007). Differentiation of femoral versus inguinal hernia: CT findings. AJR. American Journal of Roentgenology, 189(2), W78-83. doi: 10.2214/AJR.07.2085

U.S. Preventative Services Task Force. (2004). Screening for testicular cancer. Retrieved from www.uspreventiveservicestaskforce.org/uspstf/uspstest.htm

Wagenlehner, F. M., Weidner, W., & Naber, K. G. (2007). Therapy for prostatitis, with emphasis on bacterial prostatitis. Expert Opin Pharmacother, 8(11), 1667-1674. doi: 10.1517/14656566.8.11.1667

Walsh, T. J., Grady, R. W., Porter, M. P., Lin, D. W., & Weiss, N. S. (2006). Incidence of testicular germ cell cancers in U.S. children: SEER program experience 1973 to 2000. Urology, 68(2), 402-405; discussion 405. doi: 10.1016/j.urology.2006.02.045

Workowski, K. A., & Berman, S. M. (2006). Sexually transmitted diseases treatment guidelines, 2006. MMWR Recomm Rep, 55(RR-11), 1-94. doi: rr5511a1 [pii]

Zhu, Y. S., & Imperato-McGinley, J. L. (2009). 5alpha-reductase isozymes and androgen actions in the prostate. Annals of the New York Academy of Sciences, 1155, 43-56. doi: 10.1111/j.1749-6632.2009.04115.x

11

NEUROLOGIC DISORDERS

Neurologic Disorders

Headaches 425

Trigeminal Neuralgia 431

Syncope 433

Transient Ischemic Attack 435

Seizure Disorders 437

* Febrile Seizures 440

Meningitis 441

Multiple Sclerosis 443

Parkinson's Disease 445

Alzheimer's Disease 449

ADD/ADHD 452

Bell's palsy 454

Carpal Tunnel Syndrome 455

References 457

** Denotes pediatric diagnosis*

HEADACHES

DESCRIPTION

Pain in the head caused by multiple etiologies.

ETIOLOGY

Due to stimulation, traction, tension, pressure on any pain sensitive structures of the head

- Abnormal metabolism of serotonin, norepinephrine, dopamine
- Hypertension
- Sinus infections
- Tooth abscesses
- Lesions of the oral cavity
- Ear infections
- Eye strain or other eye lesions
- Dilation of cerebral blood vessels by drugs
- Space-occupying tumors
- Increased intracranial pressure from hematomas
- Hemorrhage within the cranium
- Temporal arteritis
- Uremia
- Meningitis
- Tuberculosis
- Syphilis
- Carbon monoxide poisoning
- Anxiety, hysteria, etc.

INCIDENCE

- Very common
- Cluster headaches: 0.5-1.0% of adults, rarely occur in children, very rare during pregnancy
- Tension headaches: 60% have onset after age 20 years, rarely have onset after age 50 years, 15% of pediatric patients will have onset before age 10 years, no documented relationship between tension headaches and pregnancy
- Migraine headaches: 17.6% of females, 5.6% of males in U.S.
- Pediatric migraines: 3-5% of all children in U.S. increase to 10-20% during the second decade

Headaches of new onset in the elderly tend to have a secondary cause: tumor, bleed, etc.

RISK FACTORS

Cluster headaches

- Male gender (6:1)
- Age > 30 years
- Alcohol intake
- Use of nitroglycerine
- Tension headaches
- Excessive intake of caffeine, nicotine
- Stressful situations

Migraine headaches

- Family history (> 80% have positive family history)
- Female gender
- First headache in early childhood but grossly under reported
- Excessive sleep
- Ingestion of certain foods
    - ◊ Tryptophan or tyramine rich foods: ripe cheeses, red wine, or chocolate
- Alcohol
- Estrogen replacement
- Missing meals

Tension Headaches

- Stress
- Worry
- Jaw clenching

A cluster headache is sometimes referred to as a suicide headache because there is a high rate of suicide or self-harm in these individuals during the headache cycle.

ASSESSMENT FINDINGS

- *Cluster headache*
    - ◊ Pain peaks within 15 minutes, usually lasts < 3 hours
    - ◊ Sudden, severe and unilateral
    - ◊ Eye, temple, face, or neck involvement
    - ◊ Lacrimation and/or rhinorrhea
    - ◊ Ptosis
    - ◊ Injected conjunctiva
    - ◊ Nasal stuffiness
    - ◊ Attacks may occur at the same time for several days

- ◊ Attack may occur within 90 minutes of falling asleep
- Tension Headaches
  - ◊ Bilateral in 90% of cases
  - ◊ Dull, vice-like, pressure around head
  - ◊ May be frontal-occipital
  - ◊ May be intermittent; may be present all day ranging in intensity from mild to severe
  - ◊ Palpable muscle tightness, soreness, or stiffness in neck, upper shoulders, or scalp
- Migraine: 5 phases may occur
  - ◊ Prodrome
    - * Mood swings
    - * Fatigue
    - * Food craving
    - * Yawning
  - ◊ Aura
    - * Visual disturbances: visual field cuts, flashing lights, zigzag patterns, floaters
    - * Headache begins within one hour and is usually generalized
  - ◊ Headache (lasts 4-72 hours)
    - * Unilateral, bilateral, or generalized
    - * Throbbing (or not)
    - * Anorexia, nausea, vomiting
    - * Photophobia, phonophobia, lightheadedness
    - * Vertigo
  - ◊ Termination of headache
    - * Usually occurs with sleep or medication
  - ◊ Postdrome
    - * Lingering symptoms: fatigue, malaise, inability to problem solve

Most patients with migraine will NOT experience all 5 phases.

ASSESSMENT FINDINGS

Characteristics of secondary headaches:

- "Worst headache of my life": subarachnoid hemorrhage
- Headache worse in the morning, deep pain, aggravated by coughing, sneezing: brain tumor
- Morning headaches worse in the occipital region: hypertension
- Headaches worse with bending over, nasal congestion, facial tenderness: sinusitis
- Severe headache, tachycardia, diaphoresis: pheochromocytoma
- Orbital headache: acute angle glaucoma

DIFFERENTIAL DIAGNOSIS

- Headache disorders
- Secondary headaches
- Giant cell arteritis
- Drug-seeking patients
- Psychiatric disease

DIAGNOSTIC STUDIES

- Depends on patient's symptoms and presumed etiology
- CT and/or MRI (reserve for patients with neurological deficits, sudden onset of severe headache, or change in frequency and occurrence of headaches)
- Consider sinus series
- CBC, complete metabolic panel, TSH
- Cervical x-rays
- EEG
- Lumbar puncture
- Sedimentation rate

PREVENTION/AVOIDANCE

Cluster headache	• Avoid triggering substance (e.g., alcohol, nictotine) • Temper strong emotions • Maintain usual sleep/wake hours • Pharmacologic interventions for prophylaxis (see Pharmacologic Management) • Avoidance of vasodilators (NTG, alcohol)
Tension headache	• Relaxation therapy • Stress management
Migraine headache	• Avoid precipitating factors • Avoid foods which may precipitate headaches: ◊ Nitrite-containing foods (e.g., hot dogs) ◊ Monosodium glutamate-containing foods (e.g., Chinese food) ◊ Tyramine-containing foods (e.g., chocolate, cheese, red wine, caffeine containing beverages) • Pharmacologic prophylaxis (see Pharmacologic Management)

NONPHARMACOLOGIC MANAGEMENT

- See Prevention/Avoidance
- Application of ice, cool compresses to head, face, scalp, or neck
- Darkened room
- Quiet atmosphere

PHARMACOLOGIC MANAGEMENT

Cluster headache	Tension headache	Migraine headache
• Abortive: 100% oxygen 7-10 liters for 10-15 minutes at onset, "triptans", ergotamine (Cafergot®), intranasal lidocaine 4% topical on same side as symptoms • Prophylaxis (calcium channel blocker): verapamil (Calan®), lithium (Lithobid®), indomethacin (Indocin®), nifedipine (Procardia®), nimodipine (Nimotop®) • Prednisone used while waiting for other therapy (oral medications) to become effective	• Abortive (NSAIDs): naproxen sodium, ibuprofen, ketoprofen, aspirin • Prophylaxis: amitriptyline (Elavil®), imipramine (Tofranil®), non-specific beta blockers	• Abortive: "triptans", ergotamine-caffeine (Cafergot®), isometheptene-dichloralphenazone-acetaminophen (Midrin®), butalbital-acetaminophen (Fioicet®), NSAIDs (aspirin, ibuprofen, naproxen, ketoprofen) • Prophylaxis: topiramate (Topamax®), propanolol, timolol, calcium channel blockers • TCA off label use for prophylaxis

MIGRAINE HEADACHE PHARMACOLOGIC MANAGEMENT

Acetaminophen, aspirin, and caffeine in combination are as effective as triptans for mild and moderate migraine with fewer adverse events if given at onset of symptoms. Consider anti-emetics (metoclopramide, prochlorperazine) for accompanying nausea. Many drug classes are used for prophylaxis but are off-label.

Class	Drug Generic name (Trade name®)	Dosage How supplied	Comments
Abortive agents Serotonin 5HT1 receptor agonists ("Triptans") **General Comments** Monitor for angina, cerebro-vascular events, gastrointestinal ischemic events	**almotriptan** Axert	**Adults and > 12 years**: 6.25 mg or 12.5 mg single dose. May repeat in 2 hours if needed. *Max*: 25 mg/24 hours *Tabs: 6.25 mg, 12.5 mg*	• Pregnancy Category C • Dosage adjustment for hepatic or severe renal impairment or concomitant 3A4 inhibitors • Watch for drug interactions, especially with SSRIs • Cautious use in patients who are sensitive to sulfonamides • Unknown safety in treating more than 4 headaches in 30 days
Do not use within 24 hours of ergotamine type medications or other triptans Take as soon as possible after onset of migraine	**naratriptan**	**Adults > 18 years**: 1 mg or 2.5 mg with fluids; may repeat once after 4 hours if needed *Max*: 5 mg/24 hours	• Pregnancy Category C • Dosage adjustment for hepatic or renal impairment • Consider EKG monitoring in patients with likelihood of unrecognized coronary disease • Watch for drug interactions, especially with SSRIs

continued

MIGRAINE HEADACHE PHARMACOLOGIC MANAGEMENT

Acetaminophen, aspirin, and caffeine in combination are as effective as triptans for mild and moderate migraine with fewer adverse events if given at onset of symptoms. Consider anti-emetics (metoclopramide, prochlorperazine) for accompanying nausea. Many drug classes are used for prophylaxis but are off-label.

Class	Drug Generic name (Trade name®)	Dosage How supplied	Comments
Contraindicated in ischemic heart disease, vasospastic coronary artery disease, uncontrolled hypertension, peripheral vascular disease, cerebrovascular disease, basilar or hemiplegic migraine Frequent use may lead to reduced efficacy	Amerge	*Tabs: 1 mg, 2.5 mg*	
	sumatriptan	**Adults**: 25-100 mg once with fluids; may repeat dose at intervals of 2 hours *Max*: 200 mg/day Hepatic impairment: 50 mg/ dose	• Pregnancy Category C • Consider EKG monitoring in patients with likelihood of unrecognized coronary disease • Watch for drug interactions, especially with SSRIs • Unknown safety in treating more than 4 headaches in 30 days
	Imitrex	*Tabs: 25 mg, 50 mg, 100 mg*	
	Injection: 4 mg/0.5 mL, 6 mg/0.5 mL	**Adults**: 6 mg subcutaneously May repeat in 1 hour *Max*: two 6 mg doses in 24 hours	
	Nasal Spray: 5 mg/spray, 20 mg/spray	**Adults**: 5 mg, 10 mg, 20 mg once. May repeat once after 2 hours *Max*: 40 mg/day	
	zolmitriptan	**Adults**: 2.5 mg single dose. May repeat after 2 hours *Max*: 10 mg/24 hours	• Pregnancy Category C • Consider EKG monitoring in patients with likelihood of unrecognized coronary disease • Watch for drug interactions, especially with SSRIs • OK to break 2.5 mg tab in half if lower dose relieves headache • Dosage adjustment needed for hepatic dysfunction • Unknown safety in treating more than 3 headaches in 30 days
	Zomig	*Tabs: 2.5 mg, 5 mg*	
	Zomig ZMT	**Adults**: 2.5 mg single dose Place on tongue and allow to dissolve. Swallow with saliva. May repeat after 2 hours *Max*: 10 mg/24 hours *ZMT Tabs: 2.5 mg, 5 mg*	• Pregnancy Category C • ZMT tabs: dissolve under tongue and swallow without water • Do not remove tablet from blister until immediately before using • Do not break ZMT in half • Dosage adjustment needed for hepatic dysfunction

continued

MIGRAINE HEADACHE PHARMACOLOGIC MANAGEMENT

Acetaminophen, aspirin, and caffeine in combination are as effective as triptans for mild and moderate migraine with fewer adverse events if given at onset of symptoms. Consider anti-emetics (metoclopramide, prochlorperazine) for accompanying nausea. Many drug classes are used for prophylaxis but are off-label.

Class	Drug Generic name (Trade name®)	Dosage How supplied	Comments
Abortive Agents Ergotamine *Selectively bind to serotonin 5-HT1A, 5-HT2A, and 5-HT2C* **General Comments** Serious and/or life-threatening peripheral ischemia has been associated with coadministration of potent CYP 3A4 inhibitors and ergotamines Do not use in patients with documented or suspected ischemic or vasospastic coronary artery disease, unrecognized coronary artery disease Frequent use may lead to reduced efficacy	**dihydroergotamine** mesylate nasal spray (4 mg/mL) Migranal	**Adults**: Administer one spray (0.5 mg) in each nostril. 15 minutes later, administer one spray in each nostril for a total of 4 sprays *Nasal spray: 8 spray vials containing 4 mg of DHE mesylate*	• Pregnancy Category X • Many drug interactions with CYP 3A4 inhibitors: protease inhibitors, macrolide antibiotics, ketoconozaole, others resulting in cerebral and peripheral ischemia • Other drug interactions with sumatriptan, beta blockers, nicotine, SSRIs • Contraindicated in patients with uncontrolled hypertension, hemiplegic or basilar migraine • Prior to administration, pump must be primed before use. Discard after 8 hours • Do not sniff after spraying
Prophylactic Agents **General Comments** Anticonvulsant Mechanism of action is unknown but thought to block voltage dependent sodium channels, augments activity of GABA-A receptor Increased risk of suicidal behavior or ideation May cause cognitive dysfunction. Cautious use when engaging in activities requiring mental alertness	**topiramate** Topamax	**Adults**: 25 mg administered nightly for the first week. Second week, administer 25 mg twice daily. Third week, administer 25 mg in AM, 50 mg in PM. Fourth week, administer 50 mg twice daily. Titrate by clinical outcome *Usual*: 100 mg/d administered in two divided doses *Tabs: 25 mg, 50 mg, 100 mg, 200 mg* *Topamax Sprinkle Capsules: 15 mg, 25 mg*	• Pregnancy Category C • Contraindicated in untreated elevated intraocular pressure • Baseline and periodic measurement of serum bicarbonate is recommended • Depression and mood problems may occur • Increased risk of kidney stones • Monitor for drug interactions especially with oral contraceptives, metformin, lithium, carbonic anhydrase inhibitors • Dosage adjustment required for renal and hepatic dysfunction, elderly • Dosing for sprinkle caps exactly as for tablets

continued

MIGRAINE HEADACHE PHARMACOLOGIC MANAGEMENT

Acetaminophen, aspirin, and caffeine in combination are as effective as triptans for mild and moderate migraine with fewer adverse events if given at onset of symptoms. Consider anti-emetics (metoclopramide, prochlorperazine) for accompanying nausea. Many drug classes are used for prophylaxis but are off-label.

Class	Drug Generic name (Trade name®)	Dosage How supplied	Comments
Prophylactic Agents **General Comments** Beta Blockers Mechanism of action is unknown Contraindicated in bradycardia, asthma May mask signs and symptoms of hypoglycemia in diabetics Cautious use in patients with impaired renal or hepatic dysfunction Patients with history of severe anaphylactic reaction may be unresponsive to usual doses of epinephrine used to treat allergic reaction Monitor for symptoms of ischemic heart disease after withdrawing	**propanolol**	**Adult**: 80 mg once daily Gradually increase at 3-7 day intervals until optimal response is obtained *Usual*: 160 mg- 240 mg *Max*: 320 mg daily	• Pregnancy Category C • If insufficient response is seen after 4-6 weeks of optimal dose, discontinue by gradually withdrawing drug over several weeks • Many possible drug interactions. Check compatibilities
	Inderal LA	*Caps: 60 mg, 80 mg, 120 mg, 160 mg*	
	timolol	**Adult**: 10 mg twice daily During maintenance, 20 mg may be administered as a single dose *Max*: 30 mg given in divided doses	• Pregnancy Category C • If satisfactory response is not noted in 6-8 weeks of maximum daily dosage, discontinue by withdrawing over several weeks
	various generics	*Tabs: 5 mg, 10 mg, 20 mg*	

SPECIAL CONSIDERATIONS

- Avoid triptans in patients with coronary artery disease, poorly controlled hypertension
- Triptans most effective if given during early headache phase
- Avoid concomitant use of triptans and ergotamine within a 24-hour period
- Reserve narcotics for infrequent use due to addiction potential

PREGNANCY/LACTATION CONSIDERATIONS

- Triptan Pregnancy Category C drug
- Avoid use of ergotamine
- Number and intensity of migraine headaches may decrease during 2nd and 3rd trimester

CONSULTATION/REFERRAL

- Refer to neurologist for severe headaches or those that are unresponsive to drug therapy

FOLLOW-UP

- Return to clinic or emergency department if headache unresolved after treatment, becomes more severe, or varies from the usual pattern

EXPECTED COURSE

- Cluster headache: recurrent attacks are usual until cycle can be interrupted
- Tension headache: most follow a chronic course if stressors are not eliminated
- Migraine headache: most resolve within 72 hours; decrease in frequency and duration as patient ages

POSSIBLE COMPLICATIONS

- Cluster headache: suicide or self-injury during an attack, risk of addiction to narcotic analgesics
- Tension headache: GI bleed from continued use of NSAIDs
- Migraine headache: risk of addiction to narcotic analgesics, iatrogenic complications from treatment (e.g., angina from triptans)

TRIGEMINAL NEURALGIA
(Tic Douloureux)

DESCRIPTION

A disorder of the 5th cranial nerve (trigeminal nerve) which produces severe pain in the lip, gum, cheek, and/or face.

ETIOLOGY

- Compression of the 5th cranial nerve from unknown causes, tumors, or vascular malformations

INCIDENCE

- 16/100,000 in U.S.
- Females > Males (2:1)
- Peak age is 60 years

RISK FACTORS

- None known

ASSESSMENT FINDINGS

- Severe pain in the lip, face, mouth, gum, cheek
- Wincing
- Pain may be in "bursts" with pain free period after burst
- Pain may be elicited by touch, changes in temperature, or a light breeze on the cheek
- Lacrimation, flushing, salivation

Pain can be reported as "unbearable" and initially thought to be of dental origin.

DIFFERENTIAL DIAGNOSIS

- Other form of neuralgia
- Migraine

DIAGNOSTIC STUDIES

- MRI or CT scan to rule out neoplasm

PREVENTION/AVOIDANCE

- Withdraw medications used for management slowly (4-6 weeks)
- Restart at highest level if pain resumes
- Avoidance of breeze, heat, cold on facial areas

NONPHARMACOLOGIC MANAGEMENT

- Avoidance of breeze, heat, cold on facial areas
- Surgical decompression or nerve ablation
- Peripheral nerve block of the 5th cranial nerve

PHARMACOLOGIC MANAGEMENT

- Carbamazepine is used first line; 70-90% of patients respond initially
- Many drugs are used off label: oxcarbazepine (Trileptal®), pheynytoin (Dilantin®), baclofen (Lioresal®), gabapentin (Neurontin®), lamotrigine

TRIGEMINAL NEEURALGIA PHARMACOLOGIC MANAGEMENT

Class	Drug Generic name (Trade name®)	Dosage How supplied	Comments
Anticonvulsants **General Comments** Mechanism of action is unknown but reduces polysynaptic responses and blocks post-tetanic potentiation. Reduces or abolishes pain induced by stimulation of the infraorbital nerve Aplastic anemia and agranulocytosis have been reported with use of carbamazapine	**carbamazepine** Various generics	**Immediate Release** **Adults**: 100 mg twice daily in increments of 100 mg every 12 hours *Max*: 1200 mg/24 hours *Tabs: 100 mg, 200 mg, 300 mg, 400 mg*	• Pregnancy Category D • Baseline and periodic CBC, renal and liver function tests, eye exam, UA, lipids, TSH, sodium • Monitor for hyponatremia • Monitor for decreased WBC or platelet counts. Discontinue if any evidence of bone marrow depression occurs. Do not use in patients with a history of bone marrow depression or hepatic porphyria • Cautious use in patients with increased intraocular pressure • Carbamazepine can interact with many CYP 3A4 drugs. Check compatibilities • Concurrent MAOIs is contraindicated • Elderly more likely to exhibit confusion or agitation • May cause sedation especially in combination with CNS depressants • Attempt to reduce dose at least every 3 months
	carbamazepine (CBZ) Carbatrol	**Extended Release** **Adults**: 200 mg every 12 hours May increase by 200 mg every 12 hours only as needed to achieve freedom from pain *Usual*: 400-800 mg/day *Max*: 1200 mg daily *Ext Release Caps: 100 mg, 200 mg, 300 mg*	• Pregnancy Category D • Baseline and periodic CBC, renal and liver function tests, eye exam, UA, lipids, TSH, sodium • Monitor for hyponatremia • Monitor for decreased WBC or platelet counts. Discontinue if any evidence of bone marrow depression occurs. Do not use in patients with a history of bone marrow depression or hepatic porphyria • Cautious use in patients with increased intraocular pressure • Carbamazepine can interact with many CYP 3A4 drugs. Check compatibilities • Elderly more likely to exhibit confusion or agitation • May cause sedation especially in combination with CNS depressants • Attempt to reduce dose at least every 3 months

CONSULTATION/REFERRAL

- Neurologist

FOLLOW-UP

- Check carbamazepine and phenytoin levels
- Check liver and hematopoietic (LFT and CBC) functions if carbamazepine prescribed

EXPECTED COURSE

- Prognosis good
- Exacerbations in spring and fall

POSSIBLE COMPLICATIONS

- Sedation from medications
- Vertigo from carbamazepine

SYNCOPE
(Faint)

DESCRIPTION

A sudden, brief loss of consciousness with a spontaneous recovery.

ETIOLOGY

Vasovagal	Due to decreased cardiac output from peripheral vasodilation and bradycardia
Orthostatic hypotension	Due to medications, hypovolemia, autonomic dysfunction
Situational syncope	Due to coughing, micturition, or defecation
Cardiac	Due to sudden decrease in cardiac output ◊ Aortic stenosis ◊ Arrhythmias (heart blocks, ventricular tachycardia)
Carotid sinus syncope	Due to manual pressure/ stimulation of the carotid arteries
Cerebrovascular disease	Due to decreased perfusion of the vertebrobasilar system
Other causes	Depression, alcohol ingestion, drug abuse, psychogenic, subclavian steal syndrome, cardiomyopathy

INCIDENCE

- 6% in persons over age 75 years
- More common in the elderly
- Unidentifiable cause in 48% of patients

RISK FACTORS

- Underlying cardiac disease
- Patients on antihypertensive agents, antiarrhythmics, antidepressants, diuretics, phenothiazines, vasodilators
- Malfunctioning pacemaker

ASSESSMENT FINDINGS

- General findings
  - ◊ Feelings of lightheadedness, weakness, nausea, vomiting, diaphoresis
  - ◊ Loss of consciousness
  - ◊ Loss of postural tone
  - ◊ Spontaneous recovery
- Vasovagal
  - ◊ Fear, anxiety, or sudden emotion may precipitate syncopal episode
  - ◊ Sudden onset of weakness, sweating, nausea
- Orthostatic hypotension
  - ◊ Occurs when patient stands
- Situational syncope
  - ◊ May be precipitated by swallowing, coughing, micturition, defecation
- Cardiac arrhythmias
  - ◊ Usually abrupt onset without warning
  - ◊ Related to physical activity
  - ◊ May be precipitated by electrolyte imbalance (especially potassium, calcium, or magnesium), malfunction of prosthetic heart valve or pacemaker, hypoxia, coronary artery disease
- Carotid sinus syncope
  - ◊ Bradycardia often precipitates syncope
  - ◊ Turning of neck may precipitate syncope

- Cerebrovascular disease
  - ◊ May experience auditory, visual, or vestibular symptoms prior to syncope
  - ◊ May have history of previous transient ischemic attack

DIFFERENTIAL DIAGNOSIS

- Vertigo
- Seizure activity
- Cerebellar disease
- Space-occupying lesion in the cranial cavity
- Psychological stress
- Cardiac vs. noncardiac syncope

DIAGNOSTIC STUDIES

- Complete metabolic panel: Sodium, calcium, glucose needed
- 24-hour ECG monitoring (helpful 4-15% of the time)
- Blood pressure measurements in both arms: difference of 20 mm Hg or more is considered abnormal
- Blood pressure measurements lying and standing: normal findings are systolic pressure decrease of less than 10 mm Hg, increase in diastolic 2-5 mm Hg, and increase in heart rate 5-20 beats. If heart rate does not increase, consider cardiac origin
- Flexion/extension of neck 10 times to simulate vertebrobasilar insufficiency
- Flexion/extension of arms to simulate symptoms of subclavian steal syndrome
- Complete neurological examination; if abnormal, consider CT, MRI, EEG
- Complete cardiac examination
- Carotid auscultation/studies for suspected carotid artery disease: bruit indicates probable blockage
- Echocardiogram if valvular or cardiomyopathy is suspected
- Tilt testing

After thorough examination, only 50-60% of patients will have an identifiable cause.

PREVENTION

- Rise slowly from lying or sitting to standing

NONPHARMACOLOGIC MANAGEMENT

- Elevate patient's legs if due to vasovagal or hypotension
- Elastic support stockings to prevent orthostatic hypotension
- Changing positions slowly, especially to an upright position
- Teach patient about measures to take to ensure safety (e.g., do not climb on stools, or operate dangerous machinery, avoid bathing in tub of very hot water, etc.), especially if a particular activity may precipitate syncopal episode
- Other actions dependent on underlying cause of syncope
- Increased sodium intake to help expand volume

PHARMACOLOGIC MANAGEMENT

- Depends on underlying cause
- β-blockers may prevent recurrent vasovagal symptoms
- Antiarrhythmic drugs for documented arrhythmias

PREGNANCY/LACTATION CONSIDERATIONS

- Vasovagal syncope may present in pregnant women from compression of the vena cava and aorta
- Positioning the pregnant woman on her left side should relieve the compression and the symptoms

CONSULTATION/REFERRAL

- Refer to cardiologist, neurologist, depending on etiology

FOLLOW-UP

- Depends on etiology

EXPECTED COURSE

- Depends on etiology

POSSIBLE COMPLICATIONS

- Head injury from falls during episode
- Sudden death (more common if cardiac etiology)

TRANSIENT ISCHEMIC ATTACK
(TIA)

DESCRIPTION

A sudden onset of neurological deficits which is caused by cerebral ischemia and lasts < 24 hours

ETIOLOGY

- Atherosclerotic disease within the brain and/or carotid arteries
- Microemboli from atrial fibrillation, cardiac valve disorders
- Hypercoagulable states
- Spontaneous
- Cerebral artery vasospasm
- Use of oral contraceptive

INCIDENCE

- 30/100,000 in U.S.
- Males > Females 3:1

RISK FACTORS

- Hypertension
- Advanced age
- Prior TIA
- Smoking
- Diabetes
- Hyperlipidemia
- Cardiac disease
- Atrial fibrillation
- Family history of TIA or stroke
- Oral contraceptive use

ASSESSMENT FINDINGS

- Aphasia
- Visual field defects
- Confusion
- Amnesia
- Diplopia
- Dysphagia
- Dysarthria
- Unilateral weakness
- Neurological deficits usually last < 24 hours

Any sudden onset of neurological symptoms should prompt an evaluation for stroke.

DIFFERENTIAL DIAGNOSIS

- Stroke
- Seizure
- Hypoglycemia
- Vestibular disease
- Migraine
- Subdural hemorrhage

DIAGNOSTIC STUDIES

- CT, MRI of head: rule out hemorrhage, CVA
- Carotid studies (ultrasound and/or angiography): > 70% blockage may cause symptoms
- Cerebral angiography: may demonstrate atherosclerosis
- ECG, 24-hour Holter monitor, echocardiogram if underlying cardiac problem suspected
- EEG if seizure suspected
- Lab to rule out medical causes: CBC with platelets, INR, ESR, glucose, lipid profile, urinalysis

PREVENTION

- Control blood pressure, lipids, diabetes
- Antiplatelet therapy
- ACE inhibitors
- Statins
- Aspirin or ticlopidine (Ticlid®)

NONPHARMACOLOGIC MANAGEMENT

- Control risk factors: hypertension, hyperlipidemia, diabetes
- Patient education regarding importance of stopping smoking, taking medications as prescribed (e.g., antihypertensives, lipid lowering agents, anticoagulants)
- Endarterectomy

PREGNANCY/LACTATION CONSIDERATIONS

- Pregnancy may produce a state of hypercoagulation

CONSULTATION/REFERRAL

- Cardiologist if underlying cardiac disorders
- Neurologist

FOLLOW-UP

- Depends on etiology

EXPECTED COURSE

- Increased risk of stroke with presence of additional risk factors (e.g., hypertension, hypercholesterolemia, smoking)

POSSIBLE COMPLICATIONS

- Stroke
- Injury from fall

TRANS ISCHEMIC ATTACK PHARMACOLOGIC MANAGEMENT

Class	Drug Generic name (Trade name®)	Dosage How supplied	Comments
Platelet Aggregation Inhibitors *inhibit platelet aggregation and have been shown to decrease morbid events in people with established cardiovascular atherosclerotic disease* General Comment Observe for bleeding	**clopidogrel** Plavix	**Adults**: 75 mg once daily *Tabs: 75 mg*	• Pregnancy Category B • Prolongs bleeding time. Cautious use in patient at risk of increased bleeding • Teach patient to notify all health care providers of clopidogrel use • Platelet aggregation is observed 2 hours after initial dose. Gradually returns to baseline about 5 days after treatment is discontinued • No dosage adjustment needed for elderly, hepatic, or mild/moderate renal impairment • Increased rates of occult bleeding when used in conjunction with NSAIDs • Monitor for drug interactions with 2C19 medications. They diminish response to clopidogrel, especially omeprazole
Aspirin *Prevents platelet aggregation and exerts anti-inflammatory effect in vessels by inhibiting prostaglandin synthesis*	**acetylsalicylic acid (ASA)** Various generics	**Adult**: 50-325 mg once daily *Max*: 325 mg daily *Tabs: 81 mg, 162 mg 325 mg* *Caplets: 81 mg, 325 mg* *Gel caps: 325 mg*	• Pregnancy Category D • Use in caution with patients with reactive airway disease (asthma) • Consider enteric coated in patients with prior gastric irritation • Avoid in patients with NSAID allergies • May need to reduce dose in severe hepatic or renal dysfunction

continued

TRANS ISCHEMIC ATTACK PHARMACOLOGIC MANAGEMENT

Class	Drug Generic name (Trade name®)	Dosage How supplied	Comments
	ticlopidine Ticlid, various generics	**Adult**: 250 mg twice daily with food *Max*: 250 mg daily *Tabs: 250 mg*	• Pregnancy Category B • Can cause life-threatening hematological adverse reactions. Contraindicated in hematopoetic disorders, history of TTP, active bleeding • Dosage adjustment needed for renal, hepatic dysfunction • After discontinuation of ticlopidine, bleeding time and other platelet function tests return to normal within 2 weeks • Drug reactions will occur with NSAIDs, aspirin, cimetidine, digoxin, theophylline, food

SEIZURE DISORDERS
(Convulsions, Epilepsy)

DESCRIPTION

A transient alteration in behavior with or without loss of consciousness, sensory perception, motor function, and/or autonomic function. Seizures are due to excessive rate of neuronal discharges. Seizures which are recurrent are termed epilepsy.

Status epilepticus is a medical emergency.

TYPES OF SEIZURES

Seizures are classified by the location of their onset

Partial (begins with motor symptoms characterized by recurrent contractions of muscles in one part of the body
- ◊ Simple (consciousness not impaired) Jacksonian-type seizures begin in one part of the body and progress to contiguous body parts over seconds or minutes
- ◊ Complex (consciousness impaired)
- ◊ Mixed (begin as simple or partial and evolve into generalized tonic/clonic; consciousness impaired)

Seizures are classified by the location of their onset

Generalized (bilaterally symmetrical but without local onset)
- ◊ Absence (Petit mal): brief arrest of activity and loss of consciousness
- ◊ Atypical absence
- ◊ Myoclonic: muscle movements are repetitive
- ◊ Tonic-clonic
- ◊ Tonic, clonic or atonic seizures

ETIOLOGY

- Idiopathic
- Alcohol intoxication or withdrawal
- Brain tumor
- Hypoxia
- Brain attack (formerly called stroke)
- Breath holding spells
- Exposure to toxic agents
- Eclampsia
- Fever (*see Febrile Seizures, page 440*)
- Head injury
- Hyperthermia
- Hyperventilation
- Meningitis
- Migraine

INCIDENCE

- Highest incidence is in children
- 4-6% of children will have a seizure before age 16 years
- 1.5 million people in U.S. have epilepsy
- 1.2/1000 in U.S. for all types of seizures
- 10% of general population has isolated seizures

Patients most likely to have seizures are pediatric and geriatric patients.

RISK FACTORS

- Previous history of seizure
- Family history
- Brain tumor
- History of neurological insult (e.g., brain attack, intracranial hemorrhage, head trauma, meningitis)
- Withdrawal from anticonvulsant medications

ASSESSMENT FINDINGS

- Seizure with or without loss of consciousness, with or without loss of posture

DIAGNOSTIC CLUES

- Fever: infectious etiology
- Headache: infectious etiology, hemorrhage, tumor
- Meningismus (irritation of the brain and spinal cord without meningitis): CNS infection
- Papilledema: increased intracranial pressure from tumor, bleed
- Focal neurologic finding: tumor or localized injury to specific site in brain

DIFFERENTIAL DIAGNOSIS

Age	Causes
Newborn to 2 years of age	Metabolic (hypoglycemia, hypocalcemia, hypo-magnesemia, phenylketonuria) Infection Birth injury Febrile seizure Congenital anomaly
2 to 10 years of age	Febrile seizure Tumor CNS infection Trauma Idiopathic
10 to 18 years of age	Tumor Trauma Arteriovenous malformation Drug or alcohol related Idiopathic
18 to 25 years of age	Tumor Trauma Infection, meningitis Drug or alcohol intoxication or withdrawal Idiopathic
25 to 60 years of age	Tumor Trauma Infection, meningitis Drug or alcohol related Syncope Cardiac dysrhythmias
Over 60 years of age	Infection, meningitis, vascular diseases Syncope Cardiac dysrhythmias Drug or alcohol related Tumor Metabolic (hypoglycemia, hypocalcemia, hypomagnesemia, uremia)

DIAGNOSTIC STUDIES

- Complete metabolic panel to assess for glucose, electrolytes, BUN, ammonia
- Toxicology screens: presence of drugs or alcohol
- Complete blood count: elevated WBC if infection present
- Anticonvulsant levels if patient is on anticonvulsant
- MRI or CT of brain: MRI preferred because it provides more detailed information, but CT is faster, may be more easily accessible, and easier to obtain if patient is medically unstable
- EEG usually indicated for all children with a first nonfebrile seizure
- Lumbar puncture indicated for most children under 2 years of age or if CNS infection is suspected in any age

PREVENTION

- Usually none
- Fever management
- Maintain medication regimen if on anticonvulsants

NONPHARMACOLOGIC MANAGEMENT

- Monitor anticonvulsant levels if appropriate
- Patient education particular to type of anticonvulsant patient is taking
- Provide safe environment during seizure
- Discussion regarding driving, swimming, other activities

	Commonly Used Drugs for Treatment	
Type of Seizure*	Traditional AED#	Newer AED#
Partial • Simple partial • Complex partial • Secondarily generalized	Carbamazepine Phenobarbital Phenytoin Primidone Valproic acid	Oxcarbazepine Gabapentin Lamotrigine Levetiracetam Pregabalin Topiramate Tiagabine
Primary Generalized • Absence (petit mal) • Atypical Absence • Myolonic • Tonic-clonic (grand mal) • Status epileptical	Carbamazepine Phenobarbital Phenytoin Primidone Valproic acid	Lamotrigine Levetiracetam Topiramate

*defined by International League Against Epilepsy # Anti-epileptic drug

	Dosing parameters			
Selected AED#	Adult (mg)	Children [(1)] (mg/kg)	Target serum (mcg/mL)	General comments [(2)]
Carbamazepine	600-1600	10-35	4-12	Adverse CNS effects, hyperplasia of gums, affects hormonal contraception
Gabapentin	1200-3600	25-50	12-20	Adverse CNS effects, nystagamus, weight loss
Lamotrigine	400	5	3-14	Sedation, ataxia, affects hormonal contraception
Levetiracetam	2000-3000	40-100	10-40	Adverse CNS effects
Oxcarbazepine	900-2400	30-46	3-40	Adverse CNS effects, hyperplasia of gums, affects hormonal contraception
Phenobarbital	60-120	3-6	15-45	Adverse CNS effects
Phenytoin	200-300	4-8	10-20	Adverse CNS effects, hyperplasia of gums, affects hormonal contraception
Primodone	500-750	10-25	5-15	Adverse CNS effects, skin rashes, megaloblastic anemia
Topiramate	100-400	3-9	5-25	Adverse CNS effects, weight loss, renal calculi
Valproic acid	750-3000	15-45	40-100	Drowsiness, nausea, vomiting, weight gain, alopecia

Anti-epileptic drug
(1) Prescriber must ensure pediatric indications and doses
(2) Prescriber should be familiar with various dosage forms, strengths, contraindications and precautions specific to each product

PREGNANCY/LACTATION CONSIDERATIONS

- Monitor levels closely if on anticonvulsants
- Increased risk of congenital malformations in babies born to mothers on anticonvulsant therapy
- Breastfeeding is NOT a contraindication if mother is taking anticonvulsant (may necessitate checking levels in baby). Observe for sedation in baby

CONSULTATION/REFERRAL

- Consult neurologist for all patients with first-time seizure

FOLLOW-UP

- Depends on etiology and severity
- Monitor anticonvulsant levels periodically

EXPECTED COURSE

- Depends on etiology

POSSIBLE COMPLICATIONS

- Drug toxicity from anticonvulsants
- Hypoxia from repetitive seizures with resultant neurological manifestations

FEBRILE SEIZURES

DESCRIPTION

Seizures which occur during a febrile episode. The seizure is not associated with any underlying disorder. They usually occur within the first 24 hours of an illness and do not necessarily occur when the fever is highest.

ETIOLOGY

- Fever lowers the seizure threshold
- Elevated temperature (usually > 102.2 °F, 39 °C)

Rapidity with which body temperature rises or falls seems to be a greater predictor of seizure than the actual body temperature.

INCIDENCE

- Highest incidence occurs between one and two years of age
- 85% occur before the age of 4 years
- 2-5% incidence overall
- Males slightly greater than females

RISK FACTORS

- Very rapid rise in temperature within 24 hours of a febrile illness (most common illnesses are viral upper respiratory and otitis media)
- Febrile seizure in a sibling (risk increased by 2-3 times)
- Recent MMR immunization (within 7-10 days) or DPT (previous 48 hours)

ASSESSMENT FINDINGS

- Fever of > 102.2 °F (39 °C)
- First 24 hours of a febrile illness
- Seizure may be first sign of illness in child

DIFFERENTIAL DIAGNOSIS

- Syncopal episode
- Night terrors
- Breath-holding spells
- Febrile associated shivering or delirium
- Afebrile seizure which coincidentally occurs during a febrile event
- Sudden discontinuance of anticonvulsants
- Underlying CNS infection

DIAGNOSTIC STUDIES

- Lumbar puncture if child is younger than 12 months old
- Laboratory testing not done routinely for simple, febrile seizure
- Consider CBC, electrolytes, chemistries, urinalysis
- CBC, electrolytes, chemistries, EEG, MRI, CT if child appears toxic, has neurological deficits, multiple seizures, prolonged recovery, etc.

PREVENTION

- Antipyretics for fever > 100.6 °F (38.1 °C)
- Tepid sponge bath for high fever

NONPHARMACOLOGIC MANAGEMENT

- Supportive care after seizure has occurred
- Patient/family education regarding
  - ◊ Emergency measures if seizures occur in the future
  - ◊ Fever management at home
  - ◊ Educate parents that febrile seizures do not cause developmental delays, learning problems or behavior problems

PHARMACOLOGIC MANAGEMENT

- Treatment for initial simple febrile seizure is not indicated. Cost-benefit ratio does not justify treatment
- Only 33% of children with initial seizure have a recurrence
- Treat high fever with acetaminophen, ibuprofen or other antipyretic
- Children's ibuprofen may be administered to children > 6 months of age

Alternating ibuprofen and acetaminophen every 2 hours for fever management leads to medication errors and is not recommended by American Academy of Pediatrics.

CONSULTATION/REFERRAL

- Consult neurologist for suspected underlying cause (e.g., CNS infection, afebrile seizure)

FOLLOW-UP

- Depends on etiology of febrile illness and whether seizure was a simple febrile seizure
- If assessment indicates questionable underlying cause of seizure, follow-up by neurologist needed

EXPECTED COURSE

- 33% will develop recurrent seizures
- 95% of those that will have a recurrence do so within one year of initial episode

POSSIBLE COMPLICATIONS

- Slight increase in risk of development of epilepsy later in life

MENINGITIS

DESCRIPTION

Inflammation of the brain and spinal cord caused by infection with bacteria, viruses, and fungi. Occasionally parasites are responsible for meningitis.

ETIOLOGY

- Bacterial meningitis
  - ◊ Group B or D *Streptococcus*
  - ◊ *Streptococcus pneumoniae* (most common in adults)
  - ◊ *Neisseria meningitidis*
  - ◊ Other organisms
- Viral meningitis
  - ◊ Enterovirus is the most common cause, includes Coxsackie A and B, polioviruses, echoviruses
- Fungal meningitis
  - ◊ *Candida* species
  - ◊ *Aspergillus*
  - ◊ *Cryptococcus neoformans*

INCIDENCE

- Bacterial
  - ◊ Predominant age: extremes of age (very young, very old)
  - ◊ 80% occur in children under age 24 months
  - ◊ Males = Females
  - ◊ 3-10/100,000 in U.S.

- Viral
  - ◊ Most common in young adults
  - ◊ Effects all ages
  - ◊ About 10,000 cases annually in U.S.
  - ◊ Common in summer and early fall
- Fungal
  - ◊ Cryptococcal meningitis is most common in immunocompromised adults, especially those with AIDS
  - ◊ Candida species most common in premature infants and other immunocompromised adults

RISK FACTORS

- Bacterial
  - ◊ Immunocompromised hosts
  - ◊ Alcoholics
  - ◊ Neurosurgical patients
- Viral
  - ◊ Immunocompromised hosts
- Fungal
  - ◊ Immunocompromised hosts
  - ◊ Exposure to pigeon or bird droppings

ASSESSMENT FINDINGS

- Bacterial
  - ◊ Recent URI
  - ◊ Neck pain/stiff neck
  - ◊ Headache, fever
  - ◊ Nausea and vomiting, especially in children
  - ◊ Decreased level of consciousness, seizures
  - ◊ Meningococcemia rash
  - ◊ Nuchal rigidity
  - ◊ Positive Kernig and Brudzinski signs:
    - * Kernig sign: complete extension of leg causes neck pain and flexion
    - * Brudzinski sign: flexion of legs if neck is passively flexed
  - ◊ In infants:
    - * Irritable
    - * Sleeping more than usual
    - * Cries when moved
    - * Cries inconsolably
- Viral
  - ◊ Headache
  - ◊ Fever
  - ◊ Stiff neck
  - ◊ Photophobia
  - ◊ Rash
  - ◊ Seizures
  - ◊ Illness lasts 2-6 days
- Fungal
  - ◊ Worsening headaches over a period of days
  - ◊ Vomiting for days or weeks

Positive Kernig and Brudzinski signs are highly suggestive of meningitis.

DIFFERENTIAL DIAGNOSIS

- Bacterial vs. viral vs. fungal vs. tuberculous meningitis
- Meningitis caused by other infectious agents (e.g., syphilis, ameba)
- Seizure disorder
- Encephalopathy
- Brain abscess

Viral meningitis is rarely seen in the elderly. Strongly consider other differential diagnoses in the elderly.

DIAGNOSTIC STUDIES

- Lumbar puncture: cerebrospinal fluid (CSF) may be turbid, presence of WBCs, elevated protein levels
- CSF: decreased glucose if bacterial
- CSF Gram stain and cultures: presence of infectious agent
- CBC: elevated WBC
- Blood cultures: positive in 80% of bacterial meningitis patients
- Consider CT/MRI

PREVENTION

- Strict aseptic technique during neurosurgical dressing changes
- Treat URI infections promptly
- Administer meningococcal immunization as part of routine immunizations

NONPHARMACOLOGIC MANAGEMENT

- Vigorous supportive care
- Measures to prevent dehydration
- Good handwashing
- Anticipatory guidance for family

PHARMACOLOGIC MANAGEMENT

- Antibiotic specific for culture if available
- Empiric treatment with ampicillin PLUS third-generation cephalosporin; may need to add aminoglycoside

- Dexamethasone: may decrease morbidity and mortality
- Antipyretics
- Analgesics for headache
- Antiemetics
- Antiviral agents not recommended

Depending on etiology: prophylaxis for contacts.

CONSULTATION/REFERRAL

- Refer to emergency department/neurologist immediately

FOLLOW-UP

- Depends on severity

EXPECTED COURSE

- Bacterial
  - ◊ Overall fatality is 14%
  - ◊ Afebrile by 7-10 days
  - ◊ Headache and other symptoms may persist intermittently for 2 weeks
- Viral
  - ◊ Recovery in 2-7 days
  - ◊ Headache and other symptoms may persist intermittently for 2 weeks
- Fungal
  - ◊ poor prognosis usually related to overall health of patient

POSSIBLE COMPLICATIONS

- Seizures (common in bacterial meningitis, rare in viral)
- Unresolved neurologic deficits
- Sensorineural hearing loss
- Irritability
- Hydrocephaly

MULTIPLE SCLEROSIS
(MS)

DESCRIPTION

A disease of the central nervous system (CNS) which is slow and progressive. It is characterized by demyelination of nerve cells in the brain and spinal cord which produces a variety of neurologic deficits.

ETIOLOGY

- Cause is unknown
  - ◊ Viral origin: supported by clusters in families, geographical clusters of cases
  - ◊ Immunologic: supported by presence of immunocytes in plaques
  - ◊ Environmental: supported by higher incidence in colder climates

INCIDENCE

- Age at onset 16-40 years
- Female > Male
- Approximately 25,000 new cases each year

RISK FACTORS

- Family history
- Northern European descent

ASSESSMENT FINDINGS

- Any of the following findings may present at various times during the illness
- Onset is insidious. Complaints may be present for months or years before diagnosis made
- CNS complaints are intermittent with remissions and exacerbations. May be minor complaints or may be incapacitating
- Paresthesias in extremities, weakness or clumsiness of a hand or leg
- Stiffness or unusual fatigability of a limb
- Transient blindness or pain in an eye
- Nystagmus common

- Speech may be slow with hesitancy at beginning of word (scanning speech)
- Mild emotional disturbances (e.g., apathy, lack of judgment, emotional lability) may be due to scattered CNS involvement
- Difficulty with bladder control (e.g., urgency, hesitancy, incontinence) may be present
- Deep tendon reflexes increased; superficial reflexes diminished
- Charcot's triad (i.e., scanning speech, nystagmus, tremor) common in later stages of disease

DIFFERENTIAL DIAGNOSIS

- Spinal cord or brain stem tumors
- Amyotrophic lateral sclerosis (ALS)
- CNS infections
- Compressed/ruptured intervertebral disk
- Multiple cerebral infarcts
- Inflammatory: SLE, Sjogrens, Behcet's disease, vasculitis, sarcoidosis, celiac disease
- Neoplasms, lymphoma

DIAGNOSTIC STUDIES

- No specific test confirms diagnosis
- Diagnosis is from clinical exam and laboratory findings
- CSF: demonstrates total elevated IgG; protein and lymphocytes may be elevated
- Evoked potentials: recorded electrical responses to stimulation of a sensory system are abnormal in 75-97% of cases. May be an early finding
- MRI (preferred) or CT: most sensitive technique; may show plaques or demyelination
- Syphilis serology: used to exclude this diagnosis
- With initial diagnosis, get CBC, Chemistry-7, liver function, ANA, ESR, thyroid function tests, vitamin B12 level

NONPHARMACOLOGIC MANAGEMENT

- Avoid factors which precipitate attack (e.g., hot weather, fatigue)
- Attempt to maintain as much patient independence as long as possible
- Extensive patient and family education regarding nature of disease
- Emotional support from family, health care provider
- Monitor for depression
- Occupational, physical therapy to help maintain range of motion, muscle flexibility, etc.
- Massage and passive movement of spastic limbs
- Teach self-catheterization if urinary retention is a problem
- High fiber diet to prevent constipation
- Possible custodial care for severe physical or cognitive impairments

PHARMACOLOGIC MANAGEMENT

- Goals of pharmacologic treatment are to slow disease progression, improve symptoms and decrease relapses. No current therapy is completely effective
- Immune modulators are helpful in suppressing the inflammatory effect of MS (Avonex®, Betaseron®, Copaxone®)
- Some medications are used to manage symptoms: antispasmodics for spasticity; NSAIDs, gabapentin, others for pain; anticholinergics for bladder dysfunction, incontinence; stool softeners, fiber for constipation; antidepressants for depression and emotional lability; others

PREGNANCY/LACTATION CONSIDERATIONS

- May be a triggering factor

CONSULTATION/REFERRAL

- Consult neurologist for suspected initial diagnosis and long-term management plan
- Physical, occupational therapy

Patients with MS should receive care from a neurologist.

FOLLOW-UP

- Depends on severity and frequency of exacerbations

EXPECTED COURSE

- Highly variable and unpredictable
- May have frequent exacerbations and remissions
- About 70% of patients lead very active lives but should avoid extreme fatigue
- Average illness lasts greater than 25 years

POSSIBLE COMPLICATIONS

- Urinary tract infections
- Depression
- Sexual impotence
- Decubitus ulcers if bedridden

- Severe depression
- Coma
- Optic nerve atrophy
- Paraplegia

PARKINSON'S DISEASE

DESCRIPTION

Idiopathic, neurodegenerative movement disorder characterized by 4 prominent features:
- Bradykinesia
- Muscular rigidity
- Resting tremor
- Postural instability

Diagnosis of PD supported by therapeutic response to levodopa.

ETIOLOGY

- There is a gradual loss of neurons in the substantia nigra which results in a decrease in production of the neurotransmitter dopamine

INCIDENCE

- 50,000 cases annually in U.S.
- Males > Females (1.4:1)
- Mean age of onset is 60 years
- Onset in childhood or adolescence is rare

RISK FACTORS

- Family history
- Ingestion of toxins, drugs, may produce a secondary Parkinson's disease

ASSESSMENT FINDINGS

- "Pill-rolling" tremor is presenting sign of 50-80% of patients (30% do not present with tremor)
- Tremor is maximal at rest, minimal with activity, and absent during sleep
- Bradykinesia (movement initiation is difficult for patient): often the most disabling symptom and must be present for diagnosis
- Cogwheel rigidity with tremor
- Stooped posture
- Gait disturbances evidenced by shuffling with short steps and lack of arm swinging
- Steps may become quickened to keep from falling (festination)
- Loss of postural reflexes results in tendency to fall forward or backward
- Face becomes mask-like and there is decreased blinking in later stages
- Seborrhea
- Constipation, incontinence, sexual dysfunction
- Drooling from inability to swallow in later stages
- Dysphonia
- Depression

A patient who presents with tremor at rest, rigidity, and bradykinesia should be suspected of having Parkinson's disease.

DIFFERENTIAL DIAGNOSIS

- Benign essential tremor
- Other movement disorders
- Parkinson's disease from secondary causes (e.g., side effects from neuroleptic medications)

Benign essential tremor is relieved by alcohol ingestion and usually associated with a positive family history.

DIAGNOSTIC STUDIES

- CT or MRI can eliminate other causes of symptoms (e.g., brain tumor)

PREVENTION

- See *Risk Factors*

NONPHARMACOLOGIC MANAGEMENT

- Patient and family education
- Anticipatory guidance regarding progression of disease
- Encourage compliance with medication
- Physical, occupational, and speech therapy
- Adjustments in home environment to accommodate physical limitations (e.g., elevated toilet seat, elimination of floor objects which would increase likelihood of falls, elevated chair, elimination of stairs when possible, wheel chair ramp for later stages of disease)

PARKINSON'S DISEASE PHARMACOLOGIC MANAGEMENT

Class	Drug Generic name (Trade name®)	Dosage How supplied	Comments
Dopamine Agonists *Directly activates dopamine receptors in the striatum* **General comments** First line therapy in Parkinson's disease Associated with serious effects, especially hallucinations, day time sleepiness and postural hypotension More commonly used in younger patients due to side effects	**amantadine**	**Used as Monotherapy** **Adult:** *Initial*: 100 mg twice daily *Usual*: 100 mg twice daily *Max*: 200 mg twice daily **Used with Levodopa** **Adult:** *Initial*: 100 mg twice daily *Usual*: 100 mg twice daily *Max*: 100 mg twice daily	• Pregnancy Category C • Reduce dose in patients with chronic heart failure, edema, hypotension, or impaired renal function, impaired hepatic function • Increases risk of melanoma • May cause blurry vision • May impair mental activity • Avoid alcohol usage
	Symmetrel	*Tab: 100 mg;* *Syrup: 50 mg/5mL*	
	pramipexole	**Immediate Release** **Normal Renal Function** **Adult:** Week 1: 0.125 mg TID Week 2: 0.25 mg TID Week 3: 0.5 mg TID Week 4: 0.75 mg TID Week 5: 1 mg TID Week 6: 1.25 mg TID Week 7: 1.50 mg TID	
		Adult: **Impaired Renal Function** *Mildly*: 0.125 mg TID *Moderately*: 0.125 mg BID *Severely*: 0.125 daily **Dialysis**: Avoid	• Pregnancy Category C • May cause sudden drowsiness and falling asleep, even while engaging in activities of daily living • May cause orthostatic hypotension • Adjust dose in impaired renal function • Side effects may include dyskinesia, hallucinations

continued

PARKINSON'S DISEASE PHARMACOLOGIC MANAGEMENT

Class	Drug Generic name (Trade name®)	Dosage How supplied	Comments
		Extended Release **Adult:** 0.375 mg daily; may increase after 5-7 days to 0.75 mg; and then by weekly increments 0.75 mg until maximum of 4.5 mg/day	• Do not crush or chew ER tablets • Avoid ER formulations with impaired renal function patients • Can switch between Immediate release and Extended Release on a mg for mg basis
	Mirapex	*Tabs: 0.125 mg, 0.25 mg, 0.5 mg, 0.75 mg, 1 mg, 1.5 mg*	
	Mirapex ER	*Ext. Rel. Tabs: 0.375 mg, 0.75 mg, 1.5 mg, 3 mg, 4.5 mg*	
	ropinirole	**Immediate Release** **Adult**: Week 1: 0.25 mg three times daily Week 2: 0.50 mg three times daily Week 3: 0.75 mg three times daily Week 4: 1 mg three times daily **Extended Release** 2 mg once daily for 14 days; then increase by 2 mg/day at 7 day intervals until max dose of 24 mg/day	• Pregnancy Category C • May be taken without regard to meal • If drug is to be discontinued, should be tapered • May cause sudden drowsiness and falling asleep, even while engage in activities of daily living • May cause hypotension, dyskinesia • See package inserts for conversion from immediate release to extended release conversions
	Requip	*Tabs: 0.25 mg, 0.5 mg, 1 mg*	
	Requip XL	*Ext. Rel. Tabs: 2 mg, 4 mg, 8 mg*	
Dopaminergic Agents	**carbidopa/levodopa**	**1:4 ratio (Preferred)** **Adult:** 25/100 three times a day, may increase by one tablet every day or every other day until 8 tablets of 25/100 is reached **1:10 ratio (Less effective)** 10/100 tablet three or four times a day. May increase by one tablet every day or every other day until two tablets four times a day is reached	• Pregnancy Category C • Must discontinue levodopa at least 12 hours before starting carbidopa/levodopa • May cause dyskinesias, mental disturbances, hypotension • Note dose ratios • Avoid abrupt cessation of CR formulations

continued

PARKINSON'S DISEASE PHARMACOLOGIC MANAGEMENT

Class	Drug Generic name (Trade name®)	Dosage How supplied	Comments
	Sinemet	*Tabs: 25/100, 10/100, 25/250*	
	Sinemet CR	*Ext. Rel. Tabs: 50/100, 25/100*	
MAO Inhibitors *inhibit the breakdown of dopamine in the brain and prolongs the action of levodopa*	**selegiline** Eldepryl	**Adult**: 5 mg twice daily *Caps: 5 mg* *Tabs: 5 mg*	• Pregnancy Category C • Used as adjunct therapy with levodopa/carbidopa • May reduce dose of levodopa/carbidopa as tolerated • May cause dry mouth, blurred vision, hypotension

A sudden worsening in the patient's status may indicate depression or non-compliance with medication.

CONSULTATION/REFERRAL

- Consult neurologist for Parkinson's disease
- Allied health professionals: physical, occupational, and speech therapy
- Support groups

FOLLOW-UP

- Lifelong follow-up and medication adjustment will be needed

EXPECTED COURSE

- Chronic and progressive neurological disorder

POSSIBLE COMPLICATIONS

- Multiple falls
- Aspiration pneumonia
- Dementia
- Depression
- Accidents from falls

ALZHEIMER'S DISEASE

DESCRIPTION

The permanent or progressive decline in the intellectual functioning of a person that substantially interferes with his social and/or economic welfare. The decline in functioning is due to damage to the hippocampus, amygdala, or other areas of the brain.

INCIDENCE

- 50% of Alzheimer's patients have a family history of Alzheimer's disease
- 40% of all patients over 85 years are affected
- Usually occurs after age 60

RISK FACTORS

- Aging
- Smoking (2-4x increase)
- Genetic markers on Chromosomes 1, 12, 14, 19, 21
- Family history

ASSESSMENT FINDINGS

- Recent memory loss (early finding)
- Impaired judgment, abstract thinking, memory, reasoning, orientation, attention
- Difficulty with speech and other forms of communication
- Inability to interpret sounds, speech, and use of objects
- Arousal disturbances: insomnia, daytime sleepiness
- Hyperactivity, wandering, restlessness
- Mood disturbances and emotional outbursts
- Urinary and/or fecal incontinence
- Paranoia, hallucinations, delusions (late findings)

DIFFERENTIAL DIAGNOSIS

- Normal aging process
- Hypothyroidism
- Depression
- Brain tumor
- Alcoholism
- Metabolic abnormalities
- Schizophrenia
- Delirium
- Other neurological conditions
- Side effects from medications

DIAGNOSTIC STUDIES

- To rule out reversible causes:
  - ◊ CBC
  - ◊ Electrolytes
  - ◊ Complete metabolic panel to include BUN, creatinine
  - ◊ Urinalysis
  - ◊ Liver function tests
  - ◊ Thyroid function tests
  - ◊ Vitamin B12 and folate levels
  - ◊ Syphilis serology
  - ◊ Consider CT or MRI
  - ◊ Others by history
- Mini Mental State Exam

PREVENTION

- None at this time

NONPHARMACOLOGIC MANAGEMENT

- Maintain routine and familiar environment for patient
- Attempt to maintain nutritional status by offering and encouraging regular meals of high nutritive value
- Display family pictures, calendars, clocks in prominent places
- Provide as much "accident-proofing" in the living environment as possible
- Emotional support and encouragement to family members
- Respite care for the caregivers
- Discuss advanced directives with family
- Offer information on support group for family

ALZHEIMER'S DISEASE PHARMACOLOGIC MANAGEMENT

Class	Drug Generic name (Trade name®)	Dosage How supplied	Comments
Cholinesterase Inhibitors *Prevents breakdown of acetylcholine by acetylcholinesterase, thereby increasing the availability of acetylcholine at cholinergic synapses* **General comments** These products have potential to demonstrate vagotonic effects on cardiac conduction If patient to have surgery, must notify anesthesia provider and seek guidance for holding medication Dose escalations are based upon assessment of clinical benefit	*donepezil*	**Mild to Moderate Disease** **Adult:** *Initial*: 5 mg nightly *Max*: 10 mg nightly **Moderate to Severe Disease** **Adult**: *Initial*: 10 mg nightly *Max*: 23 mg nightly	• Pregnancy Category C • Take at bedtime, without regard to food • Do not split, crush, or chew 23 mg strength tablet • Higher doses associated with weight loss • Monitor for gastrointestinal bleeding • Use higher dose with caution in low body weight patients
	Aricept	*Tabs: 5 mg, 10 mg, 23 mg*	
	Aricept ODT	*Oral Disolve Tabs: 5 mg, 10 mg*	
	galantamine	**Immediate Release Dose** **Adult:** *Initial*: 4 mg twice daily, increase after 4 weeks to 8 mg twice daily; may increase after 4 weeks to 12 mg twice daily *Max*: 24 mg/day **Extended Release Dose** **Adult:** *Initial*: 8 mg/day, increase after 4 weeks to 16 mg/day, increase after 4 weeks to 24 mg/day *Max*: 24 mg/day	• Pregnancy Category B • Carries indication for treatment of mild to moderate dementia • Note various dosage forms • Immediate release dose should be taken with meals and maintain adequate hydration • Extended release dose should be given in AM • Do not exceed 16 mg/day in patients with renal impairment • Avoid in patients with hepatic impairment • Use caution if patient has asthma or chronic pulmonary disease • Dose increases are based upon assessment of clinical benefit
	Razadyne	*Tabs: 4 mg, 8 mg, 12 mg* *Ext. Rel. Caps: 8 mg, 16 mg, 24 mg*	
	rivastigmine	**Adult**: *Initial*: 1.5 mg twice daily, may increase after 2 weeks to 3 mg twice daily. Subsequent dose adjustments after 2 weeks to 4.5 mg twice daily then to 6 mg twice daily *Max*: 6 mg twice daily	• Pregnancy Category B • Carries indication for treatment of mild to moderate dementia • Associated with warnings of gastrointestinal adverse reactions • If treatment interrupted, must resume at lower dose • Dose with morning and evening meals
	Exelon	*Caps: 1.5 mg, 3 mg, 4.5 mg, 6 mg*	

continued

ALZHEIMER'S DISEASE PHARMACOLOGIC MANAGEMENT

Class	Drug Generic name (Trade name®)	Dosage How supplied	Comments
NMDA (N-methyl-D-aspartate) receptor antagonist General comments Dose escalations are based upon assessment of clinical benefit	**memantine**	**Adult:** *Initial*: 5 mg once daily, may increase after 7 days to 5 mg twice daily. After 7 days increase to 5 mg AM and 10 mg PM dose (total 15), after 7 days may increase to 10 mg twice daily *Max*: 10 mg twice daily	• Pregnancy Category B • Indicated for moderate to severe dementia • May be taken without regard to meals • For significant renal impairment, max dose is 5 mg twice daily
	Namenda	*Tabs: 5 mg, 10 mg* *Soln: 2 mg/mL*	

Depression develops in 33% of patients who are diagnosed with AD; therefore, remain alert for symptoms. Start treatment at low doses.

CONSULTATION/REFERRAL

- Consult neurologist for new-onset dementia
- Consult social services as needed for family
- Other consults as needed

FOLLOW-UP

- Depends on severity
- Periodic follow-up needed to assess rate of decline, predict prognosis, and assess caregiver coping

EXPECTED COURSE

- Alzheimer's disease: variable rates of progression
- Average survival after diagnosis is 7-9 years

POSSIBLE COMPLICATIONS

- Accidents
- Malnutrition
- Caregiver exhaustion

ATTENTION DEFICIT DISORDER (ADD)
ATTENTION DEFICIT HYPERACTIVITY DISORDER (ADHD)

DESCRIPTION

Developmental disorder characterized by shortened attention span, impulsivity, and distractibility. Hyperactivity may or may not be present. When it is present, it is termed attention deficit hyperactivity disorder (ADHD).

ETIOLOGY

- Unknown
- Many factors seem to contribute: behavioral, biochemical, physiologic, and sensory and motor influences

INCIDENCE

- Estimated to affect 5-10% of school aged children
- Males > Females (5:1)
- Onset < 7 year of age
- Exists in adolescence and adulthood

RISK FACTORS

- Family history
- Possible association with poor prenatal health (e.g., alcohol or drug abuse, smoking, pre-eclampsia)

ASSESSMENT FINDINGS

- DSM-IV Criteria: symptoms must be present by age 7, last > 6 months, and be evident in 2 different settings (home, school)

ADHD **(hyperactivity with inattention)** *6 or more of the following must be present for diagnosis:*
◊ Fidgets, squirms, restless ◊ Difficulty remaining in seat ◊ Excessive activity ◊ Quiet play is difficult for child ◊ Acts as if "motorized" ◊ Excessive talking ◊ Impatient when forced to wait for turn ◊ Blurts out answers to questions before time ◊ Interrupts conversation

Note: Adapted from DSM-IV, 1994.

ADD **(Inattention)** *6 or more must be present for diagnosis:*
◊ Realizes careless mistakes when pointed out ◊ Exhibits difficulty maintaining attention ◊ Difficulty listening ◊ Does not finish tasks ◊ Organization skills are poor ◊ Tasks requiring sustained attention are difficult ◊ Forgetful ◊ Loses items (shoes, socks, school assignment) ◊ Easily distracted

Note: Adapted from DSM-IV, 1994.

DIFFERENTIAL DIAGNOSIS

- Learning disability
- Hearing/vision disorder
- Dysfunctional family situation
- Conduct disorder
- Poor parenting
- Inappropriate discipline
- Medication reaction (e.g., decongestants)
- Absence seizures

DIAGNOSTIC STUDIES

- Diagnosis by DSM-IV criteria
- Other studies may be done to rule out other diagnoses, but no test is diagnostic

NONPHARMACOLOGIC MANAGEMENT

- Parent/teacher/patient education
- No dietary eliminations or additions are known to help. Some benefit may be gained for individual patients with elimination of sugar, dyes, and some additives
- Educate parents about disorder
- Reinforce good behavior
- Singular task requests are more likely to be completed than multiple task requests
- Make eye contact when assigning tasks
- Time out
- Stop dangerous and threatening behavior before it reaches unmanageable levels
- Educate parents about risks and benefits of drug therapy
- Immediate consequences for broken rules
- Close monitoring of school activities and consistent reinforcement
- Education and support groups for parents and teachers

PHARMACOLOGIC MANAGEMENT

- 6 broad classes of agents are used to treat ADD/ADHD: methylphenidate, dextroamphetamine, lisdexamfetamine, dexmethylphenidate, atomoxetine, mixed dextroamphetamine/amphetamine salts
- Prescribers must conform to state's prescribing laws
- Potential for abuse and addiction
- May exacerbate pre-existing psychiatric illnesses
- Use in caution in patients with seizure disorder

PREGNANCY/LACTATION CONSIDERATIONS

- Avoid stimulant medications during pregnancy

CONSULTATION/REFERRAL

- Refer to personnel who can perform a psychometric evaluation for diagnosis
- Refer to neurologist if poor response to medication

FOLLOW-UP

- Close phone contact during initial and subsequent titration periods
- Monthly, quarterly, or every 6 months depending on severity and response
- Provide parents and teachers with regular support and encouragement
- Consult teachers regarding effectiveness of therapy
- Monitor growth and blood pressure, CBC periodically

EXPECTED COURSE

- More easily controlled as patient ages
- May last into and through adulthood

POSSIBLE COMPLICATIONS

- Children are at increased risk for abuse, social isolation, and depression
- Poor self-esteem and diminished self-confidence
- Failure in school

BELL'S PALSY
(Idiopathic Facial Paralysis)

DESCRIPTION

Facial nerve (Cranial Nerve VII) weakness or paralysis usually unilateral and idiopathic.

ETIOLOGY

- Idiopathic
- Viral
- Exposure to cold
- Facial trauma causing inflammation of the facial canal (as in herpes zoster lesions)
- Can be a manifestation of Lyme disease

INCIDENCE

- 16 per 100,000 people in U.S.
- Age > 30 years
- Males = Females

RISK FACTORS

- Lyme Disease
- 3rd trimester of pregnancy
- Family history
- Diabetes mellitus
- Herpes zoster

ASSESSMENT FINDINGS

- Numbness on affected side
- Sagging of eyebrow
- Mouth drawn to affected side
- Partial or total paralysis of facial muscles
- Hypersensitivity to sound
- Excessive tearing
- Inadequate tearing
- Ipsilateral loss of taste
- Ipsilateral ear pain, cheek pain
- Loss of nasolabial fold

DIFFERENTIAL DIAGNOSIS

- Stroke
- Lyme Disease
- Tumor
- Trauma
- Otitis media

DIAGNOSTIC STUDIES

- Usually diagnosed on clinical symptoms unless diagnosis is questionable
- Lyme titer if history of tick bite
- CT to rule out stroke or neoplasm
- Electromyographic (EMG) testing

PREVENTION

- None
- See *Risk Factors*

NONPHARMACOLOGIC MANAGEMENT

- Patient education regarding condition, expected outcomes, management
- Eyedrops to maintain lubrication (if inadequate tearing)
- Close and patch affected eye (especially at night)
- Warm, moist heat to affected side of face

PHARMACOLOGIC MANAGEMENT

- Tapered dosage of corticosteroids (must be initiated within 4 days of onset or corticosteroids are of little benefit)
- 80 mg prednisone daily for 3 days, then 60 mg daily for 3 days, then 40 mg daily for 3 days, then 20 mg daily for 3 days
- Oral antiviral agents (acyclovir, famciclovir, valacyclovir) in conjunction with oral steroids found to be more beneficial than steroid alone

PREGNANCY/LACTATION CONSIDERATIONS

- Cautious use of steroids in pregnancy

CONSULTATION/REFERRAL

- Obstetrician for pregnant patients
- Refer to neurologist for serious comorbid conditions
- Ophthalmologist for actual or suspected corneal abrasions

FOLLOW-UP

- Re-evaluate in 3-5 days, then 2-4 weeks until resolved

EXPECTED COURSE

- Usually complete or partial recovery

POSSIBLE COMPLICATIONS

- Emergence of a subclinical infection from high dose steroid
- Corneal abrasion or ulceration if unable to blink eye

CARPAL TUNNEL SYNDROME

DESCRIPTION

Entrapment neuropathy of the median nerve at the wrist due to inflammation of wrist tendons, transverse carpal ligament, and/or surrounding soft tissue.

This is also called "wake and shake syndrome".

ETIOLOGY

- The median nerve is entrapped or compressed as it passes through a tunnel composed of the carpal bones and the transverse carpal ligament
- Any condition that results in edema may precipitate carpal tunnel syndrome (CTS)

INCIDENCE

- Common
- Females > Males (3-10:1)
- Predominant age is 40 to 60 years

RISK FACTORS

- Repetitive flexion, pronation, and supination of the wrist
- Tenosynovitis of the flexor tendons of the fingers
- Local trauma
- Prolonged improper positioning
- Weight gain
- Pregnancy or premenstrual edema
- Arthritis
- Hypothyroidism

ASSESSMENT FINDINGS

- Median paresthesias affecting the thumb, index finger, middle finger, and radial side of the ring finger
- Nocturnal paresthesias
- Positive Phalen's test
    - ◊ Hold flexed fingers against each other with wrists flexed at a 90° angle for 60 seconds
    - ◊ Considered positive if paresthesia occurs
    - ◊ Not highly sensitive
- Positive Tinel's test
    - ◊ Percuss over the median nerve on the volar aspect of the wrist
    - ◊ Considered positive if paresthesia occurs
    - ◊ Not highly sensitive
- Dull, aching sensation in hand, wrist, forearm, or upper arm
- Weakness and sensory loss, dropping objects from affected hand
- Affected hand may be cool to touch, pale in color, with dry skin
- Atrophy of thenar muscle

A blood pressure cuff blown up on the affected arm may precipitate symptoms.

DIFFERENTIAL DIAGNOSIS

- De Quervain's disease
- Cervical radiculopathy
- Lesion of the brachial plexus
- Peripheral neuropathy
- Thoracic outlet syndrome
- Multiple sclerosis

- CVA

DIAGNOSTIC STUDIES

- Nerve conduction studies of the median nerve: delayed latency across the wrist confirms diagnosis
- Consider EMG especially if nerve conduction studies are negative

PREVENTION

- Frequent rest periods when repetitive wrist motions are performed
- Proper hand/wrist positioning

NONPHARMACOLOGIC MANAGEMENT

- Correct underlying disorder
- Avoid aggravating factors
- Splinting of wrists in extension
- Surgical decompression of the carpal tunnel with release of the transverse carpal ligament and debridement

PHARMACOLOGIC MANAGEMENT

- Nonsteroidal anti-inflammatory agents in doses sufficient for anti-inflammatory effect
- Local anesthetic and hydrocortisone injection provides temporary relief (40 mg Medrol and 1% lidocaine)

PREGNANCY/LACTATION CONSIDERATIONS

- Pregnancy is a risk factor due to edema
- Local injection of anesthetic and hydrocortisone useful during pregnancy

CONSULTATION/REFERRAL

- Surgeon if severe or persistent despite conservative therapy

FOLLOW-UP

- Evaluate effect of conservative therapy (i.e., splints, NSAIDs and cortisone injections)
- Postoperative evaluation by surgeon

EXPECTED COURSE

- If untreated, there is a risk of permanent loss of function of affected hand
- Recurrence likely with nonsurgical interventions
- Recurrence is unusual following surgery

POSSIBLE COMPLICATIONS

- Postoperative infection
- Surgical complications
- Permanent damage from prolonged median nerve compression

References

Adelman, A. M., & Daly, M. P. (2005). Initial evaluation of the patient with suspected dementia. American Family Physician, 71(9), 1745-1750.

American Academy of Pediatrics. (2009). Red book: 2009 report of the committee on infectious diseases (28th ed.). Elk Grove Village, IL: American Academy of Pediatrics.

American Psychiatric Association. (2000a). Diagnostic and statistical manual of mental disorders (4th ed.). Washington, DC: American Psychiatric Association.

American Psychiatric Association. (2000b). Diagnostic and statistical manual of mental disorders Attention-deficit and disruptive behavior disorders (4th ed.). Washington, DC: American Psychiatric Association.

Ashraf, A. R., Jali, R., Moghtaderi, A. R., & Yazdani, A. H. (2009). The diagnostic value of ultrasonography in patients with electrophysiologicaly confirmed carpal tunnel syndrome. Electromyography and Clinical Neurophysiology, 49(1), 3-8.

Barone, P., Antonini, A., Colosimo, C., Marconi, R., Morgante, L., Avarello, T. P., . . . Dotto, P. D. (2009). The priamo study: A multicenter assessment of nonmotor symptoms and their impact on quality of life in parkinson's disease. Movement Disorders, 24(11), 1641-1649. doi: 10.1002/mds.22643

Beghi, E., Carpio, A., Forsgren, L., Hesdorffer, D. C., Malmgren, K., Sander, J. W., . . . Hauser, W. A. (2010). Recommendation for a definition of acute symptomatic seizure. Epilepsia, 51(4), 671-675. doi: 10.1111/j.1528-1167.2009.02285.x

Benditt, D. G. (2006). Syncope management guidelines at work: First steps towards assessing clinical utility. European Heart Journal, 27(1), 7-9. doi: 10.1093/eurheartj/ehi626

Bennetto, L., Patel, N. K., & Fuller, G. (2007). Trigeminal neuralgia and its management. BMJ, 334(7586), 201-205. doi: 10.1136/bmj.39085.614792.BE

Biederman, J., Petty, C. R., Evans, M., Small, J., & Faraone, S. V. (2010). How persistent is adhd? A controlled 10-year follow-up study of boys with adhd. Psychiatry Research, 177(3), 299-304. doi: 10.1016/j.psychres.2009.12.010

Bland, J. D. (2007). Carpal tunnel syndrome. BMJ, 335(7615), 343-346. doi: 10.1136/bmj.39282.623553.AD

Busse, A., Hensel, A., Guhne, U., Angermeyer, M. C., & Riedel-Heller, S. G. (2006). Mild cognitive impairment: Long-term course of four clinical subtypes. Neurology, 67(12), 2176-2185. doi: 10.1212/01.wnl.0000249117.23318.e1

Chung, B., & Wong, V. (2007). Relationship between five common viruses and febrile seizure in children. Archives of Disease in Childhood, 92(7), 589-593. doi: 10.1136/adc.2006.110221

Compston, A., & Coles, A. (2008). Multiple sclerosis. Lancet, 372(9648), 1502-1517. doi: 10.1016/S0140-6736(08)61620-7

de Almeida, J. R., Al Khabori, M., Guyatt, G. H., Witterick, I. J., Lin, V. Y., Nedzelski, J. M., & Chen, J. M. (2009). Combined corticosteroid and antiviral treatment for bell palsy: A systematic review and meta-analysis. JAMA, 302(9), 985-993. doi: 10.1001/jama.2009.1243

De Jager, P. L., Jia, X., Wang, J., de Bakker, P. I., Ottoboni, L., Aggarwal, N. T., . . . Oksenberg, J. R. (2009). Meta-analysis of genome scans and replication identify cd6, irf8 and tnfrsf1a as new multiple sclerosis susceptibility loci. Nature Genetics, 41(7), 776-782. doi: 10.1038/ng.401

Denisco, S., Tiago, C., & Kravitz, C. (2005). Evaluation and treatment of pediatric adhd. Nurse Practitioner, 30(8), 14-17, 19-23; quiz 24-15. doi: 00006205-200508000-00004 [pii]

Domino, F., Baldor, R., Golding, J., Grimes, J., & Taylor, J. (2011). The 5-minute clinical consult 2011. Philadelphia: Lippincott Williams & Wilkins.

Drug facts and comparisons 2010. (2010). St. Louis: Wolters Kluwer Health.

Easton, J. D., Saver, J. L., Albers, G. W., Alberts, M. J., Chaturvedi, S., Feldmann, E., . . . Sacco, R. L. (2009). Definition and evaluation of transient ischemic attack: A scientific statement for healthcare professionals from the american heart association/american stroke association stroke council; council on cardiovascular surgery and anesthesia; council on cardiovascular radiology and intervention; council on cardiovascular nursing; and the interdisciplinary council on peripheral vascular disease. The american academy of neurology affirms the value of this statement as an educational tool for neurologists. Stroke, 40(6), 2276-2293. doi: 10.1161/STROKEAHA.108.192218

Ernst, D., & Lee, A. (2010). Nurse practitioners prescribing reference. New York: Haymarket Media Publication.

Febrile seizures: Clinical practice guideline for the long-term management of the child with simple febrile seizures. (2008). Pediatrics, 121(6), 1281-1286. doi: 10.1542/peds.2008-0939

Fitch, M. T., & van de Beek, D. (2007). Emergency diagnosis and treatment of adult meningitis. Lancet Infect Dis, 7(3), 191-200. doi: 10.1016/S1473-3099(07)70050-6

Gronseth, G., Cruccu, G., Alksne, J., Argoff, C., Brainin, M., Burchiel, K., . . . Zakrzewska, J. M. (2008). Practice parameter: The diagnostic evaluation and treatment of trigeminal neuralgia (an evidence-based review): Report of the quality standards subcommittee of the american academy of neurology and the european federation of neurological societies. Neurology, 71(15), 1183-1190. doi: 10.1212/01.wnl.0000326598.83183.04

Jain, S., Lo, S. E., & Louis, E. D. (2006). Common misdiagnosis of a common neurological disorder: How are we misdiagnosing essential tremor? Archives of Neurology, 63(8), 1100-1104. doi: 10.1001/archneur.63.8.1100

Koch-Henriksen, N., & Sorensen, P. S. (2010). The changing demographic pattern of multiple sclerosis epidemiology. Lancet Neurol, 9(5), 520-532. doi: 10.1016/S1474-4422(10)70064-8

Krumholz, A., Wiebe, S., Gronseth, G., Shinnar, S., Levisohn, P., Ting, T., . . . French, J. (2007). Practice parameter: Evaluating an apparent unprovoked first seizure in adults (an evidence-based review): Report of the quality standards subcommittee of the american academy of neurology and the american epilepsy society. Neurology, 69(21), 1996-2007. doi: 10.1212/01.wnl.0000285084.93652.43

Langston, J. W. (2006). The parkinson's complex: Parkinsonism is just the tip of the iceberg. Annals of Neurology, 59(4), 591-596. doi: 10.1002/ana.20834

Lim, S. Y., Fox, S. H., & Lang, A. E. (2009). Overview of the extranigral aspects of parkinson disease. Archives of Neurology, 66(2), 167-172. doi: 10.1001/archneurol.2008.561

Menactra: A meningococcal conjugate vaccine. (2005). Medical Letter on Drugs and Therapeutics, 47(1206), 29-31.

Muslimovic, D., Post, B., Speelman, J. D., Schmand, B., & de Haan, R. J. (2008). Determinants of disability and quality of life in mild to moderate parkinson disease. Neurology, 70(23), 2241-2247. doi: 10.1212/01.wnl.0000313835.33830.80

Obermann, M., Yoon, M. S., Ese, D., Maschke, M., Kaube, H., Diener, H. C., & Katsarava, Z. (2007). Impaired trigeminal nociceptive processing in patients with trigeminal neuralgia. Neurology, 69(9), 835-841. doi: 10.1212/01.wnl.0000269670.30045.6b

Ois, A., Gomis, M., Rodriguez-Campello, A., Cuadrado-Godia, E., Jimenez-Conde, J., Pont-Sunyer, C., . . . Roquer, J. (2008). Factors associated with a high risk of recurrence in patients with transient ischemic attack or minor stroke. Stroke, 39(6), 1717-1721. doi: 10.1161/STROKEAHA.107.505438

Ortega-Sanchez, I. R., Meltzer, M. I., Shepard, C., Zell, E., Messonnier, M. L., Bilukha, O., . . . Messonnier, N. E. (2008). Economics of an adolescent meningococcal conjugate vaccination catch-up campaign in the United States. Clinical Infectious Diseases, 46(1), 1-13. doi: 10.1086/524041

Pavlidou, E., Tzitiridou, M., Kontopoulos, E., & Panteliadis, C. P. (2008). Which factors determine febrile seizure recurrence? A prospective study. Brain and Development, 30(1), 7-13. doi: 10.1016/j.braindev.2007.05.001

Pliszka, S. (2007). Practice parameter for the assessment and treatment of children and adolescents with attention-deficit/hyperactivity disorder. Journal of the American Academy of Child and Adolescent Psychiatry, 46(7), 894-921. doi: 10.1097/chi.0b013e318054e724

Portet, F., Scarmeas, N., Cosentino, S., Helzner, E. P., & Stern, Y. (2009). Extrapyramidal signs before and after diagnosis of incident alzheimer disease in a prospective population study. Archives of Neurology, 66(9), 1120-1126. doi: 10.1001/archneurol.2009.196

Qaseem, A., Snow, V., Cross, J. T., Jr., Forciea, M. A., Hopkins, R., Jr., Shekelle, P., . . . Owens, D. K. (2008). Current pharmacologic treatment of dementia: A clinical practice guideline from the american college of physicians and the american academy of family physicians. Annals of Internal Medicine, 148(5), 370-378. doi: 148/5/370 [pii]

Recommended adult immunization schedule - United States, 2009. (2009). MMWR. Morbidity and Mortality Weekly Report, 57(53).

Revised recommendations of the advisory committee on immunization practices to vaccinate all persons aged 11-18 years with meningococcal conjugage vaccine. (2007). MMWR. Morbidity and Mortality Weekly Report, 56.

Roberts, R. O., Geda, Y. E., Knopman, D. S., Cha, R. H., Pankratz, V. S., Boeve, B. F., . . . Rocca, W. A. (2008). The mayo clinic study of aging: Design and sampling, participation, baseline measures and sample characteristics. Neuroepidemiology, 30(1), 58-69. doi: 10.1159/000115751

Sadleir, L. G., & Scheffer, I. E. (2007). Febrile seizures. BMJ, 334(7588), 307-311. doi: 10.1136/bmj.39087.691817.AE

Santiago-Rosado, L. (2005). Syncope: Step-by-step through the workup. Consultant, 45, 759-768.

Stowe, R. L., Ives, N. J., Clarke, C., van Hilten, J., Ferreira, J., Hawker, R. J., . . . Gray, R. (2008). Dopamine agonist therapy in early parkinson's disease. Cochrane Database Syst Rev(2), CD006564. doi: 10.1002/14651858.CD006564.pub2

Strickberger, S. A., Benson, D. W., Biaggioni, I., Callans, D. J., Cohen, M. I., Ellenbogen, K. A., . . . Sila, C. A. (2006). Aha/accf scientific statement on the evaluation of syncope: From the american heart association councils on clinical cardiology, cardiovascular nursing, cardiovascular disease in the young, and stroke, and the quality of care and outcomes research interdisciplinary working group; and the american college of cardiology foundation: In collaboration with the heart rhythm society: Endorsed by the american autonomic society. Circulation, 113(2), 316-327. doi: 10.1161/CIRCULATIONAHA.105.170274

Suchowersky, O., Reich, S., Perlmutter, J., Zesiewicz, T., Gronseth, G., & Weiner, W. J. (2006). Practice parameter: Diagnosis and prognosis of new onset parkinson disease (an evidence-based review): Report of the quality standards subcommittee of the american academy of neurology. Neurology, 66(7), 968-975. doi: 10.1212/01.wnl.0000215437.80053.d0

Thomas, K. E., Hasbun, R., Jekel, J., & Quagliarello, V. J. (2002). The diagnostic accuracy of kernig's sign, brudzinski's sign, and nuchal rigidity in adults with suspected meningitis. Clinical Infectious Diseases, 35(1), 46-52. doi: 10.1086/340979

Tolosa, E., Wenning, G., & Poewe, W. (2006). The diagnosis of parkinson's disease. Lancet Neurol, 5(1), 75-86. doi: 10.1016/S1474-4422(05)70285-4

Zoons, E., Weisfelt, M., de Gans, J., Spanjaard, L., Koelman, J. H., Reitsma, J. B., & van de Beek, D. (2008). Seizures in adults with bacterial meningitis. Neurology, 70(22 Pt 2), 2109-2115. doi: 10.1212/01.wnl.0000288178.91614.5d

12

OPHTHALMIC DISORDERS

Ophthalmic Disorders

Ocular Foreign Body....... 465

Corneal Abrasion 466

Ocular Chemical Burn 467

Hyphema....... 468

Conjunctivitis....... 469

* Neonatal Conjunctivitis....... 473

* Strabismus....... 474

Refractive Errors/Color Blindness 475

Cataract....... 476

Glaucoma....... 477

Chalazion 480

Blepharitis 481

* Dacryostenosis....... 483

References....... 484

* Denotes pediatric diagnosis

Ophthalmic Disorders

OCULAR FOREIGN BODY

DESCRIPTION

Presence of substance, material, objects adhering to the eye or penetrating trauma in the eye.

INCIDENCE

- Unknown

RISK FACTORS

- Improper use of protective eyewear
- Lack of protective eye wear

ASSESSMENT FINDINGS

- Feeling that "something is in my eye"
- Red eye
- Tearing
- Pain or photophobia
- Frequent eye rubbing
- Appearance of dark specks against the iris
- Corneal "rust ring" indicates steel or iron foreign body
- Fluorescein staining may also indicate corneal abrasion

Any patient with blood in the anterior chamber should be examined by an ophthalmologist the same day.

DIFFERENTIAL DIAGNOSIS

- Corneal abrasion, ulceration, or laceration
- Intraocular penetration of foreign body
- Herpes ulcers
- Glaucoma

DIAGNOSTIC STUDIES

- Assessment of visual acuity (e.g., Snellen chart)
- Examination with slit lamp or binocular loupe after Snellen examination
- Fluorescein staining is used to assess for corneal defects (should be done as last part of examination)
- Consider X-ray of orbits if history dictates
- May consider MRI if unable to locate foreign object, MRI contraindicated if metallic objects involved

PREVENTION

- Use of protective eyewear devices
- Use of protective eyewear during situations where it is reasonable to expect that eye injury might occur

NONPHARMACOLOGIC MANAGEMENT

- Removal of the foreign body/object/material if it is superficial and NOT impaled
- A patch or metal shield to protect the eye if object is visible in eye
- Keep patient NPO if patient is referred to ophthalmologist in case surgery is needed to remove impaled object
- Referral to ophthalmologist for follow-up
- Inspect entire eye for damage/additional foreign bodies

As a general rule, an eye patch has NOT been found to improve the rate of healing or comfort in patients with traumatic eye injuries.

PHARMACOLOGIC MANAGEMENT

- Antibiotic instillation
- Tetanus prophylaxis for penetrating eye injuries

Corticosteroids are CONTRAINDICATED because they may foster bacterial/fungal growth.

CONSULTATION/REFERRAL

- A penetrating injury is a medical emergency and must be referred immediately
- Referral to ophthalmologist for all but simple nonpenetrating injuries
- Referral after any eye injury if changes in visual acuity occur

FOLLOW-UP

- Depends on degree of injury

EXPECTED COURSE

- Depends on extent of injury

POSSIBLE COMPLICATIONS

- Secondary bacterial infection (endophthalmitis)
- Corneal abrasion
- Traumatic cataract due to foreign body induced shock wave or direct puncture of the lenticular capsule
- Glaucoma due to intraocular inflammation

CORNEAL ABRASION

DESCRIPTION

Complete or partial tear of the epithelium of the cornea.

ETIOLOGY

- Disruption of the outermost layer of the cornea, the epithelium, by either chemical or mechanical means, including contact lens
- A good history is critical to help determine the etiology
- Contact lens induced roughing
- Damaged contact lens

INCIDENCE

- More common in young, active patients
- Common in contact lens wearers
- Uncommon in the elderly

Most abrasions are caused by fingernails, paws, tree branches, rust, wood, glass, and fiberglass.

ASSESSMENT FINDINGS

- Complaint of "gritty" feeling or "something" in eye
- Eye pain usually proportional to degree of epithelial damage
- Photophobia
- Constricted pupil
- Red eye
- May identify foreign body embedded in eye
- Lacrimation

Most common complaint of a patient with a corneal abrasion is excruciating eye pain and an inability to open the eye due to a foreign body sensation.

DIFFERENTIAL DIAGNOSIS

- Presence of foreign body
- Keratitis, uveitis, iritis
- Corneal ulceration

DIAGNOSTIC STUDIES

- Assess visual acuity: should be normal unless abrasion is large or affects the visual axis
- Fluorescein is instilled only after penlight and fundus exam (it is confirmatory, not diagnostic)
- Fluorescein staining to assess corneal integrity: fluorescein is instilled in the eye and areas of epithelial disruption will fluoresce green when exposed to a Wood's lamp

The eyelid should be flipped after abrasion is confirmed to rule out a foreign body under the lid.

PREVENTION

- Protective eye wear for potentially dangerous activities
- Contact lenses may provide some minor protection

NONPHARMACOLOGIC MANAGEMENT

- Evaluate for presence of foreign body
- Eye patch to protect eye not found to decrease pain or speed healing
- Use normal saline to irrigate eye

PHARMACOLOGIC MANAGEMENT

- Antibiotic ointment or drops for 5-7 days to prevent bacterial infection
- Analgesics for pain
- Topical anesthetic for evaluation but warn patient not to rub or touch eye until anesthetic effect resolves
- Tetanus prophylaxis

Ointment is better to instill in eye than drops because it acts as a lubricant and may help facilitate regeneration of epithelium.

CONSULTATION/REFERRAL

- Ophthalmologist if injury involved thermal or chemical materials; blunt or sharp objects, or penetration into the eye by any object
- Referral for any distortion of vision
- Refer any injury which does not improve in 24 hours

A corneal abrasion should never be treated with an ophthalmic steroid.

FOLLOW-UP

- 24 hours to assess healing and status
- Usually followed up daily by ophthalmologist
- Dependent on patient condition

EXPECTED COURSE

- Dependent on severity of injury

POSSIBLE COMPLICATIONS

- Loss of vision
- Widespread corneal roughing due to patient's attempts to remove
- Corneal erosion (recurrent roughness at site of original corneal injury)

OCULAR CHEMICAL BURN

DESCRIPTION

Introduction of an acidic or alkaline agent into the eye that results in damage to the eye or its outer structures. This is an ophthalmologic emergency.

ETIOLOGY

- Acidic and alkaline agents can both cause injury, but alkaline agents may be more destructive

INCIDENCE

- Unknown

RISK FACTORS

- Improper eye protection when handling potentially injurious products

ASSESSMENT FINDINGS

- Eye pain, burning, and distorted vision
- Decreased vision due to corneal roughing
- Photophobia
- Eyelid skin burns may be present

DIFFERENTIAL DIAGNOSIS

- Foreign object embedded in eye

DIAGNOSTIC STUDIES

- Defer pending ophthalmology evaluation

PREVENTION

- Protective eye equipment
- Tetanus prophylaxis

NONPHARMACOLOGIC MANAGEMENT

- Flush affected eye with 0.9% sodium chloride for 30 minutes; always irrigate away from unaffected eye
- Always inquire whether contact lenses are in use
- Immediate referral to ophthalmologist

PHARMACOLOGIC MANAGEMENT

- Consider analgesic for eye pain

CONSULTATION/REFERRAL

- Immediate referral to ophthalmologist

EXPECTED COURSE

- Depends on extent of injury

POSSIBLE COMPLICATIONS

- Loss of vision due to scarring
- Traumatic cataract formation
- Chronic ocular discomfort
- Symblepharon: adhesion between the conjunctiva of lid and the eyeball

HYPHEMA

DESCRIPTION

Hemorrhage into the anterior chamber of the eye as a result of iris or ciliary body rupture; may be spontaneous, but usually a result of trauma. This is an ophthalmologic emergency.

ETIOLOGY

- Usually results from a blunt or penetrating trauma to the eye

INCIDENCE

- Unknown

RISK FACTORS

- Blunt trauma to the eye
- Penetrating injury to the eye
- Hemophilia
- Diabetes
- Anticoagulant therapy

ASSESSMENT FINDINGS

- Blood in the anterior chamber
- Visible fluid line in the pupil

DIFFERENTIAL DIAGNOSIS

- Globe trauma
- Eye contusion
- Systemic disease (e.g., hemophilia, diabetes)

DIAGNOSTIC STUDIES

- Consider hematology studies (e.g., clotting factors) based on history and exam

PREVENTION

- Protective eye devices
- Control of diabetes and hemophilia

NONPHARMACOLOGIC MANAGEMENT

- Binocular bandaging
- Head elevated 30-40°
- Complete bedrest

PHARMACOLOGIC MANAGEMENT

- Do not administer any aspirin products, miotics, or mydriatics in the acute setting, however, mydriatics are commonly used by ophthalmologists

CONSULTATION/REFERRAL

- Immediate referral to ophthalmologist

EXPECTED COURSE

- Hospitalization often not necessary
- Hospitalization based on additional injuries (e.g., head trauma)
- Possible evacuation of blood by ophthalmologist

POSSIBLE COMPLICATIONS

- Recurrent bleeding and development of glaucoma
- Loss of vision possible due to corneal staining This potential complication is more likely in a total hyphema (complete filling of the anterior chamber, also referred to as an "8-ball hyphema")

CONJUNCTIVITIS
(Pink Eye)

DESCRIPTION

An inflammation or irritation of the conjunctiva.

ETIOLOGY

Causes of Conjunctivitis	
Bacterial	*Staphylococcus aureus* *Streptococcus pneumoniae* *Haemophilus influenza* *Pseudomonas sp.* (common in contact lens wearers) *Neisseria gonorrhoeae* *Neisseria meningitidis*
Viral	Adenovirus Coxsackie virus Herpes simplex
Chlamydial	*Chlamydia trachomatis*
Allergic	Environmental (trees, weeds, spores, pollen) Cosmetics
Chemical	Thimerosal Erythromycin Silver nitrate

INCIDENCE

- Very common

RISK FACTORS

- Bacterial or viral: contact lens use, rubbing eyes, contact with the infecting organism, trauma
- Allergic: wind exposure, contact with allergic substance, often with allergic rhinitis
- Chemical: exposure to irritating chemical substance

ASSESSMENT FINDINGS

- Conjunctival erythema
- Burning
- Profuse exudate
- Itching
- Sensation of foreign body
- Ocular exudate with matting, especially upon awakening
- Preauricular adenopathy
- Tearing
- Normal visual acuity

Assessment Findings	
Bacterial	Exudates, initially unilateral, then often bilateral
Viral	Profuse tearing, burning, concurrent upper respiratory infections
Chlamydial	Profuse exudate, associated genitourinary symptoms *Onset of symptoms*: 1-2 weeks after birth
Gonococcal	Profuse exudate, associated genitourinary symptoms *Onset of symptoms*: 2-4 days after birth
Allergic	Severe itching, tearing, sneezing & rhinitis
Chemical	Conjunctival erythema, conjunctival discharge *Onset of symptoms*: 30 minutes after prophylactic antibiotic drops; usually resolves by 48 hours

A sensation of having a foreign body in the eye is common with bacterial conjunctivitis.

DIFFERENTIAL DIAGNOSIS

- Foreign body
- Uveitis, iritis, scleritis
- Corneal abrasion
- Dacryocystitis

Conjunctivitis never accompanies a change in vision. If there is a change in vision with conjunctival symptoms, this is a red flag.

DIAGNOSTIC STUDIES

- Usually none
- Consider culture of exudates, but rarely indicated
- Immunofluorescence test for herpes simplex or chlamydia

PREVENTION

- See *Risk Factors*

NONPHARMACOLOGIC MANAGEMENT

- Good hand-eye hygiene (wash hands frequently to prevent spread to other eye)
- Use clean wash cloths each time face is washed
- Change pillowcase on bed daily until resolved (if bacterial or viral)
- Warm compresses if origin is infectious
- Cool compresses if origin is allergic or chemical
- Irrigation if chemical or allergic etiology
- Teach patient how to instill eye drops/ointment
- Do not wear contact lenses until conjunctival inflammation resolved (usually one week)
- Discard or disinfect contact lenses prior to wearing contact lenses again
- Discard any eye makeup, especially mascara
- Assess visual acuity
- Consider fluorescein staining

PHARMACOLOGIC MANAGEMENT

Agent	Treatment
Bacterial	Eyedrops or ointment: Tobramycin, gentamicin, sodium sulfacetamide, or ciprofloxacin
Viral	Trifluridine
Chlamydial	Oral doxycycline (Vibramycin®) (tetracyclines increase photosensitivity)
Allergic	Topical antihistamine, oral antihistamine, or topical vasoconstrictor (vasoconstrictors may mask severity), topical steroid*
Chemical	Avoid contact Usually none, but consider steroid use

**Cautious use of topical steroids*

CONJUNCTIVITIS PHARMACOLOGIC MANAGEMENT

Class	Drug Generic name (Trade name®)	Dosage How supplied	Comments
Topical Ophthalmic Antibiotics	**azithromycin**	**All patients**: One drop twice daily for two days then daily for additional 5 days	• Pregnancy Category B
General comments	Azasite	*Soln: 2.5 mL*	
Patients should be advised not to wear contact lens during acute infections Patients should be advised that ointments may cause blurry vision Ophthalmic ointments may retard corneal healing Overuse of these products may predispose patients to fungal infections	**blephamide**	**Adult:** 2 drops every four hours **Children < 6 yrs:** not recommended **> 6 yrs:** 2 drops every four hours	• Pregnancy Category C • Product indicated for short term use; if over 10 days, most measure ocular pressure
	Bleph 10	*Susp: 5 mL, 10 mL* *Oint: 3.5 g*	
	ciprofloxacin	**Adult:** 1-2 drops every two hours for 2 days; then 1-2 drops every 4 hours for 5 days (while awake) **Children < 1 yr:** not recommended **> 1 yr:** 1-2 drops every 2 hours for 2 days; then 1-2 drops every 4 hours for 5 days (while awake)	• Pregnancy Category C
	Ciloxan 0.3%	*Soln: 2.5 mL, 5 mL, 10 mL* *Oint: 3.5 g*	
	gatifloxacin	**Adult:** 1 drop every two hours for 2 days; then one drop 4 times daily for 5 days (while awake) **Children < 1 yr**: not recommended **> 1 yr:** 1 drop every 2 hours for 2 days; then 1 drop 4 times daily for 5 days (while awake)	• Pregnancy Category C
	Zymar	*Soln: 5 mL*	

continued

CONJUNCTIVITIS PHARMACOLOGIC MANAGEMENT

Class	Drug Generic name (Trade name®)	Dosage How supplied	Comments
	gentamicin	**Adult:** *Soln*: 1-2 gtt every 4-6 hours *Oint*: 1/2 inch in conjunctival sac; 2-3 times daily **Children:** not recommended	• Pregnancy Category C
	Genoptic various generics	*Soln: 2.5 mL,* *15 mL* *Oint: 3.5 g*	
	levofloxacin	**Adult**: 1-2 drops every 2 hours while awake for 2 days; then 1-2 drops 4 times a day for 3-7 days **Children < 1 yr**: not recommended **> 1 yr:** 1-2 drops every 2 hours while awake for 2 days; then 1-2 drops 4 times a day for 3-7 days	• Pregnancy Category C • Has been associated with ocular burning sensation, photophobia
	Quixin	*Soln: 5 mL*	

PREGNANCY/LACTATION CONSIDERATIONS

- Tetracycline should not be used in pregnant or lactating patients

CONSULTATION/REFERRAL

- Refer to ophthalmologist if herpes, hemorrhagic conjunctivitis, or ulcerations present
- Refer to ophthalmologist for any worsening in vision

FOLLOW-UP

- Telephone or office follow up in 24 hours to assess effectiveness of treatment

EXPECTED COURSE

- Bacterial or viral: improvement in 2-4 days
- Viral conjunctivitis associated with pharyngitis: improvement in 5-10 days
- Herpes simplex: improvement in 2-3 weeks

POSSIBLE COMPLICATIONS

- Blepharitis
- Corneal ulcerations
- Scarring (herpes simplex)
- Bacterial superinfection (allergic or chemical)

NEONATAL CONJUNCTIVITIS
(Ophthalmia Neonatorum)

DESCRIPTION

Inflammation (aseptic) or infectious (septic) process of the mucous membrane of the eye (conjunctiva) in the newborn (< 40-60 days of age). A significant cause of worldwide blindness.

ETIOLOGY

- Chemical conjunctivitis due to silver nitrate/ erythromycin administration; aseptic
- Chlamydial conjunctivitis due to *Chlamydia trachomatis* from perinatal transmission at birth
- Gonococcal conjunctivitis due to *Neisseria gonorrhoeae* from perinatal transmission at birth
- Other pathogens: adenovirus, herpes simplex, *Staphylococcus, Streptococcus, Pseudomonas*

INCIDENCE

- Unknown

RISK FACTORS

- Maternal infection with causative agent
- Silver nitrate/erythromycin/tetracycline prophylaxis

ASSESSMENT FINDINGS

Chemical	*Onset of symptoms:* 30 minutes after prophylactic antibiotic drops; usually resolves by 48 hrs. *Characteristics:* Red eyes, usually bilateral
Chlamydial	*Onset of symptoms:* 1-2 weeks after birth *Characteristics:* Mild mucopurulent discharge, lid erythema and edema, conjunctival erythema, possible pneumonia
Gonococcal	*Onset of symptoms:* 2-4 days after birth *Characteristics:* Mucopurulent discharge, lid edema, possible central nervous system symptoms

DIFFERENTIAL DIAGNOSIS

- Birth trauma
- Forceps delivery
- Preseptal cellulitis
- Nasolacrimal duct obstruction
- Bacterial vs. viral vs. chemical conjunctivitis
- Congenital glaucoma

DIAGNOSTIC STUDIES

- Gram stain of discharge
- Culture
- Immunofluorescence may be helpful to identify *Chlamydia trachomatis*

PREVENTION

- Treat maternal infection prior to pregnancy and birth
- Instillation of antibiotic drops after birth for prophylaxis

NONPHARMACOLOGIC MANAGEMENT

- Explanation to parents of condition
- Warm compresses
- Good hand washing
- Passage of time for chemical conjunctivitis

PHARMACOLOGIC MANAGEMENT

- Chlamydia: oral erythromycin for 14 days, plus topical erythromycin or tetracycline/ointment
- Gonococcal: intravenous ceftriaxone (Rocephin®), one-time dose, plus topical erythromycin or tetracycline ointment QID for 14 days

CONSULTATION/REFERRAL

- Refer to ophthalmologist for chlamydial infection which may lead to corneal scarring and opacification
- Refer to ophthalmologist for HSV which may lead to loss of vision and corneal scarring
- Refer to ophthalmologist for gonococcal conjunctivitis
- Refer any which is slow to respond to treatment

FOLLOW-UP

- Dependent on etiology, but daily for gonorrhea, chlamydia and HSV

EXPECTED COURSE

- Chlamydia and HSV have highest incidence of corneal scarring
- Gonorrhea, if treated early, has relatively benign course, but can be devastating if not recognized or is undertreated

POSSIBLE COMPLICATIONS

- Loss of vision
- Corneal scarring

STRABISMUS
(Crossed Eyes)

DESCRIPTION

Non parallelism of the visual axis of the eyes so that they do not focus on the same object at the same time. A complication can be amblyopia, a reduction in visual acuity caused by strabismus (or other causes).

ETIOLOGY

- Due to a disorder of the intraocular muscles or their cranial nerves
- Due to an arrest or delay in normal ocular development
- Can be caused by ocular tumors (retinoblastoma)
- 66% of patients with strabismus are affected as children

INCIDENCE

- 4% of population has some form of strabismus

RISK FACTORS

- Positive family history (30% have a family member with strabismus)
- Ocular tumors
- History of forceps delivery
- Presence of cerebral palsy
- Diabetics in poor control due to lateral rectus paralysis. This impairs abduction of one or both eyes

ASSESSMENT FINDINGS

- Disconjugate gaze
- Possible diminished visual acuity; legal blindness (20/200) not uncommon
- Displaced corneal light reflexes (Hirschberg test)
- Inability to focus on an object without tilting head possible
- Nystagmus may be present
- Abnormal cover/uncover test
- Positive red reflex unless cataracts, retinoblastoma

Esotropia	Eye drifts inward
Exotropia	Eye drifts outward
Hypertropia	Eye drifts upward
Hypotropia	Eye drifts downward

A primary care provider's exam of a patient with suspected strabismus should focus on general health of the patient, neurologic status, and the presence of a head tilt.

DIFFERENTIAL DIAGNOSIS

- Pseudostrabismus: false impression that eyes are malaligned when they really are aligned properly; may be due to craniofacial features such as prominent epicanthal folds or a wide nasal bridge
- Neurological abnormalities (e.g., cerebral palsy)

DIAGNOSTIC STUDIES

- Hirschberg test
- Cover/uncover test
- CT/MRI to rule out ocular tumors
- Vision assessment to determine amblyopia

PREVENTION

- Careful monitoring and evaluation of patients with a family history of strabismus
- Referral for patients with true strabismus to ophthalmologist

NONPHARMACOLOGIC MANAGEMENT

- Patching (by ophthalmologist) of strong eye to allow weak eye to work and become stronger
- Visual training exercises are of limited help and can prolong amblyopia if surgical realignment is delayed
- Surgical interventions helpful to physically move the eyes into closer alignment

PHARMACOLOGIC MANAGEMENT

- None

CONSULTATION/REFERRAL

- Immediate referral to ophthalmologist when strabismus is suspected (normal eye alignment usually established by 3 months of age)

FOLLOW-UP

- By ophthalmologist

EXPECTED COURSE

- Goal is improving vision, then correcting alignment
- Most patients will need long-term ophthalmologic care because of recurrence of ocular deviation

POSSIBLE COMPLICATIONS

- Amblyopia can result in loss of vision

REFRACTIVE ERRORS/COLOR BLINDNESS

DESCRIPTION

An inability to see near, far, peripherally, certain colors, or a combination of any of these

TERMS

Nearsightedness (myopia)	Light is focused anterior to the retina, often hereditary, may also be due to prematurity, progressive with age
Farsightedness (hyperopia)	Light is focused behind the retina, often hereditary, normal in young children less than age 6 years
Astigmatism	Due to an irregularly shaped cornea or lens, often hereditary; may prohibit use of contact lenses
Color blindness	Due to an inherited disorder
Presbyopia	Age-related decline in focusing ability due to the loss of elasticity of the lens

INCIDENCE

- Refractive errors: Very common
- Color blindness: Males > Females

RISK FACTORS

- Family history
- Eye trauma (refractive errors)

ASSESSMENT FINDINGS

- Nearsightedness: poor distant vision
- Farsightedness: poor near vision
- Astigmatism: poor vision, headache, eye pain, night-

Ophthalmic Disorders

time "blindness" common
- Color blindness: inability to see certain combinations of colors, or in rare cases, inability to see any colors

Screening for refractive errors should be assessed throughout the lifespan, but patients need to be examined by an ophthalmologist or optometrist.

DIFFERENTIAL DIAGNOSIS

- Other refractive disorders
- Ocular tumors
- Cataract growth may alter refractive error
- Diabetes, if uncontrolled, may significantly impact refractive error

DIAGNOSTIC STUDIES

- Test each eye separately, then together
- Record values with and without correction
- Visual acuity of near vision (reading card)
- Visual acuity of distant vision (Snellen test)
- Color recognition testing (Ishihara test)

CONSULTATION/REFERRAL

- Optometrist or ophthalmologist

FOLLOW-UP

- Lifelong for refractive errors
- None needed for color blindness

CATARACT

DESCRIPTION

An opacification of the lens of the eye; and the leading cause of blindness in the U.S.

ETIOLOGY

Age related (senile)	Most common > 90%
Congenital	1 per 250 newborns
Secondary to: Trauma	Heat, penetration of eye by foreign object, electricity
Other eye diseases	Wilson's disease, hypocalcemia
Medications	Long-term steroid use (e.g., arthritis, asthma)

INCIDENCE

- Age-related (most common): about 90%
- Congenital: 0.4% of live births

RISK FACTORS

- Advancing age
- Diabetes
- Familial disorders
- Ocular trauma, sunlight, smoking
- Presence of retinoblastoma or other ocular tumors
- Maternal malnutrition/infectious disorders
- Maternal use of corticosteroids in congenital cataracts
- Steroid use

ASSESSMENT FINDINGS

- Opacification of the lens
- Diminished red reflex
- Leukocoria (white reflex)
- Blurred vision
- Diminished night vision
- Diminished visual acuity (especially at night or sensitivity to glare)

Any gradual decline in vision in an older patient should prompt the health care provider to examine the eye for cataract formation.

DIFFERENTIAL DIAGNOSIS

- Ocular tumors

- Retinal detachment
- Macular degeneration
- Other ocular disorders
  - ◊ Pterygium (often mistaken for a cataract)
  - ◊ Corneal scars, lesions

DIAGNOSTIC STUDIES

- Ocular exam, slit lamp exam
- Fundoscopic exam
- Glare testing

PREVENTION

- Depends on the cause
- Wearing of UV protectant eyewear may help slow development
- Tight control of glycemia in diabetics (also helps discourage progression of diabetic retinopathy)

NONPHARMACOLOGIC MANAGEMENT

- Protection from injury caused by diminished visual acuity
- Surgical removal by ophthalmologist (often with lens implant)

PHARMACOLOGIC MANAGEMENT

- None

CONSULTATION/REFERRAL

- Referral to ophthalmologist

FOLLOW-UP

- Postsurgical removal by ophthalmologist
- Assist family in finding resources if needs exist

EXPECTED COURSE

- Prognosis is good if identified and treated early and if no permanent ocular damage existed prior to removal
- Poor prognosis if presence of nystagmus or amblyopia prior to surgery
- Better prognosis for congenital cataracts if surgery performed prior to 3 months to discourage amblyopia. However, intraocular lens implants are not placed in very young patients, requiring use of contact lenses

POSSIBLE COMPLICATIONS

- Blindness
- If cataract not removed, hypermaturity of the cataract can result in a leaking lens capsule

GLAUCOMA

DESCRIPTION

A group of disorders characterized by an elevated intraocular pressure. All can lead to blindness. There are 3 predominant forms:

- Primary open-angle (POAG)
- Acute closed-angle (closed-angle, narrow-angle)
- Congenital (infantile)

ETIOLOGY

- Primary open-angle: slow rise in intraocular pressure
- Acute closed-angle: sudden increase in intraocular pressure
- Congenital: structural abnormalities in the trabecular network which prevent outflow of aqueous humor

INCIDENCE

- Chronic open-angle: most common, approximately 85%
- Acute closed-angle: approximately 15%
- Congenital: 1-2/10,000 births

RISK FACTORS

- Chronic open-angle: age > 35 years, diabetes mellitus, myopia, African-American (4-5 times higher), family history
- Acute closed-angle: age > 30 years, hyperopia (thickened "magnifying" eyeglass lenses)

ASSESSMENT FINDINGS

Primary open-angle	Usually asymptomatic Increased intraocular pressure (usually bilateral) Frequent prescription lens changes Halos around lights Headaches Impaired dark perception Visual disturbances Notching of the optic cup
Acute closed-angle	Increased intraocular pressure (usually unilateral) Severe throbbing eye pain or headache Rapid loss of vision Poorly reacting pupil Patient may present acutely ill with vomiting and may be misdiagnosed as suffering from appendicitis
Congenital	Tearing Photophobia Corneal haziness Corneal clouding or enlargement

DIFFERENTIAL DIAGNOSIS

- Conjunctivitis
- Macular degeneration
- Foreign body
- Keratitis, uveitis, scleritis

DIAGNOSTIC STUDIES

- Tonometry (normal intraocular pressure = 10-23 mm Hg)
- Corneal inspection (hazy cornea)
- Inspection of the optic nerves: unequal cups, or cupping >30, should be referred to ophthalmologist
- Visual field testing

PREVENTION

- Monitor intraocular pressure at regular eye exams (more frequent eye exams for high-risk individuals: positive family history, unequal cups)
- Avoid/limit use of OTC vasoconstrictive (oral and ocular) agents, or anticholinergic medications (e.g., scopolamine), especially in patients with narrow-angle anatomy

NONPHARMACOLOGIC MANAGEMENT

- Surgery or laser treatment to reduce intraocular pressure

PHARMACOLOGIC MANAGEMENT

- Topical β-adrenergic blockers
- Miotics: pilocarpine (Pilocar®)
- Systemic agents: carbonic anhydrase inhibitors

Use topical β-adrenergic blockers with caution in patients already on oral β-adrenergic blockers and in patients with COPD, asthma.

CONSULTATION/REFERRAL

- Ophthalmologist for suspected disease
- Emergency department for acute symptoms of glaucoma
- Potential for glaucoma in family, therefore, recommend having family members screened

FOLLOW-UP

- By ophthalmologist

EXPECTED COURSE

- Excellent prognosis if identified early and before optic damage occurs
- Need lifelong treatment and monitoring

POSSIBLE COMPLICATIONS

- Blindness
- Decreased peripheral vision (may be classified as visually disabled if severe)

Do not recommend antihistamines in patients with narrow angle glaucoma patients.

GLAUCOMA PHARMACOLOGIC MANAGEMENT

Class	Drug Generic name (Trade name®)	Dosage How supplied	Comments
Topical β-adrenergic blockers General comments Ophthalmic administration of beta blocker may have systemic effects, such as cardiac conduction defect May be associated with transient discomfort	**levobunolol** Betagan	**Adult:** 0.5%, 1-2 drops, 1-2 times per day OR 0.25% 1-2 drops twice daily *Soln: 0.25%, 5 mL, 10 mL* *Soln: 0.5%, 2 mL, 5 mL, 10 mL, 15 mL*	• Pregnancy Category C • Contraindicated in second and third degree heart block, sinus bradycardia, cardiogenic shock • Avoid in patients with COPD, asthma
	betaxolol Betopic-S	**Adult:** *Initial*: 1-2 drops twice daily *Max*: 1-2 drops twice daily *Soln: 0.25%, 2.5 mL, 5 mL, 10 mL, 15 mL* *Soln: 0.5%, 2 mL, 5 mL, 10 mL, 15 mL*	• Pregnancy Category C • Contraindicated in second and third degree heart block, sinus bradycardia, cardiogenic shock • Avoid in patients with COPD, asthma
	isopto carpine Pilocarpine	**Adult:** *Initial*: 2 drops 3-4 times daily *Max*: 2 drops 3-4 times daily **Children:** not recommended *Soln: 1%, 2%, 4% 15 mL*	• Pregnancy Category C • Contraindicated in history (or risk) of retinal detachment • Heavily pigmented irises may require higher concentrations • May lead to transient night blindness
	timoptic Timolol	**Adult:** *Initial*: 1 drop 0.25% twice daily *Max*: 1 drop 0.5% twice daily **Children:** not recommended *Soln: 0.25%, 0.5% 5 mL, 10 mL, 15 mL*	• Pregnancy Category C • Contraindicated in second and third degree heart block, sinus bradycardia, cardiogenic shock • Avoid contact lens wearing • Avoid in patients with COPD, asthma
Carbonic anhydrase inhibitors	**brinzolamide** Azopt	**Adult:** 1 drop, 3 times daily **Children**: not recommended *Soln: 2.5 mL, 5 mL, 10 mL, 15 mL*	• Pregnancy Category C • Contraindicated in patients with hepatic impairment or severe renal failure • May wear soft contact lens if inserted 15 minutes or later after medication

continued

GLAUCOMA PHARMACOLOGIC MANAGEMENT

Class	Drug Generic name (Trade name®)	Dosage How supplied	Comments
	acetazolamide Diamox Sequels	**Adult:** 1 capsule twice daily **Children:** not recommended *Caps: 50 mg*	• Pregnancy Category C • Use caution if hypokalemia, hyponatremia, severe renal impairment, severe hepatic impairment • Contraindicated in sulfonamide allergy
	dorzolamide Trusopt	**Adult:** 1 drop 3 times daily **Children:** not recommended *Soln: 2%, 10 mL*	• Pregnancy Category C • Use caution in severe renal impairment, severe hepatic impairment • Avoid soft contact lens
Alpha agonists	**brimondine tartrate** Alphagan P	**Adult:** 1 drop every 8 hours **Children < 2 yrs:** not recommended 2 yrs: 1 drop every 8 hours *Soln: 5 mL, 10 mL, 15 mL*	• Pregnancy Category B • Contraindicated in patients with MAO inhibitors • Remove soft contact lens before administration; may reinsert 15 minutes after • Use with caution if patient concurrently taking CNS depressants

CHALAZION

DESCRIPTION

Benign, nodular lesion of the meibomian gland. Plural form: chalazia

ETIOLOGY

- Obstruction of the meibomian gland duct with occasional secondary infection

INCIDENCE

- Common

RISK FACTORS

- Hordeolum or any condition which may impede flow through the meibomian tear gland

ASSESSMENT FINDINGS

- May be indistinguishable from a stye on exam, but is usually painless
- Lid edema or palpable mass: often best seen with the lids closed
- Red or gray mass on the inner aspect of the lid margin
- Possible astigmatism from pressure placed on the eyeball, rare

DIFFERENTIAL DIAGNOSIS

- Hordeolum
- Tumor
- Blepharitis
- Embedded foreign body

DIAGNOSTIC STUDIES

- None usually needed

PREVENTION

- Good eye hygiene

NONPHARMACOLOGIC MANAGEMENT

- Warm, moist compresses on effected lid area 5-6 times per day
- Incision and curettage if no resolution with conservative treatment
- May be spontaneous resolution with time

PHARMACOLOGIC MANAGEMENT

- Usually NOT necessary
- If secondarily infected, consider sulfacetamide, erythromycin or other topical ophthalmic antibiotic
- See complete list under conjunctivitis heading
- Oral antibiotics (dicloxacillin/Dynapen®) may be used for larger/persistent lesions or for multiple infected chalazia 500 mg po every 6 hours on empty stomach for 7 days
- Pediatrics:
  < 40 kg: 3.125 - 6.25 mg/kg every 6 hours
  > 40 kg: 125 mg - 250 mg every 6 hours

Antibiotics are not indicated because a chalazion is a granulomatous condition.

CONSULTATION/REFERRAL

- Ophthalmologist if no response to treatment after 6 weeks

FOLLOW-UP

- 2-4 weeks if small and uncomplicated
- If infected, depends on severity

EXPECTED COURSE

- Prognosis excellent
- Small chalazia usually resolve spontaneously

POSSIBLE COMPLICATIONS

- Some chalazia may become secondarily infected and cause cellulitis of the lid
- Loss of eyelashes
- Deformity of the eyelid

BLEPHARITIS

DESCRIPTION

Inflammation/infection of the lid margins which is often a chronic problem. There are two basic types:

- Seborrheic (non-ulcerative)
- Ulcerative (usually staphylococcal)

ETIOLOGY

- Seborrheic: irritants (e.g., smoke, eye make-up, chemicals), secondary to scalp or facial seborrhea, or infection (usually *Staphylococcus* or *Streptococcus*)
- Ulcerative: infection with *Staphylococcus* or *Streptococcus*
- Common skin microflora includes: *S. epidermis* and *P. Acnes*

INCIDENCE

- Common (most frequent ocular disease)

RISK FACTORS

- Frequent hordeola or chalazia
- Facial or scalp seborrhea
- Immunocompromised state
- Acne rosacea
- Diabetes mellitus

ASSESSMENT FINDINGS

Ulcerative	Itching Tearing Recurrent styes Chalazia Photophobia Small ulcerations at eyelid margin Broken or absence of eyelashes
Seborrheic	Chronic inflammation of the eyelid Erythema Scaling, loss of eyelashes

The most frequent complaint is ongoing eye irritation and conjunctival redness.

DIFFERENTIAL DIAGNOSIS

- Sebaceous cell/basal cell, squamous cell carcinoma
- Chalazion
- Lice infestation

DIAGNOSTIC STUDIES

- Usually none
- Can do eyelid culture if infection present

PREVENTION

- Good eye hygiene
- Discourage eye rubbing

NONPHARMACOLOGIC MANAGEMENT

- Clean eyelid margins 2-4 times per day with baby shampoo depending on severity
- Warm, moist compresses several times per day
- Lid massage to empty meibomian glands; best time to perform is immediately after warm compresses
- Remove contact lenses and disinfect

PHARMACOLOGIC MANAGEMENT

- For infected eyelids, antibiotic ointment (bacitracin, erythromycin ointment, and quinolone ointments)
- See *conjunctivitis page 471* for list of medications
- For infections resistant to topical treatment, consider oral tetracycline for several weeks
- Tetracycline 250 mg 4 times daily
- Doxycycline 100 mg twice daily

CONSULTATION/REFERRAL

- Ophthalmologist for severe infections
- Ophthalmologist for conditions which do not improve after treatment

FOLLOW-UP

- None usually needed for simple cases
- Re-evaluate depending on severity

EXPECTED COURSE

- Frequent recurrences expected for seborrheic blepharitis

POSSIBLE COMPLICATIONS

- Corneal infection
- Hordeolum
- Scarring of lids
- Trichiasis: misdirection of eye lashes

DACRYOSTENOSIS

DESCRIPTION

Obstruction in the nasolacrimal duct.

This is the most common cause of persistent tearing in children.

ETIOLOGY

- Congenital: due to failure of the nasolacrimal duct to canalize
- Infection: chronic inflammation of the duct caused by staphylococcal or streptococcal infection may lead to obstruction

INCIDENCE

- Common in neonates (usually resolves by 6 months of age due to maturing facial anatomy)

RISK FACTORS

- Unknown; nasolacrimal ducts develop during the 3rd to 5th week of embryologic development

ASSESSMENT FINDINGS

- Epiphora: persistent overflow of tears over the lower lid margin
- Mild crusting of lashes
- Red eye due to conjunctivitis
- Mucus reflux through the punctum when pressure is applied

DIFFERENTIAL DIAGNOSIS

- Dacryocystitis
- Conjunctivitis

DIAGNOSTIC STUDIES

- None usually indicated

PREVENTION

- Maintain patency by applying pressure/massaging nasolacrimal duct several times daily

NONPHARMACOLOGIC MANAGEMENT

- Maintain patency by applying pressure/massaging nasolacrimal duct at least twice daily if chronic
- Surgery to probe the tear duct and facilitate permanent drainage

PHARMACOLOGIC MANAGEMENT

- None needed unless there is purulent drainage from the duct or evidence of conjunctivitis
- Symptoms often subside while antibiotic eyedrops in use

CONSULTATION/REFERRAL

- Ophthalmologist for dacryostenosis beyond 9-12 months of age
- Ophthalmologist for severe obstruction prior to 6 months of age

Correction of dacryostenosis surgically is usually reserved until at least 12 months of age because of high rates of spontaneous resolution.

FOLLOW-UP

- As needed depending on severity

EXPECTED COURSE

- Excellent prognosis

POSSIBLE COMPLICATIONS

- Conjunctivitis

Akbari, M., Akbari, S., & Pasquale, L. R. (2009). The association of primary open-angle glaucoma with mortality: a meta-analysis of observational studies. Archives of Ophthalmology, 127(2), 204-210. doi: 10.1001/archophthalmol.2008.571

American Academy of Opthalmology. (2002). Preferred practice pattern guidelines: Esotropia and exotropia. San Francisco: American Academy of Opthalmology.

American Academy of Opthalmology Pediatric Ophthalmology/Strabismus Panel. (2007). Preferred practice pattern guideline: Amblyopia. San Francisco: American Academy of Opthalmology.

Asbell, P. A., Dualan, I., Mindel, J., Brocks, D., Ahmad, M., & Epstein, S. (2005). Age-related cataract. Lancet, 365(9459), 599-609. doi: 10.1016/S0140-6736(05)17911-2

Ben Simon, G. J., Huang, L., Nakra, T., Schwarcz, R. M., McCann, J. D., & Goldberg, R. A. (2005). Intralesional triamcinolone acetonide injection for primary and recurrent chalazia: is it really effective? Ophthalmology, 112(5), 913-917. doi: 10.1016/j.ophtha.2004.11.037

Burns, C. E., Dunn, A. M., Brady, M. A., Starr, N. B., & Blosser, C. (2008). Pediatric primary care: A handbook for nurse practitioners. Philadelphia: W. B. Saunders.

Congdon, N., O'Colmain, B., Klaver, C. C., Klein, R., Munoz, B., Friedman, D. S., . . . Mitchell, P. (2004). Causes and prevalence of visual impairment among adults in the United States. Archives of Ophthalmology, 122(4), 477-485. doi: 10.1001/archopht.122.4.477

Domino, F., Baldor, R., Golding, J., Grimes, J., & Taylor, J. (2011). The 5-minute clinical consult 2011. Philadelphia: Lippincott Williams & Wilkins.

Ernst, D., & Lee, A. (2010). Nurse practitioners prescribing reference. New York: Haymarket Media Publication.

Everitt, H. A., Little, P. S., & Smith, P. W. (2006). A randomised controlled trial of management strategies for acute infective conjunctivitis in general practice. BMJ, 333(7563), 321. doi: 10.1136/bmj.38891.551088.7C

Friedman, D. S., Repka, M. X., Katz, J., Giordano, L., Ibironke, J., Hawse, P., & Tielsch, J. M. (2009). Prevalence of amblyopia and strabismus in white and African American children aged 6 through 71 months the Baltimore Pediatric Eye Disease Study. Ophthalmology, 116(11), 2128-2134 e2121-2122. doi: 10.1016/j.ophtha.2009.04.034

Huang, T., Wang, Y., Liu, Z., Wang, T., & Chen, J. (2007). Investigation of tear film change after recovery from acute conjunctivitis. Cornea, 26(7), 778-781. doi: 10.1097/ICO.0b013e31806457f8

Kaiser, P. K. (1995). A comparison of pressure patching versus no patching for corneal abrasions due to trauma or foreign body removal. Corneal Abrasion Patching Study Group. Ophthalmology, 102(12), 1936-1942.

Kuckelkorn, R., Schrage, N., Keller, G., & Redbrake, C. (2002). Emergency treatment of chemical and thermal eye burns. Acta Ophthalmologica Scandinavica, 80(1), 4-10. doi: aos800102 [pii]

Kwon, Y. H., Fingert, J. H., Kuehn, M. H., & Alward, W. L. (2009). Primary open-angle glaucoma. New England Journal of Medicine, 360(11), 1113-1124. doi: 10.1056/NEJMra0804630

Le Sage, N., Verreault, R., & Rochette, L. (2001). Efficacy of eye patching for traumatic corneal abrasions: a controlled clinical trial. Annals of Emergency Medicine, 38(2), 129-134. doi: 10.1067/mem.2001.115443

Lindblad, B. E., Hakansson, N., Philipson, B., & Wolk, A. (2008). Metabolic syndrome components in relation to risk of cataract extraction: a prospective cohort study of women. Ophthalmology, 115(10), 1687-1692. doi: 10.1016/j.ophtha.2008.04.004

Luchs, J. (2008). Efficacy of topical azithromycin ophthalmic solution 1% in the treatment of posterior blepharitis. Advances in Therapy, 25(9), 858-870. doi: 10.1007/s12325-008-0096-9

McCulley, J. P., & Shine, W. E. (2004). The lipid layer of tears: dependent on meibomian gland function. Experimental Eye Research,

78(3), 361-365.

Robb, R. M. (2001). Congenital nasolacrimal duct obstruction. Ophthalmology Clinics of North America, 14(3), 443-446, viii.

Sheikh, A., & Hurwitz, B. (2006). Antibiotics versus placebo for acute bacterial conjunctivitis. Cochrane Database Systematic Review(2), CD001211. doi: 10.1002/14651858.CD001211.pub2

Turner, A., & Rabiu, M. (2006). Patching for corneal abrasion. Cochrane Database Systematic Review(2), CD004764. doi: 10.1002/14651858.CD004764.pub2

Viswalingam, M., Rauz, S., Morlet, N., & Dart, J. K. (2005). Blepharokeratoconjunctivitis in children: diagnosis and treatment. British Journal of Ophthalmology, 89(4), 400-403. doi: 10.1136/bjo.2004.052134

Wagner, R. S. (2001). Management of congenital nasolacrimal duct obstruction. Pediatric Annals, 30(8), 481-488.

Weinreb, R. N., & Khaw, P. T. (2004). Primary open-angle glaucoma. Lancet, 363(9422), 1711-1720. doi: 10.1016/S0140-6736(04)16257-0

Williams, C., Northstone, K., Howard, M., Harvey, I., Harrad, R. A., & Sparrow, J. M. (2008). Prevalence and risk factors for common vision problems in children: data from the ALSPAC study. British Journal of Ophthalmology, 92(7), 959-964. doi: 10.1136/bjo.2007.134700

Wirbelauer, C. (2006). Management of the red eye for the primary care physician. American Journal of Medicine, 119(4), 302-306. doi: 10.1016/j.amjmed.2005.07.065

Wong, R. K., & VanderVeen, D. K. (2008). Presentation and management of congenital dacryocystocele. Pediatrics, 122(5), e1108-1112. doi: 10.1542/peds.2008-0934

13

ORTHOPEDIC DISORDERS

Orthopedic Disorders

Osteoarthritis 491

Rheumatoid Arthritis 494

Gout 497

Low Back Pain 502

Bursitis 505

Epicondylitis 507

* Upper Extremity Joint Derangement 509

* Subluxation of the Radial Head 510

Sprain 511

Fractures 512

Stress Fracture 514

Clavicular Fracture 515

Rotator Cuff Syndrome 516

Osteoporosis 517

Osgood-Schlatter Disease 522

* Developmental Dysplasia of the Hip 523

* Legg-Calve-Perthes Disease 524

Slipped Capital Femoral Epiphysis 525

* Transient Synovitis of the Hip 526

Scoliosis 527

* Talipes Equinovarus 529

* Metatarsus Adductus 530

Plantar Fasciitis 531

References *532*

** Denotes pediatric diagnosis*

OSTEOARTHRITIS
(OA)

DESCRIPTION

Progressive destruction of the articular cartilage and subchondral bone accompanied by osteophyte formation and sclerosis. OA is confined to the joints. There is an absence of constitutional symptoms.

Osteoarthritis is the most common joint disease in the U.S.

ETIOLOGY

- Primary OA is a localized or generalized disease with no known cause
- Secondary OA is associated with trauma, infection, or metabolic disorders

INCIDENCE

- Males = Females
- Predominantly > age 40 years
- Common

RISK FACTORS

- Obesity
- Age
- Trauma
- Prolonged use or overuse of joints related to occupation or activity
- Family history
- History of developmental dysplasia of the hip or slipped femoral epiphysis
- Hemophilia
- Paget's disease

ASSESSMENT FINDINGS

- Joint pain, usually asymmetrical, develops insidiously and accompanies or follows physical activity
- Morning stiffness lasting < 1 hour
- Joints are cool with possible crepitus and limited range of motion
- Overgrowth of osteophytes results in bony enlargement, especially bunions (MTP joint), Heberden's nodes (DIP joints), and Bouchard's nodes (PIP joints)

Commonly involved joints:
Distal interphalangeal (DIP)
Proximal interphalangeal (PIP)
First carpometacarpal (CMC)
First metatarsophalangeal (MTP)
Hips, knees, cervical and lumbar spine

DIFFERENTIAL DIAGNOSIS

- Gout, pseudogout
- Infective arthritis
- Rheumatoid arthritis
- Joint injury
- Soft tissue injury
- Peripheral vascular disease
- Giant cell arteritis
- Bursitis
- Tendonitis
- Osteopenia, osteoarthritis
- Neuropathy

DIAGNOSTIC STUDIES

- No diagnostic laboratory tests are available for osteoarthritis; diagnosis is based on history, physical, and x-ray findings
- X-rays: osteophytes, joint space narrowing
- Inflammation markers: negative
  - ◊ Erythrocyte sedimentation rate (ESR)
  - ◊ Rheumatoid factor (RF)
  - ◊ Antinuclear antibodies (ANA)
- In younger patients, consider iron saturation or ferritin levels to rule out hemochromatosis

PREVENTION

- Weight control
- Management of underlying causes of secondary disease

NONPHARMACOLOGIC MANAGEMENT

- Emphasis must be given to nonpharmacologic management to delay or minimize use of medications which have adverse effects
- Weight loss, if indicated
- Education that OA is a chronic disorder requiring patient participation in therapy

- Organized program of supervised exercise
- Rest
- Knee or elbow braces to stabilize joints during exercise
- Orthotic shoes, cane, collar, sling, corset, wedged insoles
- Apply heat and/or cold to affected joints
- Wedge osteotomy, arthroplasty
- Acupuncture may be beneficial
- Local cream/liniments for counter irritant effect

PHARMACOLOGIC MANAGEMENT

- Drugs are usually needed long-term and their use is associated with many possible side effects
- Acetaminophen recommended as first-line therapy by the American College of Rheumatology
- Add NSAID for pain that persists despite acetaminophen at adequate doses
- Short-acting NSAIDs are associated with fewer side effects
- Concomitant use of misoprostol (Cytotec®) to prevent gastric ulcer development caused by NSAIDs
- Consider COX-2 inhibitors for GI protection (risk of GI bleeds decreased but still present)
- Narcotic analgesics indicated briefly for severe exacerbation
- Intra-articular corticosteroid injections, limited to 4 times a year, and not recommended for the hip

Risk of vascular events such as myocardial infarction or stroke is increased with use of NSAIDs.

OSTEOARTHRITIS PHARMACOLOGIC MANAGEMENT

Class	Drug Generic name (Trade name®)	Dosage How supplied	Comments
NSAIDs *inhibit cyclooxygenase (COX-1 and COX-2) activity and prostaglandin synthesis* <u>General comments:</u> May cause serious gastrointestinal events including bleeding, ulceration, perforation, and occur with or without warning Use with caution in patients with known or suspected cardiovascular risk factors May lead to or worsen hypertension May lead to fluid retention or worsen heart failure	**celecoxib** Celebrex	**Adult:** either 200 mg once daily **OR** 100 mg twice daily *Caps: 50 mg, 100 mg, 200 mg*	• Pregnancy Category C if < 30 weeks; Category D if > 30 weeks • Mostly COX2 selective • Avoid in patients with sulfonamide hypersensitivity • Reduce dose by 50% if hepatic impairment
	diclofenac Voltaren	**Adult**: total daily dose of 100-150 mg in two or three divided doses *Tabs: 25 mg, 50 mg, 75 mg*	• Pregnancy Category C • Avoid in late pregnancy due to inhibition of uterine contractions
	etodolac Lodine	**Adult**: *Initial*: Titrate for effect, **either**: 300 mg two or three times daily 400 mg twice daily 500 mg twice daily *Usual*: 300 mg twice daily *Max*: 1000 mg/day *Caps: 200 mg, 300 mg* *Tabs: 400 mg, 500 mg*	• Pregnancy Category C • Avoid late in pregnancy due to premature closure of the ductus arteriosus • May diminish effect of ACE inhibitors

continued

OSTEOARTHRITIS PHARMACOLOGIC MANAGEMENT

Class	Drug Generic name (Trade name®)	Dosage How supplied	Comments
Avoid concomitant use with salicylates Use with caution in patients with asthma Avoid use in patients with renal disease Patients must receive accompanying medication guide when product dispensed	**ibuprofen**	**Adult**: *Initial*: Titrate for effect, 400 mg, 600 mg, 800 mg three or four times daily *Usual*: 2,400-3,200 mg daily *Max*: 3200 mg /day	• Pregnancy Category C • Avoid late in pregnancy due to premature closure of the ductus arteriosus • May diminish effect of ACE inhibitors • Available by either prescription or various over-the counter products
	Motrin	*Tabs: 400 mg, 600 mg, 800 mg*	
	ketoprofen	**Immediate Release** **Adult**: *Initial*: either 50 mg four times daily **OR** 75 mg three times daily *Max*: 300 mg daily **Sustained Release** **Adult**: *Initial*: 200 mg daily *Max*: 200 mg daily	• Pregnancy Category C • Avoid use late in pregnancy • Do not mix dose forms • Reduce dose in patients > 75 years
	Orudis	*Caps: 50 mg, 75 mg* *Ext. Rel. Caps: 200 mg*	
	meloxicam	**Adult**: *Initial:* 7.5 mg daily *Usual:* 7.5 mg daily *Max:* 15 mg daily	• Pregnancy Category C • May be taken without regard to meals
	Mobic	*Tabs: 7.5 mg, 15 mg* *Susp: 7.5 mg/5 mL*	

CONSULTATION/REFERRAL

- Orthopedist
- Physical therapist
- Supervised exercise program
- Nutritionist for weight loss

FOLLOW-UP

- Regularly scheduled return visits for evaluation, support and education
- NSAID therapy requirements (includes COX-2): periodic CBC, renal function studies, and stool for occult blood

EXPECTED COURSE

- Usually progressive with more pain at rest, joint effusions, and bony enlargement

POSSIBLE COMPLICATIONS

- Adverse effects from NSAIDs
- Corticosteroid adverse effects
- Depression associated with chronic illness

RHEUMATOID ARTHRITIS
(RA)

DESCRIPTION

An autoimmune disease that is systemic, frequently progressive, and is characterized by joint inflammation and constitutional symptoms. There is inflammation and thickening of the synovial membrane and inflammation in the blood vessels.

ETIOLOGY

- Unknown
- Possible genetic predisposition coupled with an environmental trigger
- Antigen-antibody reaction results in inflammatory response

INCIDENCE

- 1% of U.S. population
- Females > Males
- Common in Caucasians, Native Americans; rare in African Americans
- Occurs between ages 30 and 50 years; peak onset is age 40 years
- Juvenile RA mean age onset 1-3 yr; 30% have severe long term effects

RISK FACTORS

- Family history

ASSESSMENT FINDINGS

- May be acute onset over 24 hours, or gradual and insidious
- Constitutional symptoms:
  - ◊ Weakness, malaise, fatigue, anorexia, weight loss, depression
  - ◊ Lymphadenopathy, aches, low-grade fever
- Joint pain/stiffness at rest and with movement; can disturb sleep and lasts > 1 hour in morning upon arising
  - ◊ Polyarticular: proximal interphalangeal (PIP), metacarpophalangeal (MCP), wrist, elbow, knee, ankle
  - ◊ Symmetrical
- Rheumatoid nodules may occur on extensor surfaces of elbows and fingers

Symptoms are usually present for 9 months prior to diagnosis.

DIFFERENTIAL DIAGNOSIS

- Septic arthritis
- Gout
- Trauma
- Bursitis
- Systemic lupus erythematosus: multisystem inflammatory illness with positive antinuclear antibody (ANA)
- Osteoarthritis

DIAGNOSTIC CRITERIA

- Five of the 7 criteria must be present; and the first 4 must be present for at least 6 weeks:
  - ◊ Morning stiffness > 1 hour
  - ◊ Soft tissue swelling of 3 or more joints (PIP, MCP, wrist, elbow, knee, ankle, metatarsophalangeal (MTP)
  - ◊ Swelling of at least 1 joint in the hand or wrist
  - ◊ Symmetrical joint swelling
  - ◊ Rheumatoid nodules
  - ◊ Serum rheumatoid factor (RF)
  - ◊ Bony erosions demonstrable by x-ray
  - ◊ Juvenile RA diagnostic criteria:
    - Before age 16 yr
    - 1 or more joints with swelling or effusion
    - Decreased ROM, tenderness, localized heat
    - Duration 6 weeks to 3 months

DIAGNOSTIC STUDIES

- X-ray studies: joint space narrowing, bony erosion in joints, reduced bone density surrounding joints
- Rheumatoid factor (RF): elevated (20% of patients are negative despite having other symptoms of RA)
- Erythrocyte sedimentation rate (ESR): elevated, nonspecific for RA
- Antinuclear antibodies (ANA): usually negative, but can be positive in 20-30% of patients)

- C-reactive protein: if positive, indicates acute nonspecific inflammation
- Joint aspiration to rule out infectious arthritis and gout

ESR is a good measure of the disease's activity.

PREVENTION

- Unknown

Prompt diagnosis and treatment will minimize harmful sequelae. Goals are to prevent damage to joints if possible and to maintain mobility.

NONPHARMACOLOGIC MANAGEMENT

- Exercise program
  - ◊ Increase in pain or swelling indicates excessive exercise
  - ◊ Should not involve joints that are acutely inflamed
- Splinting reduces inflammation and deformities
- Orthotics can relieve pain and prevent deformities
- Cold therapy for analgesic, anti-inflammatory effect
- Heat therapy for relaxation and circulatory stimulation
- Weight loss, if indicated, reduces joint pain; avoidance of allergens that precipitate symptoms
- Surgery: arthroscopy with synovectomy, arthroplasty
- Education regarding illness and therapies improves patient's ability to form appropriate goals and participate in treatment plan

RHEUMATOID ARTHRITIS PHARMACOLOGIC MANAGEMENT

Initial pharmacologic interventions for early, moderately active RA include use of nonsteroidal antiinflammatory drugs, and single agents or combinations of nonbiologic disease-modifying antirheumatic drugs (DMARDs).The dose of nonsteroidal antiinflammatory drugs (NSAIDs) is titrated to the optimum tolerated level.

Class	Drug Generic name (Trade name®)	Dosage How supplied	Comments
Disease-modifying antirheumatic drugs (DMARDs)	**etanercept**	**Adult:** 50 mg weekly (SC injection) **Children:** < 63 kg: 0.8 mg/kg/week > 63 kg: 50 mg weekly	• Pregnancy Category B • Predisposes patient to viral, bacterial and fungal infections • May lead to hypoglycemia
	Enbrel	*Inj: Prefilled syringe, sure click autoinject*	
	hydroxychloroquine	**Adult:** *Initial*: 400 mg daily, may increase in 5-10 day intervals to 600 mg; then reduce to usual dose in 4-12 weeks *Usual*: 200-400 mg **Children**: not recommended	• Pregnancy Category C • If objective improvement not seen within 6 months, discontinue • Patients must receive periodic retinal examinations
	Plaquenil	*Tabs: 200 mg*	

continued

RHEUMATOID ARTHRITIS PHARMACOLOGIC MANAGEMENT

Initial pharmacologic interventions for early, moderately active RA include use of nonsteroidal antiinflammatory drugs, and single agents or combinations of nonbiologic disease-modifying antirheumatic drugs (DMARDs).The dose of nonsteroidal antiinflammatory drugs (NSAIDs) is titrated to the optimum tolerated level.

Class	Drug Generic name (Trade name®)	Dosage How supplied	Comments
	methotrexate	**Adult:** 7.5 mg once weekly **OR** 2.5 mg every 12 hours for 3 doses/ week *Tabs: 2.5 mg, 5 mg, 7.5 mg*	• Pregnancy Category X • Carries **Black Box** warning

Methotrexate has the most predictable effect. Always prescribe folate with methotrexate to reduce risk of liver toxicity.

Juvenile RA Pharmacology:

- NSAIDS for mild cases
  - ◊ Naprosyn 10 mg/kg/d in 2 divided doses (susp 125 mg/5 mL)
  - ◊ Ibuprofen 30-40 mg/kg/day in 3-4 divided doses (susp 100 mg/5 mL)
  - ◊ COX-2 may be beneficial to children with GI problems
- If DMARDs indicated, get specialist consultation

PREGNANCY/LACTATION CONSIDERATIONS

- Methotrexate has teratogenic potential. Pregnancy should be avoided if either the male or the female partner is taking the drug. Women should wait at least one ovulatory cycle after stopping methotrexate before conceiving; men at least 3 months

CONSULTATION/REFERRAL

- Rheumatologist for confirmation of diagnosis, treatment plan, and for initiation of disease-modifying antirheumatic drugs (DMARDs)
- Occupational therapist, physical therapist
- Nutritionist
- Supervised exercise program
- Arthritis Foundation
- Social services due to personal, social, and financial implications
- Surgeon, if indicated
- In children, get ophthalmologist referral at time of diagnosis and periodically

FOLLOW-UP

- CBC, chemistry profile, renal and liver functions as baseline before initiating anti-inflammatory or antirheumatic therapy
- Eye exam if on Plaquenil®
- Appropriate monitoring of laboratory values depending on therapeutic agents used
- Ongoing assessment of disease symptoms, ESR, CRP

Ongoing laboratory follow up is critical for patients on DMARDs because of potential toxicity of these agents.

EXPECTED COURSE

- Persistent swelling of PIP joints, early onset (young age) with involvement of >20 joints, high RF, and high ESR have poorest prognosis
- Course may be insidious or acute
- Complete remission is rare, but with appropriate therapy, pain and disability may be minimized
- Average life expectancy is decreased by 7 years for men and 3 years for women

POSSIBLE COMPLICATIONS

- Depression
- Drug toxicity
- Joint destruction
- Sjögren syndrome
- Social and occupational disability

GOUT

DESCRIPTION

Deposition of monosodium urate (MSU) crystals in joints and other connective tissue causing acute or chronic inflammation manifested as acute or chronic arthritis, tophi, nephropathy, and/or renal stones.

ETIOLOGY

- Elevated serum and total body uric acid is a result of either its overproduction or underexcretion
- Underexcretion may be due to renal insufficiency, acidosis, or use of diuretics, aspirin, or cyclosporine
- Overproduction may be due to enzyme deficiencies, psoriasis, or hematologic malignancies
- Dietary excess of purines
- Alcoholism is a contributing factor in both overproduction and underexcretion of urate

INCIDENCE

- Increasing in U.S.
- Males > Females (20:1)
- More common in age > 45 years

RISK FACTORS

- Alcohol abuse
- Medication use
  - ◊ Aspirin
  - ◊ Nicotinic acid
  - ◊ Diuretics
  - ◊ Cyclosporine
- Renal insufficiency
- Acidosis
- Enzyme deficiencies
- Psoriasis
- Hematologic malignancies
- Family history
- Obesity
- Hypertension

Alcohol use or abuse may trigger an episode of gout.

ASSESSMENT FINDINGS

- Acute joint pain and swelling, with warmth and erythema, beginning abruptly, usually involving a single joint (75% of time)
  - ◊ Metatarsophalangeal joint of first toe is involved most often
  - ◊ Ankle, tarsal area, wrist or finger joint may be involved
- Acute attacks usually subside without treatment in approximately 1-2 weeks
- Skin may desquamate over the affected joint after the inflammation subsides
- Subsequent episodes may involve several joints, and persist longer
- There may be a history of a stressful event that triggered the first attack
  - ◊ Trauma
  - ◊ Alcohol
  - ◊ Drugs
  - ◊ Surgery
  - ◊ Acute medical illness
- Tophi, monosodium urate (MSU) crystal-containing deposits in subcutaneous tissue of antihelix of ears and extensor aspect of elbow, occur in fairly advanced gout
- Fever
- Kidney stones

DIFFERENTIAL DIAGNOSIS

- Arterial insufficiency
- Muscular or ligamentous strain

- Traumatic arthritis
- Rheumatoid arthritis
- Septic arthritis
- Pseudogout
- Cellulitis

DIAGNOSTIC STUDIES

- WBC: usually elevated during acute attack
- ESR: usually elevated during acute attack
- X-ray studies of joints: soft tissue swelling, otherwise, normal initially; after multiple episodes, may see tophi and joint changes
- Serum uric acid levels not helpful in diagnosis, but are important in following treatment
- Synovial fluid aspiration (not usually performed):
  - ◊ Presence of monosodium urate crystals is diagnostic
  - ◊ Elevated white blood cells

Normal uric acid levels are common during an acute attack. Elevated uric acid levels are not diagnostic of gout. Therefore, always look at the clinical presentation in conjunction with diagnostic studies.

PREVENTION

- Avoid contributing substances (e.g., alcohol, medications)
- Good hydration
- Maintain ideal body weight

NONPHARMACOLOGIC MEASURES

- Rest acutely inflamed joint
- Educate patient about avoidance of contributing substances
- Weight reduction if indicated, low purine diet
- Fluid intake of 3 liters/day

PHARMACOLOGIC MANAGEMENT

Acute attacks:
- High dose NSAIDs for 2-5 days and reduce dose as soon as symptoms allow
- Corticosteroids may be effective if patient cannot tolerate NSAIDs
- Intra-articular injection of corticosteroids can provide rapid relief

Infection in joint must be ruled out before intra-articular injection of corticosteroids.

Preventive therapy:
- Used for recurrent attacks or if tophi present
- Urate-lowering agents taken long term
  - ◊ Uricosurics increase execretion of uric acid: probenecid, colchicine
  - ◊ Allopurinol (Zyloprim®): decreases production of uric acid
- Monitor CBC, renal and hepatic function at 1 week, 6 weeks, and every 3 months while on allopurinol. Bone marrow suppression, as well as, renal and hepatic impairment can occur

GOUT PHARMACOLOGIC MANAGEMENT

Class	Drug Generic name (Trade name®)	Dosage How supplied	Comments
NSAIDs *inhibit cyclooxygenase (COX-1 and COX-2) activity and prostaglandin synthesis* **General comments**: May cause serious gastrointestinal events including bleeding, ulceration, perforation, and occur with or without warning Avoid in patients with sulfonamide hypersensitivity Use with caution in patients with known or suspected cardiovascular risk factors May lead to or worsen hypertension May lead to fluid retention or worsen heart failure Avoid concomitant use with salicylates Use with caution in patients with asthma Avoid use in patients with renal disease Patients must receive accompanying medication guide when product dispensed	**indomethacin** Indocin	**Adult**: *Initial*: Titrate for effect, 50 mg three times daily until pain resolved *Usual*: 150 mg daily divided into 3 doses for short term use *Max*: 150 mg/day *Caps: 25 mg, 50 mg*	• Pregnancy Category C • Avoid late in pregnancy due to premature closure of the ductus arteriosus • May diminish effect of ACE inhibitors • Available by either prescription or various over-the-counter products
	naproxen Naprosyn	**Adult**: *Initial:* 500 mg twice daily Titrate for effect *Tabs: 250 mg, 375 mg, 500 mg*	• Pregnancy Category C • Avoid late in pregnancy due to premature closure of the ductus arteriosus • Different dose strengths and formulations (i.e., tablets, suspension) of the drug are not necessarily bioequivalent. This difference should be taken into consideration when changing formulation

continued

GOUT PHARMACOLOGIC MANAGEMENT

Class	Drug Generic name (Trade name®)	Dosage How supplied	Comments
Urate-lowering agents Uricosurics **General comments**: All should be accompanied by adequate daily fluid intake	**allopurinol**	**Adult:** MILD *Initial*: 100-200 mg/day *Usual*: 200-300 mg/day *Max*: 800 mg/day MODERATELY SEVERE *Initial*: 400-600 mg/day *Usual*: 200-300 mg/day *Max*: 800 mg/day PREVENTION OF ACUTE ATTACK *Initial*: 100 mg/day; increase at weekly intervals to target serum uric acid level of 6 mg/dL (do not exceed max dose) **Children**: not recommended	• Pregnancy Category C • Doses above 300 mg should be administered in divided doses • Maintain adequate fluid hydration • Alkaline urine state preferred
	Zyloprim	*Tabs: 100 mg, 300 mg*	
	colchicine	**Adults**: INITIAL FLARE 1.2 mg initially, then 0.6 mg one hour later; wait 12 hours then 0.6 mg twice daily PREVENTION 0.6 mg twice daily **Children**: not recommended	• Pregnancy Category C • May take without regard to meals • If moderate or severe renal or hepatic dysfunction, treatment course can be repeated no more than once every two weeks • If on dialysis, maximum dose is 0.6 mg • Gastrointestinal side effects are common
	Colcrys	*Tabs: 0.6 mg*	
	probenecid	**Adults**: *Initial (Post-Attack):* 250 mg twice daily (with food) for 7 days; advance to 500 mg twice daily; may increase every 4 weeks thereafter *Max:* 2 grams	• Pregnancy Category B • Do not initiate therapy during acute gouty attack • Patients should be adequately hydrated • If gout attack free for > 6 months, may decrease daily dose (monitor serum urate levels)
	Benemid	*Tabs: 500 mg*	

continued

GOUT PHARMACOLOGIC MANAGEMENT

Class	Drug Generic name (Trade name®)	Dosage How supplied	Comments
	sulfinpyrazone Anturane	**Adults**: *Initial:* 200-400 mg daily in two divided doses, with food *Usual:* 400 mg daily, in two divided doses, with food *Max:* 800 mg daily *Tabs: 100 mg* *Caps: 200 mg*	• Pregnancy Category unknown • Avoid in patients with active peptic ulcer, gastrointestinal inflammation • Monitor periodic blood count • Monitor blood urate level • Gastrointestinal disturbances most common side effect

CONSULTATION/REFERRAL

- Patients with complications requiring nephrologist, hematologist, oncologist, or urologist

FOLLOW-UP

- Evaluate response to therapy for acute attack within several days
- Assess serum uric acid levels monthly until desirable level (< 7 mg/dL) is reached, then annually

EXPECTED COURSE

- Good control can be achieved with early detection and treatment and patient compliance with lifestyle changes
- Recurrent attacks require long-term use of preventive medications and monitoring of laboratory values
- Over half of patients develop chronic disease within 20 years of initial attack

POSSIBLE COMPLICATIONS

- Nephropathy
- Kidney stones
- Joint destruction
- Infection

LOW BACK PAIN
(Secondary to Disc Disorders)

DESCRIPTION

Activity intolerance due to lumbar pain that involves an intervertebral disc; frequently there is referral of pain to the buttocks and posterior thighs, and/or down one or both legs.
Radiculopathy describes a disorder of the roots of the spinal nerves due to compression, inflammation, or tearing of nerve roots at the site of entry into the vertebral canal.

ETIOLOGY

- Often unclear; stretching or tearing of nerves, muscles, tendons, ligaments, or fascia of back secondary to trauma or chronic mechanical stress
- Compression or irritation of a nerve root is a common cause

The discs most commonly affected are L4-L5 and L5-S1.

INCIDENCE

- > 80% of U.S. population affected at some time in their lives
- 31 million people affected in U.S.
- Males = Females

RISK FACTORS

- Obesity
- Sedentary lifestyle, inadequate conditioning, cigarette smoking
- Chronic occupational strain, improper lifting techniques
- Exaggerated lumbar lordosis, chronic poor posture
- Leg length discrepancy

ASSESSMENT FINDINGS

- Pain in back, buttocks, and/or one or both thighs, aggravated by movement, rising from sitting position, standing, and flexion, and may be relieved by rest, repositioning, or reclining
- Muscle spasm may be present over lumbosacral area because of soft tissue involvement (ligaments, muscles)
- Pain usually radiates down leg and below the knee

***Sciatic stretch test*: elevation of affected leg in supine position will elicit pain at 15-30 degrees for severe disease; 30-60 degrees for moderate disease**

***Crossed leg raise*: elevating unaffected leg produces pain in affected leg**

- Bowel and bladder function preserved
- Motor, sensory, and reflex examination
- Observe gait, assess lower extremity strength and bulk of muscles, pulses
- Listen for abdominal bruits and assess rectal sphincter tone
- Deep tendon reflexes (DTR)
  - ◊ Biceps: tests nerves at roots C5-C6
  - ◊ Brachioradialis: tests nerves at roots C5-C6
  - ◊ Triceps: tests nerves at roots T2-T4
  - ◊ Patellar: tests nerves at roots L2-L4
  - ◊ Achilles: tests nerves at roots S1-S2
- DTR responses are graded as follows:
  - ◊ 0: no response
  - ◊ +1: diminished response
  - ◊ +2: normal response
  - ◊ +3: increased response
  - ◊ +4: hyperactive response

Responses below normal may imply myopathies, decreased muscle mass, nerve root impairment. Responses above normal are characteristic of pyramidal tract disease, electrolyte imbalance, hyperthyroidism, or other endocrine abnormalities.

New onset radicular pain in older patients is frequently spinal stenosis.

DIFFERENTIAL DIAGNOSIS

- Low back strain
- Herniated intervertebral disc
- Prostatitis, pyelonephritis
- Vascular occlusion at level of bifurcation, abdominal aneurysm
- Carcinoma if bony metastasis occurs

- Endometriosis, fibromyoma
- Depression, hysteria
- Malingering
- Compression fracture, osteoporosis
- Osteoarthritis
- Ankylosing spondylitis
- Cauda equina syndrome

DIAGNOSTIC STUDIES

- X-rays may identify tumor or a structural abnormality. Consider imaging in the following situations with a complaint of low back pain:
  - ◊ Age over 50 years
  - ◊ Neurologic deficits
  - ◊ History of cancer
  - ◊ Accompanying unexplained weight loss
  - ◊ Substance abuse: steroids, alcohol, drugs
  - ◊ Recurrent or chronic back pain, or unresponsive to treatment after 1 month
  - ◊ History of significant trauma
  - ◊ Patient involved in litigation, desiring compensation
- Studies that may be done to exclude disc disease and tumors:
  - ◊ CT, MRI (study of choice for evaluation of disc disease), bone scan
  - ◊ CBC, ESR, serum calcium, alkaline phosphatase, serum immunoelectrophoresis
  - ◊ Urinalysis

Many asymptomatic patients have bulging discs.

PREVENTION

- Education regarding proper lifting techniques, body mechanics
- Conditioning exercises
- Maintenance of appropriate weight for height
- Avoid cigarette smoking

NONPHARMACOLOGIC MANAGEMENT

- Modify activities for 3 to 6 weeks
  - ◊ Limit bedrest to 2-4 days, then restrict activities to avoid heavy lifting and aggravating activities
  - ◊ Assume position that maximizes comfort
  - ◊ Gradually resume activities as tolerated and include gradually increasing low-stress aerobic exercises
- Physical modalities
  - ◊ Cryotherapy for 20-30 minutes several times up to 48 hours after onset
  - ◊ Apply heat for 20-30 minutes several times a day after the first 48 hours
  - ◊ Exercise: isometric tightening of abdominal and gluteal muscles after acute pain subsides; lumbar hyperextension exercises
  - ◊ Spinal manipulation may be helpful during the first month of back pain, but neurologic involvement must first be ruled out
- Education regarding preventive measures
- Shoe insoles, shoe lifts recommended for leg length discrepancies > 2 cm

Conservative measures are usually recommended for the first 6 weeks unless there are neurological deficits or severe pain.

PHARMACOLOGIC MANAGEMENT

- NSAIDs reduce pain and inflammation and promote healing
- Acetaminophen reduces pain but is more effective in combination with a narcotic analgesic or NSAID
- Muscle relaxants have not been proven more effective than NSAIDs, either alone, or used concomitantly, but are helpful for spastic conditions
- Short term use of opioid analgesics for pain relief, but have not been proven more effective than NSAIDs and have potential for physical dependence
- Epidural steroid injections to reduce inflammation and pain if more conservative treatments fail

LOW BACK PAIN PHARMACOLOGIC MANAGEMENT

Class	Drug Generic name (Trade name®)	Dosage How supplied	Comments
Muscle Relaxants *act on the central nervous system to decrease input to the alpha neurons*	**cyclobenzaprine**	**Adult**: *Initial*: 5 mg up to three times daily *Max*: 10 mg up to three times daily **Children**: not recommended	• Pregnancy Category B • Therapy should not exceed 2-3 weeks • Use lower doses in elderly or those with hepatic impairment • May cause disorientation, drowsiness, falls • Avoid concomitant use of MAO inhibitor • Avoid following acute myocardial infarction, heart block, or heart failure • Cautious use in patients with history of urinary retention, glaucoma • Avoid concurrent anticholinergic medications • Avoid concurrent use of alcohol products
	Flexeril	*Tabs: 5 mg, 10 mg*	
	metaxalone	**Adult**: 800 mg three or four times per day **Children**: not recommended	• Pregnancy Category C • Avoid in patients with hepatic dysfunction • May enhance central nervous system depression • Avoid concurrent use of alcohol products
	Skelaxin	*Tabs: 800 mg*	
	methocarbamol	**Adult**: *Initial*: 1,500 mg four times per day for 2-3 days *Usual*: 4 grams/day over four divided doses **Children**: not recommended	• Pregnancy Category C • May enhance central nervous system depression • Avoid concurrent use of alcohol products
	Robaxin	*Tabs: 500 mg, 750 mg*	

CONSULTATION/REFERRAL

- Findings that indicate neurological involvement
- Recurrent or chronic pain unresponsive to therapy
- Physical therapy initially if pain is moderate and conservative treatment has not provided relief

FOLLOW-UP

- Return for repeat evaluation in 24-48 hours if pain is severe, and in 7-10 days if pain is moderate; follow every 2-4 weeks until able to resume lifestyle
- Ongoing education and support regarding lifestyle changes
- If there is inability to tolerate activities in the face of no serious underlying pathology, explore psychosocial factors

EXPECTED COURSE

- In 80% of cases, symptoms resolve in 4-6 weeks

POSSIBLE COMPLICATIONS

- Prolonged disability associated with physical, psychologic, social, and economic factors

BURSITIS

DESCRIPTION

Inflammation of a bursa, a flattened sac of synovial membrane which contains synovial fluid. These are found in areas where friction is likely to occur, such as, where a tendon overrides bony structures. They may be deep, (e.g., hip, ischial tuberosity), or superficial (e.g., shoulder, knee, heel, elbow).

ETIOLOGY

- Bursitis is often secondary to calcific tendinitis. An acutely inflamed tendon irritates the overlying bursa.
- Contributing factors are overuse and structural and functional abnormalities
- May also be a result of bacterial infection

INCIDENCE

- Common
- Males > Females

RISK FACTORS

- Local trauma
- Repetitive motion
- Sudden increase in level of activity
- Gout
- Rheumatoid arthritis
- Aging
- Obesity
- Leg length discrepancy
- Osteoarthritis
- Penetrating injury

ASSESSMENT FINDINGS

Types of Bursitis	
Infective Bursitis	Elevated temperature, red, exquisitely tender overlying tissue
Anserine Bursitis	Painful knee, worse with stair climbing
Achilles Bursitis	Painful heel, subcutaneous swelling at back of Achilles tendon ("pump bump")
Calcaneal Bursitis	Painful plantar surface of heel
Infrapatellar Bursitis	Swelling and tenderness below patella
Iliopsoas Bursitis	Painful groin and anterior thigh
Ischial Bursitis	Pain with sitting or lying, may radiate down back of thigh, point tenderness over ischium
Olecranon Bursitis	Elbow pain with subcutaneous swelling, no loss of motion to elbow
Prepatellar Bursitis	Pain over medial aspect of knee
Subdeltoid Bursitis	Shoulder pain with subcutaneous swelling
Trochanteric Bursitis	Gradual onset of lateral hip and thigh pain

DIFFERENTIAL DIAGNOSIS

- Sprain, strain
- Tendonitis
- Osteoarthritis, rheumatoid arthritis
- Gout
- Degenerative joint disease

DIAGNOSTIC STUDIES

- Aspiration and culture of synovial fluid if infective bursitis suspected
- Bursitis seldom shown on x-ray, but may see calcium deposits
- MRI, CT (not initially done)
- ESR to differentiate soft tissue disease from connective tissue disease
- Blood culture indicated for multiple systemic features: methicillin-resistant *Staphylococcus aureus* is frequent finding
- CBC
- Consider RPR to rule out syphilis

PREVENTION

- Avoid overuse of joints without adequate rest periods
- Maintain physical fitness

NONPHARMACOLOGIC MANAGEMENT

- Identify and avoid aggravating factors
- Slings, shoe lifts, splints, or canes to correct biomechanical disruption
- Physical therapy program of stretching and strengthening
- Ice to inflamed area
- Rest, immobility of affected extremity
- Weight loss if indicated
- Application of ice/heat

PHARMACOLOGIC MANAGEMENT

Inflammatory bursitis:

- Administer NSAIDs at full anti-inflammatory dose (see NSAID table in Osteoarthritis)
- Intrabursal aspiration and injection of an anesthetic and a corticosteroid
    - ◊ Avoid injecting Achilles bursitis due to risk of Achilles tendon rupture

CONSULTATION/REFERRAL

- Orthopedist for surgical excision of involved area if chronic bursitis develops or for incision and drainage if infected

FOLLOW-UP

- Use NSAID until symptoms have subsided for 1 week
- Up to 3 corticosteroid injections may be given 4-6 weeks apart
- Recurrence of bursitis within 7 days of injection should raise suspicion of septic bursitis and indicate a need for re-aspiration

EXPECTED COURSE

- Once aggravating factors are removed, bursitis usually heals without complications or progression to chronic condition

POSSIBLE COMPLICATIONS

- Progression to chronic bursitis with limitation of range of motion

EPICONDYLITIS
(Tennis Elbow, Golfer's Elbow)

DESCRIPTION

Lateral epicondylitis, or "tennis elbow", is inflammation of the common tendinous origin of the extensor muscles of the forearm on the humeral lateral epicondyle. *Medial epicondylitis,* or "golfer's elbow", is inflammation of the common tendinous origin of the extensor muscles of the forearm at the humeral medial epicondyle. The principles outlined in epicondylitis apply to other types of tendonitis.

ETIOLOGY

- Repetitive overuse of the involved muscle without sufficient rest to allow rebuilding of muscle tissue

INCIDENCE

- Common over age 40 years

RISK FACTORS

Lateral epicondylitis:
- Overuse activities requiring a strong grasp during wrist extension
  - ◊ Typing
  - ◊ Weight lifting
  - ◊ Knitting
  - ◊ Backhand tennis stroke
  - ◊ Carpentry
  - ◊ Factory work

Medial epicondylitis:
- Activities which require forcefully extending the elbow against resistance with the forearm supinated and the wrist dorsiflexed
- Golf
- Pitching

ASSESSMENT FINDINGS

Lateral epicondylitis:
- Gradual onset of dull, aching pain over a period of weeks or months on the lateral aspect of the elbow; may be present at rest, but usually worse with activity
- Pain may radiate down the back of the forearm
- Shaking hands, lifting a cup, or turning a door knob may elicit sharp pain
- Point tenderness over lateral epicondyle; full range of motion; no swelling, and no erythema
- Pain to the lateral aspect of the elbow when resistance is applied against wrist extension

Medial epicondylitis:
- Pain to the region of the medial epicondyle, reproducible by forcefully extending the elbow against resistance with the forearm supinated and the wrist dorsiflexed
- Pain may radiate down the flexor surface of the forearm
- Point tenderness over medial epicondyle; no swelling or erythema

DIFFERENTIAL DIAGNOSIS

- Olecranon bursitis (may coexist)
- Tendon avulsion or rupture
- Osteoarthritis
- Radial nerve entrapment syndrome
- Radial head dislocation
- Synovitis of the elbow
- Interarticular loose bodies
- Cervical spine disorder
- Carpal tunnel syndrome
- Radial tunnel syndrome
- Fracture

Tendonitis and arthritis may be difficult to differentiate clinically. Arthritis produces pain in the joint. Tendinitis produces pain at the insertion point of the affected tendon (not in the joint).

DIAGNOSTIC STUDIES

- X-rays of the elbow are usually normal and are unnecessary unless there is a history of trauma, or therapy failure
- Diagnosis is made on basis of characteristic presentation
- MRI is preferred diagnostic tool when conservative measures have failed (will identify tears, ruptures)

PREVENTION

- Educate about need to balance repetitive movement with rest
- Educate that all changes in intensity, duration, or frequency of physical activity should be gradual to allow for conditioning
- Ergonomic evaluation if contributory

NONPHARMACOLOGIC MANAGEMENT

- Rest, cessation of exacerbating activity for 2 weeks, with gradual return to full activity
- Ice massage to area: apply ice, with pressure, directly to the skin over the epicondyle and surrounding area for 20 minutes three times a day
- Once acute symptoms have abated, patient should begin forearm strengthening and muscle stretching exercises
- Tennis elbow counterforce brace may help to relieve pain while playing
- Changing size of grip or string tension of tennis racket may be helpful
- Deep massage of the tendinous insertions of the epicondyle is theorized to help regenerate damaged tendons
- Surgical intervention is an option if unresponsive to 6-12 months of therapy

PHARMACOLOGIC MANAGEMENT

- Nonsteroidal anti-inflammatory (NSAID) medication (see NSAID table in Osteoarthritis)
- Intra-articular corticosteroid injection, best reserved for cases unresponsive to more conservative therapies

CONSULTATION/REFERRAL

- Orthopedist if unresponsive to therapy
- Physical therapist for instruction on strengthening and stretching exercise
- Occupational therapist for work-related etiology and ergonomic evaluation

FOLLOW-UP

- 2 weeks after initial intervention to evaluate effect of therapy
- Once acute pain abates, a conditioning program should be initiated

EXPECTED COURSE

- Acute symptoms usually resolve in 2 weeks with conservative treatment
- Return to previous activities without sufficient conditioning may result in recurrence

POSSIBLE COMPLICATIONS

- Reduction in occupational productivity (lost work days)

UPPER EXTREMITY JOINT DERANGEMENT
(LITTLE LEAGUE ELBOW)

DESCRIPTION

An overuse injury of the elbow that occurs in children.

ETIOLOGY

- Repeated forceful pulls of the flexor/pronator muscle group results in post traumatic changes in the medial condylar apophysis

INCIDENCE

- Occurs predominantly in children ages 9-15 years

RISK FACTORS

- Playing baseball, particularly pitching
- Previous elbow trauma

ASSESSMENT FINDINGS

- Pain about the elbow, worse after throwing
- Loss of motion, especially supination and full extension of the elbow
- Pain with passive wrist extension
- Weak grip
- Ulnar nerve paresthesia

DIFFERENTIAL DIAGNOSIS

- Ulnar collateral ligament sprain
- Cervical radiculopathy
- Ulnar neuritis

DIAGNOSTIC STUDIES

- Anterior/posterior, lateral, medial, and lateral oblique x-ray of the elbow: widening of the apophyseal plate, medial epicondylar apophyseal avulsion

PREVENTION

- Education regarding conditioning, proper technique of throwing motion, adequate rest
- Avoid repetitious throwing (limit number of games pitched)

NONPHARMACOLOGIC MANAGEMENT

- Rest
- Children who are heavily emotionally involved in sports may tolerate playing in other positions
- Avoid pitching until symptoms are resolved and range of motion is normal
- Counsel overzealous parents or coaches
- Application of ice for 15 minutes three times a day and after activity

PHARMACOLOGIC MANAGEMENT

- NSAIDs (ibuprofen most commonly used in children)

CONSULTATION/REFERRAL

- Orthopedist if not resolved with rest, ice, and therapy
- Physical therapist for conditioning and strengthening

FOLLOW-UP

- Gradual program of increased activity is necessary to prevent recurrence

EXPECTED COURSE

- May return to full activity once free of pain and full range of motion has returned

POSSIBLE COMPLICATIONS

- Avulsion-fragmentation of the apophysis

SUBLUXATION OF THE RADIAL HEAD
(Nursemaid's Elbow, Pulled Elbow)

DESCRIPTION

A radial head subluxation is a partial dislocation but contact between joints remains intact.

ETIOLOGY

- Infants and young children's radial heads are not as bulbous as that of an older child or adult
- Subluxation of the annular ligament can be initiated if longitudinal traction is applied to the arm while the elbow is extended
- A jerk of the arm while a child's hand is being held by an adult is a common cause
- Another cause is the child being forcibly lifted by the hand

INCIDENCE

- Occurs in children < 4 years of age usually

RISK FACTORS

- History of previous subluxation

ASSESSMENT FINDINGS

- Child holds hand in a pronated position, may refuse to use the hand, and cries when the elbow is moved

As long as pronated position is maintained, child usually does not complain of pain.

DIFFERENTIAL DIAGNOSIS

- Fracture

DIAGNOSTIC STUDIES

- X-rays are not usually necessary for diagnosis

PREVENTION

- Educate parents to avoid lifting or pulling child (especially forcefully) by the hands/arms

MANAGEMENT

- Apply pressure over the radial head while rotating the hand and forearm to a supinated position until a palpable click is felt along the elbow's lateral aspect

EXPECTED COURSE

- Once a subluxation has occurred, there is an increased likelihood of recurrence until age 4 years at which time the radial head is sufficiently developed

SPRAIN

DESCRIPTION

Stretching or partial tearing of ligaments. Ligaments are dense connective tissue arranged in a parallel fashion that connect one bone to another.

Sprains Graded According To Severity	
Grade I	Minimally torn ligament, stable joint
Grade II	More severely torn ligament, stable joint
Grade III	Completely torn ligament, unstable joint

A strain is an injury to a muscle or tendon usually associated with improper use or overuse.

ETIOLOGY

- The relative weakness of the ligament, along with the bony characteristics of the joint, result in susceptibility to injury
- Eversion ankle sprains, resulting from tears in the deltoid ligament, are less common, but tend to be more severe

INCIDENCE

- A common musculoskeletal injury, often sports-related
- 85% of ankle injuries are sprains
- Prevalent in all ages in which patient engages in physical activity
- Males > Females

RISK FACTORS

- Sports participation, especially volleyball, football, or basketball
- Prior sprain
- Trauma, falls
- Excessive exercise
- Inadequate warmup
- Poor strength, flexibility, or proprioception
- Wearing inappropriate shoes for activity

ASSESSMENT FINDINGS

- Pain and edema over and around injured joint
- Erythema
- Ecchymosis
- Audible pop heard at time of injury
- Discomfort upon weight-bearing
- Abnormal gait if affects lower extremity (ankle, knee)
- Decreased range of motion (Grade 1 and 2 sprains)
- No focal point of exquisite tenderness

If increased range of motion occurs at any injured joint, suspect severe tear or rupture of ligament.

DIFFERENTIAL DIAGNOSIS

- Fracture
- Ruptured tendon
- Tendinitis
- Bursitis

Often difficult clinically to distinguish between strain and sprain and so a common diagnosis is strain/sprain.

DIAGNOSTIC STUDIES

- X-rays indicated if there is suspicion of fracture:
  - ◊ Point of exquisite tenderness
  - ◊ Pain near the bone of the injured joint
  - ◊ Inability to bear weight immediately after injury or at time of exam

PREVENTION

- During pre-participation sports examination, discuss importance of training and flexibility
- Consider external supports for patients with poor flexibility, weakness, or decreased proprioception
- Ankle/knee training programs to improve strength, flexibility, and proprioception, and for those with previous history of ankle/knee injury
- Taping or bracing the ankle/knee of those participating in high-risk activities
- Appropriate conditioning and maintenance of physical conditioning

NONPHARMACOLOGIC MANAGEMENT

R I C E **Therapy**
Rest, stop all weight-bearing immediately after injury
Ice applied to injured area for 20 minutes every hour (while awake) for the first 24 hours after injury
Compression of injured area, accomplished by wrapping with an elastic bandage
Elevation of injured joint above heart level

- Apply heat for 20 minute periods 4 times a day after the first 24-48 hours
- Crutches while unable to bear weight
- Air casts provide pain relief and usually allow patient to resume mobility and weight bearing

PHARMACOLOGIC MANAGEMENT

- Children: acetaminophen as needed to relieve pain
- Adults: nonsteroidal anti-inflammatory (NSAID) agents used to relieve pain and reduce inflammation (see NSAID table in Osteoarthritis, page 493)
- Short course narcotic analgesics for moderate to severe pain

CONSULTATION/REFERRAL

- Orthopedist if Grade III sprain or eversion sprain
- Orthopedist if not significantly improved in 3 weeks
- Orthotist for support devices

FOLLOW-UP

- Return in 2 weeks:
    - Educate regarding preventive measures (e.g., ankle strengthening exercises and supportive footwear)
    - Evaluate for pain, swelling, and weight-bearing ability

EXPECTED COURSE

- Recovery expected in 2-6 weeks, depending on severity of sprain/strain

POSSIBLE COMPLICATIONS

- Arthritis
- Recurrence due to joint instability

FRACTURES

DESCRIPTION

A complete or incomplete break in the continuity of a bone.

ETIOLOGY

- Usually associated with a direct blow, fall, crushing injury, snapping force, or twisting motion

INCIDENCE

- Common
- Age of prevalence dependent on fracture location
- 75% of fractures in children occur in the upper extremities

RISK FACTORS

- Osteoporosis, alcohol use, cigarette smoking
- Use of sedatives in the elderly
- Neurological impairment, impaired vision
- Malignancy
- Frequent falls, frailty
- Participation in contact sports, deconditioning

ASSESSMENT FINDINGS

- Swelling
- Point tenderness at fracture site
- Decreased or abnormal mobility of affected extremity; pain with motion
- Open wound
- Asymmetry of extremities
- Gross deformity of extremity

A hip fracture may be present in the absence of hip pain. The pain may be referred to the knee. This may be the patient's only complaint after trauma or a fall.

DIFFERENTIAL DIAGNOSIS

- Fracture with associated neurovascular damage
- Fracture with associated injuries to joints above and below
- Open fracture vs. closed fracture
- Growth center vs. avulsion fracture
- Nursemaid's elbow
- Sprain, strain, soft tissue injury
- Dislocation of joint
- Presence of malignancy

DIAGNOSTIC STUDIES

- Neurovascular examination to rule out damage to nerves or blood vessels
  - ◊ A cool, pulseless extremity signals an emergency
- AP and lateral x-ray of affected extremity, but consider x-ray above and below affected joint
  - ◊ With inclusion of joints above and below suspected fracture site
  - ◊ Comparison views if growth plate involvement is suspected
- Assessment of underlying organs, (e.g., heart, lungs)
- Skeletal survey if child abuse suspected

PREVENTION

- Prophylaxis for osteoporosis
- Avoidance of long-acting sedatives in elderly
- Encourage use of walkers, and other devices that assist with mobility for the neurologically impaired or elderly
- Proper protective gear for athletes

NONPHARMACOLOGIC MANAGEMENT

- Splinting for immobilization should precede x-ray evaluation in order to prevent damage due to sharp bony ends
  - ◊ Adequate padding should precede splint
  - ◊ Joint above and below suspected fracture site should be included
- Application of ice for 48-72 hours
- Elevation of extremity if possible

PHARMACOLOGIC MANAGEMENT

- Analgesia
  - ◊ NSAIDs (use is controversial because the inflammatory process is thought to speed healing)
  - ◊ Acetaminophen
  - ◊ Narcotic analgesics (avoid if head injury is suspected)
- Tetanus toxoid for open wounds, if indicated
- Antibiotics if infection is a likely complication

CONSULTATION/REFERRAL

- Orthopedist for casting of nondisplaced fracture or surgical reduction and pinning as needed
- Neurosurgeon for head, spinal injuries, or neurological injuries
- Otorhinolaryngologist/oral surgeon for facial injuries
- Orthotist
- Physical therapist
- Occupational therapist

FOLLOW-UP

- Cast care
  - ◊ Keep dry
  - ◊ Seek attention for pain or severe pressure within cast, or color change (blue), temperature change (cold), tingling, swelling, or decreased motion to fingers or toes
  - ◊ Obvious malodor should be evaluated by healthcare provider
  - ◊ Avoid sticking objects into cast, often used for scratching
- X-ray studies should be obtained after reduction
- Long-term monitoring of growth if growth plate affected

EXPECTED COURSE

- Callus formation expected by 6 weeks
- Remodeling occurs in 1 year
- Growth is likely to be affected if the fracture extends through the epiphysis

POSSIBLE COMPLICATIONS

- Untreated compartment syndrome resulting in ischemic contracture
- Phlebitis

- Deformities related to malreduction or loss of reduction
- Permanent nerve injury
- Infection
- Posttraumatic arthritis
- Growth arrest due to involvement of growth plate

STRESS FRACTURE

DESCRIPTION

Fractures that occur in the tibia, fibula, metatarsals, and femoral neck.

ETIOLOGY

- Repetitive force applied to the lower leg during strenuous activity

INCIDENCE

- Females > Males
- Incidence increases with age

RISK FACTORS

- Long-distance running
- Sudden increase in intensity or level of activity
- Age
- Female gender
- Osteoporosis
- Malalignment of the leg

ASSESSMENT FINDINGS

- Vague hip or leg pain, in early stages present only with activity, in later stages present even at rest
- Full range of motion on examination

DIFFERENTIAL DIAGNOSIS

- Bursitis
- Lumbosacral radiculopathy
- Slipped capital femoral epiphysis
- Tibial stress syndrome (shin splints)
- Abdominal or pelvic mass
- Abdominal aortic aneurysm

DIAGNOSTIC STUDIES

- X-ray: may be negative, hairline radiolucency or periosteal callus
- Triple phase bone scan: increased uptake at fracture site

PREVENTION

- Cross-training (engagement in a different type of activity)
- Prevention of osteoporosis
- Education regarding foot gear, technique, and terrain

MANAGEMENT

- Cross-train for 3-6 weeks (e.g., swimming, cycling, running in water)
- Use cane, crutches, or apply air cast, if weight-bearing causes pain

CONSULTATION/REFERRAL

- Orthopedist for fractures at increased risk of nonunion:
  - ◊ Anterior medial third of tibia
  - ◊ Tarsal navicular and diaphyseal-metaphyseal junction of the fifth metatarsal (Jones's fracture)
  - ◊ Fracture in hypovascular area

FOLLOW-UP

- Perform x-ray after 3-6 weeks, prior to returning to running: should demonstrate callus formation and alignment
- Runner should be free of pain with walking for 1-2 weeks before beginning to run
- If symptoms recur, decrease activity for 1 week to a level that is pain-free

EXPECTED COURSE

- Full recovery is expected in 2 months

POSSIBLE COMPLICATIONS

- Avascular necrosis
- Refracture
- Pseudoarthrosis

CLAVICULAR FRACTURE

DESCRIPTION

Disruption of the junction of the middle and lateral aspects of the clavicle. Fractures are differentiated by location and severity:

- Type I: distal third of clavicle; supporting ligaments remain intact
- Type II: distal third of clavicle; coracoclavicular ligaments remain attached to the distal fragment and the proximal fragment is displaced upward
- Type III: intra-articular fracture through the acromioclavicular joint; no displacement

ETIOLOGY

- Trauma: can result from birth injury, a fall on an extended arm, or a blow to the shoulder or chest

INCIDENCE

- The clavicle is the bone most frequently fractured at birth
- Common in childhood secondary to trauma

RISK FACTORS

- Macrosomic infant
- Falls

ASSESSMENT FINDINGS

- Fracture of the distal clavicle may present with no deformity
- Pain with shoulder movement; holding arm against chest to prevent motion
- Edema, crepitus, and/or point tenderness over fracture site
- Ecchymosis or tenting of the skin over the fracture site
- History of difficult delivery, especially if there was shoulder dystocia
- Noticeable bump at fracture site
- Gentle pressure elicits pain
- Grinding sensation with attempts to raise arm

DIFFERENTIAL DIAGNOSIS

- Sternoclavicular ligamentous tear
- Acromioclavicular separation
- Brachial palsy

DIAGNOSTIC STUDIES

- X-rays are usually not necessary in infants
- Standard clavicle x-ray series, which includes anteroposterior and apical lordotic views
- If there is strong clinical suspicion in light of negative x-rays, MRI may be indicated

PREVENTION

- Include palpation of clavicles in all newborn examinations for early detection
- Seatbelt use

NONPHARMACOLOGIC MANAGEMENT

- Neonate usually requires only gentle movement until formation of callus, by 2-3 weeks
- Apply ice first 24 hours after injury
- Sling for 3-6 weeks is usually adequate for nondisplaced fracture; figure-8 clavicle strap for 4-8 weeks may be preferable for adults
- Instruct patient to use arm as pain permits; avoid

contact sports for 2-3 months, and gradually increase activity as symptoms allow
- Open reduction internal fixation (ORIF) for Type II distal clavicle fracture with significant displacement, or for neurovascular or intrathoracic injury

PHARMACOLOGIC MANAGEMENT

- Analgesics as needed during acute stage

CONSULTATION/REFERRAL

- Orthopedist
  - ◊ Neurovascular compromise
  - ◊ Severe tenting of skin
  - ◊ Open fracture
  - ◊ Multiple injuries
  - ◊ If improved cosmetic results are needed
  - ◊ Nonunion symptoms after 3-4 months
  - ◊ Posterior displacement significant with risk of intrathoracic injury
  - ◊ Type II fracture for possible ORIF

FOLLOW-UP

- 1-2 weeks after injury, then every 2-3 weeks until asymptomatic
- Repeat x-rays may be performed once patient is asymptomatic to assess callus formation

EXPECTED COURSE

- Clinical union occurs by 12 weeks in adults and by 6 weeks in children
- Callus can be felt over site of fracture in neonate within a few days
- Remodeling occurs by 6-12 months

POSSIBLE COMPLICATIONS

- Malunion, resulting in angulation, shortening, and poor cosmetic appearance
- Degenerative arthritis of the acromioclavicular joint
- Underlying intrathoracic injury

ROTATOR CUFF SYNDROME

DESCRIPTION

- A spectrum of injuries involving any of the 4 rotator cuff muscles (most commonly the supraspinatus). Injuries range from sprains, tendinitis, to complete rupture with cuff-tear arthroplasty.

ETIOLOGY

- Cuff tears may occur with acute injury or may be age related due to degeneration, chronic muscle impingement, or inadequate blood supply to the tendons

INCIDENCE

- 5-10% of general population, more common in males

RISK FACTORS

- Repetitive use
- Overhead throwing motion
- Shoulder instability

ASSESSMENT FINDINGS

- Pain, often at night
- Pain may be referred down deltoid; may be increased with overhead movement
- Tenderness over rotator cuff area
- Weakness with abduction or forward flexion
- Atrophy of supraspinatus and infraspinatus muscles resulting in sunken area in back of shoulder
- Limited active range of motion (ROM)
- Grating sensation at tip of shoulder when lifting the arm
- Positive “drop arm” test (weakness with abduction against downward pressure at 90°)
- Cross Arm test to identify acromioclavicular joint disease

DIFFERENTIAL DIAGNOSES

- Shoulder instability, frozen shoulder
- Degenerative arthritis
- Cervical radiculopathy
- Avascular necrosis
- Suprascapular nerve entrapment
- Thoracic outlet syndrome

DIAGNOSTIC STUDIES

- Plain shoulder x-ray, with visualization of acromion at 30° caudal tilt
- Ultrasound may be helpful with large tears
- MRI to diagnose full or partial thickness tears or other causes of shoulder pain

NONPHARMACOLOGIC MANAGEMENT

- Rest to avoid overhead activity
- Ice or heat for comfort
- Strengthening exercises

PHARMACOLOGIC MANAGEMENT

- NSAIDS
- Shoulder injection 1-2 times at 2 week intervals
- Note: Avoid shoulder injections in presence of local infection
- Injections may weaken the tendon, and with repeated injections my accelerate rotator cuff tear

CONSULT/REFERRALS

- Surgical intervention considered if not responsive to rehabilitation over 3-6 months, exception to this rule: patient with an acute traumatic cuff tear
- Failure of 6 weeks nonsurgical treatment is indicative of further evaluation

FOLLOW UP

- With conservative treatments, follow up in 2 weeks to evaluate effectiveness

POSSIBLE COMPLICATIONS

- Loss of shoulder function
- Chronic pain
- Joint degeneration with long standing tears

OSTEOPOROSIS

DESCRIPTION

Deterioration of bone tissue results in low bone density, bone fragility, and consequent increased risk of fractures.

Post menopausal fractures occur because of resorption of bone due to lack of estrogen secretion.

ETIOLOGY

- Genetics influences bone mass by 50%
- Estrogen deficiency
- Calcium deficiency
- Use of alcohol and nicotine
- Immobilization
- Certain medications

INCIDENCE

- 1.2 million fractures each year in the U.S. are attributable to osteoporosis
- 1/3 of women > age 65 years sustain vertebral fractures
- Females > Males
- Common in Caucasians and Orientals
- Uncommon in African-Americans and Latinos

After age 75, osteoporotic fractures occur at the same rate in men and women.

RISK FACTORS

- Age (bone loss is a consequence of aging)
- Medication use: corticosteroids, anticonvulsants, thyroid supplements

- Estrogen deficiency related to menopause
- Testosterone deficiency related to hypogonadism
- Eating disorders
- Calcium/Vitamin D deficiency
- Excessive phosphate, protein intake
- Immobilization, sedentary lifestyle
- Cigarette smoking, chronic alcohol use, caffeine intake
- Family history

ASSESSMENT FINDINGS

- Often asymptomatic until present with fractures of the hip, vertebra, proximal humerus, proximal tibia, or pelvis
- Painless dorsal kyphosis (dowager's hump)
- Back pain
- Loss of height

DIFFERENTIAL DIAGNOSIS

- Primary osteoporosis: idiopathic or postmenopausal
- Secondary osteoporosis related to:
  - ◊ Chronic endocrine (hyperthyroidism especially), rheumatic, neurologic, or malabsorptive disease
  - ◊ Chronic renal failure
  - ◊ Liver disease
  - ◊ Anticonvulsant therapy
  - ◊ Malignancy (multiple myeloma and others)

DIAGNOSTIC STUDIES

- Bone mineral density (BMD) of both the spine and proximal femur
- T scores indicative of severity of bone loss:
  - ◊ Normal: + 1 SD (standard deviation)
  - ◊ Osteopenia: 1-2 SD
  - ◊ Osteoporosis: > 2 SD
- Z scores indicate number of SD compared to age matched controls
- Biochemical profile and CBC to exclude causes of secondary osteoporosis
- TSH to determine presence of hyperthyroidism or excessive thyroid supplementation
- 24-hour urine collection for calcium excretion: hypercalcuria indicates need to change calcium supplementation; low calcium excretion indicates vitamin D deficiency

PREVENTION

- Weight-bearing exercise daily
- Diet and supplements to achieve sufficient calcium and vitamin D
  - ◊ Young adults: calcium 800 mg/day and vitamin D 800 IU/day
  - ◊ Pregnant or lactating women: calcium 1500 mg/day and vitamin D 1000 IU/day
  - ◊ Postmenopausal women: calcium 1500 mg/day and vitamin D 1000 IU/day
  - ◊ Older male adults: calcium 1000 mg/day and vitamin D 1000 IU/day
- Parenteral testosterone for hypogonadal men (benefit may be offset by testosterone's hypertrophic effect on prostate and by its adverse effect on lipoproteins)
- Avoidance of nicotine, alcohol in excess, and if possible, medications known to contribute to bone loss
- Avoid falls and medications which may increase risk of falls

NONPHARMACOLOGIC MANAGEMENT

- Diet, exercise and avoidance of contributing risk factors
- Education regarding appropriate foot wear and lighting for fall prevention

PHARMACOLOGIC MANAGEMENT

- Daily calcium supplementation of 1500 mg/day and vitamin D 1000 IU/day
- Humans are only able to absorb about 500 mg of calcium at one time. Therefore, 1500 mg/day must be divided into 3 doses
- Testosterone replacement, if indicated, in hypogonadal men

Orthopedic Disorders

OSTEOPOROSIS PHARMACOLOGIC MANAGEMENT

Class	Drug Generic name (Trade name®)	Dosage How supplied	Comments
Calcium Supplements	**calcium carbonate**	**Adult:** chew 2 tabs twice daily with meals	• Pregnancy Category not available
<u>General comments</u> Vitamin D is required for calcium absorption Absorption is enhanced when taken with food Calcium may be irritating to the GI tract and may cause constipation	Tums	*Tabs: 200 mg* *Tums EX: 300 mg* *Tums Ultra: 400 mg*	
	calcium citrate	**Adult**: 1-2 tab daily	• Pregnancy category not available • Calcium citrate is more easily absorbed by the human body than calcium carbonate
	Citracal	*Tabs: 315 mg calcium* *200 IU vitamin D*	
Selective Estrogen Receptor Modulators (SERMS)	**raloxifene**	**Adult**: 60 mg daily **Children**: not recommended	• Pregnancy Category X • Increased risk of DVT especially during first 4 months of treatment • Reduce resorption of bone and decrease overall bone turnover • Taken without regard to meals
	Evista	*Tabs: 60 mg*	
Oral biphosphates <u>General comments</u> Supplement diet with additional calcium and vitamin D May cause local irritation of upper gastrointestinal mucosa Use caution in patients with Barrett's esophagus, dysphagia, gastritis	**alendronate**	<u>Post menopausal women and men with osteoporosis</u> **Adult**: Must take in AM at least 30 min prior to meal with 6-8 oz. water Either 10 mg daily or 70 mg weekly <u>Prevention of osteoporosis</u> Either 5 mg daily or 35 mg weekly	• Pregnancy Category C • Must remain upright for at least 30 minutes after dose • Avoid in patients with renal insufficiency • Concurrent use of aspirin products increases risk of adverse gastrointestinal events
	Fosamax	*Tabs: 5 mg, 10 mg, 35 mg, 70 mg* *Soln: 70 mg/75 mL*	

continued

OSTEOPOROSIS PHARMACOLOGIC MANAGEMENT

Class	Drug Generic name (Trade name®)	Dosage How supplied	Comments
	ibandronate	Post menopausal women and men with osteoporosis **Adult**: Either: 2.5 mg daily or 150 mg once monthly Prevention of osteoporosis **Adult:** Either: 2.5 mg daily **OR** 35 mg weekly	• Pregnancy Category C • Must remain upright for at least 60 minutes after dose • Swallow whole tablet • Take on the same day of each month
	Boniva	*Tabs: 2.5 mg, 150 mg*	
	risedronate	Post menopausal women and men with osteoporosis **Adult**: Either: 5 mg daily; OR 35 mg weekly OR 75 mg taken on two consecutive days each month OR 150 mg tablet once a month Prevention of osteoporosis **Adult**: Either: 5 mg daily; OR 35 mg weekly OR 75 mg taken on two consecutive days each month OR 150 mg tablet once a month	• Pregnancy Category C • Must remain upright for at least 30 minutes after dose • Avoid in patients with delayed esophageal emptying or stricture
	Actonel	*Tabs: 5 mg, 30 mg, 35 mg, 75 mg, 150 mg*	
	zoledronic acid	**Adult**: 5 mg IV yearly, administered over at least 15 minutes	• Pregnancy Category D • Supplement with calcium 1500 mg daily and vitamin D 1000 IU daily, especially 2 weeks prior to treatment • Avoid in patients with renal insufficiency
	Reclast	*Inj: 5 mg in 100 mL*	

continued

OSTEOPOROSIS PHARMACOLOGIC MANAGEMENT

Class	Drug Generic name (Trade name®)	Dosage How supplied	Comments
Hormone treatment	**calcitonin-salmon** Miacalcin	**Adult Female:** 1 spray in alternating nare daily *Spray: 200 I.U./spray*	• Pregnancy Category C • Monitor number of doses administered; discard bottle after 30 doses • Supplement diet with additional calcium and vitamin D

CONSULTATION/REFERRAL

- Appropriate specialist for management of underlying disease
- Exercise program to improve strength, balance, and flexibility
- Occupational therapist for assistance with activities of daily living
- Physical therapist for gait training and transfer skills

FOLLOW-UP

- Evaluate effects of medication at 1 month, then periodically thereafter
- Ongoing education and support regarding lifestyle changes
- Annual bone mineral density assessment
- X-rays as indicated for acute pain (to rule out fractures)
- Consider serum biochemical markers to monitor bone formation response to therapy at 3 months
  - ◊ Serum osteocalcin
  - ◊ Serum bone-specific alkaline phosphatase

EXPECTED COURSE

- In > 50% of cases, compliance with treatment will at least stabilize bone mass, and in some cases will increase it to a small degree, resulting in improved mobility and reduced pain
- In < 50% of cases, fractures occur despite treatment

POSSIBLE COMPLICATIONS

- Fractures resulting in musculoskeletal and sometimes neurologic deficits
- Disabling pain

OSGOOD-SCHLATTER DISEASE
(Apophysitis of the Tibial Tuberosity)

DESCRIPTION

An abnormality of the epiphyseal ossification of the tibial tubercle

ETIOLOGY

- During periods of rapid bone growth increased traction is placed upon the insertion of the patellar tendon at the tibial tubercle

INCIDENCE

- A common cause of knee pain in children ages 10-18 years
- Males > Females

RISK FACTORS

- Periods of rapid growth
- Repetitive jumping

ASSESSMENT FINDINGS

- Painful swelling of the tibial tubercle at the insertion of the patellar tendon, exacerbated by activity, squatting, or crouching, and relieved by rest
- Pain worsens with contraction of the quadriceps against resistance
- Unilateral or bilateral

DIFFERENTIAL DIAGNOSIS

- Fracture of the tibial plateau or proximal tibia
- Avulsion of the quadriceps tendon
- Patellofemoral syndrome
- Bursitis, synovitis
- Neoplasm of the proximal tibia

DIAGNOSTIC STUDIES

- None usually needed
- X-ray of the proximal tibia and knee: calcified thickening of tibial tuberosity
- Bone scan is not a good choice because there will be increased uptake because of age

NONPHARMACOLOGIC MANAGEMENT

- Rest, avoid activities that increase pain or swelling
- Quadriceps strengthening and stretching
- Application of ice
- Educate that participation in activities is reasonable as long as pain is minimal

PHARMACOLOGIC MANAGEMENT

- Analgesics (acetaminophen) or ibuprofen

CONSULTATION/REFERRAL

- Usually none

FOLLOW-UP

- As needed

EXPECTED COURSE

- Self-limiting condition resolves with skeletal maturation

POSSIBLE COMPLICATIONS

- Avulsion injury of the anterior tibial spine
- Chondromalacia
- Patellofemoral degenerative arthritis

DEVELOPMENTAL DYSPLASIA OF THE HIP
(DDH - Congenital Dislocation of the Hip)

DESCRIPTION

Partial or complete subluxation/dislocation of the femoral head from the pelvic acetabulum. Originally named congenital hip dislocation, but is now known to occur postnatally rather than congenitally.

ETIOLOGY

- Multifactorial
- Generalized laxity of ligaments
- Maternal estrogen and relaxin contribute to pelvic relaxation
- Breech position results in exaggerated hip flexion with limited hip motion and stretching of the ligaments. The limited motion of the hips leads to underdevelopment of the cartilaginous acetabulum
- Postnatal maintenance of the infant in an adducted, extended position rather than the natural abducted, flexed position

INCIDENCE

- Uncertain, ranges from 1/60 to 1/1000 births
- Females > Males
- 30-50% develop in breech positions
- 20% positive family history

RISK FACTORS

- Breech position, especially frank breech
- Use of swaddling or cradle board maintaining extended adducted position
- Underlying neuromuscular disorders
  - ◊ Myelodysplasia
  - ◊ Arthrogryposis multiplex congenita
- Positive family history
- Congenital muscular torticollis
- Metatarsus adductus
- Down syndrome

ASSESSMENT FINDINGS

- Limited abduction of the affected hip (< 60%)
- Asymmetric gluteal or inguinal folds
- Unequal leg length (shorter on affected side)
- Positive Barlow's sign (ability to dislocate an unstable hip)
  - ◊ Stabilize the pelvis with one hand and flex and adduct the opposite hip while applying a posterior force
  - ◊ The unstable hip will easily dislocate, then will relocate once the posterior force is removed
- Positive Ortolani's sign (useful between age 1 month and 3 months only)
  - ◊ Flex and abduct the thigh with the infant in the supine position
  - ◊ Lift the femoral head into the acetabulum
  - ◊ If reduction occurs, there is a palpable "clunk"
- Positive Galeazzi's sign: unequal knee heights when infant is placed in supine position with the hips and knees flexed and feet placed side by side on the table
- Limping, waddling, lumbar lordosis, toe-walking and leg length discrepancy are indications in older children

DIFFERENTIAL DIAGNOSIS

- Nonpathologic hip clicks

DIAGNOSTIC STUDIES

- Pelvic ultrasound is especially useful in neonates: unstable hip with limited acetabular development
- Anterior/posterior and Lauenstein x-rays are helpful after age 3 months. The newborn hip joint is too cartilaginous for x-ray to be reliable
- Arthrography, MRI and tomography are useful in cases that are difficult to diagnose

PREVENTION

- Educate about possible deleterious effect of maintaining the infant in the hip adducted and extended position (e.g., in swaddling or cradle board)
- Include hip examination in all infant and child assessments up to two years of age for early detection

MANAGEMENT

- Early treatment is crucial for good prognosis
- The earlier the therapy is begun, the less likely surgical reduction will be necessary

- Abduction orthoses hold the hip in the flexed abducted position for 1-2 months
  - ◊ Pavlik harness
  - ◊ Frejka splint
- Surgical closed reduction is primary treatment after age 6 months
- After age 18 months, open reduction with osteotomy is the only effective treatment

CONSULTATION/REFERRAL

- Immediate referral to orthopedist for orthosis or surgery

FOLLOW-UP

- Therapy is continued until there is clinical hip stability and radiographic evidence of resolution
- After surgical reduction, a spica cast is worn for 6-8 weeks
- Child and family require frequent support and education regarding cast care, skin care, car safety, and developmental stimulation while immobilized

EXPECTED COURSE

- Best outcomes achieved with early detection and treatment

POSSIBLE COMPLICATIONS

- Permanent dislocation of the femoral head with consequent limited mobility is the result of failure to treat
- Aseptic and avascular necrosis of the capital femoral epiphysis
- Redislocation or persistent dysplasia
- Postoperative complications (e.g., infection)

LEGG-CALVE-PERTHES DISEASE
(Legg-Perthes Disease)

DESCRIPTION

Osteonecrosis of the capital femoral epiphysis due to interrupted vascular supply results in ischemia and alteration in cartilage growth. The area eventually revascularizes and new bone begins to grow, but there is the likelihood of fracture due to fragility of bone. If a fracture occurs, the shape of the femoral head changes, causing interruption in articulation of the femoral head in the hip joint.

ETIOLOGY

- Pathology of the compromised blood flow to the femoral head is unclear
- Familial tendency

INCIDENCE

- Predominant age is 7 years; occurs from age 3-12 years
- Males > Females (4:1)

RISK FACTORS

- Slipped capital femoral epiphysis
- Developmental dysplasia of the hip
- Corticosteroid use
- Sickle cell disease
- Family history

ASSESSMENT FINDINGS

- Pain to the hip or referral to the medial aspect of the knee (pain has usually been present for 2-3 weeks before child complains)
- Limp
- Limited internal rotation and abduction of femur
- Unequal leg lengths, antalgic gait
- Atrophy of thigh muscles, muscle spasm
- History of hip trauma

- Positive Trendelenburg's sign:
  - ◊ Child stands and raises one foot off the ground
  - ◊ The pelvis drops on the raised foot side

DIFFERENTIAL DIAGNOSIS

- Toxic synovitis
- Lymphoma
- Osteomyelitis
- Juvenile rheumatoid arthritis
- Spondyloepiphyseal dysplasia
- Slipped capital femoral epiphysis

DIAGNOSTIC STUDIES

- CBC: normal
- ESR: normal
- Anterior/posterior and Lauenstein x-rays: altered epiphysis, subluxation
- MRI: necrosis
- Aspiration of synovial fluid: normal

The goal of treatment is to avoid severe arthritis.

NONPHARMACOLOGIC MANAGEMENT

- Initially, bedrest with possible femoral traction for 1-2 weeks
- Maintain range of motion
- Education regarding disease process

PHARMACOLOGIC MANAGEMENT

- Nonsteroidal anti-inflammatory agents

CONSULTATION/REFERRAL

- Immediate orthopedic surgeon referral
- Physical therapist

FOLLOW-UP

- Serial anterior/posterior and Lauenstein x-rays to determine progression

EXPECTED COURSE

- Self-limiting, revascularization occurs in 2-3 years
- Older children have a poorer prognosis; less growth period allows for decreased remodeling time

POSSIBLE COMPLICATIONS

- Osteoarthritis
- Decreased use of hip joint due to femoral head distortion

SLIPPED CAPITAL FEMORAL EPIPHYSIS
(SCFE)

DESCRIPTION

A fracture through the proximal femoral epiphysis. Shear force placed on the growth plate can cause osteonecrosis as the bone moves because at this age, blood supply to this part of the bone is tenuous.

ETIOLOGY

- Unknown
- Basis is believed to be endocrine because it is often accompanied by growth abnormalities

INCIDENCE

- The most common adolescent hip disorder
- 1 per 100,000 children
- Seen in adolescents
- Males > Females
- More common in African American boys

RISK FACTORS

- Obese adolescents with delayed skeletal maturation
- Tall, thin adolescents with a recent growth spurt
- Hypothyroidism

- Pituitary disorder
- Pseudohypoparathyroidism

ASSESSMENT FINDINGS

- Pre slip: mild discomfort of the hip, frequently noticed in the opposite hip of a previous slipped capital femorral epiphysis (SCFE)
- Acute: mild pain or limp lasting < 3 weeks followed by sudden hip pain so severe that the child is unable to bear weight, even with support; severe pain with any attempted hip motion
- Acute or chronic: child has had moderate pain, limp, and externally rotated gait lasting several months, then the epiphysis slips acutely, resulting in severe pain and inability to bear weight
- Chronic: several months of progressively worsening hip pain (child may walk with an antalgic, externally rotated gait; lack of internal rotation and increased external rotation noted on examination

SCFE is often misdiagnosed because only 50% of patients have hip pain and 25% have knee pain.

DIFFERENTIAL DIAGNOSIS

- Osgood-Schlatter disease
- Patellofemoral stress syndrome
- Legg-Calve-Perthes disease
- Transient synovitis of the hip
- Toxic synovitis
- Femoral neck stress fracture
- Septic arthritis
- Osteomyelitis

DIAGNOSTIC STUDIES

- AP x-ray of the pelvis
- Lauenstein leg x-ray
- MRI and CT are rarely needed for diagnosis

CONSULTATION/REFERRAL

- Urgent orthopedic referral for pinning (epiphysiodesis)

FOLLOW-UP

- By orthopedist; screw removal following closure of the capital femoral epiphysis (CFE) is controversial

EXPECTED COURSE

- Pinning prevents progression

POSSIBLE COMPLICATIONS

- Long-term disability from progression of the slip if pinning is not performed
- Osteonecrosis
- Chondrolysis

TRANSIENT SYNOVITIS OF THE HIP

DESCRIPTION

A self-limited, usually benign condition causing acute onset of limp and hip pain in children; it occurs rarely in adults

ETIOLOGY

- Uncertain
- Possibly related to a recent virus, trauma, or hypersensitivity reaction

INCIDENCE

- The most common cause of hip pain in children 3-10 years of age
- Mean age of onset is 6 years, but can occur at any age
- Males > Females

RISK FACTORS

- History of upper respiratory infection 7-14 days before onset of symptoms in 70% of affected children
- History of trauma

ASSESSMENT FINDINGS

- Acute onset of groin, anterior thigh, or knee pain

- Child remains ambulatory but walks with a limp to avoid pain (antalgic gait)
- May have low grade temperature
- Does not hold hip flexed or abducted; abduction and internal rotation are restricted
- Hip may be tender to palpation
- Most sensitive test is log roll: with child supine, roll affected hip from side to side; may see guarding or decreased range of motion
- May have decreased range of motion in knee on affected side
- Usually unilateral

In young children, the only symptom may be crying at night time.

DIFFERENTIAL DIAGNOSIS

- Legg-Calve-Perthes disease
- Septic arthritis
- Osteomyelitis
- Slipped capital femoral epiphysis
- Femoral neck stress fracture

DIAGNOSTIC STUDIES

- ESR: mildly elevated
- CBC: normal
- Fluoroscopic arthrocentesis: negative except for possibly a 1-3 mL synovial effusion
- Anterior/posterior & Lauenstein x-rays of the pelvis: normal
- Ultrasound of the hip: effusion
- Bone scan or MRI to rule out infection or Legg-Calve-Perthes disease

NONPHARMACOLOGIC MANAGEMENT

- Bedrest and non-weight-bearing until pain resolves, usually 7 days
- Limited activities for 2 weeks thereafter
- Check temperature regularly to exclude possibility of septic arthritis

PHARMACOLOGIC MANAGEMENT

- Nonsteroidal anti-inflammatory agents

CONSULTATION/REFERRAL

- Orthopedist if not resolved in 2 weeks with appropriate rest

POSSIBLE COMPLICATIONS

- Recurrence if activities are not sufficiently limited
- Coxa magna: enlargement and deformity of the femoral head and neck
- Legg-Calve-Perthes disease

SCOLIOSIS

DESCRIPTION

Lateral curvature of the spine

- *Idiopathic*: curve is > 10° and occurs in an otherwise healthy child > 10 years of age
- *Functional scoliosis*: appearance of a lateral curvature without structural changes in the vertebral column
- *Structural scoliosis*: true deformity of the vertebrae rather than a postural problem

ETIOLOGY

- Usually idiopathic
- Can be associated with anomalies of the spinal column, neuromuscular disease, or genetic disease
- Sometimes related to infection, tumor, or metabolic disease

INCIDENCE

- Females > Males (4-5:1)
- 3% of U.S. population affected

RISK FACTORS

- Legs of unequal length
- Anomalies of spinal column
- Cerebral palsy
- Neurofibromatosis
- Marfan syndrome
- Poliomyelitis

- Muscular dystrophy
- Friedreich's ataxia
- Charcot-Marie-Tooth disease
- Family history of scoliosis

ASSESSMENT FINDINGS

- Nonpainful, insidious onset of lateral curvature of the spine
- Unequal shoulder heights
- Unequal scapula prominences and heights
- Unequal waist angles
- Unequal rib prominences
- Chest asymmetry

DIFFERENTIAL DIAGNOSIS

- Neurofibromatosis
- Cerebral palsy
- Juvenile idiopathic scoliosis
- Multiple sclerosis
- Rett syndrome
- Rickets
- Tuberculosis
- Tumor
- Functional scoliosis disappears when child is placed in Adam's position (bending forward at the waist); structural scoliosis is accentuated

DIAGNOSTIC STUDIES

- Posteroanterior and standing x-rays of the entire spine identify the degree of curvature
- MRI to rule out tumor if there is associated back pain

Diagnosis is made when lateral curvature is 10° or greater.

PREVENTION

- Screening and early identification helps prevent need for more invasive treatment

Scoliosis is seen most often at the beginning of growth spurts and during adolescence and so screening should take place PRIOR to this time (around age 10 years).

MANAGEMENT

- Infants with curve > 25° usually require casting followed by a brace
- Spinal fusion may be necessary in adolescence (usually recommended once curve is 40°)
- Curves up to 25° are observed for 4-6 months
- Curves > 25°: refer
- Patient and family support

CONSULTATION/REFERRAL

- Orthopedic or neurosurgeon for surgical evaluation

FOLLOW-UP

- Monitoring and treatment continues until growth is complete

EXPECTED COURSE

- Depends on degree of curvature and how quickly treatment is initiated
- Full correction of deformity is not usually expected

POSSIBLE COMPLICATIONS

- Severe deformity may limit physical activities
- Cardiovascular and respiratory impairment
- Psychological sequelae: anger, low self-esteem

TALIPES EQUINOVARUS
(Club Foot)

DESCRIPTION

A congenital deformity of the foot, involves plantar flexion of the foot at the ankle joint, inversion deformity of the heel, and adduction of the forefoot. Unlike positioning deformities, correction requires active treatment. The foot cannot be manually corrected with the heel down. The condition can range from mild to severe.

ETIOLOGY

- Congenital
- Usually idiopathic
- May be associated with neurological problems or muscular disease
- Uterine positioning may also be a factor

INCIDENCE

- Occurs in 1/1000 births
- Males > Females (2:1)

RISK FACTORS

- Myelomeningocele
- Cerebral palsy
- Family history

ASSESSMENT FINDINGS

- Present at birth, ranging from mild to severe
- Foot in pointed toe position, plantar flexed
- Sole of foot is inverted
- Convex shape to foot, markedly adducted
- Position cannot be manually corrected with the heel down, heel cord not flexible
- Unilateral or bilateral
- In the older child, there is foot and calf atrophy

DIFFERENTIAL DIAGNOSIS

- Metatarsus adductus

DIAGNOSTIC STUDIES

- AP and lateral standing or simulated weight-bearing x-rays with line measurements to determine the navicular bone position and overall foot alignment

PREVENTION

- Early intervention results in easier correction due to greater flexibility of joints of the newborn

MANAGEMENT

- Orthopedist may attempt casting, but surgery (soft tissue release, naviculectomy, or arthrodesis) is usually required for correction

CONSULTATION/REFERRAL

- Urgent orthopedic referral

FOLLOW-UP

- Prolonged orthopedic follow-up is necessary

EXPECTED COURSE

- Possible recurrence
- Goal is a pain-free foot and ability to wear shoes
- Lifelong orthosis is frequently necessary

POSSIBLE COMPLICATIONS

- Surgery complications

METATARSUS ADDUCTUS

DESCRIPTION

A condition which occurs at birth and is characterized by a straight hindfoot and an adducted forefoot. The result is a curved, intoeing shape to the foot.

ETIOLOGY

- Intrauterine positioning

INCIDENCE

- Commonly occurs at birth

RISK FACTORS

- Family history

ASSESSMENT FINDINGS

- Convexity of the lateral border of the foot in contrast to the normal straight appearance
- If a line drawn from the center of the heel through the center of the metatarsal-tarsal line bisects lateral to the space between the second and third toes, the forefoot is adducted in relation to the hindfoot
- If the foot is flexible, the forefoot can be abducted past midline; in rigid metatarsus adductus, the forefoot cannot be abducted past midline
- Foot turns inward whether child is weight-bearing or not

DIFFERENTIAL DIAGNOSIS

- Congenital vertical talus
- Talipes equinovarus

DIAGNOSTIC STUDIES

- X-rays of the foot are indicated in rigid metatarsus adductus

MANAGEMENT

- Flexible foot: teach parent to perform passive stretching of the forefoot into the straight position several times a day
- Rigid foot: may require serial casting or surgery for correction

CONSULTATION/REFERRAL

- Rigid foot: orthopedist at time condition is identified
- Condition unresponsive after 4-6 months: orthopedist
- Following casting, orthotist for out flaring or reverse last shoes

FOLLOW-UP

- Evaluate response to passive exercise every 2 months

EXPECTED COURSE

- 85% of cases resolve spontaneously
- Resolution occurs most rapidly with a flexible foot
- Children older than 2-3 years of age are more likely to require corrective surgery

POSSIBLE COMPLICATIONS

- Surgery complications

PLANTAR FASCIITIS

DESCRIPTION

Painful, inflammatory and/or degenerative overuse injury of the plantar fascia caused by collagen degeneration secondary to repetitive microtrauma of the plantar fascia.

ETIOLOGY

- Uncertain
- Inflammation, microscopic tears and degeneration
- May also have tight heel cord

INCIDENCE

- Middle age
- Bilateral in 10-20% of cases

RISK FACTORS

- Overuse (runners, occupational hazard)
- Flat feet, high arches
- Functional
- Obesity
- Age
- Females > Males
- Improper shoes

ASSESSMENT FINDINGS

- Heel pain worse with first steps in morning or after sitting for several minutes, decreases with activity
- Can be triggered by standing for long period of time
- Sharp pain in heel of foot
- Point tenderness in anteromedial region of calcaneous
- Pain increases with dorsiflexion of toes

DIFFERENTIAL DIAGNOSES

- Tarsal tunnel syndrome
- Stress fracture
- Entrapment syndrome
- Calcaneal fracture
- Paget's disease
- Soft tissue disorder
- Neuropathy
- Gout

DIAGNOSTICS

- X-ray to rule out suspected tumors, fractures, or spurs

MANAGEMENT

- Rest
- Stretching/strengthening exercises
- NSAIDS
- Ice massage 15-20 minutes four times daily
- Intractable pain, may consider injection of cortisone or lidocaine
- Avoid flat shoes, walking barefoot
- Weight loss if indicated
- Night splints
- Orthotics, arch supports

CONSULTATION/REFERRAL

- If no improvement after 6 weeks, refer to podiatrist

EXPECTED COURSE

- Generally self limiting within 12-18 months

References

Anderson, B. C. (2006a). Office orthopedics for primary care: Diagnosis. Philadelphia: Saunders.

Anderson, B. C. (2006b). Office orthopedics for primary care: Treatment. Philadelphia: Saunders.

Baim, S., Binkley, N., Bilezikian, J. P., Kendler, D. L., Hans, D. B., Lewiecki, E. M., & Silverman, S. (2008). Official positions of the Interational Society for Clnical Densitometry and Executive Summary of the 2007 ISCD position development conference. Journal of Clinical Densitometry, 11, 75-91.

Beker, M. (2010). Low-dose oral colchicine in the treatment of patients with acute gout flares. U.S. Musculoskeletal Review, 5, 23-28.

Bridgens, J., & Kiely, N. (2010). Current management of clubfoot (congenital talipes equinovarus). BMJ, 340, c355. doi: 10.1136/bmj.c355

Bruce, M. L., & Peck, B. (2005). New rheumatoid arthritis treatments. Nurse Practitioner, 30(4), 28-29, 32-27, 39; quiz 39-41. doi: 00006205-200504000-00006 [pii]

Burns, C. E., Brady, M. A., Blosser, C., Starr, N. B., & Dunn, A. M. (2009). Pediatric primary care: A handbook for nurse practitioners (4th ed.). Philadelphia: W.B. Saunders.

Buszewicz, M., Rait, G., Griffin, M., Nazareth, I., Patel, A., Atkinson, A., . . . Haines, A. (2006). Self management of arthritis in primary care: randomised controlled trial. BMJ, 333(7574), 879. doi: 10.1136/bmj.38965.375718.80

Carr, A. J., & Hamilton, W. (2005). Orthopediacs in primary care. St. Louis: Elsevier.

Cole, C., Seto, C., & Gazewood, J. (2005). Plantar fasciitis: evidence-based review of diagnosis and therapy. American Family Physician, 72(11), 2237-2242.

Devos-Comby, L., Cronan, T., & Roesch, S. C. (2006). Do exercise and self-management interventions benefit patients with osteoarthritis of the knee? A metaanalytic review. Journal of Rheumatology, 33(4), 744-756. doi: 0315162X-33-744 [pii]

Dezateux, C., & Rosendahl, K. (2007). Developmental dysplasia of the hip. Lancet, 369(9572), 1541-1552. doi: 10.1016/S0140-6736(07)60710-7

Domino, F., Baldor, R., Golding, J., Grimes, J., & Taylor, J. (2011). The 5-minute clinical consult 2011. Philadelphia: Lippincott Williams & Wilkins.

Drug Facts and Comparisons. (2010). St. Louis: Wolters Kluwer Health. Facts & Comparisons.

Ernst, D., & Lee, A. (2010). Nurse practitioners prescribing reference. New York: Haymarket Media Publication.

Felson, D. T., Niu, J., Clancy, M., Sack, B., Aliabadi, P., & Zhang, Y. (2007). Effect of recreational physical activities on the development of knee osteoarthritis in older adults of different weights: the Framingham Study. Arthritis and Rheumatism, 57(1), 6-12. doi: 10.1002/art.22464

Ferri, F. (2010). Ferri's 2010 clinical advisor. Philadelphia: Mosby Elsevier.

Fransen, M., & McConnell, S. (2009). Land-based exercise for osteoarthritis of the knee: a metaanalysis of randomized controlled trials. Journal of Rheumatology, 36(6), 1109-1117. doi: 10.3899/jrheum.090058

Freburger, J. K., Holmes, G. M., Agans, R. P., Jackman, A. M., Darter, J. D., Wallace, A. S., . . . Carey, T. S. (2009). The rising prevalence of chronic low back pain. Archives of Internal Medicine, 169(3), 251-258. doi: 10.1001/archinternmed.2008.543

Gholve, P. A., Scher, D. M., Khakharia, S., Widmann, R. F., & Green, D. W. (2007). Osgood Schlatter syndrome. Current Opinion in Pediatrics, 19(1), 44-50. doi: 10.1097/MOP.0b013e328013dbea

Gough-Palmer, A., & McHugh, K. (2007). Investigating hip pain in a well child. BMJ, 334(7605), 1216-1217. doi: 10.1136/bmj.39188.515741.47

Griffin, L. (Ed.). (2005). Essentials of musculoskeletal care. Rosemont, IL: American Academy of Orthopedic Surgeons.

Janssens, H. J., Janssen, M., van de Lisdonk, E. H., van Riel, P. L., & van Weel, C. (2008). Use of oral prednisolone or naproxen for the treatment of gout arthritis: a double-blind, randomised equivalence trial. Lancet, 371(9627), 1854-1860. doi: 10.1016/S0140-6736(08)60799-0

Kemmler, W., von Stengel, S., Engelke, K., Haberle, L., & Kalender, W. A. (2010). Exercise effects on bone mineral density, falls, coronary risk factors, and health care costs in older women: the randomized controlled senior fitness and prevention (SEFIP) study. Archives of Internal Medicine, 170(2), 179-185. doi: 10.1001/archinternmed.2009.499

Klareskog, L., Catrina, A. I., & Paget, S. (2009). Rheumatoid arthritis. Lancet, 373(9664), 659-672. doi: 10.1016/S0140-6736(09)60008-8

Konstantinou, K., & Dunn, K. M. (2008). Sciatica: review of epidemiological studies and prevalence estimates. Spine (Phila Pa 1976), 33(22), 2464-2472. doi: 10.1097/BRS.0b013e318183a4a2

Kornaat, P. R., Bloem, J. L., Ceulemans, R. Y., Riyazi, N., Rosendaal, F. R., Nelissen, R. G., . . . Kloppenburg, M. (2006). Osteoarthritis of the knee: association between clinical features and MR imaging findings. Radiology, 239(3), 811-817. doi: 10.1148/radiol.2393050253

Lenssinck, M. L., Frijlink, A. C., Berger, M. Y., Bierman-Zeinstra, S. M., Verkerk, K., & Verhagen, A. P. (2005). Effect of bracing and other conservative interventions in the treatment of idiopathic scoliosis in adolescents: a systematic review of clinical trials. Physical Therapy, 85(12), 1329-1339.

MacLean, C., Newberry, S., Maglione, M., McMahon, M., Ranganath, V., Suttorp, M., . . . Grossman, J. (2008). Systematic review: comparative effectiveness of treatments to prevent fractures in men and women with low bone density or osteoporosis. Annals of Internal Medicine, 148(3), 197-213. doi: 0000605-200802050-00198 [pii]

Mattila, V. M., Niva, M., Kiuru, M., & Pihlajamaki, H. (2007). Risk factors for bone stress injuries: a follow-up study of 102,515 person-years. Medicine and Science in Sports and Exercise, 39(7), 1061-1066. doi: 10.1249/01.mss.0b013e318053721d

Nattiv, A., Loucks, A. B., Manore, M. M., Sanborn, C. F., Sundgot-Borgen, J., & Warren, M. P. (2007). American College of Sports Medicine position stand. The female athlete triad. Medicine and Science in Sports and Exercise, 39(10), 1867-1882. doi: 10.1249/mss.0b013e318149f111

Olsen, S. J., 2nd, Fleisig, G. S., Dun, S., Loftice, J., & Andrews, J. R. (2006). Risk factors for shoulder and elbow injuries in adolescent baseball pitchers. American Journal of Sports Medicine, 34(6), 905-912. doi: 10.1177/0363546505284188

Saag, K. G., Teng, G. G., Patkar, N. M., Anuntiyo, J., Finney, C., Curtis, J. R., . . . Furst, D. E. (2008). American College of Rheumatology 2008 recommendations for the use of nonbiologic and biologic disease-modifying antirheumatic drugs in rheumatoid arthritis. Arthritis and Rheumatism, 59(6), 762-784. doi: 10.1002/art.23721

Sanders, J. O., Khoury, J. G., Kishan, S., Browne, R. H., Mooney, J. F., 3rd, Arnold, K. D., . . . Finegold, D. N. (2008). Predicting scoliosis progression from skeletal maturity: a simplified classification during adolescence. Journal of Bone and Joint Surgery, 90(3), 540-553. doi: 10.2106/JBJS.G.00004

Shiri, R., Viikari-Juntura, E., Varonen, H., & Heliovaara, M. (2006). Prevalence and determinants of lateral and medial epicondylitis: a population study. American Journal of Epidemiology, 164(11), 1065-1074. doi: 10.1093/aje/kwj325

Sutaria, S., Katbamna, R., & Underwood, M. (2006). Effectiveness of interventions for the treatment of acute and prevention of recurrent gout--a systematic review. Rheumatology, 45(11), 1422-1431. doi: 10.1093/rheumatology/kel071

The National Osteoporsis Foundation. (2010). Clinician's guide to prevention and treatment of osteoporosis. Retrieved from http://www.nof.org/professionals/clinical-guidelines

U.S. Preventative Services Task Force. (2006). Screening for developmental dysplasia of the hip Retrieved from http://www.uspreventiveservicestaskforce.org/uspstf/uspshipd.htm

Visser, K., Katchamart, W., Loza, E., Martinez-Lopez, J. A., Salliot, C., Trudeau, J., . . . Dougados, M. (2009). Multinational evidence-based recommendations for the use of methotrexate in rheumatic disorders with a focus on rheumatoid arthritis: integrating systematic literature research and expert opinion of a broad international panel of rheumatologists in the 3E Initiative. Annals of the Rheumatic Diseases, 68(7), 1086-1093. doi: 10.1136/ard.2008.094474

Orthopedic Disorders

14

PREGNANCY

Pregnancy

Pregnancy

Preconceptual Care 539

Physiologic and Psychologic Changes of Pregnancy 541

Prenatal Care 542

Common Discomforts of Pregnancy 545
- Ankle Edema 545
- Nausea and Vomiting 545
- Backache 546
- Constipation 546
- Heartburn 546
- Hemorrhoids 547
- Leg Cramps 547
- Leukorrhea 547
- Nasal Congestion and Epistaxis 547
- Round Ligament Pain 548
- Urinary Frequency 548
- Varicose Veins 548

Assessment of Fetal Well-Being 549
- Amniocentesis 549
- Biophysical Profile 549
- Maternal Assessment of Fetal Activity 550
- Nonstress Testing 550
- Contraction Stress Test 550
- Ultrasound 551

Complications Associated with Pregnancy 552
- Abruptio Placentae 552
- Ectopic Pregnancy 553
- Genetic Disorders 554
- Down Syndrome 555
- Gestational Trophoblastic Disease 555
- Hyperemesis Gravidarum 556
- Incompetent Cervix 557
- Multiple Gestation 558
- Placenta Previa 559
- Pre-eclampsia, Eclampsia 559

Pre-term Labor 561
Post-term Labor 562
Prolapsed Umbilical Cord 563
Spontaneous Abortion 563
Substance Abuse in Pregnancy 564

Adolescent Pregnancy 566

References *567*

Pregnancy

PRECONCEPTUAL CARE

DEFINITION

Interventions aimed at promoting the health and well-being of a woman before pregnancy.

TERMS

Nulligravida	a woman who has never been pregnant
Primigravida	a woman in her first pregnancy
Primipara	a woman who has had or who is giving birth to her first child
Multigravida	a woman who has been pregnant two or more times
Multipara	a woman who has borne more than one offspring

HEALTH ASSESSMENT

- Complete physical examination
- Past medical history
- GYN surgery history (especially if cervical or uterine)
- Obstetric history
  - ◊ Menstrual history
  - ◊ Contraceptive history
  - ◊ Sexual history
  - ◊ Reproductive history (vaginal deliveries, c-sections)
  - ◊ Complications during previous pregnancies
- Nutrition assessment
- Cultural history
- Support systems

Assessment of Risk Factors
◊ Maternal age (increased risk at age extremes)
◊ Ethnic origin
◊ Presence of chronic disease (e.g., diabetes mellitus, essential hypertension, heart disease, renal disease, seizure disorder, thyroid abnormality, asthma, rheumatoid arthritis, or tuberculosis) may affect pregnancy through pathophysiological mechanisms or as a result of medications used in their treatment
◊ In utero exposure to DES
◊ Previous preterm labor and/or delivery
◊ Repeated early miscarriages
◊ Presence of infectious disease or exposure to infectious disease
◊ Domestic violence risk
◊ Substance abuse
◊ Tobacco use

DISCONTINUATION OF CONTRACEPTION

- Oral contraceptives should be discontinued 2-3 months before attempting pregnancy
- Intrauterine devices should be removed and pregnancy delayed one month after removal
- Barrier methods of contraception may be used (e.g., condoms, diaphragm) in the interim

GENETIC ISSUES

- Complete genetic history should be taken including genogram
- Couple should be referred for genetic counseling if history of genetic disorders in family, especially Tay-Sachs, thalassemia, hemophilia, phenylketonuria, cystic fibrosis, sickle cell disease or trait, birth defects, or mental retardation

IMMUNIZATIONS

- Bring all immunizations up to date
- Rubella vaccine if not immune
- Influenza immunization for all pregnant patients

Pregnancy should not be attempted for 28 days after rubella vaccine.

DIAGNOSTIC STUDIES

- Hematocrit and hemoglobin/CBC
- Blood type and Rh factor
- Coombs' test
- Urinalysis
- Pap smear
- HIV screening
- Screening for sexually transmitted diseases (e.g., syphilis, gonorrhea, chlamydia)
- Rubella titer
- Screening for hepatitis B

A pregnant patient should be screened for anemia. Variation in practice exists. CBC and hemoglobin/hematocrit are commonly used for assessment.

NUTRITION

- Maintain or attain average body weight for height
- Folic acid 0.4 mg/day (minimally) to decrease risk of neural tube defects
- Assess for cultural nutrition practices which may affect pregnancy

EXERCISE

- Establish a regular exercise program at least 3 months before attempting to become pregnant. Should include aerobic and toning exercises

Even if no exercise was engaged in prior to pregnancy, walking can be safely encouraged during pregnancy. Swimming is also recommended due to water's buoyancy and decreased risk of injury during exercise.

SMOKING CESSATION

- Assist couples with smoking cessation before pregnancy
- Educate about risk of cigarette smoking during pregnancy
  - ◊ Lower birth weight
  - ◊ Stillbirth
  - ◊ Spontaneous abortion
  - ◊ Sudden infant death syndrome

Second hand smoke has adverse effects on the fetus.

ALCOHOL

- Educate about risk of alcohol use in pregnancy
  - ◊ Decreased birth weight
  - ◊ Stillbirth
  - ◊ Spontaneous abortion
  - ◊ Fetal alcohol syndrome
- Safety level for alcohol use during pregnancy has not been established
- Total avoidance is recommended

MEDICATIONS

- Avoidance of medications which could have negative effect on pregnancy

Categories of Medications According to the Risk in Pregnancy

Category	Explanation	Drug Examples
A	Controlled studies show no human risk	Folic acid, thyroid supplement
B	Animal studies show no risk, but no good human studies have been done	Penicillin, cephalosporins
C	No adequate studies exist in either animals or humans	Pseudoephedrine, quinolones
D	Evidence of fetal risk is clear-cut, but the benefits may outweigh the risks	Phenytoin Lithium Tetracycline
X	Proven fetal risks clearly outweigh any benefit	Alcohol Warfarin Diethylstilbestrol Isotretinoin Methotrexate Valproic acid

Note: FDA Pregnancy Categories

OCCUPATIONAL ISSUES

- Assess potential teratogenic occupational environment of the woman and her partner

SEXUAL ACTIVITY

- Safe sex practices

PHYSIOLOGIC AND PSYCHOLOGIC CHANGES OF PREGNANCY

BREASTS

- Increased in size
- Darkening and enlargement of areolae and nipples occur
- Prominent superficial veins
- Hypertrophy of Montgomery's glands
- Striae may develop
- Leakage of colostrum can occur

CARDIOVASCULAR SYSTEM

- Heart is pushed upward, to the left and rotated forward
- Decreased peripheral and pulmonary vascular resistance
- Cardiac output increased
- Pulse rate increased 10-15 beats per minute
- Blood pressure decreased slightly

Blood pressure is lowest in the second trimester.

ENDOCRINE SYSTEM

- Thyroid
  - ◊ TSH decreases; T_4 level increases
  - ◊ Basal metabolic rate increases
- Parathyroid
  - ◊ Increased size
  - ◊ Increased parathormone levels
- Pituitary
  - ◊ Enlarges
- Adrenals
  - ◊ Increased cortisol levels
  - ◊ Increased aldosterone
- Pancreas
  - ◊ Increased insulin needs

EYES

- Decreased intraocular pressure
- Increased corneal thickness
- Transient loss of accommodation

GASTROINTESTINAL SYSTEM

- Increased human chorionic gonadotropin (HCG) is associated with nausea and vomiting during first trimester
- Hyperemic gum tissue
- Increased salivation
- Increased acidity of gastric contents
- Intestines are displaced as the uterus grows
- Relaxation of lower esophageal sphincter
- Gastric emptying and intestinal motility are delayed
- Decreased plasma albumin
- Prolonged emptying time of the gallbladder

Elevated estrogen levels make gallstones more likely during pregnancy.

HEMATOLOGICAL SYSTEM

- Blood volume progressively increased secondary to increased plasma volume and erythrocytes
- Hemoglobin and hematocrit decrease slightly
- Increased leukocyte production
- Increased fibrin level, fibrinogen, blood factors VII, VIII, IX, and X
- Increased erythrocyte sedimentation rate (ESR)
- Physiologic anemia occurs in response to the increased plasma volume

INTEGUMENTARY SYSTEM

- Hyperpigmentation of areolae, nipples, vulva, perianal area
- Linea nigra
- Facial chloasma (mask of pregnancy)
- Striae gravidarum (stretch marks) of abdomen, breasts, thighs
- Vascular spider nevi
- Decreased rate of hair growth

MUSCULOSKELETAL SYSTEM

- Relaxation of sacroiliac, sacrococcygeal, and pubic joints of the pelvis due to the effects of the hormones progesterone and relaxin
- Progressive lordosis

REPRODUCTIVE SYSTEM

Uterus Increase in size to accommodate growing fetus	
10-12 weeks	Fundus slightly above symphysis pubis
16 weeks	Fundus midway between symphysis pubis and umbilicus
20-22 weeks	Fundus at level of umbilicus
28 weeks	Fundus three finger breadths above umbilicus
36 weeks	Fundus just below xiphoid

- Cervix
  - ◊ Production of thick, tenacious mucus plug in the endocervical canal
  - ◊ Softening (Goodell's sign)
  - ◊ Increased vascularity causing the cervix to appear blue
- Ovaries
  - ◊ Ovulation ceases
  - ◊ Corpus luteum produces progesterone and other hormones in early pregnancy
- Vagina
  - ◊ Hypertrophy
  - ◊ Increased vascularity and hyperemia causing the vagina to appear bluish-purple (Chadwick's sign)
  - ◊ Increased vaginal secretion
  - ◊ Vaginal pH becomes more acidic

RESPIRATORY SYSTEM

- Increased tidal volume
- Increased oxygen consumption
- Decreased functional residual capacity and residual volume
- Decreased airway resistance
- Elevation of diaphragm as pregnancy progresses
- Increased subcostal angle
- Increased AP: lateral diameter
- Increased vascular congestion and edema of nasal mucosa

URINARY TRACT

- Decreased capacity of bladder due to uterine pressure
- Dilation of kidney and ureter due to pressure of uterus
- Increased glomerular filtration rate and renal plasma flow

PSYCHOLOGICAL ADJUSTMENT

- Developmental tasks of each trimester
  - ◊ First: accept biologic fact of pregnancy; ambivalence common
  - ◊ Second: accept fetus as distinct entity
  - ◊ Third: preparation for separation from fetus, labor, and parenthood

Pregnancy

PRENATAL CARE

INITIAL PRENATAL VISIT

DIAGNOSIS OF PREGNANCY

Subjective (*Presumptive*) signs:
* Amenorrhea
* Nausea and vomiting
* Urinary frequency
* Breast tenderness
* Perception of fetal movement (quickening: usually felt between 16-18 weeks gestation)
* Fatigue

Objective (*Probable*) signs:
* *Goodell's sign*: softening of the cervix
* *Chadwick's sign*: dark blue to purplish-red color of vaginal mucosa
* *Hegar's sign*: softening of the isthmus of the uterus
* Uterine enlargement
* *Braxton-Hicks contractions*: painless uterine contractions that occur every 10-20 minutes after the third month of pregnancy and do not represent true labor
* Uterine souffle
* Hyperpigmentation of skin
* Abdominal striae
* Ballottement
* Positive pregnancy test
* Palpation of fetal outline

Diagnostic (*Positive*) signs:
* Auscultation of fetal heartbeat * Fetal movements palpated by examiner * Ultrasound recognition of pregnancy

DETERMINATION OF ESTIMATED DATE OF CONFINEMENT (EDC)

- *Naegele's Rule* (Due Date)
  - ◊ Subtract 3 months from last menstrual period then add 7 days and one year
  - ◊ Naegele's Rule is only accurate with regular 28 day cycles

HISTORY

- Menstrual history
- Previous pregnancy history
- Family history of pre-eclampsia (more likely if mother or sister had pre-eclampsia)
- Current medications
- Contraception used prior to pregnancy
- Assessment of risk factors which may complicate pregnancy

PHYSICAL EXAMINATION

- Blood Pressure
- Height
- Weight
- Thyroid gland: hypo and hyperthyroidism often diagnosed during pregnancy
- Uterus: uterine fundal height

Between 18 and 32 weeks there is good correlation between fundal height and gestational age of the fetus (*McDonald's rule*).

- Vagina: anomalies, lesions
- Cervix: consistency, length, and dilation; lesions
- Pelvis: clinical measurement of pelvis and its general configuration
- Breast: presence of nipple abnormalities, masses
- Extremities: varicosities
- Fetal heart sounds

DIAGNOSTIC STUDIES

- Pregnancy test unless pregnancy already established
- CBC preferred to evaluate for anemia
- Urinalysis
- Urine culture
- Blood type, Rh, and antibody screen
- Rubella titer
- Syphilis serology
- HIV screen
- Hepatitis B screen
- Sickle cell screen
- Tuberculosis skin test
- Consider glucose screen if patient at high risk for gestational diabetes
- Screen for gonorrhea, Chlamydia
- Wet prep for *Trichomonas vaginalis* and *Candida albicans* and bacterial vaginosis
- Cervical cytology screen

Post-coital bleeding is common because blood flow to the vagina and cervix are increased during pregnancy. During sexual activity, small blood vessels can break and are the usual cause of small amounts of post-coital bleeding.

Ultrasound is commonly performed if patient is unsure of last menses or if she became pregnant while on an oral or injectable contraceptive.

NUTRITION

- Recommended weight gain for normal weight women: 25-35 lbs; more for women who are underweight and less for women who are overweight
- Recommended nutrition during pregnancy
  - ◊ Calories: increase of 300 kcal/day over prepregnancy requirement
  - ◊ Folic acid: 0.4 mg/day (some experts recommend 1 mg)
  - ◊ Elemental iron: 30 mg/day
  - ◊ Calcium: 1200 mg/day
- Avoid raw or undercooked foods, especially seafood, unpasteurized dairy products, etc.
- Pica may be a problem, especially in some cultures

ACTIVITIES

- Not necessary for pregnant woman to limit activity if she does not become excessively fatigued or risk injury to herself or fetus
- Women who are accustomed to aerobic exercise may continue, but new aerobic exercise program (except walking) should not be started
- Scuba diving, roller coasters, and bungee jumping are contraindicated

SEXUAL ACTIVITY

- Generally accepted that in healthy pregnant women sexual intercourse causes no harm
- Sexual intercourse should be avoided in the presence of threatening abortion or preterm labor

DANGER SIGNS OF PREGNANCY

- Any vaginal bleeding
- Swelling of face or fingers
- Severe or continuous headache
- Dimness or blurring of vision
- Abdominal or epigastric pain
- Persistent vomiting
- Chills or fever
- Dysuria
- Escape of fluid from the vagina
- Marked changes in frequency or intensity of fetal movements

OCCUPATIONAL ISSUES

- Avoidance of potential teratogens in workplace (e.g., radiation, chemotherapy, anesthesia, chemicals)
- Frequent rest periods during the work day

TRAVEL

- Travel in properly pressurized aircraft offers no unusual risk to the pregnant woman and her fetus
- While traveling, the woman should walk at least every 2 hours
- Lap and shoulder belts should be used at all times. The lap belt should be placed under the abdomen and across the upper thighs. The shoulder belt should be placed snugly across the abdomen and between the breasts.

Pregnancy produces a state of hypercoagulability, so, pregnant women should walk at least every 2 hours after having been immobile to help prevent DVT.

AVOIDANCE OF POTENTIAL TERATOGENS

- Teach women to avoid medications unless specifically prescribed by health care provider
- Avoid hot tubs
- Avoid douching
- Avoid working with chemicals, paint, etc., especially in poorly ventilated area

CHILDBIRTH PREPARATION

- Introduce subject of childbirth preparation and childbirth options

SUBSEQUENT PRENATAL VISITS

TRADITIONAL SCHEDULE OF VISITS IN UNCOMPLICATED PREGNANCY

- Every 4 weeks until 28 weeks gestation
- Every 2 weeks between 28 and 36 weeks gestation
- Every week after 36 weeks of gestation

ASSESSMENT

- Blood pressure
- Weight
- Urinalysis as indicated
- Review of symptoms indicating danger signs of pregnancy
- Fundal height
- Later in pregnancy: vaginal examination to determine cervical dilation and effacement, station of presenting part
- Fetal heart sounds: normal is 120-160 beats/minute
- Presenting fetal part (later in pregnancy)
- Fetal activity

DIAGNOSTIC STUDIES

8-18 weeks:
- Ultrasound to assess gross anomalies
- Amniocentesis if indicated

16-18 weeks:
- Maternal serum α-fetoprotein (AFP)
- Quad/triple screen depending on risk

24-28 weeks:
- Diabetes screening if plasma glucose (measured one hour after 50 gram oral glucose challenge) is ≥ 130-140 mg/dL, additional testing should be performed on a different day
- Positive screen: 100 g glucose load is administered and glucose values are measured fasting, at 1 hour, 2 hours, and 3 hours. If 2 of the 4 values are abnormal, a diagnosis of gestational diabetes is made
- Repeat CBC

32-36 weeks:

- Ultrasound if medically warranted
- Repeat gonorrhea and chlamydia cultures
- Culture for Group A Beta Hemolytic Strep
- Repeat CBC

LEOPOLD'S MANEUVERS

- Used to assess presentation/ position
- Composed of four maneuvers by examiner
  - ◊ Palpate fundus
  - ◊ Palpate to identify fetal back and extremities
  - ◊ Palpate presenting part
  - ◊ Palpate down sides of abdomen to locate cephalic prominence or brow

EDUCATION

- Reinforce previous teaching
- Follow-up on plans for childbirth and breastfeeding
- Signs and symptoms of labor
  - ◊ Lower back pain
  - ◊ Passage of "bloody show"
  - ◊ Regular contractions
  - ◊ Rupture of membranes

Differentiation of True vs. False Labor	
True Labor	**False Labor**
Contractions occur at regular intervals	Contractions are irregular
Intervals between contractions gradually shorten Contractions increase in duration and intensity	Usually no change Usually no change
Discomfort begins in back and radiates around to abdomen	Discomfort usually in abdomen
Intensity usually increases with walking	Walking has no effect on, or lessens contractions
Progressive cervical dilation and effacement	No cervical changes

COMMON DISCOMFORTS OF PREGNANCY

ANKLE EDEMA

CAUSES

- Prolonged standing or sitting
- Increased sodium levels due to hormonal influences
- Increased capillary permeability
- Varicose veins

USUAL TIMING IN PREGNANCY

- Second and third trimesters

DIFFERENTIAL DIAGNOSIS

- Thrombophlebitis
- Preeclampsia

MANAGEMENT

- Frequent dorsiflexion of feet when sitting or standing
- Elevate legs when sitting or resting
- Avoid restrictive bands around legs

NAUSEA AND VOMITING

CAUSES

- Chorionic gonadotropin (hCG) is likely cause of nausea and vomiting during pregnancy
- Changes in carbohydrate metabolism
- Emotional factors
- Fatigue

USUAL TIMING IN PREGNANCY

- First trimester of pregnancy

DIFFERENTIAL DIAGNOSIS

- Hyperemesis gravidarum
- Gastroenteritis

MANAGEMENT

- Reassurance and support
- Avoidance of medications if possible
- Eat small frequent meals
- Avoid foods with strong odor
- Eat dry crackers or toast before arising in morning
- Increase carbohydrate percentage in diet
- Decrease fat in diet
- Eating ginger in soda, tea, or ginger snaps
- Supplemental vitamin B6 (pyridoxine)
- If severe, hospitalization may be considered for rehydration and parenteral nutrition

BACKACHE

CAUSES

- Increased curvature of the lumbosacral vertebrae as the uterus enlarges
- Increased weight
- General relaxation of pelvic ligaments and motion of the symphysis pubis and lumbosacral joints
- Fatigue
- Poor body mechanics

USUAL TIMING IN PREGNANCY

- Second and third trimesters

DIFFERENTIAL DIAGNOSIS

- Herniated disc
- Sciatica
- Muscle strain
- Urinary tract infection
- Pyelonephritis

MANAGEMENT

- Rest
- Lumbar support
- Avoidance of straining and lifting
- Proper body mechanics
- Pelvic tilt exercises
- Avoid uncomfortable working heights, high-heeled shoes, and fatigue

CONSTIPATION

CAUSES

- Generalized relaxation of smooth muscle and decreased motility of the gastrointestinal tract in response to increased level of progesterone
- Compression of the lower bowel by the enlarging uterus and presenting part
- May be exacerbated by iron and calcium supplementation
- Lack of exercise
- Decreased fluid intake

USUAL TIMING IN PREGNANCY

- Any time during pregnancy

MANAGEMENT

- Increase daily fiber intake
- Increase fluid intake
- Daily exercise
- Mild laxative (e.g., prune juice, milk of magnesia), bulk-producing agents, or stool-softening agents
- Harsh laxatives and enemas are not recommended
- Regular bowel habits

HEARTBURN

CAUSE

- Reflux of gastric contents into the lower esophagus due to:
  - ◊ Increased production of progesterone decreasing gastrointestinal motility and increasing relaxation of cardiac sphincter
  - ◊ Displacement of stomach by enlarging uterus

USUAL TIMING IN PREGNANCY

- Second and third trimesters

MANAGEMENT

- Small frequent meals
- Avoidance of bending over
- Elevation of head of bed
- Avoidance of tight and binding clothing
- Antacid preparations (avoid sodium containing products)
- Avoid overeating, fatty foods

HEMORRHOIDS

CAUSES

- Increased pressure in the rectal veins due to obstruction of venous return
- Constipation

USUAL TIMING IN PREGNANCY

- Second and third trimesters

MANAGEMENT

- Increased fiber and fluids in diet to keep stool soft
- Stool softeners may be needed
- Topical ointments
- Warm sitz baths
- Ice packs

LEG CRAMPS

CAUSES

- Imbalance of calcium/phosphorous ratio
- Increased pressure of uterus on nerves
- Fatigue
- Decreased venous circulation in legs

USUAL TIMING IN PREGNANCY

- Second and third trimesters

DIFFERENTIAL DIAGNOSIS

- Thrombophlebitis
- Electrolyte imbalance

MANAGEMENT

- Avoid pointing toes
- Dorsiflexion of foot to stretch affected muscles
- Apply heat to affected muscles

LEUKORRHEA

CAUSE

- Increased mucus formation by the cervix in response to elevated estrogen levels

USUAL TIMING IN PREGNANCY

- First trimester

DIFFERENTIAL DIAGNOSIS

- Trichomoniasis
- Candidal vaginitis
- Bacterial vaginosis
- Gonorrhea
- Chlamydia

MANAGEMENT

- Wearing of perineal pad with frequent change
- Daily bathing
- Good perineal hygiene
- Avoid douching
- Wear cotton underwear
- Avoid panty hose

NASAL CONGESTION AND EPISTAXIS

CAUSE

- Elevated estrogen levels

USUAL TIMING IN PREGNANCY

- First trimester

DIFFERENTIAL DIAGNOSIS

- Allergic rhinitis
- Upper respiratory infection

MANAGEMENT

- Cool air vaporizer
- Avoid use of nasal sprays and decongestants
- Consider topical nasal steroid for nasal congestion

ROUND LIGAMENT PAIN

CAUSE

- Stretching of the round ligaments as the uterus enlarges

USUAL TIMING IN PREGNANCY

- Second and third trimesters

DIFFERENTIAL DIAGNOSIS

- Appendicitis
- Cholecystitis
- Labor

MANAGEMENT

- Heating pad to abdomen
- Position with knees into chest
- Acetaminophen

URINARY FREQUENCY

CAUSE

- Pressure of uterus resting on bladder

USUAL TIMING IN PREGNANCY

- First and third trimester

DIFFERENTIAL DIAGNOSIS

- Urinary tract infection

MANAGEMENT

- Void when urge is felt
- Increase fluid intake during day
- Decrease fluid intake in evenings to decrease nocturia

VARICOSE VEINS

CAUSES

- Increased pressure in femoral veins due to obstruction of venous return
- Hereditary factors
- Weight gain
- Increased age

USUAL TIMING IN PREGNANCY

- Second and third trimesters

MANAGEMENT

- Avoid prolonged standing or sitting
- Elevate legs frequently
- Support stockings
- Avoid crossing legs at the knees or wearing knee-hi stockings which restrict venous return

ASSESSMENT OF FETAL WELL-BEING

AMNIOCENTESIS

DESCRIPTION

Involves inserting a needle through the maternal abdomen into the uterine cavity to withdraw a sample of amniotic fluid

INDICATIONS

16-18 weeks gestation:

- Pregnancies in women aged 35 or older
- Previous pregnancy resulting in the birth of a child with a chromosomal abnormality
- Down syndrome or other chromosome abnormality in either parent or a close family member
- Mother who is a carrier of any X-linked disease
- Neural tube defect in either parent or a first-degree relative
- Previous child born with a neural tube defect
- Abnormal serum maternal α-fetoprotein level
- Either parent being a carrier of a genetically transmitted metabolic disease
- Pregnancy after three or more spontaneous abortions

Late pregnancy:

- Determine fetal lung maturity based on phospholipids
- Detect isoimmunization

PROCEDURE

- Woman positioned with left lateral tilt to prevent vena cava compression
- Done under ultrasound guidance for location of fetus and placenta
- Needle is inserted into an adequate pocket of fluid under sterile conditions
- Fetal heart rate is monitored for 15 minutes after procedure
- Rh-negative women should be given Rh immune globulin (RhoGAM®) after procedure

AMNIOTIC FLUID TESTS

- α-fetoprotein: elevated in open neural tube defect, abdominal wall defect, congenital nephrosis, cystic hygroma, multiple gestation, fetal death (only done after a positive α-fetoprotein screen of the serum)
- Lecithin-to-sphingomyelin (L/S) ratio: If L/S is greater than 2.0, there is a low risk of respiratory distress secondary to prematurity
- Phosphatidylglycerol (PG): PG first appears at 35 weeks gestation and increases in concentration until 40 weeks; if present, it provides reassurance of fetal lung maturity
- Identification of meconium staining

POSSIBLE COMPLICATIONS

- Complications occur in $< 1\%$ of cases
- Fetus, umbilical cord, or placenta may be punctured inadvertently
- Hemorrhage
- Fetal anemia
- Intraamniotic infection
- Induction of preterm labor

BIOPHYSICAL PROFILE

DESCRIPTION

Ultrasonographic assessment and nonstress test to evaluate five fetal biophysical variables:

- Fetal heart rate reactivity
- Amniotic fluid volume measurement
- Fetal breathing movements
- Fetal body movements
- Fetal tone

INDICATIONS

- Hypertension
- Diabetes mellitus
- Multiple gestation
- Suspected oligohydramnios/intrauterine growth restriction (IUGR)
- Known placental abnormality
- Maternal heart or renal disease
- Hemoglobinopathy
- Postdate pregnancies
- Previous unexplained fetal demise
- Maternal perceptions of decreased fetal movement
- Assessment of fetus at risk for intrauterine compromise

FINDINGS

- Each component is worth 2 points, with a maximum possible score of 10
- 8-10: reassuring
- 6: suspicious and indicates need for further evaluation and possible intervention
- 4 or less: ominous and indicates need for immediate intervention

MATERNAL ASSESSMENT OF FETAL ACTIVITY

DESCRIPTION

Maternal perception of fetal activity; has been shown to be an effective screening method of fetal well-being

INDICATION

- All pregnant patients should monitor fetal activity daily

PROCEDURE

- Patient lies on her left side 30 minutes after eating
- She records the time she starts the test and notes each time the fetus moves or kicks

FINDINGS

- A healthy fetus should move 3-5 times within one hour.

Pregnancy

NONSTRESS TESTING (NST)

DESCRIPTION

Indirect measurement of uteroplacental function

INDICATIONS

- Hypertension
- Diabetes mellitus
- Multiple gestation
- Suspected oligohydramnios/IUGR
- Known placental abnormality
- Maternal heart or renal disease
- Hemoglobinopathy
- Postdate pregnancies
- Previous unexplained fetal demise
- Maternal perceptions of decreased fetal movement
- Assessment of fetus at risk for intrauterine compromise

PROCEDURE

- Patient should either sit or lie on her left side
- Electronic fetal monitor is used to monitor fetal heart rate and uterine activity
- The patient presses a button on the monitor that marks the tracing every time she feels fetal movement

FINDINGS

- Reassuring or reactive test: shows at least two 15 beats/minute accelerations in fetal heart rate lasting at least 15 seconds in a 20 minute period
- Nonreassuring or nonreactive test: does not meet the above criteria; suggests that fetus may be compromised
- Unsatisfactory test: inadequate tracing of fetal heart rate
- 65% of healthy fetuses will have a reactive nonstress test at 28 weeks gestation; 85% at 32 weeks and 95% at 34 weeks.

CONTRACTION STRESS TEST
(Oxytocin Challenge Test)

DESCRIPTION

Method used to evaluate respiratory function (oxygen and carbon dioxide exchange) of the placenta

INDICATIONS

- Identifies the fetus at risk for intrauterine asphyxia
- Intrauterine growth restriction (IUGR)
- Diabetes mellitus
- Postdates (≥42 weeks gestation)
- Abnormal or suspicious biophysical profile

CONTRAINDICATIONS

- Patients at high risk for premature labor
- Patients who have a classic uterine scar from uterine

surgery or cesarean section
- Patients with a placenta previa or marginal abruptio placentae

PROCEDURE

- The goal of the test is for the patient to have three uterine contractions during a 10 minute time period
- The contractions may occur spontaneously, with nipple stimulation, or with oxytocin infusion
- An electronic fetal monitor is used to monitor fetal heart rate and uterine activity
- Woman assumes semi-Fowler's or side-lying position to avoid vena cava compression

FINDINGS

- Negative: no late decelerations observed
- Positive: late decelerations detected with more than 50% of contractions

POSSIBLE COMPLICATIONS

- Uterine hyperstimulation

ULTRASOUND

INDICATIONS

- Determine the presence or absence of an intrauterine pregnancy
- Determine the gestational age
- Measure fetal growth and identify intrauterine growth restriction
- Identify multiple gestation pregnancies
- Detect fetal anomalies (nearly 100% sensitive for the detection of neural tube defects)
- Detect oligohydramnios or polyhydramnios
- Demonstrate placental abnormalities
- Identify maternal uterine and pelvic anomalies

PROCEDURE

- May be done transabdominally or endovaginally
- Woman should have partially full or full bladder

FINDINGS

- The following data may be obtained from ultrasound:
    - ◊ Cardiac activity
    - ◊ Crown-rump length of fetus for accurate dating of pregnancy before 12 weeks of gestation
    - ◊ Fetal biparietal diameter (BPD)
    - ◊ Femur length
    - ◊ Abdominal and head circumference

COMPLICATIONS ASSOCIATED WITH PREGNANCY

ABRUPTIO PLACENTAE

DESCRIPTION

Premature separation of the placenta from the uterine wall.

TERMS

Marginal	Separation at the periphery of the placenta; vaginal bleeding present
Central	Placenta separates centrally and blood is trapped between placenta and uterine wall; vaginal bleeding absent
Complete	Total separation of the placenta from the uterine wall with resultant massive vaginal bleeding

ETIOLOGY

- Primary cause unknown

INCIDENCE

- Occurs in 10% of all births, but severe abruptio is rare
- Accounts for 15% of fetal deaths
- More common in African-American women

RISK FACTORS

- Maternal age > 35 years
- Grand multiparity
- Pregnancy-induced hypertension
- Essential hypertension
- Prematurely ruptured membranes
- Abdominal trauma
- Cigarette smoking
- Cocaine use
- Uterine fibroids
- Maternal coagulopathies
- Malnutrition or severe folate deficiency
- Abdominal trauma
- Short umbilical cord

ASSESSMENT FINDINGS

- Profuse to absent vaginal bleeding
- Amount of bleeding has no correlation with degree of separation
- Uterine tenderness
- Board-like uterus on palpation
- Abdominal pain
- Back pain
- Fetal distress
- Hypertonus
- Preterm labor
- Shock

DIFFERENTIAL DIAGNOSIS

- Placenta previa

DIAGNOSTIC STUDIES

- Ultrasound
- Fetal monitoring
- Fibrinogen level: decreased
- Platelet count: decreased
- Prothrombin time and partial thromboplastin time: normal to prolonged
- Fibrin degradation products: increased
- Hematocrit and hemoglobin

MANAGEMENT

- Refer to person who will deliver patient (midwife, OB/GYN)
- Prompt delivery. If separation mild, labor induction may be attempted; if severe separation, immediate cesarean section is indicated
- Blood transfusions if bleeding severe
- Fluid replacement therapy
- Correction of coagulation defects with cryoprecipitate or plasma
- Hysterectomy may be needed in extreme cases

EXPECTED COURSE

- Risk of recurrence in subsequent pregnancy is high
- Fetal/neonatal mortality 20-35% overall; is near 100% in complete separations

POSSIBLE COMPLICATIONS

Fetal risks:

- Fetal demise
- Fetal hypoxia
- Preterm birth
- Anemia
- Neurological damage

Maternal risks:

- Disseminated intravascular coagulation
- Couvelaire uterus (infiltration of blood into uterine musculature)
- Renal failure
- Shock
- Death (rare)

ECTOPIC PREGNANCY

DESCRIPTION

Pregnancy which implants outside the uterus; most common site is the ampulla of the fallopian tube.

ETIOLOGY

- Tubal damage secondary to PID
- Previous pelvic or tubal surgery
- Presence of an IUD
- High levels of estrogen and progesterone which alter the motility of the egg in the fallopian tube
- Congenital anomalies of the tube
- Blighted ovum

INCIDENCE

- > 1/100 pregnancies
- 85% of these occur in the fallopian tubes

RISK FACTORS

- History of pelvic inflammatory disease
- Multiple sexual partners
- History of endometriosis
- Previous ectopic pregnancy
- Present or past use of intrauterine device
- History of pelvic or tubal surgery
- Cigarette smoking
- In vitro fertilization

ASSESSMENT FINDINGS

- Initially may have normal signs of pregnancy
- Vaginal bleeding
- Fainting or dizziness
- Lower abdominal pain
- Palpable adnexal mass
- If tube has ruptured, has acute onset of a sharp lower abdominal pain
- Right-sided shoulder pain due to irritation of the subdiaphragmatic phrenic nerve by blood
- Shock if bleeding profuse and rapid
- Abdomen may gradually become rigid and very tender
- Abdominal tenderness
- Cervical motion pain

DIFFERENTIAL DIAGNOSIS

- Intrauterine pregnancy
- Appendicitis
- Cholecystitis
- Pelvic inflammatory disease
- Spontaneous abortion
- Ruptured ovarian cyst
- Torsion of the ovary
- Urinary tract infection

DIAGNOSTIC STUDIES

- Serial quantitative β-hCG determinations
- Pelvic ultrasound
- Serum progesterone: < 5 ng/mL exclude viable pregnancy; < 25 ng/mL exclude ectopic pregnancy
- Culdocentesis: presence of nonclotting blood
- Laparoscopy

MANAGEMENT

- Refer immediately to ER or obstetrician/gynecologist
- Laparotomy and surgical removal of fallopian tube
- If tube has not ruptured: methotrexate or microsurgery may save the tube
- If woman is Rh-negative: Rh immune globulin (RhoGAM®) should be administered
- Intravenous fluids
- Blood transfusion may be needed
- Anticipatory guidance regarding reaction to loss of pregnancy
- Assess support systems

POSSIBLE COMPLICATIONS

- Second leading cause of maternal mortality
- Loss of fertility

GENETIC DISORDERS

CATEGORIES OF GENETIC DISORDERS

Chromosomal Abnormalities:

- Numerical autosomal abnormalities: result of uneven distribution of chromosomes during cell division. Most common are trisomy (presence of an extra chromosome)
  - ◊ Examples: trisomy 21 (Down syndrome), trisomy 13, trisomy 18
- Structural autosomal abnormalities: variety of structural chromosomal alterations including deletions and rearrangements (e.g., rings, inversions, and translocations).
  - ◊ Examples: *Cri du chat* syndrome, Robertsonian translocations
- Mosaicism: presence of two or more distinct cell lines in the same individual
- Sex chromosome abnormalities: involve abnormalities in number of X and Y chromosomes
  - ◊ Examples: Turner's syndrome (female who has one X and a partial second X or a partial Y chromosome), Klinefelter's syndrome (male who has ≥ one X chromosome, usually XXY)

Single Gene Defects:

- Autosomal dominant inheritance: expressed when only one copy of a mutant gene is inherited. Nearly 1200 have been identified
  - ◊ Examples: Huntington's chorea, Marfan's syndrome, neurofibromatosis, von Willebrand disease
- Autosomal recessive inheritance: expressed when two copies of a mutant gene are inherited. More than 600 have been identified.
  - ◊ Examples: cystic fibrosis, sickle cell anemia, thalassemia, PKU, Tay-Sachs
- Sex-linked or X-linked inheritance: classified as dominant, recessive, or fragile with the majority being recessive. X-linked recessive disorders are carried by females and only males are affected. One half of male offspring of a carrier mother will be affected and half of the daughters will be carriers.
  - ◊ Examples: color blindness, hemophilia A, Duchenne muscular dystrophy

Multifactorial Inheritance:

- Multifactorial inheritance: characteristic inherited patterns are not found, but there is an increased frequency of the disorder in families. Thought to involve multiple genes and environmental factors.
  - ◊ Examples: neural tube defects, congenital heart disease, orthopedic anomalies, cleft lip and palate, pyloric stenosis

Unknown:

- The etiology of a number of congenital anomalies is unknown
  - ◊ Examples: hydrocephaly, urinary tract anomalies, diaphragmatic hernia

INCIDENCE

- Up to 5% of all newborns have a recognizable birth defect, 20-25% of these are caused by a genetic disorder
- 1 in 170 newborns are affected by some type of chromosomal abnormality
- 1% have a single gene defect

RISK FACTORS

- Family history of genetic disorder
- Preterm infant
- Increased maternal age (> 35 years)
- Recurrent spontaneous abortion
- Infertility
- Exposure to ionizing radiation

DIAGNOSTIC STUDIES

- Maternal α-fetoprotein
- Ultrasound
- Amniocentesis
- Chromosomal analysis

MANAGEMENT

- Preconceptual counseling for couples with a family history of genetic disorders
- Refer for genetic counseling and testing
- Surgical repair of structural defects
- Dietary modifications necessary in some disorders

DOWN SYNDROME
(Trisomy 21)

DESCRIPTION

Chromosomal abnormality in which there is an extra chromosome 21, resulting in a characteristic combination of birth defects.

ETIOLOGY

- Unknown

INCIDENCE

- Incidence of 1/1000 births
- 20 year old woman: 1 in 1200 chance
- 40 year old woman: 1 in 70 chance
- Occurs slightly more in Caucasians than African-Americans, Asians, Hispanics

RISK FACTORS

- Mother older than 35 years of age
- Previous child with Down syndrome

ASSESSMENT FINDINGS

- Simian crease on one or both palms
- Fingers short and stubby
- Fifth fingers are often incurved (clinodactyly)
- Epicanthal folds
- Flattened nasal bridge
- Head relatively small with flattened occiput
- Loose skin at nape of neck
- Poor muscle tone
- Protruding tongue
- Low-set ears
- Mental retardation of varying severity

ASSOCIATED MAJOR MALFORMATIONS

- Congenital heart defects
- Gastrointestinal atresias

DIAGNOSTIC STUDIES

- In utero diagnosis by amniocentesis
- Chromosomal analysis

MANAGEMENT

- Immunizations according to schedule
- Genetic counseling
- Surgical correction of anomalies
- Educate parents regarding syndrome
- Refer to support groups and community resources

EXPECTED COURSE

- Life expectancy 50 years of age

POSSIBLE COMPLICATIONS

- Frequent respiratory infections
- Increased risk of leukemia
- Feeding problems related to protruding tongue and hypotonia

GESTATIONAL TROPHOBLASTIC DISEASE
(Hydatidiform Mole, Molar Pregnancy)

DESCRIPTION

Includes hydatidiform mole, invasive mole (chorioadenoma destruens), and choriocarcinoma. Hydatidiform mole is the most common form; there is abnormal development of the placenta, resulting in fluid-filled, grapelike clusters with trophoblastic tissue proliferation. There is a risk of development of choriocarcinoma from the trophoblastic tissue.

ETIOLOGY

- Develops from ovum which has lost its genetic material
- Reason for this loss is unknown

INCIDENCE

- 1/2000 pregnancies in the U.S.

RISK FACTORS

- Extremes of maternal age
- Familial tendency
- Previous molar pregnancy

ASSESSMENT FINDINGS

- Severe nausea and vomiting at 12-16 weeks gestation
- Continuous or intermittent brown discharge for several weeks
- Heavy vaginal bleeding
- Uterus may be soft
- Uterine size greater than expected for gestational age
- Absent fetal heart tones
- Anemia
- Hydropic vesicles may be passed vaginally
- Pregnancy-induced hypertension may be present in the first half of the pregnancy

DIFFERENTIAL DIAGNOSIS

- Multiple gestation
- Spontaneous abortion

DIAGNOSTIC STUDIES

- Quantitative β-hCG levels higher than expected for gestational age
- Ultrasound: characteristic "starburst" pattern

MANAGEMENT

- Immediate evacuation of uterus
- Hysterectomy may be the treatment of choice in an older woman who has completed her childbearing
- Biweekly serum β-hCG until values return to normal, then monthly for 6 months, then every other month for 6 months for a total of one year
- Pregnancy should be avoided for at least one year
- If woman is Rh-negative: Rh immune globulin (RhoGAM®) should be administered

CONSULTATION/REFERRAL

- Treatment at a center specializing in gestational trophoblastic disease is recommended if hCG levels remain high or continue to rise

POSSIBLE COMPLICATIONS

- Choriocarcinoma develops following evacuation of a molar pregnancy in 20% of women
- Anemia
- Hyperthyroidism
- Infection
- Disseminated intravascular coagulation (DIC)
- Trophoblastic embolization of the lung
- Ovarian cysts

HYPEREMESIS GRAVIDARUM

DESCRIPTION

Persistent, intractable vomiting during pregnancy.

ETIOLOGY

- Not completely known
- Multifactorial: hormonal, neurologic, metabolic, psychosomatic factors
- May be related to increased levels of human chorionic gonadotropin (hCG) and estradiol

INCIDENCE

- Relatively rare condition

RISK FACTORS

- Multiple gestation
- Hydatidiform mole

ASSESSMENT FINDINGS

- Weight loss
- Persistent nausea and vomiting
- Signs of dehydration
- Jaundice
- Hemorrhage
- Peripheral neuropathy

DIFFERENTIAL DIAGNOSIS

- Gastroenteritis
- Appendicitis
- Cholecystitis
- Viral hepatitis
- Hydatidiform mole
- Peptic ulcer disease
- Intestinal obstruction

DIAGNOSTIC STUDIES

- Electrolytes: hypokalemia
- Urinalysis: ketonuria
- Hematocrit: elevated
- BUN: elevated
- Total protein: decreased

DIAGNOSTIC CRITERIA

- Intractable vomiting in the first half of pregnancy
- Dehydration
- Ketonuria
- Weight loss of 5% of prepregnancy weight

MANAGEMENT

- Hospitalization may be necessary with intravenous fluids and parenteral nutrition
- Conservative management as with nausea and vomiting
- Medications may be needed
- Antiemetics
  - ◊ Doxylamine (Unisom®)
  - ◊ Trimethobenzamide (Tigan®) suppository
  - ◊ Ondansetron (Xofran®)

POSSIBLE COMPLICATIONS

- Starvation
- Ketosis
- Electrolyte imbalance
- Dehydration
- Embryonal or fetal death

INCOMPETENT CERVIX

DESCRIPTION

Premature dilatation of the cervix, usually in the fourth or fifth month of pregnancy; is associated with repeated second trimester spontaneous abortion.

ETIOLOGY

Congenital causes:
- Cervical structural defects
- Uterine anomalies
- Abnormal cervical development secondary to in utero exposure to DES

Acquired causes:
- Previous traumatic birth
- Trauma to cervix during dilation and curettage
- Cervical conization
- Cervical cauterization

INCIDENCE

- Occurs in 0.5-1.0% of pregnancies
- Responsible for 15-20% of second trimester pregnancy losses

RISK FACTORS

- History of repeated second trimester spontaneous abortions

ASSESSMENT FINDINGS

- Progressive effacement and dilation of the cervix
- Bulging of membranes through cervical os
- Uterine contractions absent until late in process

DIFFERENTIAL DIAGNOSIS

- Spontaneous abortion

DIAGNOSTIC STUDIES

- Serial ultrasound
- Cervical cultures for gonorrhea and group B *Streptococcus* before placement of cerclage

MANAGEMENT

- Cervical cerclage placed at 14-18 weeks gestation in women with history of incompetent cervix
- Bedrest
- Abstinence of coitus
- Education regarding rupture of membranes

EXPECTED COURSE

- Success rate for carrying a pregnancy to term is 80-90% with appropriate treatment

POSSIBLE COMPLICATIONS

- Premature rupture of membranes
- Failure to stop fetal loss
- Tearing of cervix

MULTIPLE GESTATION

DEFINITION

Pregnancy with multiple fetuses.

ETIOLOGY

- Results from fertilization of separate ova (fraternal) or from a single fertilized ovum that divides into separate structures (identical)

INCIDENCE

- Incidence of twins in U.S. is 1/80 pregnancies

RISK FACTORS

- African-American
- Women who were twins are more likely to have twins
- Increased maternal age
- Increased parity
- More common in large and tall women than in small women
- Use of fertility agents
- In vitro fertilization

ASSESSMENT FINDINGS

- Uterus size is larger than expected for gestational age
- Auscultation of two separate fetal heart sounds

DIAGNOSTIC STUDIES

- Serial ultrasound to determine growth of each fetus
- Maternal α-fetoprotein: elevated
- Chorionic gonadotropin: elevated
- Biophysical profile and nonstress testing beginning at 30-34 weeks gestation

DIFFERENTIAL DIAGNOSIS

- Inaccurate menstrual history
- Hydramnios
- Hydatidiform mole
- Uterine fibroids
- Adenomyosis
- Adnexal mass
- Fetal macrosomia

MANAGEMENT

- More frequent prenatal visits
- Dietary intake increased an additional 300 kcal/day
- Iron intake increased to 60-100 mg/day
- Folic acid intake increased to 1 mg/day
- Bedrest may be necessary toward end of pregnancy or at any time if preterm labor threatens
- Cesarean section indicated for birth of three or more fetuses

EXPECTED COURSE

- Morbidity and mortality are considerably increased in pregnancy with multiple fetuses

POSSIBLE COMPLICATIONS

Maternal risks:
- Anemia
- Pregnancy-induced hypertension
- Placenta previa
- Abruptio placenta
- Uterine dysfunction
- Preterm labor
- Increased physical discomfort

Fetal risks:
- Spontaneous abortion
- Increased perinatal mortality
- Low birthweight
- Congenital anomalies
- Fetal-fetal hemorrhage
- Cord accidents
- Hydramnios
- Abnormal fetal presentation
- The more fetuses conceived, the smaller they tend to be at birth
- Death of one or more fetuses

PLACENTA PREVIA

DESCRIPTION

Improper implantation of the placenta in the lower uterine segment. Four common classifications:

- *Complete*: placental tissue completely covers cervical os
- *Partial*: only a portion of os is covered
- Marginal: the edge of the placenta is at the margin of the os
- *Low-lying*: placenta does not cover os, but is low in the uterine segment

ETIOLOGY

- Unknown

INCIDENCE

- 1/250 births

RISK FACTORS

- History of previous placenta previa
- Grand multiparity
- Maternal age over 35 years
- Previous cesarean section
- Previous induced abortion
- Cigarette smoking
- Multiple gestation
- History of dilatation and curettage
- History of myomectomy
- Large placenta

ASSESSMENT FINDINGS

- Painless vaginal bleeding usually beginning at the end of the second trimester
- A vaginal examination should not be performed if placenta previa is suspected

DIFFERENTIAL DIAGNOSIS

- Abruptio placentae
- Coagulation defects
- Bloody show
- Vaginal/cervical lesion
- Trauma
- Trophoblastic disease

DIAGNOSTIC STUDIES

- Ultrasound

MANAGEMENT

- Dependent on gestational age of fetus and degree of bleeding
- Expectant management if pregnancy < 37 weeks gestation and bleeding not severe
    - ◊ Bedrest
    - ◊ No rectal or vaginal examinations
    - ◊ Electronic fetal monitoring
    - ◊ Intravenous fluids
- Cesarean section before 37 weeks is required if frequent, recurrent, or profuse bleeding persists or if fetal well-being jeopardized
- Refer for physician management

POSSIBLE COMPLICATIONS

- Shock
- Preterm delivery
- Placenta accreta

PRE-ECLAMPSIA, ECLAMPSIA

DESCRIPTION

Hypertensive condition that occurs during pregnancy and resolves after pregnancy; occurs after 20 weeks.

TERMS

Preeclampsia	Pregnancy-induced hypertension which may progress to eclampsia if untreated
Eclampsia	Seizures or coma in a patient with pre-eclampsia

ETIOLOGY

- Unknown

INCIDENCE

- Most common hypertensive disorder in pregnancy
- Occurs in 6-8% of all pregnancies

- Among African-American primigravidas the incidence is 15-20%
- In young primigravidas with twin pregnancy, the incidence is 30%

RISK FACTORS

- Primigravida
- Family history of preeclampsia
- History of preeclampsia in a previous pregnancy
- Adolescents of lower socioeconomic status
- Women over 35 years
- Multiple gestation
- Polyhydramnios
- Malnutrition
- Preexisting hypertension or renal disease
- Hydatidiform mole
- Rh incompatibility
- Diabetes mellitus

DIAGNOSTIC CRITERIA

- BP > 140/90 in a previously normotensive patient; BP elevated on 2 occasions at least 6 hours a part, no more than 7 days apart
- Excretion of > 300 mg/dL of protein over 24 hours; dipstick reading of 1 + (30 mg/dL) or greater
- No longer a criterion but must assess for pedal edema 1+ or greater that does not resolve with overnight rest, edema of the face and hands, and edema associated with more than a 2 kg weight gain in one week

ASSESSMENT FINDINGS

- Hypertension, tachycardia
- Hyperreflexia
- Oliguria or anuria in severe preeclampsia
- Proteinuria, hematuria, edema
- Dizziness, headache
- Blurred vision, diplopia
- Scotomata (spots before the eyes)
- Retinal edema
- Dyspnea
- Crackles in lung fields
- Epigastric pain
- Hepatomegaly

DIFFERENTIAL DIAGNOSIS

- Essential hypertension
- Renal disease

DIAGNOSTIC STUDIES

- Hematocrit: increased
- Platelet counts: decreased
- Prothrombin time and activated partial thromboplastin time: prolonged
- BUN and serum creatinine: increased in worsening disease
- Urinalysis: high specific gravity, proteinuria
- Liver enzymes: increased if HELLP syndrome present
- 24-hour urine specimen for creatinine clearance and total protein
- Uric acid: increased
- Total protein: decreased
- Lactate dehydrogenase: increased
- Nonstress testing
- Ultrasound for determination of fetal growth
- Biophysical profile
- Amniocentesis to determine fetal lung maturity

MANAGEMENT

- Hospitalization recommended if proteinuria present and/or outpatient management has not been successful
- Bed rest in left lateral recumbent position to decrease pressure on vena cava
- Quiet, low stimulus environment
- Seizure precautions
- Well-balanced diet with moderate to high intake of protein
- Excessive salt intake should be avoided, but strict sodium restriction not recommended
- Diuretics not recommended for treatment
- Magnesium sulfate intravenous for prevention or treatment of seizures
- Antihypertensives
    - ◊ Methyldopa (Aldomet®) is the drug of choice
    - ◊ Hydralazine (Apresoline®)
- Beta blockers, calcium channel blockers commonly used
- Education regarding signs and symptoms or worsening preeclampsia
- Delivery of infant is definitive treatment

CONSULTATION/REFERRAL

- Obstetrician consultation or referral
- Women with HELLP syndrome should be referred to tertiary care center
- Refer to hospital if BP > 160/110 mm Hg

EXPECTED COURSE

- Perinatal mortality associated with preeclampsia is 10%; with eclampsia 20%
- Risk for eclampsia continues until 48 hours postpartum

POSSIBLE COMPLICATIONS

- Cerebral edema
- Cerebral hemorrhage
- Seizures
- Coma
- Intrauterine growth restriction of fetus
- Chronic fetal hypoxia
- Fetal distress
- Premature delivery
- Increased intraocular pressure leading to retinal detachment
- HELLP syndrome: involves **H**emolysis, **E**levated **L**iver enzymes, and **L**ow **P**latelet count; associated with severe preeclampsia

PRE-TERM LABOR

DESCRIPTION

Onset of regular uterine contractions which effect cervical change occurring between 20 and 37 weeks of pregnancy

ETIOLOGY

- Actual cause unknown

Maternal factors:
- Cardiovascular disease
- Renal disease
- Diabetes
- Pregnancy-induced hypertension
- Abdominal surgery
- Uterine anomalies
- Incompetent cervix
- In utero DES exposure
- Infection
- Retained IUD

Fetal factors:
- Multiple gestation
- Hydramnios
- Fetal or amniotic fluid infection
- Fetal death
- Premature rupture of membranes
- Fetal or placental anomaly

Placental factors:
- Placenta previa
- Abruptio placentae

INCIDENCE

- 7-10% of all live births occur prematurely in the U.S.

RISK FACTORS

- Low socioeconomic status
- History of preterm births
- Poor prenatal care
- Maternal smoking
- See *Etiology*

ASSESSMENT FINDINGS

- Painful or painless uterine contractions at least every 10 minutes with a duration of 30 seconds
- Pelvic pressure
- Menstrual-like cramping
- Watery or bloody vaginal discharge
- Low back pain
- Cervical effacement and dilatation

DIFFERENTIAL DIAGNOSIS

- Braxton-Hicks contractions
- Leukorrhea

DIAGNOSTIC STUDIES

- Biophysical profile to assist with determination of gestational age of fetus

PREVENTION

- Early identification of women at risk using risk-scoring system
- Education of high-risk women regarding signs and symptoms of preterm labor
- Appropriate prenatal care

MANAGEMENT

- Fetal heart monitoring
- Uterine contraction monitoring
- Bedrest

- Hydration
- Sedation
- Tocolytics
    - ◊ Magnesium sulfate or β-adrenergic agonists (e.g., ritodrine, terbutaline) administered intravenously
    - ◊ Oral tocolytics once contractions stop
    - ◊ Subcutaneous terbutaline via infusion pump may be used if needed for long-term maintenance
- Administration of corticosteroids (e.g., betamethasone, dexamethasone) to accelerate fetal lung maturation
- Care of the woman at home may be accomplished once stable utilizing home monitoring
- Contraindications of interrupting labor: severe PIH, eclampsia, maternal hemodynamic instability, fetal anomalies incompatible with life, chorioamnionitis, fetal maturity, severe abruptio placentae, acute fetal distress

POSSIBLE COMPLICATIONS

- Delivery of premature infant
- Complications from tocolytics (e.g., magnesium and β-adrenergic agonists)

POST-TERM PREGNANCY

DESCRIPTION

Pregnancy that persists beyond 42 weeks gestation and is associated with placental changes that cause a decrease in the uterine-placental-fetal circulation. This reduces the blood supply, oxygen, and nutrition for the fetus.

ETIOLOGY

- Not completely understood
- Associated with lack of usually high estrogen level in normal pregnancy
- Extrauterine pregnancy

INCIDENCE

- 7-12% of all pregnancies

RISK FACTORS

- Nullipara between 15-20 years of age
- Multipara over age 35 years
- Fetal adrenal hypoplasia
- Anencephalic fetus

ASSESSMENT FINDINGS

- Oligohydramnios
- Macrosomic infant
- High incidence of fetal heart rate baseline changes (e.g., tachycardia, variable decelerations)
- Meconium stained amniotic fluid
- Neonatal depression

DIFFERENTIAL DIAGNOSIS

- Inaccurate assessment of gestational age

DIAGNOSTIC STUDIES

- Biophysical profile
- Nonstress testing 2-3 times/week after 40 weeks of gestation

MANAGEMENT

- Electronic fetal monitoring during labor
- Induction of labor after 42 weeks of gestation if cervix favorable (soft, with some effacement)
- Birth accomplished at 43 weeks by induction or cesarean section if vaginal delivery not possible

EXPECTED COURSE

- Induction of labor is usually 95% successful at delivery
- Perinatal mortality doubles by 43 weeks gestation and triples by 44 weeks

POSSIBLE COMPLICATIONS

- Macrosomia (large for gestation age infant)
- Shoulder dystocia
- Postmature infant
    - ◊ Long, thin infant with loss of subcutaneous tissue
    - ◊ Desquamation present
    - ◊ Meconium stained skin and nails
    - ◊ Long nails
    - ◊ Wrinkled hands and feet
- Fetal distress
- Oligohydramnios
- Asphyxia
- Birth trauma
- Umbilical cord compression
- Infant hypoglycemia

PROLAPSED UMBILICAL CORD

DESCRIPTION

The umbilical cord precedes the fetal presenting part causing pressure on the cord and vessels as it is trapped between the maternal pelvis and the presenting part.

ETIOLOGY

- The cord can fall or be washed through the cervix into the vagina anytime the pelvic inlet is not completely filled by the fetus

INCIDENCE

- 0.2-0.6% of births

RISK FACTORS

- Malpresentation of fetus
- Low birth weight
- Multipara with more than 5 previous births
- Multiple gestation
- Presence of a long cord
- Premature rupture of membranes
- Amniotomy

ASSESSMENT FINDINGS

- Visualization of cord protruding from vagina
- Palpation of cord in vagina or protruding through cervical os
- Fetal bradycardia
- Persistent variable decelerations

DIFFERENTIAL DIAGNOSIS

- Fetal distress from another cause

MANAGEMENT

- Relief of pressure on cord by positioning patient in knee-chest or Trendelenburg position and pushing presenting part upward off of cord
- Electronic fetal monitoring
- Oxygen to mother
- Immediate cesarean section

POSSIBLE COMPLICATIONS

- Fetal hypoxia
- Neurological damage
- Fetal death

SPONTANEOUS ABORTION

DESCRIPTION

Involuntary expulsion of the products of conception during the first 20 weeks of gestation.

ETIOLOGY

- Incompetent cervix
- Fetal chromosomal abnormalities
- Cigarette smoking
- Immunologic rejection
- Uterine structural abnormalities
- Teratogenic drugs
- Endocrine imbalance
- Maternal infections

TERMS

Threatened Abortion	Unexplained bleeding, cramping, or backache; cervix is closed; may be followed by partial or complete expulsion of pregnancy or continuance of viable pregnancy; 50% progress to inevitable abortion
Imminent or inevitable abortion	Bleeding and cramping increase; internal cervical os dilates; membranes may rupture
Complete Abortion	Complete abortion: complete products of conception are expelled
Incomplete Abortion	Part of the products of conception are retained, usually the placenta
Missed Abortion	Fetus dies in utero, but is not expelled
Habitual Abortion	Abortion occurs in three or more consecutive pregnancies with no apparent cause
Septic	Any of the above scenarios plus a temperature >100.4° F (38° C) without another source of fever may be septic abortion. Associated with IUD or instrumentation in attempted induced abortion

INCIDENCE

- May be as high as 31%, including recognized and unrecognized pregnancy

RISK FACTORS

- Previous spontaneous abortion

ASSESSMENT FINDINGS

- Vaginal bleeding
- Lower abdominal cramping
- Backache
- Dilation of cervix

DIFFERENTIAL DIAGNOSIS

- Spontaneous abortion
- Ectopic pregnancy
- Abruptio placentae
- Placenta previa
- Vaginal and/or cervical lesions
- Trauma
- Trophoblastic disease

DIAGNOSTIC STUDIES

- Ultrasound: absence of fetal cardiac activity
- Quantitative β-human chorionic gonadotropin (β-hCG): levels fall shortly after fetal death
- Serum progesterone level: < 5 ng/mL is indicative of a nonviable pregnancy
- Hemoglobin and hematocrit to assess blood loss

MANAGEMENT

- Bedrest
- Abstinence from coitus
- Hospitalization may be required if bleeding persists
- Intravenous fluids and blood replacement may be required
- Evacuation of the uterus once fetal death has occurred, usually by dilation and curettage or suction evacuation
- If woman is Rh-negative: Rh immune globulin (RhoGAM®) should be administered
- Anticipatory guidance regarding reaction to loss of pregnancy
- Educate regarding support groups and other available resources

POSSIBLE COMPLICATIONS

- Disseminated intravascular coagulation
- Endometritis
- Sepsis
- Retained products of conception
- Hemorrhage
- Shock

SUBSTANCE ABUSE IN PREGNANCY

INCIDENCE

- 12-14% of pregnant women consume some alcohol during pregnancy with binge drinking reported by 1-2%
- 5.5% of pregnant women use illicit drugs during pregnancy with the most common being cocaine and marijuana

SUBSTANCES COMMONLY ABUSED DURING PREGNANCY

- Alcohol
- Cocaine
- Marijuana
- Amphetamines
- Barbiturates
- Hallucinogens
- Heroin and other narcotics

DIAGNOSTIC STUDIES

- Urine drug screening throughout pregnancy
- Screening for sexually transmitted diseases

MANAGEMENT

- Emphasis on adequate nutrition: high protein, high caloric diet; supplemental vitamins
- Assess support systems
- Referral to treatment program
- Referral to social services
- Hospitalization may be needed
- Detoxification
- Counseling regarding risk of substance abuse to self and developing fetus
- Breastfeeding is not recommended if woman continues using drugs
- Plan for frequent follow-up after delivery including home visits

POSSIBLE CONSEQUENCES

Alcohol:

- Fetal alcohol syndrome: small eyes, short, upturned nose, small, flat cheeks, heart anomalies, mental retardation, short attention span, behavioral problems, poor coordination
- Intrauterine growth restriction
- Morphologic anomalies
- Neurologic, behavior, and cognitive defects
- Folic acid and thiamine deficiencies in mother
- Increased infections in mother
- Withdrawal syndrome in mother and infant

Cocaine:

- Abruptio placentae
- Decreased blood flow to fetus
- Withdrawal syndrome in mother and infant: seizures, hallucinations, pulmonary edema, respiratory failure, cardiac problems
- Increased incidence of first trimester spontaneous abortion
- Intrauterine growth restriction
- Preterm birth
- Stillbirth
- Malformations of fetal genitourinary tract
- Lowered Apgar scores
- Increased risk of sudden infant death syndrome (SIDS)
- Neurobehavioral disturbances in infant

Marijuana:

- Decreased sperm counts in men
- Infants exposed to marijuana may have fine tremors, prolonged startles, and irritability

Heroin:

- Hepatitis
- HIV/AIDS
- Increased incidence of pregnancy-induced hypertension
- Abruptio placentae
- Preterm labor
- Premature rupture of membranes
- Meconium staining
- Intrauterine growth restriction
- Fetal hypoxia
- Withdrawal syndrome: irritability, poor consolability, high-pitched cry, vomiting, seizures

ADOLESCENT PREGNANCY

INCIDENCE

- 1 in 10 adolescent girls (approximately 1 million) become pregnant each year in the U.S.

RISK FACTORS

- Early dating
- Early onset of sexual activity
- Dating male 5-6 years older
- Low self-esteem
- Daughter of an adolescent mother
- Daughter of a single parent
- Poverty
- Minority
- Poor academic achievement
- Substance abuse
- Depression

PREVENTION

- Counseling about pregnancy prevention (e.g., abstinence, contraception)
- Early identification of at-risk children

FACTORS WHICH INCREASE RISKS TO ADOLESCENTS DURING PREGNANCY

- < 15 years of age
- Failure to seek prenatal care
- Inadequate nutrition
- Poor health before pregnancy
- Presence of sexually transmitted diseases
- Smoking
- Alcohol and drug abuse

MANAGEMENT

- Increased attention to nutrition counseling
- Smoking cessation counseling
- Assess for alcohol and substance abuse
- Counseling regarding pregnancy options
- Education regarding importance of prenatal care
- Screening for sexually transmitted diseases
- Assessment of support systems
- Education regarding physiology of pregnancy in terms adolescent can understand

RISKS TO ADOLESCENT MOTHER

- Increased death rate
- Increased rate of premature labor, prolonged labor, pregnancy-induced hypertension, cephalopelvic disproportion, and anemia
- Increased elective abortion rates
- Fewer adolescent mothers receive prenatal care
- Adolescents may have poor eating habits, and are more likely to smoke and take drugs during pregnancy
- Slowed linear growth
- Less likely to complete high school
- Chronic unemployment
- Limited job opportunities
- Social isolation
- Depression

RISKS TO INFANT OF ADOLESCENT MOTHER

- Low birth weight
- Premature delivery
- Increased neonatal death rate
- Increased risk of child abuse and neglect
- Increased rates of birth defects
- Increased risk of being raised in poverty
- Sudden infant death syndrome

References

ACOG committee opinion no. 418: Prenatal and perinatal human immunodeficiency virus testing: Expanded recommendations. (2008). Obstetrics and Gynecology, 112, 739.

American Academy of Pediatrics and the American College of Obstetricians and Gynecologists (Ed.). (2007). Guidelines for perinatal care (6th ed.). Elk Grove Village, IL: American Academy of Pediatrics.

American College of Obstetricians and Gynecologists. (2008). ACOG practice bulletin no. 95: Anemia in pregnancy. Obstetrics and gynecology, 112(1), 201-207.

Bickley, L.S., & Szilagyi, P.G. (2008). Bates' guide to physical examination and history taking (10th ed.). Philadelphia: Lippincott Williams & Wilkins.

Broussard, A. B. , & Hurst, H. M. (2009). Antepartum-intrapartum complications. In M. T. Verklan & M. Walden (Eds.), AWHONN: Core curriculum for neonatal intensive care nursing Philadelphia: Saunders.

Centers for Disease Control and Prevention. (2006). Sexually transmitted diseases treatment guidelines, 2006. MMWR 55(RR-11), 7.

Davidson, M. B., London, M., & Ladewig, P. . (2007). Old's maternal-newbrn nursing and women's health across the lifespan. Upper Saddle River, NJ: Prentice Hall.

Hurst, H. (2007). Section 2: Selected pregnancy complications (bleeding in pregnancy). In S. Perry, K. Cashion & D. Lowdermilk (Eds.), Clincial companion for maternity and women's health care. New York: Elsevier.

Prevention of varicella. Recommendations of the advisory committee on immunization practices (2007). MMWR, 56(1).

Screening for hepatitis b virus infection in pregnancy: U.S. Preventive services task force reaffirmation recommendation statement. (2009). Annals of Internal Medicine, 150(12), 869-873.

Varney, J. , Kriebs, J. M., & Gegor, C. L. . (2004). Varney's midwifery (4th ed.). Sudbury, MA: Jones and Barlett Publishers.

ACOG committee opinion [illegible] perinatal [illegible] Obstetrics and Gynecology [illegible]

American Academy of Pediatrics and the American College of Obstetricians and Gynecologists [illegible] Guidelines for perinatal care [illegible]

American College of Obstetricians and Gynecologists [illegible] Obstetrics and Gynecology [illegible]

[illegible] Drugs [illegible] Williams & Wilkins.

[illegible]

[illegible]

Davidson [illegible]

[illegible]

[illegible]

[illegible] Annals of Internal Medicine [illegible]

[illegible]

15

PULMONARY DISORDERS

Pulmonary Disorders

Acute Bronchitis 573

Chronic Bronchitis 576

Emphysema 582

Asthma 588

Pneumonia 596

Tuberculosis (TB) 602

Pertussis 606

* Bronchiolitis 608

* Croup (Laryngotracheobronchitis) 610

Foreign Body Aspiration 612

* Cystic Fibrosis 613

* Sudden Infant Death Syndrome (SIDS) 615

Primary Lung Malignancies 616

References 618

**Denotes pediatric diagnosis*

ACUTE BRONCHITIS

DESCRIPTION

Inflammation of the bronchioles, bronchi, and trachea; usually follows an upper respiratory infection or exposure to a chemical irritant.

ETIOLOGY

- Adenovirus
- Rhinovirus
- Influenza A and B
- Parainfluenza
- RSV
- Coxsackie virus
- Other viral agents
- Secondary bacterial infection from *Streptococcus pneumoniae, Haemophilus influenzae, Moraxella catarrhalis, Chlamydia pneumoniae, Bordetella pertussis*, or other bacteria

INCIDENCE

- Common

RISK FACTORS

- Upper respiratory infection
- Air pollutants
- Smoking and/or secondary exposure
- Reflux esophagitis
- Allergy
- Chronic obstructive pulmonary disease
- Acute and chronic sinusitis

ASSESSMENT FINDINGS

- Cough: dry and nonproductive, then productive, may be purulent
- Fatigue
- Fever due to infection with pathogens; more common in smokers and patients with COPD
- Burning chest
- Crackles, wheezes

DIFFERENTIAL DIAGNOSIS

- Pneumonia
- Tuberculosis
- Asthma
- Pertussis
- Influenza
- Sinusitis
- Bronchiectasis

DIAGNOSTIC STUDIES

- Consider chest x-ray: only if high index of suspicion of pneumonia or superimposed heart failure
- Consider PPD: expect negative results
- Consider sputum culture: usually not diagnostic; often contains mixed flora
- Consider CBC

PREVENTION

- Smoking cessation
- Avoid known respiratory irritants
- Treat underlying conditions which contribute to risk (asthma, gastroesophageal reflux disease, etc.)
- Influenza immunization in high-risk population

NONPHARMACOLOGIC MANAGEMENT

- Increase fluid intake
- Use humidifier
- Rest
- Smoking cessation
- Patient education regarding disease, treatment, and emergency actions

PHARMACOLOGIC MANAGEMENT

- Cough suppressants for nighttime relief
- Avoid antihistamines
- Antibiotics if organism is bacterial
- Decongestants and antihistamines are ineffective unless sinusitis or allergy are underlying
- Bronchodilators if wheezing

Antibiotics are commonly prescribed but are not recommended.

ACUTE BRONCHITIS PHARMACOLOGIC MANAGEMENT

Class	Drug Generic name (Trade name®)	Dosage How supplied	Comments
Cough Suppressants *Suppresses cough in the medullary center of the brain*	**dextromethorphan/guafensin**	**Adult**: 10 mL every 4 hr *Max*: 4 doses in 24 hours **Children 6-12 years:** 5 mL every 4-6 hours *Max*: 4 doses in 24 hours **< 6 years:** not recommended	• Pregnancy Category C • Do not use if taking an MAO inhibitor or for 2 weeks after stopping the MAO inhibitor • Contraindicated in Parkinson's disease • Potential drug intervention with some SSRIs • Avoid in patients who are having difficulty clearing secretions
	Robitussin DM Various generics	*Dextromethorphan* *10 mg/5 mL* *Guaifenesin* *100 mg/5 mL*	
	dextromethorphan	**Adult and ≥ 12 years:** 10 mL every 6-8 hours prn cough *Max*: 4 doses in 24 hours **Children 6-12 years:** 5 mL every 6-8 hours prn cough *Max*: 4 doses in 24 hours **4-6 years:** 2.5 mL every 6-8 hours prn cough *Max*: 4 doses in 24 hours	• Pregnancy Category C • Do not use if taking an MAO inhibitor or for 2 weeks after stopping the MAO inhibitor • Contraindicated in Parkinson's Disease • Potential drug intervention with some SSRIs • Avoid in patients who are having difficulty clearing secretions • Do no use if on a sodium restricted diet
	Delysm	*Dextromethorphan* *15 mg/5 mL* *Alcohol free/orange or grape flavor*	
	codeine/guaifenesin	**Adult and ≥ 12 years:** 10 mL every 4 hours prn cough; *Max*: 6 doses in 24 hours **Children 6-12 years:** 5 mL every 4 hours prn cough *Max*: 6 doses in 24 hours	• Pregnancy Category C • Do not use if taking an MAO inhibitor or for 2 weeks after stopping the MAO inhibitor • Contraindicated in Parkinson's disease • Potential drug intervention with some SSRIs • Schedule V medication • Avoid in patients who are having difficulty clearing secretions • Avoid narcotic cough suppressants in COPDers and asthmatics • **May be habit forming** • **May aggravate constipation**
	Robitussin AC	*Each 5 mL contains 100 mg guaifenesin and 10 mg codeine*	

continued

ACUTE BRONCHITIS PHARMACOLOGIC MANAGEMENT

Class	Drug Generic name (Trade name®)	Dosage How supplied	Comments
Benzonatate *Topical anesthetic effect on the respiratory stretch receptors*	**benzonatate** Tessalon	**Adult and > 10 years:** > 10 years: 100-200 mg three times/day prn cough *Max*: 600 mg daily *Caps: 100 mg, 200 mg*	• Pregnancy Category C • Do not break or chew capsule - can produce local anesthesia and may reduce patient's gag reflex • Monitor for dizziness, drowsiness and visual changes • Begins to act in 15-20 minutes and lasts for 3-8 hours • Avoid use inpatients sensitive to or taking agents with PABA- possible adverse CNS effects

CONSULTATION/REFERRAL

- Refer to pulmonologist if not improved after 4 weeks

FOLLOW-UP

- 7 days if not improved or if condition worsens
- High-risk groups (i.e., those with co-existing disease) are usually followed up sooner

EXPECTED COURSE

- Symptoms of shorter duration if causative agent is rhinovirus or coronavirus
- Symptoms may persist up to 3-4 weeks

POSSIBLE COMPLICATIONS

- Pneumonia
- Chronic cough
- Chronic bronchitis
- Secondary bacterial infection
- Bronchiectasis

CHRONIC BRONCHITIS

DESCRIPTION

The production of sputum for at least 3 months annually for 2 consecutive years accompanied by cough. Chronic mucus production results from hyperplasia of the mucous membranes (hallmark) lining the bronchial walls. This is usually an **irreversible and progressive** airway disease. The majority of patients has coexisting emphysema and is classified as having chronic obstructive pulmonary disease (COPD), an irreversible airway disease.

ETIOLOGY

- Prolonged exposure to bronchial irritants

INCIDENCE

- Common (14.2 million people have COPD)
- 12.5 million have chronic bronchitis
- Fourth leading cause of death in US
- Typical patient is male smoker in his fifties

RISK FACTORS

- Cigarette smoking (90% attributable to smoking)
- Chronic respiratory infections
- Chronic, poorly controlled respiratory allergies

Screening is not recommended for patients who do not have dyspnea, cough, sputum production or history of lung irritant exposure.

ASSESSMENT FINDINGS

- Symptoms usually begin in 6th decade
- Chronic, productive cough – worse in a.m.
- Sputum production
- Dyspnea on exertion
- Increased respiratory rate
- Crackles and wheezes
- Barrel chest
- Prolonged expiratory phase
- Secondary polycythemia
  (HCT > 52% in males, HCT > 47% in females)
- Tobacco staining of fingers and/or teeth
- Signs of right-sided heart failure

Viral or bacterial infections cause 70-80% of exacerbations of COPD.

DIFFERENTIAL DIAGNOSIS

- Asthma
- Chronic heart failure
- Pneumonia
- Asbestosis

The gold standard for diagnosis of suspected emphysema, chronic bronchitis, or COPD is pulmonary function testing.

DIAGNOSTIC STUDIES

- Spirometry defines severity and response to therapy
- FEV_1/FVC ratio (< 70% constitutes diagnosis)

FEV_1 (forced expiratory volume in one second)
FVC (forced vital capacity)

- Chest x-ray (may see hyperinflation and/or flattened diaphragm)
- Consider CBC, PPD, ABGs, pulse oximetry, ECG
- For patients 45-50 years, consider testing for α-1-protease inhibitor deficiency

Classification of Severity	
Stage I: Mild *Mild airflow limitation*	$FEV_1/FVC < 0.70$ $FEV_1 \geq 80\%$ predicted
Stage II: Moderate *Moderate airflow limitation*	$FEV_1/FVC < 0.70$ $50\% \leq FEV_1 < 80\%$ predicted
Stage III: Severe *Severe airflow limitation*	$FEV_1/FVC < 0.70$ $30\% \leq FEV_1 < 50\%$ predicted
Stage IV: Very Severe *Very severe airflow limitation*	$FEV_1/FVC < 0.70$ $FEV_1 < 30\%$ predicted or $FEV_1 < 50\%$ predicted plus chronic respiratory failure

Source: Global Initiative for Chronic Obstructive Lung Disease, 2009

PREVENTION

- Avoid cigarette smoking
- Minimize exposure to known respiratory irritants
- Once diagnosed: Pneumococcal immunization, influenza immunization annually, minimize exposure to persons with known respiratory infections

NONPHARMACOLOGIC MANAGEMENT

- Adequate fluid intake
- Postural drainage
- Smoking cessation
- Regular exercise training
- Pursed-lip breathing
- Diaphragmatic exercises
- Consider pulmonary rehabilitation
- Patient education regarding disease, treatment, early signs and symptoms of infection, pursed lip breathing, emergency treatment for respiratory distress
- Avoid travel at high altitudes

PHARMACOLOGIC MANAGEMENT

Stage	Management
Stage 1	Active reduction of risk factors Short-acting bronchodilator (SABA) PRN If SABA are not available, consider slow release theophylline
Stage 2	Active reduction of risk factors Long-acting bronchodilator (LABA) Short-acting bronchodilator (SABA) PRN Rehabilitation
Stage 3	Active reduction of risk factors Long-acting bronchodilator (LABA) Short-acting bronchodilator (SABA) PRN Add Inhaled glucosteroids if repeated exacerbations Rehabilitation
Stage 4	Active reduction of risk factors Long-acting bronchodilator (LABA) Short-acting bronchodilator (SABA) PRN Inhaled glucosteroids if repeated exacerbations Add long term oxygen if chronic respiratory failure. Consider surgical treatments Rehabilitation

Source: Global Initiative for Chronic Obstructive Lung Disease, 2009

CHRONIC BRONCHITIS PHARMACOLOGIC MANAGEMENT

Bronchodilators and anticholinergic medications improve lung function, decrease dyspnea and exacerbations. Steroids decrease exacerbations and modestly slow progression of symptoms.

Class	Drug Generic name (Trade name®)	Dosage How supplied	Comments
Bronchodilators - Short Acting *Stimulate beta 2 receptors in the lungs causing broncho-dilation* General comments Paradoxical bronchospasm can result from use of bronchodilators and may be life threatening	**albuterol** (may be inhaled or nebulized)	**Adult and > 12 yr:** *Usual*: 2 inh every 4-6 hours prn bronchospasm *Alternative*: 1 puff every 4-6 hours Each inhalation: albuterol 90 mcg	• Pregnancy Category C • Can increase heart rate, blood pressure, and cause QT prolongation and ST segment depression • Cautious use in patients with cardiac arrhythmias, convulsive disorders, hyperthyroidism • Use extreme caution in patients on MAO inhibitors, beta blockers

continued

CHRONIC BRONCHITIS PHARMACOLOGIC MANAGEMENT

Bronchodilators and anticholinergic medications improve lung function, decrease dyspnea and exacerbations. Steroids decrease exacerbations and modestly slow progression of symptoms.

Class	Drug Generic name (Trade name®)	Dosage How supplied	Comments
	Ventolin HFA	*17 g canister contains 200 inhalations*	• May cause hypokalemia especially if in conjunction with potassium wasting medications. Consider monitoring potassium levels • Possible decreases in digoxin levels • Shake well before each spray
	albuterol	**Adult and > 12 yr:** 2 inh every 4-6 hr	
	ProAir HFA	*Each inhalation: albuterol 90mcg* *8.5 g canister/200 inhalations*	
Bronchodilators - Long-acting *Stimulate beta 2 receptors in the lungs* **General comments** **Long acting bronchodilators increase the risk of asthma-related death. Do not use in patients with asthma unless accompanied by a long-term asthma control medication like an inhaled steroid** Paradoxical bronchospasm can result from use of bronchodilators and may be life threatening	**salmeterol**	**Adult**: 1 inh every 12 hr	• Pregnancy Category C • Do not use long-acting agents to treat acute symptoms. These agents take 15-20 min to produce bronchodilation • Tolerance develops with prolonged use • Significant drug interactions with ketoconazole and erythromycin, clarithromycin • Can increase heart rate, blood pressure, and cause QT prolongation and ST segment depression • Cautious use in patients with cardiac arrhythmias, convulsive disorders, hyperthyroidism • Use extreme caution in patients on MAO inhibitors, beta blockers • May cause hypokalemia especially if in conjunction with potassium wasting medications. Consider monitoring potassium levels • **DO NOT INGEST FORADIL CAPSULES!!!! Capsules should be used only with the AEROLIZER inhaler only!**
	Serevent Diskus	*Each inhalation:30 mcg salmeterol* *60 inhalations*	
	formoterol	**Adult**: 1 inh every 12 hr	
	Foradil Aerolizer	*12 mcg formoterol/ inhalation* *Box of 12, 60 (strips of 6)*	
	Perforomist	**Adult**: 20 mcg nebulizer twice daily Inhalation: 20 mcg/2 mL 60 single use vials	

continued

CHRONIC BRONCHITIS PHARMACOLOGIC MANAGEMENT

Bronchodilators and anticholinergic medications improve lung function, decrease dyspnea and exacerbations. Steroids decrease exacerbations and modestly slow progression of symptoms.

Class	Drug Generic name (Trade name®)	Dosage How supplied	Comments
Xanthines **General comments** Very helpful in some patients with COPD Used as an alternative in asthma treatment; not first line Cause bronchodilation by relaxing smooth muscle of the bronchi and pulmonary blood vessels Toxicity is a general concern with theophylline. Activated charcoal used to manage acute and chronic toxicity	**theophylline** Theo-24	**Adult**: *Initial*: 300-400 mg daily for 3 days; if tolerated, increase dose to 400-600 mg daily; after 3 more days if tolerated and needed, increase dose to blood level *Max:* for patients with impaired clearance, age > 60 years is 400 mg daily *Tabs: 100 mg, 200 mg, Ext. Rel. Caps: 300 mg, 400 mg*	• Pregnancy Category C • The xanthenes are central respiratory stimulants and reduce fatigability in COPDers • Must monitor levels (10-20 mcg/mL is desirable). Common symptom of toxicity is repetitive vomiting • Elevated levels predispose patient to ventricular arrhythmias, seizures. Use is ill advised in patients with active peptic ulcer disease, seizure disorders, cardiac arrhythmias • Monitor for tremors, anxiety, and jitteriness • Many food drug interactions involving CYP 450 system • No dosage adjustment for renal impairment; Need adjustment for hepatic insufficiency, heart failure • Smoking increases clearance of theophylline • High fat meal increases absorption of theophylline • Do not crush or chew extended release tablets • Aminophylline is converted to theophylline
Anticholinergic - Short-acting *Blocks action of acetylcholine and thus causes mild bronchodilation and prevents bronchoconstriction* **General comments** Monitor for signs of worsening narrow angle glaucoma, worsening GI/ GU obstruction	**ipratropium** Atrovent HFA	**Adult**: 2 inh four times daily *Max*: 12 inhalations/24 hours Inh Solution for Nebulizer **Adult**: 500 mcg 3-4 times/day *17 mcg/inh* *12.9 g/200 inhalations* *Soln: 2.5 mL/vial (25)*	• Pregnancy Category B • Not indicated for relief of acute bronchospasm • Works well in conjunction with a bronchodilator • Atrovent HFA canister does not require shaking, but it does need to be primed

continued

CHRONIC BRONCHITIS PHARMACOLOGIC MANAGEMENT

Bronchodilators and anticholinergic medications improve lung function, decrease dyspnea and exacerbations. Steroids decrease exacerbations and modestly slow progression of symptoms.

Class	Drug Generic name (Trade name®)	Dosage How supplied	Comments
Anticholinergic - Long-acting	**tiotropium**	**Adult**: 2 inh of one capsule contents daily using inhaler device	• Pregnancy Category C • Not indicated for relief of acute bronchospasm • Avoid if allergic to milk proteins • Avoid concurrent use with other cholinergic medications • Monitor closely if renal impairment since this is renally excreted
<u>**General comments**</u> **Paradoxical broncho-spasms can occur** Monitor for signs of worsening narrow angle glaucoma, worsening GI/ GU obstruction	Spiriva Handihaler	*18 mcg/inh* *Caps: 5, 30, 90*	
Inhaled Corticosteroids *Glucocorticoids decrease activity of inflammatory cells and mediators*	**fluticasone**	**Adult**: ***Previously on bronchodilators:*** *Initial*: 88 mcg twice daily *Max*: 440 mg twice daily ***Previously on inhaled steroids:*** *Initial*: 88-220 twice daily *Max*: 440 mcg twice daily ***Previously on oral steroids:*** *Initial*: 440 mcg twice daily *Max*: 880 mcg twice daily	• Pregnancy Category C • Slowly wean patients who are on oral steroids to inhaled steroids • Abrupt withdrawal can cause symptoms of adrenal insufficiency (fatigue, weakness, and hypotension) • Monitor for symptoms of fungal infection in the mouth and pharynx
<u>**General comments**</u> Steroid activity is local (in the lungs) and is associated with minimal systemic absorption Decreases in bone density can occur with steroids; monitor May cause immunosuppression; possible increased risk of pneumonia, worsening of existing infections.	Flovent HFA	*44 mcg/inh (10.6 g)* *110 mcg/inh (12 g)* *220 mch/inh (12 g)*	
Cautious use with concurrent use of 3A4 inhibitors Monitor for increased intraocular pressure, glaucoma and/or cataracts	**budesonide**	**Adult**: *Initial*: 360 mcg twice daily *Alternative*: Some patients may respond to 180 mcg twice daily *Max*: 720 mcg twice daily	• Pregnancy Category C • Avoid abrupt withdrawal • Cautious use in presence of any infections
Rinse mouth well after use to prevent thrush	Pulmicort Flexhaler	*180 mcg/dose, 120 doses*	

continued

CHRONIC BRONCHITIS PHARMACOLOGIC MANAGEMENT

Bronchodilators and anticholinergic medications improve lung function, decrease dyspnea and exacerbations. Steroids decrease exacerbations and modestly slow progression of symptoms.

Class	Drug Generic name (Trade name®)	Dosage How supplied	Comments
Combination Inhaled Corticosteroid - Long Acting Bronchodilator *Glucocorticoids decrease activity of inflammatory cells and mediators* *Steroid activity is local (in the lungs) and is associated with minimal systemic absorption* **General comments** Risks associated with inhaled steroids and long acting bronchodilators are identical in these combinations products **Paradoxical bronchospasm can occur with combo medications** Decreases in bone density can occur with steroids Monitor Close monitoring for glaucoma and cataracts is warranted Possible metabolic effects: hypokalemia, hyperglycemia Rinse mouth well after use to avoid thrush	**fluticasone/salmeterol** Advair Diskus	**Adult**: 1 inhalation 250 mcg/50 mcg twice daily *Max*: 2 inhalations/24 hours *250/50* *Diskus (60 blisters)*	• Pregnancy Category C • Monitor for symptoms of fungal infection in the mouth and pharynx • NOT indicated for the relief of acute bronchospasm • Increased risk of pneumonia in patients with COPD • Risks associated with inhaled steroids and long acting bronchodilators are identical in these combinations as in individual products
	budesonide/formoterol Symbicort	**Adult**: 160/4.5 2 inhalations twice daily *160/4.5 60, 120 inhalations*	• Pregnancy Category C • Monitor for symptoms of fungal infection in the mouth and pharynx • NOT indicated for the relief of acute bronchospasm • Increased risk of pneumonia in patients with COPD • Risks associated with inhaled steroids and long acting bronchodilators are identical in these combinations as in individual products

Xanthines are rarely used because of intolerable cardiac side effects like tachycardia, angina and heart failure.

CONSULTATION/REFERRAL

- Consult pulmonologist for patients with signs/symptoms of right-sided heart failure and/or respiratory distress/failure

FOLLOW-UP

- Follow-up visits every 3-6 months for stable disease
- Maintain close follow-up with patients with acute respiratory infections
- Review treatment program with patient at each visit

EXPECTED COURSE

- Irreversible, chronic disease with frequent exacerbations and remissions

POSSIBLE COMPLICATIONS

- Frequent serious pulmonary infections
- Acute bronchospasm
- Chronic heart failure
- Acute respiratory failure

EMPHYSEMA

DESCRIPTION

Lung disease characterized by enlargement of the alveolar ducts and air spaces distal to the terminal bronchioles. The mechanism by which alveolar walls are destroyed is incompletely understood, but this results in air trapping and loss of elastic recoil of the lungs. This is usually an **irreversible and progressive** airway disease. The majority of patients have coexisting chronic bronchitis and are classified as having chronic obstructive pulmonary disease (COPD), an irreversible airway disease.

ETIOLOGY

- 14.2 million people have COPD
- 1.7 million have emphysema
- 4th leading cause of death in US
- < 1% of cases due to α-1-antitrypsin deficiency (contributes to premature emphysema); consider if patient is nonsmoker and < 45-50 years old
- Remainder of cases due to alveolar wall destruction from known and unknown causes

INCIDENCE

- Major cause of disability in the U.S.
- Males > Females
- Age > 40 years

RISK FACTORS

- Cigarette smoking most common cause
- Passive smoke
- Chronic pulmonary infections, allergies
- Chronic exposure to lung irritants (e.g., asbestos)
- α-1-antitrypsin deficiency

Screening is not recommended for patients who do not have dyspnea, cough, sputum production, or history of lung irritant exposure.

ASSESSMENT FINDINGS

- Disease begins early in adult life, but symptoms usually appear in the fifties
- Smoker's cough often present
- Dyspnea on exertion most common complaint
- Cough, wheezes
- Inability to take a deep breath
- Slowed, prolonged expiration
- Barrel chest
- Diminished breath sounds
- Clubbing of fingers
- Varying degrees of respiratory distress
- Diffuse pulmonary fibrosis
- Often significant weight loss

DIFFERENTIAL DIAGNOSIS

- Congestive heart failure
- Asthma
- Combination of chronic bronchitis/emphysema
- Chronic sinusitis
- Tuberculosis
- Mesothelioma (asbestos exposure)

DIAGNOSTIC STUDIES

- Spirometry defines severity and response to therapy
- FEV_1/FVC ratio (< 70% constitutes diagnosis)
- FEV_1 (forced expiratory volume in one second)
- FVC (forced vital capacity)
- Consider CBC, PPD, ABGs, pulse oximetry, ECG
- α-1-antitrypsin level: positive in 1% of patients
- Chest x-ray: emphysematous changes,

hyperinflation, flattened diaphragm
- Hematocrit and hemoglobin to determine severity of chronic hypoxemia
- Electrocardiogram: to exclude cardiac disease

The gold standard for diagnosis of suspected emphysema, chronic bronchitis, or COPD is pulmonary function testing.

PREVENTION

- Avoid cigarette smoking
- Avoid inhaling known respiratory irritants
- Once diagnosed: Pneumococcal immunization, influenza immunization annually, minimize exposure to persons with known respiratory infections

NONPHARMACOLOGIC MANAGEMENT

- Adequate fluid intake
- Postural drainage
- Smoking cessation
- Regular exercise training
- Pursed-lip breathing
- Diaphragmatic exercises
- Consider pulmonary rehabilitation
- Teach patients early signs and symptoms of infection
- Avoid travel at high altitude

PHARMACOLOGIC MANAGEMENT

Stage 1	Active reduction of risk factors Short-acting bronchodilator (SABA) PRN If SABA are not available, consider slow release theophylline
Stage 2	Active reduction of risk factors Long-acting bronchodilator (LABA) Short-acting bronchodilator (SABA) PRN Rehabilitation
Stage 3	Active reduction of risk factors Long-acting bronchodilator (LABA) Short-acting bronchodilator (SABA) PRN Add Inhaled glucosteroids if repeated exacerbations Rehabilitation
Stage 4	Active reduction of risk factors Long-acting bronchodilator (LABA) Short-acting bronchodilator (SABA) PRN Inhaled glucosteroids if repeated exacerbations Add long term oxygen if chronic respiratory failure Consider surgical treatments Rehabilitation

Source: Global Initiative for Chronic Obstructive Lung Disease, 2009

EMPHYSEMA PHARMACOLOGIC MANAGEMENT

Bronchodilators and anticholinergic medications improve lung function, decrease dyspnea and exacerbations. Steroids decrease exacerbations and modestly slow progression of symptoms.

Class	Drug Generic name (Trade name®)	Dosage How supplied	Comments
Bronchodilators - Short Acting *Stimulate beta 2 receptors in the lungs causing broncho-dilation* General Comment Paradoxical bronchospasm can result from use of bronchodilators and may be life threatening	**albuterol** (may be inhaled or nebulized)	**Adult > 12 yr:** *Usual*: 2 inh every 4-6 hr prn bronchospasm *Alternative*: 1 puff every 4-6 hours Each inhalation: albuterol 90 mcg	• Pregnancy Category C • Can increase heart rate, blood pressure, and cause QT prolongation and ST segment depression • Cautious use in patients with cardiac arrhythmias, convulsive disorders, hyperthyroidism • Use extreme caution in patients on MAO inhibitors, beta blockers

continued

EMPHYSEMA PHARMACOLOGIC MANAGEMENT

Bronchodilators and anticholinergic medications improve lung function, decrease dyspnea and exacerbations. Steroids decrease exacerbations and modestly slow progression of symptoms.

Class	Drug Generic name (Trade name®)	Dosage How supplied	Comments
	Ventolin HFA	*17 g canister contains 200 inhalations*	• May cause hypokalemia especially if in conjunction with potassium wasting medications. Consider monitoring potassium levels • Possible decreases in digoxin levels • Shake well before each spray
	albuterol	**Adult > 12 yr:** 2 inh every 4-6 hr	
	ProAir HFA	*Each inhalation: albuterol 90mcg* *8.5 g canister/200 inhalations*	
Bronchodilators - Long-acting *Stimulate beta 2 receptors in the lungs* General comments **Long acting bronchodilators increase the risk of asthma-related death. Do not use in patients with asthma unless accompanied by a long-term asthma control medication like an inhaled steroid** Paradoxical bronchospasm can result from use of bronchodilators and may be life threatening	**salmeterol**	**Adult**: 1 inh every 12 hr	• Pregnancy Category C • Do not use long-acting agents to treat acute symptoms. These agents take 15-20 min to produce bronchodilation • Tolerance develops with prolonged use • Significant drug interactions with ketoconazole and erythromycin, clarithromycin • Can increase heart rate, blood pressure, and cause QT prolongation and ST segment depression • Cautious use in patients with cardiac arrhythmias, convulsive disorders, hyperthyroidism • Use extreme caution in patients on MAO inhibitors, beta blockers • May cause hypokalemia especially if in conjunction with potassium wasting medications. Consider monitoring potassium levels • **DO NOT INGEST FORADIL CAPSULES!!!! Capsules should be used only with the AEROLIZER inhaler only!**
	Serevent Diskus	*Each inhalation:30 mcg salmeterol* *60 inhalations*	
	formoterol	**Adult**: 1 inh every 12 hr	
	Foradil Aerolizer	*12 mcg formoterol/ inhalation* *Box of 12, 60 (strips of 6)*	
	Perforomist	**Adult**: 20 mcg nebulizer twice daily Inhalation: 20 mcg/2 mL 60 single use vials	

continued

Pulmonary Disorders

EMPHYSEMA PHARMACOLOGIC MANAGEMENT

Bronchodilators and anticholinergic medications improve lung function, decrease dyspnea and exacerbations. Steroids decrease exacerbations and modestly slow progression of symptoms.

Class	Drug Generic name (Trade name®)	Dosage How supplied	Comments
Xanthines *Cause bronchodilation by relaxing smooth muscle of the bronchi and pulmonary blood vessels* **General comments** Very helpful in some patients with COPD Used as an alternative in asthma treatment; not first line Toxicity is a general concern with theophylline. Activated charcoal used to manage acute and chronic toxicity	**theophylline** Theo-24	**Adult**: *Initial*: 300-400 mg daily for 3 days; if tolerated, increase dose to 400-600 mg daily; after 3 more days if tolerated and needed, increase dose to blood level *Max:* for patients with impaired clearance, age > 60 years is 400 mg daily *Tabs: 100 mg, 200 mg, Ext. Rel. Caps: 300 mg, 400 mg*	• Pregnancy Category C • The xanthenes are central respiratory stimulants and reduce fatigability in COPDers • Must monitor levels (10-20 mcg/mL is desirable). Common symptom of toxicity is repetitive vomiting • Elevated levels predispose patient to ventricular arrhythmias, seizures. Use is ill advised in patients with active peptic ulcer disease, seizure disorders, cardiac arrhythmias • Monitor for tremors, anxiety, and jitteriness • Many food drug interactions involving CYP 450 system • No dosage adjustment for renal impairment; Need adjustment for hepatic insufficiency, heart failure • Smoking increases clearance of theophylline • High fat meal increases absorption of theophylline • Do not crush or chew extended release tablets • Aminophylline is converted to theophylline
Anticholinergic - Short-acting *Blocks action of acetylcholine and thus causes mild bronchodilation and prevents bronchoconstriction* **General comments** Monitor for signs of worsening narrow angle glaucoma, worsening GI/ GU obstruction	**ipratropium** Atrovent HFA	**Adult**: 2 inh four times daily *Max*: 12 inhalations/24 hours Inh Solution for Nebulizer **Adult**: 500 mcg 3-4 times/day *17 mcg/inh* *12.9 g/200 inhalations* *Soln: 2.5 mL/vial (25)*	• Pregnancy Category B • Not indicated for relief of acute bronchospasm • Works well in conjunction with a bronchodilator • Atrovent HFA canister does not require shaking, but it does need to be primed

continued

Pulmonary Disorders

EMPHYSEMA PHARMACOLOGIC MANAGEMENT

Bronchodilators and anticholinergic medications improve lung function, decrease dyspnea and exacerbations. Steroids decrease exacerbations and modestly slow progression of symptoms.

Class	Drug Generic name (Trade name®)	Dosage How supplied	Comments
Anticholinergic - Long-acting	**tiotropium**	**Adult**: 2 inh of one capsule contents daily using inhaler device	• Pregnancy Category C • Not indicated for relief of acute bronchospasm • Avoid if allergic to milk proteins • Avoid concurrent use with other cholinergic medications • Monitor closely if renal impairment since this is renally excreted
General comments **Paradoxical broncho-spasms can occur** Monitor for signs of worsening narrow angle glaucoma, worsening GI/GU obstruction	Spiriva Handihaler	*18 mcg/inh* *Caps: 5, 30, 90*	
Inhaled Corticosteroids *Glucocorticoids decrease activity of inflammatory cells and mediators*	**fluticasone**	**Adult**: **Previously on bronchodilators**: *Initial*: 88 mcg twice daily *Max*: 440 mg twice daily **Previously on inhaled steroids**: *Initial*: 88-220 twice daily *Max*: 440 mcg twice daily **Previously on oral steroids:** *Initial*: 440 mcg twice daily *Max*: 880 mcg twice daily	• Pregnancy Category C • Slowly wean patients who are on oral steroids to inhaled steroids • Abrupt withdrawal can cause symptoms of adrenal insufficiency (fatigue, weakness, and hypotension) • Monitor for symptoms of fungal infection in the mouth and pharynx
General comments Steroid activity is local (in the lungs) and is associated with minimal systemic absorption Decreases in bone density can occur with steroids; monitor May cause immunosuppression; possible increased risk of pneumonia, worsening of existing infections.	Flovent HFA	*44 mcg/inh (10.6 g)* *110 mcg/inh (12 g)* *220 mch/inh (12 g)*	
Cautious use with concurrent use of 3A4 inhibitors Monitor for increased intraocular pressure, glaucoma and/or cataracts	**budesonide**	**Adult**: *Initial*: 360 mcg twice daily *Alternative*: Some patients may respond to 180 mcg twice daily *Max*: 720 mcg twice daily	• Pregnancy Category B • Avoid abrupt withdrawal • Cautious use in presence of infections
Rinse mouth well after use to prevent thrush	Pulmicort Flexhaler	*180 mcg/dose, 120 doses*	

continued

EMPHYSEMA PHARMACOLOGIC MANAGEMENT

Bronchodilators and anticholinergic medications improve lung function, decrease dyspnea and exacerbations. Steroids decrease exacerbations and modestly slow progression of symptoms.

Class	Drug Generic name (Trade name®)	Dosage How supplied	Comments
Combination Inhaled Corticosteroid - Long Acting Bronchodilator *Glucocorticoids decrease activity of inflammatory cells and mediators* *Steroid activity is local (in the lungs) and is associated with minimal systemic absorption* **General comments** Risks associated with inhaled steroids and long acting bronchodilators are identical in these combinations products **Paradoxical bronchospasm can occur with combo medications** Decreases in bone density can occur with steroids; monitor Close monitoring for glaucoma and cataracts is warranted Possible metabolic effects: hypokalemia, hyperglycemia Rinse mouth well after use to avoid thrush	**fluticasone/salmeterol** Advair Diskus	**Adult**: 1 inhalation 250 mcg/50 mcg twice daily *Max*: 2 inhalations/24 hours *250/50* *Diskus (60 blisters)*	• Pregnancy Category C • Monitor for symptoms of fungal infection in the mouth and pharynx • NOT indicated for the relief of acute bronchospasm • Increased risk of pneumonia in patients with COPD • Risks associated with inhaled steroids and long acting bronchodilators are identical in these combinations as in individual products
	budesonide/formoterol Symbicort	**Adult**: 160/4.5 2 inhalations twice daily *160/4.5 60, 120 inhalations*	• Pregnancy Category C • Monitor for symptoms of fungal infection in the mouth and pharynx • NOT indicated for the relief of acute bronchospasm • Increased risk of pneumonia in patients with COPD • Risks associated with inhaled steroids and long acting bronchodilators are identical in these combinations products

CONSULTATION/REFERRAL

- Consult specialist for any patient with signs/symptoms of right-sided heart failure and/or respiratory distress/failure

FOLLOW-UP

- Follow-up visits every 3-6 months for stable disease
- Monthly follow-up for unstable patients
- Maintain close follow-up with patients with acute respiratory infections
- Review treatment program with patient at each visit

EXPECTED COURSE

- A irreversible, chronic disease with frequent exacerbations and remissions

POSSIBLE COMPLICATIONS

- Frequent serious pulmonary infections
- Congestive heart failure
- Acute respiratory failure

ASTHMA

DESCRIPTION

A chronic, respiratory disease characterized by **reversible** airway obstruction, inflammation, and airway hyperresponsiveness. Symptoms range from occasional and mild to severe and debilitating.

A consistent definition of asthma is elusive because patients' symptoms vary and are inconsistent. It is helpful to think of asthma as an inflammatory disorder of the airways.

ETIOLOGY

- Inflammation of the bronchial mucosa and spasm of the bronchial smooth muscle leads to narrowing of the small and occasionally large airways
- Produces characteristic cough and wheezing

INCIDENCE

- About 15 million Americans have asthma
- Most common disease of early childhood
- Leading cause of missed school days

RISK FACTORS

- History of allergies
- Family history
- Cigarette smoke exposure
- Cockroaches and dust
- Gastroesophageal reflux disease (GERD)
- Viral respiratory infection in susceptible individuals (RSV)
- Exercise
- Cold air intolerance
- Chronic sinusitis

A personal or family history of asthma or other atopic diseases is suggestive of asthma in a patient with symptoms of asthma.

ASSESSMENT FINDINGS

- Cough is the earliest symptom
- Wheezes
- Hyperresonance
- Prolonged expiration
- Accessory muscle use
- Sudden nocturnal dyspnea
- Decreased exercise tolerance
- Normal growth and development in children even with frequent steroid use

Classification of Severity	
Mild intermittent	Symptoms ≤ 2 days per week **or** ≤ 2 nights per month Exacerbations brief
Mild persistent	Symptoms ≥ 2 times per week, but < 1 time per day **or** < 2 nights per month
Moderate persistent	Daily symptoms **or** more than 1 night per week
Severe persistent	Continual symptoms **or** frequent nighttime symptoms

Source: From National Heart, Lung, and Blood Institute, National Asthma Education and Prevention Program Expert Panel Report 3: Guidelines for the diagnosis and Management of Asthma, 2007

DIFFERENTIAL DIAGNOSIS

- Respiratory infections
- Congestive heart failure
- Gastroesophageal reflux disease
- Habitual cough
- Tuberculosis
- Foreign body aspiration, especially in children

A diagnosis of asthma requires the presence of respiratory symptoms like intermittent dyspnea, cough, or wheezing; and variable expiratory airflow obstruction.

DIAGNOSTIC STUDIES

- Spirometry
- Pulmonary function tests
- Consider allergy testing
- Peak flow monitoring
- Methacholine challenge test

PREVENTION

- Learn early signs and symptoms of asthma exacerbation
- Use an asthma action plan, a pre-arranged medication plan for asthma exacerbations
- Influenza and pneumococcal pneumonia immunizations
- Monitor peak flow values
- Learn correct use of inhalers, spacers, and other medications

An asthma action plan can be based on a patient's PEFR but symptom based plans appear equally effective.

NONPHARMACOLOGIC MANAGEMENT

- Peak flow monitoring
- Avoidance of asthma triggers if possible
- Patient and family education regarding disease, treatment, avoidance of triggers, asthma management plan, and emergency actions

PHARMACOLOGIC MANAGEMENT

Mild intermittent	**Short-acting bronchodilator** for exacerbations
Mild persistent	**Preferred treatment:** low dose inhaled corticosteroids **Alternative treatment:** cromolyn, leukotriene , OR sustained-release theophylline (serum concentration 5-15 mcg/mL) Short-acting bronchodilator for exacerbations Consider leukotriene blocker (Singulair®, Accolate®)
Moderate persistent	**Preferred treatment**: low to medium dose inhaled corticosteroid and long-acting inhaled bronchodilator **Alternative treatment**: low to medium dose inhaled corticosteroid and either leukotriene blocker or theophylline Short-acting bronchodilator for exacerbations
Severe persistent	**Preferred treatment**: high dose inhaled corticosteroids and long acting inhaled bronchodilators AND if needed, oral corticosteroids (2 mg/kg/day not to exceed 60 mg/day) Short-acting bronchodilator for exacerbations

Source: From National Heart, Lung, and Blood Institute, National Asthma Education and Prevention Program Expert Panel Report 3: Guidelines for the diagnosis and Management of Asthma, 2007

<table>
<tr><td colspan="2">For infants and children < 5 years of age:
Cromolyn (Intal®) preferred over steroids if provides adequate symptom management. Nebulized bronchodilator preferred over metered dose inhaler. Use spacer/holding chamber and face mask</td></tr>
<tr><td>Mild intermittent</td><td>Short-acting bronchodilator for exacerbations</td></tr>
<tr><td>Mild persistent</td><td>Preferred treatment: low dose inhaled corticosteroids

Alternative treatment: cromolyn, leukotriene

Short-acting bronchodilator for exacerbations

Consider leukotriene blocker (Singulair®)</td></tr>
<tr><td>Moderate persistent</td><td>Preferred treatment: low dose inhaled corticosteroid and long-acting inhaled bronchodilator OR medium dose inhaled corticosteroid

Alternative treatment: low dose inhaled corticosteroid and either leukotriene blocker or theophylline

Short-acting bronchodilator for exacerbations</td></tr>
<tr><td>Severe persistent</td><td>Preferred treatment: high dose inhaled corticosteroids and long acting inhaled bronchodilators AND if needed, oral corticosteroids (2 mg/kg/day not to exceed 60 mg/day)

Short-acting bronchodilator for exacerbations</td></tr>
</table>

Source: From National Heart, Lung, and Blood Institute, National Asthma Education and Prevention Program Expert Panel Report 3: Guidelines for the diagnosis and Management of Asthma, 2007

ASTHMA PHARMACOLOGIC MANAGEMENT

Inhaled steroids are used for the maintenance of asthma in patients with persistent asthma. Long-acting beta agonists (LABA) may increase the risk of asthma-related death and should NEVER be used alone in the management of asthma. LABAs should only be used with a concurrent long-acting steroid.

Class	Drug Generic name (Trade name®)	Dosage How supplied	Comments
Bronchodilators - Short Acting *Stimulate beta 2 receptors in the lungs causing bronchodilation* **General Comment** Paradoxical bronchospasm can result from use of bronchodilators and may be life threatening Increased use of albuterol can signify deteriorating asthma. Give special consideration to anti-inflammatory treatment (corticosteroids)	**albuterol** (may be inhaled or nebulized)	**Adult and ≥ 12 years:** *Usual*: 2 inh every 4-6 hr prn bronchospasm *Alternative*: 1 puff every 4-6 hours **Children < 4 years:** not recommended **≥ 4 years:** 2 inh every 4-6 hours; 1 inh every 4 hours may suffice **Prevention of exercise induced asthma:** ≥ 4 years: 2 inh every 15-30 minutes before exercise *Each inhalation: albuterol 90 mcg*	• Pregnancy Category C • Can increase heart rate, blood pressure, and cause QT prolongation and ST segment depression • Cautious use in patients with cardiac arrhythmias, convulsive disorders, hyperthyroidism • Use extreme caution in patients on MAO inhibitors, beta blockers • May cause hypokalemia especially if in conjunction with potassium wasting medications. Consider monitoring potassium levels • Possible decreases in digoxin levels • Shake well before each spray
	Ventolin HFA	*17 g canister contains 200 inhalations*	
	albuterol	**Adult and ≥ 12 years:** *Usual*: 2 inh every 4-6 hours **Children ≥ 4 years:** 2 inh every 4-6 hours; one puff every 4 hours may be sufficient for some patients *Each inhalation: albuterol 90 mcg*	
	ProAir HFA	*8.5 g canister/200 inhalations*	
Bronchodilators - Long-acting *Stimulate beta 2 receptors in the lungs* **General comments** Paradoxical bronchospasm can result from use of bronchodilators and may be life threatening	**salmeterol**	**Adult**: 1 inh every 12 hr	• **ONLY FOR USE IN CONJUNCTION WITH A LONG-TERM ASTHMA CONTROL MEDICATION LIKE AN INHALED STEROID** • Pregnancy Category C • Do not use long-acting agents to treat acute symptoms. These agents take 15-20 min to produce bronchodilation • Tolerance develops with prolonged use

continued

Pulmonary Disorders

ASTHMA PHARMACOLOGIC MANAGEMENT

Inhaled steroids are used for the maintenance of asthma in patients with persistent asthma. Long-acting beta agonists (LABA) may increase the risk of asthma-related death and should NEVER be used alone in the management of asthma. LABAs should only be used with a concurrent long-acting steroid.

Class	Drug Generic name (Trade name®)	Dosage How supplied	Comments
Long acting bronchodilators increase the risk of asthma-related death. Do not use in patients with asthma unless accompanied by a long-term asthma control medication like an inhaled steroid	Serevent Diskus	*Each inhalation:30 mcg salmeterol* *60 inhalations*	• Significant drug interactions with ketoconazole and erythromycin, clarithromycin • Can increase heart rate, blood pressure, and cause QT prolongation and ST segment depression • Cautious use in patients with cardiac arrhythmias, convulsive disorders, hyperthyroidism • Use extreme caution in patients on MAO inhibitors, beta blockers • May cause hypokalemia especially if in conjunction with potassium wasting medications. Consider monitoring potassium levels • **DO NOT INGEST FORADIL CAPSULES!!!! Capsules should be used only with the AEROLIZER inhaler!**
	formoterol	**Adult and ≥ 5 years:** 1 inh every 12 hr *Max*: 1 inh twice daily ***Prevention of exercise induced asthma:*** 1 inh at least 15 minutes before exercise *Max*: 1 inh in 12 hours	
	Foradil Aerolizer	*12 mcg formoterol/ inhalation* *Box of 12, 60 (strips of 6)*	
Xanthines *Cause bronchodilation by relaxing smooth muscle of the bronchi and pulmonary blood vessels.* **General comments** Used as an alternative in asthma treatment; not first line Toxicity is a general concern with theophylline. Activated charcoal used to manage acute and chronic toxicity	**theophylline**	**Adult**: *Initial*: 300-400 mg daily for 3 days; if tolerated, increase dose to 400-600 mg daily; after 3 more days if tolerated and needed, increase dose to blood level *Max:* 400 mg daily for patients with impaired clearance age > 60 years **12-15 years:** 16 mg/kg *Max*: 400 mg/day	• Pregnancy Category C • The xanthenes are central respiratory stimulants and reduce fatigability in COPDers • Must monitor levels (10-20 mcg/mL is desirable). Common symptom of toxicity is repetitive vomiting • Elevated levels predispose patient to ventricular arrhythmias, seizures. Use is ill advised in patients with active peptic ulcer disease, seizure disorders, cardiac arrhythmias • Monitor for tremors, anxiety, and jitteriness • Many food drug interactions involving CYP 450 system • No dosage adjustment for renal impairment; need adjustment for hepatic insufficiency, heart failure • Smoking increases clearance of theophylline
	Theo-24	*Tabs: 100 mg, 200 mg,* *Ext. Rel. Caps: 300 mg, 400 mg*	

continued

ASTHMA PHARMACOLOGIC MANAGEMENT

Inhaled steroids are used for the maintenance of asthma in patients with persistent asthma. Long-acting beta agonists (LABA) may increase the risk of asthma-related death and should NEVER be used alone in the management of asthma. LABAs should only be used with a concurrent long-acting steroid.

Class	Drug Generic name (Trade name®)	Dosage How supplied	Comments
			• High fat meal increases absorption of theophylline • Do not crush or chew extended release tablets • Aminophylline is converted to theophylline
Anticholinergic - Short-acting *Blocks action of acetylcholine and thus causes mild bronchodilation and prevents bronchoconstriction* **General comments** No used first line in asthma Monitor for signs of worsening narrow angle glaucoma, worsening GI/GU obstruction	**ipratropium** Atrovent HFA	**Adult**: 2 inh four times daily *Max*: 12 inhalations/24 hours Inh Solution for nebulizer **Adult**: 500 mcg 3-4 times/day *17 mcg/inh* *12.9 g/200 inhalations* *Soln: 2.5 mL/vial (25)*	• Pregnancy Category B • Not indicated for relief of acute bronchospasm • Works well in conjunction with a bronchodilator • Atrovent HFA canister does not require shaking, but it does need to be primed
Inhaled Corticosteroids *Glucocorticoids decrease activity of inflammatory cells and mediators* **General comments** Steroid activity is local (in the lungs) and is associated with minimal systemic absorption	**fluticasone**	**Adult**: ***Previously on bronchodilators:*** *Initial*: 88 mcg twice daily *Max*: 440 mg twice daily ***Previously on inhaled steroids:*** *Initial*: 88-220 twice daily *Max*: 440 mcg twice daily ***Previously on oral steroids:*** *Initial*: 440 mcg twice daily *Max*: 880 mcg twice daily	• Pregnancy Category C • Slowly wean patients who are on oral steroids to inhaled steroids • Abrupt withdrawal can cause symptoms of adrenal insufficiency (fatigue, weakness, and hypotension) • Monitor for symptoms of fungal infection in the mouth and pharynx

continued

ASTHMA PHARMACOLOGIC MANAGEMENT

Inhaled steroids are used for the maintenance of asthma in patients with persistent asthma. Long-acting beta agonists (LABA) may increase the risk of asthma-related death and should NEVER be used alone in the management of asthma. LABAs should only be used with a concurrent long-acting steroid.

Class	Drug Generic name (Trade name®)	Dosage How supplied	Comments
Decreases in bone density can occur with steroids; monitor. May cause immunosuppression; possible increased risk of pneumonia, worsening of existing infections. Cautious use with concurrent use of 3A4 inhibitors Monitor for increased intraocular pressure, glaucoma and/or cataracts Rinse mouth well after use to prevent thrush	Flovent HFA	*44 mcg/inh (10.6 g)* *110 mcg/inh (12 g)* *220 mch/inh (12 g)*	
	budesonide	**Adult:** *Initial*: 360 mcg twice daily *Alternative*: Some patients may respond to 180 mcg twice daily *Max*: 720 mcg twice daily	
	Pulmicort Flexhaler	*Available: 180 mcg/dose, 120 doses*	
	mometasone	**Previously on bronchodilators alone or inhaled steroids** *Initial*: 220 mcg once in the PM *Max*: 440 mcg daily either as single dose or divided **Previously on oral corticosteroids (wean gradually)** *Initial*: 440 mcg twice daily *Max*: 880 mcg daily	
	Asmanex Twisthaler	*Inh - 20 g; 240 inhalations*	
Combination Inhaled corticosteroid/ Long Acting bronchodilator *Glucocorticoids decrease activity of inflammatory cells and mediators* *Steroid activity is local (in the lungs) and is associated with minimal systemic absorption*	**fluticasone/salmeterol**	**Adult and ≥ 12 years:** **Not previously on inhaled steroid:** 1 inh 100/50 or 250/50 daily **Already on inhaled steroid**: see literature **If insufficient response after 2 weeks:** use next higher strength *Max*: 1 inh of 500/50 twice daily 4-11 years: 1 inh of 100/50 twice daily	• Pregnancy Category C • Monitor for symptoms of fungal infection in the mouth and pharynx • NOT indicated for the relief of acute bronchospasm • Increased risk of pneumonia in patients • Risks associated wtih inhaled steroids and long acting bronchodilators are identical in these combinations products as in individual products

continued

Pulmonary Disorders

ASTHMA PHARMACOLOGIC MANAGEMENT

Inhaled steroids are used for the maintenance of asthma in patients with persistent asthma. Long-acting beta agonists (LABA) may increase the risk of asthma-related death and should NEVER be used alone in the management of asthma. LABAs should only be used with a concurrent long-acting steroid.

Class	Drug Generic name (Trade name®)	Dosage How supplied	Comments
General Comments: **Paradoxical bronchospasm can occur with combo medications** Close monitoring for glaucoma and cataracts is warranted Possible metabolic effects: hypokalemia, hyperglycemia Rinse mouth well after use to avoid thrush	Advair Diskus	*100/50, 250/50, 500/50* *Diskus (60 blisters)*	• Base initial dose on asthma severity
	budesonide/formoterol Symbicort	**Adult and ≥ 12 years:** 2 inh of 80/4.5 or 160/4.5 twice daily (AM and PM) If inadequate response after 1-2 weeks of 80/4.5, increase to 2 inh of 160/4.5; *Max*: 2 inh of 160/4.5 *Available: 80/4/5, 160/4.5* *60, 120 inhalations*	• Pregnancy Category C • Monitor for symptoms of fungal infection in the mouth and pharynx • NOT indicated for the relief of acute bronchospasm • Increased risk of pneumonia in patients • Risks associated wtih inhaled steroids and long acting bronchodilators are identical in these combinations products as in individual products
Leukotriene antagonists *Block the action of leukotrienes which are released from mast cells and eosinophils and are associated with airway edema, increased inflammatory activity and smooth muscle contraction* These agents are NOT substitutes for bronchodilators or inhaled steroids Take daily Monitor for drug interactions with zafirlukast	**montelukast** Singulair	**Adult and > 15 years:** 10 mg 6-14 years: 5 mg chewtab daily; 2-5 years: one 4 mg chewtab daily; 12-23 months: one 4 mg granule packet daily **For prevention of exercise induced asthma: take at least 2 hours before exercise** *Tabs: 10 mg* *Chewtabs: 4 mg, 5 mg* *Oral granules: 4 mg*	• Pregnancy Category B • Cautious use in hepatic dysfunction • Not for use as lone product in severe asthma • Chew tab contains phenylalaine

PREGNANCY/LACTATION CONSIDERATIONS

- Stress importance of prevention
- Poor control can result in low birth weight infants, premature labor/delivery, increased risk of fetal mortality
- Aggressive treatment of symptoms with steroids, bronchodilators, and theophylline if needed

CONSULTATION/REFERRAL

- Allergist/pulmonologist for patients with severe persistent asthma

FOLLOW-UP

- As needed to educate patient, parent, caregiver about disease and management
- Every 3-6 months for stable disease

EXPECTED COURSE

- Excellent with proper use of medications and patient education
- Small percentage of patients have poor control even with proper medication use
- Risk of mortality increased by: nocturnal symptoms, history of intubation for asthma, history of hospitalization/ICU admission for asthma, > 3 emergency department visits annually for asthma, and oral steroid dependence

POSSIBLE COMPLICATIONS

- Respiratory failure/death from unrelieved bronchospasms
- Steroid dependence

PNEUMONIA

DESCRIPTION

Infection of the lung which may include the parenchyma, alveolar spaces, and/or interstitial tissue. It can be confined to a lobe (*lobar pneumonia*), a segment of a lobe (*segmental pneumonia*), the interstitial tissue (*interstitial pneumonia*), or alveolar/bronchi (*bronchopneumonia*). Pneumonia is commonly classified as community acquired (CAP) or nosocomial.

Community acquired pneumonia is an acute infection in the lung of a patient who acquired the infection "in the community".

ETIOLOGY

Adults with Community Acquired Pneumonia:

- Viruses
- Bacteria are most common cause
  - ◊ *Mycoplasma pneumoniae* (most common cause)
  - ◊ *Streptococcus pneumoniae* (second most common cause)
  - ◊ *Haemophilus influenzae* (common in smokers)
  - ◊ *Chlamydia pneumoniae*
  - ◊ *Moraxella catarrhalis*
  - ◊ *Legionella pneumophila*
  - ◊ *Klebsiella pneumoniae*
  - ◊ Anaerobic bacteria (common with aspiration)

Young adults and older children with Community Acquired Pneumonia:

- *Mycoplasma pneumoniae* (most common cause)
- Viruses
- *Chlamydia pneumoniae* (NOT the same agent that causes chlamydial pneumonia in newborns at 3-8 weeks)

Children and infants with Community Acquired Pneumonia:

- Viral agents are most common cause
- Respiratory syncytial virus
- Adenovirus
- Parainfluenza
- Influenza A and B
- Bacteria
  - ◊ *Streptococcus pneumoniae*
  - ◊ *Haemophilus influenzae*

Immunocompromised individuals with Community Acquired Pneumonia:

- *Pneumocystis carinii*

The most common etiologic agent of pneumonia worldwide is *Streptococcus pneumoniae*.

INCIDENCE

- 2-3 million people in the U.S. get pneumonia annually
- 6th leading cause of death
- Most common cause of death from infectious disease

RISK FACTORS

- Age extremes (very young, very old)
- Other respiratory viral infections
- Cigarette smoking
- Chronic diseases (e.g., diabetes, renal disease, COPD, CAD, CHF)
- Alcoholism
- Institutionalization
- Poor cough effort
- GERD

The highest rates of pneumonia are at age extremes and during the winter months.

ASSESSMENT FINDINGS

- Cough (often productive)
- Fever
- Malaise/fatigue
- Sudden chills
- Chest pain (pleuritic)
- Sputum production
- Increased respirations and pulse
- Diminished breath sounds
- Consolidation on percussion
- Egophony (e to a changes)
- Bronchophony: voice sounds are louder and clearer than normal
- Whispered pectoriloquy: whispered sounds are louder and clearer than normal
- Tactile fremitus

SPECIFIC ASSESSMENT FINDINGS/ PATIENT PROFILES/ SYMPTOMATOLOGY

Pneumococcal pneumonia:
- Preceded by a URI
- Chills, fever
- Chest pain
- Dry cough becoming productive of rusty-colored sputum
- Myalgias
- GI symptoms

Mycoplasma pneumonia *(primary atypical pneumonia):*
- Typically in < 35 year old age group
- Malaise
- Sore throat
- Dry cough
- Paroxysmal coughing
- Disease generally mild and resolution is spontaneous (though may take 6 weeks with treatment)
- Maculopapular rash (10-20% of the time)

Viral pneumonia:
- Headache
- Fever
- Myalgia
- Cough productive of mucopurulent sputum
- Overall milder symptoms than bacterial pneumonias

Klebsiella pneumoniae pneumonia:
- Upper lobe involvement
- Currant jelly sputum
- Tissue necrosis
- Mortality rate is 25-50%

Haemophilus influenzae pneumonia:
- Younger age group if not vaccinated
- Coryza as prodrome
- Underlying lung disease present in adults or other pre-existing disease

Legionella pneumophila pneumonia:
- Common in middle-aged males
- Smokers
- Alcohol abusers
- Immunosuppressed patients
- Prodrome resembles influenza
- Fever
- Headache
- Neurological manifestations
- Nonproductive cough becomes productive of mucoid sputum
- Relative bradycardia

Chlamydial pneumonia:
- Cough
- Fever
- Sputum production
- Not seriously ill

DIFFERENTIAL DIAGNOSIS

- Acute bronchitis
- Bronchiolitis

- Asthma
- Croup
- Congestive heart failure
- Bronchogenic carcinoma
- Tuberculosis

DIAGNOSTIC STUDIES

- PA and lateral chest x-ray (infiltrates present)
- CBC with differential
- Gram stain and sputum specimen (no test for an etiologic agent recommended if outpatient)

Clinical evaluation of a patient with suspected pneumonia always begins with clinical examination and chest x-ray. The presence of an infiltrate is considered the gold standard for diagnosis of pneumonia.

PREVENTION

- Influenza and pneumococcal pneumonia immunizations
- Smoking cessation
- High-risk individuals should avoid crowds

NONPHARMACOLOGIC MANAGEMENT

- Hydration with increased fluids
- Analgesia for pain
- Reduced activity during acute phase
- Patient education regarding disease, treatment, emergency actions

PHARMACOLOGIC MANAGEMENT

- Treatment based on immunocompetent patients
- Empiric antibiotic treatment based on patient age, comorbidity, immunization status, risk factors etc.

Outpatient, previously healthy, no recent antibiotic (AB)	Macrolide (azithromycin or clarithromycin) **OR** doxycycline
Outpatient, previously healthy, recent (AB)	Respiratory fluoroquinolone (FQ); **OR** advanced macrolide (azithromycin or clarithromycin) plus high dose amoxicillin; **OR** advanced macrolide plus high dose amoxicillin/ clavulanate
Outpatient, co-morbidities (COPD, diabetes, renal or CHF, or malignancy), no recent AB	Advanced macrolide **OR** respiratory FQ
Outpatient, co-morbidities, recent (AB)	Respiratory FQ **OR** advanced macrolide plus a beta-lactam (high dose amoxicillin, high dose amoxicillin/clavulanate, cefpodoxime, cefprozil or cefuroxime)

Source: From Infectious Disease Society of America/American Thoracic Society consensus guidelines for management of community acquired pneumonia, 2007

PNEUMONIA PHARMACOLOGIC MANAGEMENT

Class	Drug Generic name (Trade name®)	Dosage How supplied	Comments
Macrolides *Antibiotic binds to the 50S subunit of susceptible organisms and prevents protein synthesis* **General comments** Macrolides are particularly effective against atypical organisms (*Chlamydia pneumoniae, Mycoplasma pneumoniae, Legionella* species)	**azithromycin** Zithromax	**Adult** CAP: 500 mg day one, then 250 mg daily for 4 days **Children > 6 months**: 10 mg/kg on day one then 5 mg/kg daily for 4 days *Max*: 500 mg daily day 1; 250 mg day 2-5 *Tabs: 250 mg, 500 mg,* *Susp: 100 m/5 mL;* *200 mg/mL*	• Pregnancy Category B • Avoid concomitant use of aluminum or magnesium containing antacids • Cautious use if renal or hepatic impairment • Hypersensitivity reactions may recur after initial successful symptomatic treatment
Erythromycin is not active against *H. influenza* infections and has high rates of *Streptococcus pneumoniae* resistance. Thus, it is not recommended for most community acquired pneumonia	**clarithromycin** Biaxin XL Biaxin	Biaxin Ext Rel: **Adult**: 1 g daily for 7 days Biaxin: **Adult**: 500 mg twice a day for 7-14 days **Children**: 7.5 mg/kg every 12 hr for 10 days *Max*: 500 mg twice daily *Biaxin XL®: 500 mg ext release* *Biaxin: 250 mg, 500 mg* *Susp: 125 mg/5 mL,* *250 mg/5 mL*	• Pregnancy Category C • Monitor for drug interactions especially with clarithromycin • Do not refrigerate suspension • Take XL form with food • Monitor serum concentration of patients taking theophyllline • Take Biaxin XL with food • Inhibits CYP 3A4 enzymes: drug interactions occur with calcium channel blockers, carbamazepine, omeprazole, ranitidine, ritonavir, digoxin, terfenadine, "statins", many others • Avoid in patients with myasthenia gravis • Can produce an abnormal taste while taking medication
Tetracyclines *inhibit protein synthesis* **General comments** Tetracyclines are active against many species of Mycoplas*ma pneumoniae, Haemophilus influenzae, Klebsiella* (respiratory species) and *Streptococcus pneumoniae*	**doxycycline**	**Adult**: 100 mg twice daily for 7-10 days **Children > 8 years:** < 100 lbs: 2 mg/lb into 2 divided doses on the first day; then 1 mg/lb of body weight given as a single dose or 2 divided doses. > 100 lbs.: Use adult dosage	• Pregnancy Category D • Avoid excessive sunlight, discontinue if photosensitivity occurs. Use sunblock • Drink extra fluids to reduce risk of esophageal irritation • Avoid in pregnant and lactating women and children < 8 years old due to discoloration of teeth • Concurrent use may render oral contraceptives less effective

continued

PNEUMONIA PHARMACOLOGIC MANAGEMENT

Class	Drug Generic name (Trade name®)	Dosage How supplied	Comments
Do not use in children < 8 years or during the last half of pregnancy due to permanent discoloration of teeth Careful dosing: dosage of doxycycline differs from tetracyclines Absorption of tetracyclines is markedly reduced with calcium containing foods. It is not markedly influenced by doxycycline	Doryx Vibramycin	*Delayed release tabs: 75 mg, 100 mg* *Tabs: 100 mg* *Susp: 25 mg/5 mL* *Syrup: 50 mg/5 mL*	• Patients on anticoagulant therapy may require downward adjustment of anticoagulant dosage
Extended Spectrum Penicillin *Inhibits cell wall synthesis of Gram positive bacteria (Staph, Strep) and are most effective against organisms with rapidly dividing cell walls* **General comments**: Addition of clavulanic acid (as potassium) extends antimicrobial spectrum (covers many Gram negative organisms too) and protects penicillin molecule if the organism produces beta lactamase Clavulanic acid associated with diarrhea Monitor for penicillin hypersensitivity	**amoxicillin and potassium clavulanate** Augmentin Augmentin XR	**Adults**: *Usual*: Two 1000 mg tablets every 12 hours for 10 days *Alternate*: One 875 mg tablet every 12 hours for 10 days **Children**: *Usual*: 90 mg/kg/day in two divided doses every 12 hours for 10 days (Must use 600 mg/5 mL susp for this regimen) *Alternate*: 45 mg/kg/d in 2 divided doses every 12 hours for 10 days (Must use 200 mg/5 mL susp or 400 mg/5 mL susp for this regimen) *Alternate*: 40 mg/kg/day in three divided doses given every 8 hours for 10 days (Must use 125 mg/5 mL susp or 250 mg/5 mL susp for this regimen) *Tabs: 250 mg, 500 mg, 875 mg, 1000 mg* *Chew tabs: 125 mg, 200 mg, 250 mg, 400 mg* *Susp: ES 600 (amoxicillin component 600 mg/5 mL)*	• Pregnancy Category B • **DO NOT USE IN PATIENTS WHO HAD HIVES OR ANAPHYLAXIS TO PENICILLIN** • Two 500 mg amoxicillin/ clavulanic acid tablets are NOT equivalent to one 1000 mg amoxicillin/clavulanic acid tablet • Do not substitute Augmentin® 200mg/5mL and 400 mg/5mL suspensions for Augmentin® ES-600. These are NOT interchangeable • Children: Base dose on amoxicillin component • Children > 40 kg should be dosed as an adult • Alternate dose for severe sinusitis based on severity of infection or likelihood of drug resistant *Streptococcus pneumoniae* • Take with meals to minimize gastrointestinal side effects • Contraindicated in severe renal impairment (Cr Cl < 30 mL/min), dialysis, or history of Augmentin® associated cholestatic jaundice/hepatic dysfunction • Chewtabs contain phenylalanine

continued

PNEUMONIA PHARMACOLOGIC MANAGEMENT

Class	Drug Generic name (Trade name®)	Dosage How supplied	Comments
Quinolones *inhibit the action of DNA gyrase which is essential for the organism to be able to replicate itself* **General comments**: Broad spectrum antimicrobial agents Monitor for QT prolongation and photosensitivity Avoid in ages < 18 years, pregnant women due to potential impairment in bone and cartilage formation Monitor for hypoglycemic reactions • Absorption significantly decreased by dairy products, multivitamins, and calcium containing products (avoid by at least 2 hours)	**levofloxacin** Levaquin	**Adults > 18 years:** *Usual*: 500 mg once daily for 10-14 days *Alternative*: 750 mg daily for 5 days **Children**: not recommended *Tabs: 250 mg, 500 mg, 750 mg* *Oral Soln: 25 mg/mL*	• Pregnancy Category C • Reduce dose for impaired renal function • Possible increased risk of tendinitis or tendon rupture • Causes photosensitivity. Avoid excessive sun or UV light exposure • Maintain adequate hydration
	moxifloxacin Avelox	**Adults**: *Usual*: One tablet once daily for 7-14 days **Children**: not indicated *Tabs: 400 mg*	• Pregnancy Category C • Reduce dose for impaired renal function • Possible increased risk of tendinitis or tendon rupture • Causes photosensitivity. Avoid excessive sun or UV light exposure • Maintain adequate hydration
	gemifloxacin Factive	**Adults**: *Usual*: one tablet once daily for 5-7 days **Children**: not indicated *Tabs: 320 mg*	• Pregnancy Category C • Reduce dose for impaired renal function • Possible increased risk of tendinitis or tendon rupture • Causes photosensitivity. Avoid excessive sun or UV light exposure • Maintain adequate hydration

PREGNANCY/LACTATION CONSIDERATIONS

- Doxycycline should not be used (Pregnancy Category D)
- Doxycycline is excreted in breast milk
- Influenza immunization may be used in pregnancy
- Quinolones contraindicated in pregnant patients

CONSULTATION/REFERRAL

- Referral for patients who appear toxic, have severe shortness of breath, have worsening symptoms despite treatment

FOLLOW-UP

- Depends on severity of illness and patient's general state of health
- Within 24-72 hours as condition warrants
- Consider follow-up chest x-ray 4-6 weeks after treatment completed in patients over 40 years and smokers (bronchogenic carcinoma often presents as pneumonia)

EXPECTED COURSE

- Excellent prognosis with proper treatment
- Improvement should take place 48-72 hours after treatment initiation

- Poor prognosis for patients at age extremes, presence of comorbidities, immunocompromised states, poorly controlled diabetics

POSSIBLE COMPLICATIONS

- Empyema
- Respiratory failure
- Adult respiratory distress syndrome
- Death

TUBERCULOSIS (TB)

(Consumption)

DESCRIPTION

Chronic, recurrent infection which primarily affects the lungs (effected organ in 85% of cases) but which can affect any organ in the human body; 90-95% of primary infections go unrecognized. There are 3 stages:

- Primary or initial infection
- Latent or dormant infection
- Recrudescent

In most patients with a normal functioning immune system, the infection is contained by the host's immune system. The infection is latent.

ETIOLOGY

- *Mycobacterium tuberculosis*
- *Mycobacterium bovis*
- *Mycobacterium africanum*

INCIDENCE

- U.S. rates vary according to risk factors (age, race, gender, socioeconomic status)
- Rates range from 10-200/100,000 in the U.S. (higher rates among those with risk factors)
- Incidence decreasing in U.S.

RISK FACTORS

- Homelessness
- Substance abuse
- Poor nutritional status
- Systemic disease
- Low socioeconomic status
- Close contact with an infected individual
- Asian, African, Latin American immigrants (within 5 years)
- Institutionalization (e.g., prisons, nursing homes, mental hospitals)
- Health care workers (particularly those working with HIV-positive populations)
- Immunocompromised (particularly HIV-positive patients, steroid use, cancer patients)
- Chronic disease (HIV, DM, renal failure)

Rates of TB infection have declined since 1992.

ASSESSMENT FINDINGS

- Cough
- Night sweats
- Fever
- Hemoptysis
- Weight loss

The most common symptoms of TB infection are fever and night sweats, but cough, weight loss, and fatigue are very common.

DIFFERENTIAL DIAGNOSIS

- Pneumonia
- Bronchitis
- Pulmonary fungal infections
- Tumor

DIAGNOSTIC STUDIES

Mantoux skin test is a screening tool for TB. It is not a diagnostic test. A positive skin test must be followed up with a diagnostic test, sputum culture.

- Mantoux skin testing using purified protein derivative (PPD) is the primary screening tool: induration as described below
- False positive skin test if BCG vaccine used
- False negative skin test: steroid use, HIV infection, new-onset TB infection, anergy, age < 6 months
- Chest x-ray: may show infiltrates, cavitary lesions and/or hilar adenopathy
- Sputum culture/sensitivity (obtain at least 3 early morning specimens): positive for organism (takes 2-6 weeks for results)
- Acid-fast bacillus (AFB) stain: red rods

TB SKIN TESTS CONSIDERED POSITIVE IF at 48-72 hours:
Induration ≥ 5 mm and:
◊ Recent close contact with person with active TB ◊ HIV patient or someone immunocompromised ◊ Clinical evidence of disease
Induration ≥ 10 mm and:
◊ Injecting drug user ◊ Contact with high-risk groups (e.g., health care workers) ◊ Immigrants from countries where TB is prevalent ◊ Children < 4 years, children, and adolescents exposed to adults at high risk ◊ Members of high-risk populations
Induration ≥ 15 mm and:
◊ Anyone who is not a member of the above populations

Source: From U.S. Department of Health and Human Services, Core curriculum on tuberculosis, 2000

Anyone with a positive PPD is considered infected until proven otherwise. Anyone with a positive PPD AND signs and symptoms is defined as having active disease.

PREVENTION

- Avoid contact with known infected persons
- Careful tracking of known patients to insure proper treatment
- PPD screening annually for persons with risk factors
- Complete course of therapy once initiated

Tuberculosis is a reportable disease and should be reported to state agency charged with tracking incidence.

NONPHARMACOLOGIC MANAGEMENT

- Notification of local health department
- Identification of contacts
- Respiratory precautions as long as patient is contagious
- Activity as tolerated for patient
- Patient education regarding disease, treatment, importance of completion of drug regimen, treatment of contacts, etc

TUBERCULOSIS PHARMACOLOGIC MANAGEMENT

Class	Drug Generic name (Trade name®)	Dosage How supplied	Comments
Isonicotinic acid *for active disease, multi drug regimens are recommended* **General comments** HIV positive patients: treat with minimum of 3 drugs For severe disease: use of 4 drugs for first 2-3 months is indicated Patients are typically referred to tuberculosis specialty care and are not managed in primary care	**isoniazid**	**Adult:** prophylactic: 300 mg daily *Active infection*: 5 mg/kg/day *Max*: 300 mg daily **Children:** prophylactic: 10 mg/kg/day *Active infection:* 10-20 mg/kg/day *Max:* 300 mg daily	• Do not interrupt therapy • Monitor hepatic and ocular function • Contraindicated in previous isoniazid associated hepatic injury, acute hepatitis • Alcohol consumption increases risk of hepatitis. Pyridoxine given concurrently reduces risk of neuropathy
	All generic isoniazid	*Tabs: 100, 300 mg scored* *Susp: 50 mg/5 mL*	
	rifampin	**Adult**: 600 mg daily, 1 hour prior or 2 hr after meals **Children**: 10-20 mg/kg/day *Max*: 600 mg/day	• Use with other antituberculars • Monitor hepatic function • May stain body secretions and contact lenses • Watch for drug interactions!
	Rifadin	*Tabs: 150 mg, 300 mg*	
	pyrazinamide	**Adult & Children**: 15-30 mg/kg/day *Max*: 2 g daily *Alternative*: 50-70 mg/kg twice weekly, based on lean weight	• Use with other antituberculars • Do not use in gout or severe hepatic disease • Monitor hepatic and serum uric acid levels before, during, and after therapy
	PZA	*Tabs: 500 mg scored*	
	streptomycin	**Adult**: 15-30 mg/kg/day IM 5-7 times/week *Max*: 1 g/dose *Alternative*: 25-30 mg/kg IM 2-3 times/week *Max*: 1.5 g/dose **Elderly:** 750 mg/dose **After 2-4 months or culture conversion:** 15-30 mg/kg IM 2-3 times weekly **Children 2-12 years**: 20-40 mg/kg/day *Max*: 1 g *Alternative*: 20-40 mg/kg 2 times/week *Max*: 1.5 g/dose	• Aminoglycoside used to treat tuberculosis • Monitor for ototoxicity and neurotoxicity. Monitor renal function since toxicity increased if present • Avoid potent diuretics • Treatment duration 1 year • Decrease dose for age > 60 years, renal or hepatic impairment
	Various generics	*1 g/vial*	

continued

TUBERCULOSIS PHARMACOLOGIC MANAGEMENT

Class	Drug Generic name (Trade name®)	Dosage How supplied	Comments
	ethambutal	**Adults and > 13 yr:** 15 mg/kg/day *Retreatment*: 25 mg/kg/day; after 60 days decrease to 15 mg/kg per day	• Use with other antituberculars • Test visual acuity prior to therapy and periodically • Check vision monthly if retreatment • Decrease dose for renal patients • Cautious use in patients with gout and hepatic impairment
	Myambutal	*Tabs: 100 mg, 400 mg (scored)*	

Multi-drug regimens change frequently as resistance develops.

IMPORTANT NOTES ABOUT MEDICATIONS

- Pyridoxine for patients taking isoniazid to prevent peripheral neuritis, especially in children, adolescents, and pregnant women
- Alternative drug for regimen is ethambutol
  - ◊ Optic neuritis possible (only use in patients who can cooperate for vision and color checks)
- Streptomycin should NOT be prescribed longer than 12 weeks due to possible ototoxicity
- Rifampin colors tears, urine, perspiration orange, can stain contact lenses; may decrease effectiveness of oral contraceptives

PREGNANCY/LACTATION CONSIDERATIONS

- Drugs considered safe to use during pregnancy are: isoniazid, ethambutol (add pyridoxine) and rifampin
- Avoid streptomycin (ototoxicity, nephrotoxicity)
- Breast-feeding OK during TB treatment

CONSULTATION/REFERRAL

- Refer patients to local health department for treatment. Close contacts should be screened as well

FOLLOW-UP

- Liver function studies for patients taking INH, PZA, RIF and in HIV positive patients, pregnant patients or anyone with liver disease
- Monthly sputum cultures until 2 consecutive negative cultures
- If cultures positive after 2 months of treatment, consider poor compliance and re-assess sensitivity
- Chest x-ray every 2-3 months during treatment
- Chest x-ray for any changes in symptomatology

EXPECTED COURSE

- Good prognosis if drug treatment regimen followed
- Poor prognosis for severely infected patients or HIV patients with multi drug resistant organisms

POSSIBLE COMPLICATIONS

- Cavitary lesions
- Drug resistance
- Spread to other body organs

PERTUSSIS
(Whooping Cough)

DESCRIPTION

An acute, highly communicable respiratory disease that has 3 stages:

- Catarrhal stage: upper respiratory symptoms and mild cough (1-2 weeks)
- Paroxysmal stage: cough (2-4 weeks)
- Convalescent stage: cough is still present (1-2 weeks)

Whooping cough is a synonym for pertussis.

ETIOLOGY

- *Bordetella* pertussis spread by respiratory droplets, direct or indirect contact with secretions (highly communicable)

INCIDENCE

- Common in infants unimmunized or partially immunized
- 10-20% of adults who cough > 14 days have pertussis
- 2.7 cases per 100,000 in US
- 80% of cases occur in ages < 18 years
- Incidence among adolescents and adults has increased 60% since late 1990's
- Pertussis immunization may lose effectiveness as one ages

RISK FACTORS

- Incomplete immunizations, no immunizations
- Contact with an infected person

ASSESSMENT FINDINGS

- Depends on stage of disease
- Fever may or may not be present
- Rhinorrhea
- Characteristic paroxysmal, high-pitched "whooping" cough
- In adolescents and adults, hallmark symptom is long-standing cough

Adolescents and adults usually have partial immunity and do not present with the characteristic symptoms. However, adults exhibit a prolonged, persistent, paroxysmal cough > one month's duration.

DIFFERENTIAL DIAGNOSIS

- Upper respiratory infection
- Bronchitis
- Pneumonia
- Asthma
- Cystic fibrosis
- Foreign body aspiration
- Tuberculosis

DIAGNOSTIC STUDIES

- Nasopharyngeal culture to isolate organism
- PCR detection of *B. pertussis* DNA in nasopharyngeal secretions (not widely available)
- Recommendation by CDC for diagnosis is combination of nasopharyngeal culture and PCR within first two weeks of onset of cough
- Single serologic test if cough present > 4 weeks
- ELISA serology (not recognized by CDC for diagnosis)
- Chest x-ray: focal atelectasis
- CBC: > 20,000 WBC with lymphocytic predominance

Culture of nasopharyngeal secretions is the traditional gold standard for diagnosis of pertussis, but has a variable sensitivity (15-80%).

PREVENTION

- Immunizations for pertussis
- Avoid exposure to patients with known pertussis before immunization complete
- Erythromycin prophylaxis for exposed patients (cultures usually negative 5 days after prophylaxis, but continue for 14 days)

Tdap vaccine is intended for previously vaccinated adolescents and adults.
DTaP is used for primary vaccination of infants and children up to 6 years old.

NONPHARMACOLOGIC MANAGEMENT

- Respiratory isolation for 5 days after antibiotic initiated
- Identify household and other close contacts
- Patient education regarding disease, treatment, emergency actions, importance of immunizations

PHARMACOLOGIC MANAGEMENT

- Erythromycin for 14 days; azithromycin or clarithromycin (5-7 days)
- Erythromycin estolate preferred because of higher drug concentrations in respiratory tract
- Prophylactic antibiotics for close household contacts regardless of immunization status
- Antibiotics do not alter course of disease, only prevent transmission
- Anti-tussives are almost always ineffective for cough suppression

PERTUSSIS PHARMACOLOGIC MANAGEMENT

Class	Drug Generic name (Trade name®)	Dosage How supplied	Comments
Macrolides *binds to the 50S subunit of susceptible organisms and prevents protein synthesis* General comments Sulfonamides are second line if patient is allergic to macrolides or strain is macrolide resistant Macrolide may abort or eliminate pertussis in catarrhal stage but does not shorten paroxysmal stage	**erythromycin**	**Adult:** 1.6 g/day in 2-4 divided doses **Children:** 40-50 mg/kg/day in 4 divided doses for 14 days *Max:* 2 g/day	• Pregnancy Category B • Erythromycin often poorly tolerated because of GI symptoms • Monitor for drug interactions especially with erythromycin
	E-mycin	*Tabs: 400 mg* *Granules: 200 mg/5 mL*	
	azithromycin	**Adult:** 500 mg day one, then 250 mg daily for 4 days **Children > 6 mo:** 10 mg/kg on day one then 5 mg/kg daily for 4 days *Max*: do not exceed adult max	• Pregnancy Category B • Avoid concomitant use of aluminum or magnesium containing antacids • Cautious use if renal or hepatic impairment • Hypersensitivity reactions may recur after initial successful symptomatic treatment
	Zithromax	*Tabs: 250 mg, 500 mg* *Susp: 100 mg/5 mL, 200 mg/5 mL*	
	clarithromycin	**Adult**: 1 g in two divided doses for 7 days **Children**: 7.5 mg/kg every 12 hr for 7 days *Max*: do not exceed adult max	• Pregnancy Category C • Do not refrigerate suspension • Take XL form with food • Monitor serum concentration of patients taking theophyllline • Inhibits CYP 3A4 enzymes: drug interactions occur with calcium channel blockers, carbamazepine, omeprazole, ranitidine, ritonavir, digoxin, terfenadine, "statins", many others

continued

PERTUSSIS PHARMACOLOGIC MANAGEMENT

Class	Drug Generic name (Trade name®)	Dosage How supplied	Comments
	Biaxin Biaxin XL	*Biaxin: 250 mg, 500 mg* *Susp: 125 mg/5 mL, 250 mg/5 mL* *Biaxin XL: 500 mg ext release*	• Avoid in patients with myasthenia gravis • Can produce an abnormal taste while taking medication

CONSULTATION/REFERRAL

- Consider referral for infants <6 months of age because of severity of symptoms and increased morbidity and mortality
- Report to local health department

FOLLOW-UP

- Depends on severity of illness and age of patient

EXPECTED COURSE

- Catarrhal stage lasts 1-2 weeks
- Paroxysmal stage lasts 2-4 weeks
- Convalescent stage can last for several months accompanied by cough
- Prognosis worse in infants < 6 months
- Early treatment with antibiotics can shorten illness

POSSIBLE COMPLICATIONS

- Pneumonia with secondary bacterial infection (responsible for 90% of deaths due to pertussis)
- Encephalopathy
- Seizures may be due to high fever or hyperventilation

BRONCHIOLITIS

DESCRIPTION

Infection of the lower respiratory tract that leads to an impedance to airflow, often wheezing

ETIOLOGY

- Respiratory syncytial virus (RSV): most common cause
- Parainfluenza virus
- Adenovirus
- Influenza A virus
- *Mycoplasma pneumoniae* (more common in older children)
- Rhinovirus
- Respiratory irritants

INCIDENCE

- Common in infants and young children under age 2 years
- Many adult cases
- More common in winter and spring

RISK FACTORS

- Contact with infected person
- Daycare attendance
- In adults: exposure to respiratory irritants (cigarette smoke exposure, toxic inhalants)

ASSESSMENT FINDINGS

- Upper respiratory infection for 1-3 days which progresses to lower respiratory tract infection
- Fever
- Cough: may be hoarse before becoming very productive
- Inspiratory crackles; expiratory wheezes
- Tachypnea
- Thick, purulent nasal secretions
- Evidence of respiratory distress (i.e., use of accessory muscles, tachypnea, cyanosis)

Otitis media commonly accompanies bronchiolitis. 50-60% of children are found to have this within 10 days of diagnosis. Bacterial pathogens are found about half the time.

DIFFERENTIAL DIAGNOSIS

- Asthma
- Pneumonia
- Emphysema
- Gastroesophageal reflux disease (GERD)

DIAGNOSTIC STUDIES

- RSV swab; consider other studies as clinically warranted
- CBC
- Chest x-ray (atelectasis is common)
- Oxygenation assessment (ABGs, pulse oximetry)

PREVENTION

- Avoid direct contact with others known to be infected with RSV

NONPHARMACOLOGIC MANAGEMENT

- Maintain adequate hydration
- Patient education regarding disease, treatment, emergency actions

PHARMACOLOGIC MANAGEMENT

Goal is to keep patient well oxygenated and well hydrated.

- Oxygen for hypoxic patients
- Nebulized bronchodilators for wheezing
- Steroids for patients with reactive airway disease and adults (rarely alters course in infants)
- Antiviral agents ribavirin (Virazole®) for high-risk patients (inconsistent demonstration of clinical efficacy)

BRONCHIOLITIS PHARMACOLOGIC MANAGEMENT

Class	Drug Generic name (Trade name®)	Dosage How supplied	Comments
Bronchodilators - Short Acting *stimulates beta 2 receptors in the lungs causing bronchodilation*	**albuterol inhalation solution** Various generics	**Children 2-12 years:** 1.25 mg administered 3 or 4 times daily by nebulization *0.75 mg albuterol/3 mL, 1.25 mg/3 mL* *25 vials per carton*	• Can increase heart rate, blood pressure, and cause QT prolongation and ST segment depression • Cautious use in patients with cardiac arrhythmias, hypertension, convulsive disorders, diabetes, hyperthyroidism • Use extreme caution in patients on MAO inhibitors, beta blockers • May cause hypokalemia especially if in conjunction with potassium wasting medications. Consider monitoring potassium levels • Possible decreases in digoxin levels

PREGNANCY/LACTATION CONSIDERATIONS

- Ribavirin is Pregnancy Category C

CONSULTATION/REFERRAL

- Consider referral for infants who were premature, <3 months of age, or have underlying disease
- Refer to nearest emergency department for airway management and possible need for mechanical ventilation

FOLLOW-UP

- Depends on patient age, underlying disease, severity, but, daily telephone calls until clinical condition dictates improvement

EXPECTED COURSE

- Should begin to improve in 3-5 days
- Complete recovery 5-10 days

POSSIBLE COMPLICATIONS

- Respiratory failure requiring mechanical ventilation
- Increased incidence of asthma, reactive airway disease in children
- Apnea

CROUP
(Laryngotracheitis)

DESCRIPTION

An acute viral illness characterized by stridor, barking cough, and hoarseness. Infection of the nasopharynx, larynx, and trachea produces swelling and subglottic obstruction.

Laryngotracheobronchitis (LTB) is the term used to describe inflammation of the airway that extends in the bronchi. It is often interchanged with laryngotracheitis, croup, but can produce more severe symptoms.

ETIOLOGY

- Parainfluenza types 1 (most frequent causes)
- Adenovirus
- Influenza virus Type A
- *Mycoplasma pneumoniae*
- Respiratory syncytial virus

INCIDENCE

- Common; especially in fall and winter
- 80% occur in children < 5 years
- Most common age of occurrence is 6 months to 3 years

RISK FACTORS

- Age (6 months to 3 years)
- Exposure (spread by respiratory droplet)
- Infection with one of the causative agents

ASSESSMENT FINDINGS

- Prodrome of coryza, fever, barking cough
- Symptoms worse at night
- Usually low grade fever
- Rarely, hypoxia as characterized by lethargy, irritability, anxiety
- Respiratory distress: nasal flaring, drooling, abdominal breathing, use of accessory muscles
- Possible stridor (most common cause in children is croup)
- Supraglottic area with normal appearance

Do NOT attempt to visualize the pharynx if severe respiratory distress. This may precipitate laryngeal spasms.

DIFFERENTIAL DIAGNOSIS

- Epiglottitis
- Tracheitis
- Retropharyngeal abscess
- Foreign body aspiration
- Diphtheria
- Neck trauma
- Tumor

DIAGNOSTIC STUDIES

- Usually none
- AP radiograph of neck: "steeple" sign due to subglottic swelling is diagnostic
- Pulse oximetry

"Thumb sign" is the term used to describe swelling of the epiglottis seen on a lateral radiograph of the neck. This is visible in patients with epiglottitis.

NONPHARMACOLOGIC MANAGEMENT

- Cool mist humidifier
- Patient educations regarding disease, treatment, signs and symptoms of respiratory distress and appropriate actions (i.e., go to nearest emergency department)

CROUP PHARMACOLOGIC MANAGEMENT

Class	Drug Generic name (Trade name®)	Dosage How supplied	Comments
Corticosteroids (oral, nebulized) <u>General comments</u> Immediate nebulized epinephrine and dexamethasone are usually given Racemic epinephrine should be administered in a hospital or under very close medical supervision	**dexamethasone**	**Children**: *Initial*: 0.15-.6 mg/kg/day in single or divided doses for 5 days	• Possible drug induced adrenocortical insufficiency from too rapid withdrawal • May mask signs/symptoms of infection • May cause increases in blood sugar. Cautious use in diabetics
	Various generics	*Soln: 0.5 mg/5 mL*	
	budesonide	**Children 12 mo-8 yr**: 0.25-0.5 mg/day in 1 or 2 divided doses	• Rinse mouth well after inhalation to prevent thrush • Administer via jet nebulizer connected to an air compressor and face mask. Do not use ultrasonic nebulizers
	Pulmicort Respules	*Susp: 0.25 mg/ 2 mL; 0.5 mg/2 mL, 1 mg/2 mL*	

CONSULTATION/REFERRAL

- Refer to nearest emergency department for airway distress or if pulse oximetry < 92%

FOLLOW-UP

- Depends on patient's condition and age but 24-48 hours usually

EXPECTED COURSE

- General improvement seen by day 2-3 with resolution by day 5-7
- Good prognosis, usually no need for hospitalization

POSSIBLE COMPLICATIONS

- Need for intubation due to severe respiratory distress (occurs < 1% of time)
- Bacterial superinfection

FOREIGN BODY ASPIRATION

DESCRIPTION

The inhalation or swallowing of a foreign object which becomes lodged in some part of the respiratory system. This is potentially life-threatening.

ETIOLOGY

- Any object, substance, or part of an object which is small enough to enter the oral or nasal orifices
- Most common objects are foods (e.g., nuts, hot dog pieces, popcorn, hard candy)

INCIDENCE

- Common in infants, toddlers, and preschoolers

RISK FACTORS

- Poorly supervised or unsupervised children
- Curious toddlers
- Households with children of varied ages (older siblings leave unsafe objects lying around play area)

ASSESSMENT FINDINGS

- Abrupt onset of wheezing in otherwise healthy child
- Fixed, localized, or unilateral wheezing
- Cough
- Chronic cough
- Possible acute stridor
- Unilateral coryza (for nasal objects)
- Halitosis (for nasally lodged objects)

Signs and symptoms of aspirated foreign bodies (FBs) vary by location. FBs in the laryngotrachea produce acute symptoms. FBs in the lower airway produce milder symptoms after the initial choking episode.

DIFFERENTIAL DIAGNOSIS

- Asthma
- Allergic rhinitis
- Sinusitis
- Upper respiratory illness
- Epiglottitis
- Tracheitis

DIAGNOSTIC STUDIES

- Chest, neck, or facial x-ray
- Bronchoscopy

PREVENTION

- Create safe play environment for toddlers and preschoolers
- Provide adequate supervision for children

NONPHARMACOLOGIC MANAGEMENT

- Provide oxygen supplementation if needed until transfer to emergency department
- Remove obstruction if possible
- Heimlich maneuver if appropriate
- Patient and family education regarding infant/toddler food safety, actions to take during emergency

Identifying the presence of a foreign body is only possible if an index of suspicion is present. This is important in lower airway aspiration where symptoms are not necessarily acute initially.

PHARMACOLOGIC MANAGEMENT

- None usually needed unless secondary infection is present

CONSULTATION/REFERRAL

- Referral depending on where item is lodged (ENT physician, surgeon, pulmonologist, gastroenterologist)

FOLLOW-UP

- Depends on patient status, age, type of object aspirated, length of time before object discovered

EXPECTED COURSE

- Prognosis usually good

POSSIBLE COMPLICATIONS

- Respiratory distress
- Infection
- Death

CYSTIC FIBROSIS (CF)

DESCRIPTION

An autosomal recessive disease characterized by COPD, pancreatic exocrine deficiency, and elevated chloride concentration in sweat. Pancreas becomes atrophied, cirrhosis of the liver occurs, and the gallbladder becomes hypoplastic.

ETIOLOGY

- An abnormal variation in the cystic fibrosis transmembrane regulator blocks transport of chloride ions. Cell surface becomes inadequately hydrated, organs are damaged, and secretions become extremely viscous

INCIDENCE

- 1/2500 in Caucasian population (most common chromosomal disorder in Caucasians)
- Rarely seen in African-Americans

RISK FACTORS

- Family history
- Parents who are carriers of the gene

ASSESSMENT FINDINGS

- Early symptoms may be gastrointestinal problems (e.g., failure to thrive, foul smelling stools, steatorrhea, meconium ileus)
- Fat malabsorption
- Barrel chest
- Clubbing of fingers
- Cough with mucopurulent sputum
- Crackles and wheezes with recurrent respiratory infections
- Electrolyte imbalances
- Delayed growth and development
- Hepatosplenomegaly in patients with cirrhosis
- Elevated blood glucose

DIFFERENTIAL DIAGNOSIS

- Asthma
- Recurrent respiratory infections
- Failure to thrive
- Immunodeficiency problems

DIAGNOSTIC STUDIES

- Gold standard: Sweat test (chloride > 60 mEq/L considered abnormal)

- Genetic testing
- Stool: increased fat
- Pulmonary function tests 3-4 times annually
- Chest x-ray: hyperaeration
- Pancreatic function tests

PREVENTION

- Genetic counseling for parents with family history
- Immunizations to help prevent childhood respiratory illnesses
- Influenza and pneumococcal immunizations to prevent respiratory infections
- Avoid persons who have acute respiratory illnesses

NONPHARMACOLOGIC MANAGEMENT

- Chest physiotherapy with postural drainage to optimize mucus clearance (thick mucus precipitates respiratory distress)
- High calorie, sodium, protein, fat diet
- Extensive family and patient education
- Supportive care depending on patient and family needs

PHARMACOLOGIC MANAGEMENT

- DNase I: decreases viscosity by cleaving long strands of DNA, may use nebulizer
- Hypertonic saline: hydrates mucus in airways, administered via inhalation
- N-acetlycysteine rarely used related to potential to induce airway inflammation and bronchospasm

CONSULTATION/REFERRAL

- Refer to cystic fibrosis center if available
- Refer to cystic fibrosis support group if appropriate
- Referral to specialist for newly diagnosed patients

FOLLOW-UP

- Depends on stage of disease
- Depends on severity of illness

EXPECTED COURSE

- Poor prognosis, average age at death is 25 years if born pre -1990
- Babies born in the 1990's expect to live 40+ years
- Frequent pulmonary infections

POSSIBLE COMPLICATIONS

- Failure to thrive
- Poor growth
- Recurrent pneumonias and respiratory infections
- Respiratory failure requiring mechanical ventilation
- Pancreatic insufficiency necessitating replacement
- Diabetes mellitus
- Cirrhosis and organomegaly

SUDDEN INFANT DEATH SYNDROME
(SIDS)

DESCRIPTION

The sudden and unexpected death of an infant less than one year of age for which there is no explanation even after a complete autopsy and investigation.

ETIOLOGY

- Unknown
- Possible respiratory control abnormality

INCIDENCE

- 1 per 2000 births; more common in males
- 90% occur before 6 months of age
- Highest rate in Native Americans (1.46/1000 births)
- Peaks at 2 - 4 months of age

SIDS is the leading cause of mortality of infants between the ages of 1 month and 1 year in the U.S.

RISK FACTORS

- Low-birth weight
- Twin births
- Small for gestational age
- Maternal cigarette smoking or drug use
- Poverty
- Young maternal age during pregnancy
- Males > Females
- Infants who sleep in the prone position
- Drug addicted mothers
- Family history

ASSESSMENT FINDINGS

- Well-developed, well-nourished infant
- No evidence of abuse or trauma
- Possible previous apparent life-threatening event (ALTE) including apnea, cyanosis, choking

DIFFERENTIAL DIAGNOSIS

- Trauma or accidental death
- Child abuse
- Congenital heart disease
- Arrhythmias

DIAGNOSTIC STUDIES

- Autopsy

PREVENTION

- Avoid placement in prone position for sleeping
- Apnea monitor for prior ALTE patients

CONSULTATION/REFERRAL

- Notification of coroner's office or medical examiner
- Counseling for family if needed

PRIMARY LUNG MALIGNANCIES

DESCRIPTION

The most common primary lung malignancies are of two types: small cell and non-small cell. They may be a primary malignancy or secondary metastasis

ETIOLOGY

- Small cell malignancies
- Non-small cell malignancies include squamous cell (most common), adenocarcinoma, and large cell carcinoma

INCIDENCE

- Leading cause of cancer mortality
- 70/100,000 cases in the U.S.
- Males > Females
- Usually discovered in fifties, sixties, or seventies

Leading cause of cancer death in males and females in the U.S.

RISK FACTORS

- Smoking (greater than 90% of patients smoke or have smoked)
- Asbestos exposure (pleural mesothelioma)
- COPD
- Exposure to heavy metals, gases
- Secondary smoke

ASSESSMENT FINDINGS

- Usually asymptomatic until an advanced stage
- Cough
- Palpable supraclavicular nodes
- Hemoptysis
- Dyspnea
- Weight loss
- Fatigue

Most patients who present with lung cancer exhibit symptoms. This indicates advanced disease and is usually not amenable to cure.

DIFFERENTIAL DIAGNOSIS

- Primary lesion vs. metastatic lesion (50% are metastatic at diagnosis)
- Tuberculosis

DIAGNOSTIC STUDIES

- Chest x-ray
- CT scan
- Bronchoscopy
- Biopsy

PREVENTION

- Avoid tobacco use, especially cigarettes
- Avoid exposure to asbestos, other potentially carcinogenic agents
- Research indicates that screening provides no decrease in mortality, therefore, routine screening of asymptomatic patients is not recommended

Prevention is the most effective way to reduce the burden of lung cancer.

NONPHARMACOLOGIC MANAGEMENT

- Radiation if indicated
- Surgical resection

PHARMACOLOGIC MANAGEMENT

- Chemotherapy if indicated
- Pain medication as needed
- Oxygen supplementation as needed

CONSULTATION/REFERRAL

- Surgeon, oncologist, pulmonologist
- Consider hospice if consistent with patient's advance directives

FOLLOW-UP

- Depends on patient status, advance directives, and staging

EXPECTED COURSE

- Depends on staging at time of diagnosis, whether surgically resectable, and tumor type
- 5-year survival for all stages is 15%

POSSIBLE COMPLICATIONS

- Metastasis-brain, bones, liver common
- Death

References

Barnes, P. J., & Celli, B. R. (2009). Systemic manifestations and comorbidities of COPD. European Respiratory Journal, 33(5), 1165-1185.

Bickley, L. S., & Szilagyi, P. G. (2003). Bates' guide to physical examination and history taking (8th ed.). Philadelphia: Lippincott Williams & Wilkins.

Bjornson, C. L., & Johnson, D. W. (2008). Croup. Lancet, 371(9609), 329-339.

Blumberg, H. M., Burman, W. J., Chaisson, R. E., Daley, C. L., Etkind, S. C., Friedman, L. N., et al. (2003). American thoracic society/centers for disease control and prevention/infectious diseases society of america: Treatment of tuberculosis. American Journal of Respiratory and Critical Care Medicine, 167(4), 603-662.

Braman, S. S. (2006). Chronic cough due to acute bronchitis: Accp evidence-based clinical practice guidelines. Chest, 129(1 Suppl), 95S-103S.

Centers for Disease Control and Prevention. (2005). Pertussis. Retrieved from http://www.cdc.gov/vaccines/pubs/pinkbook/downloads/pert.pdf

Centers for Disease Control and Prevention. (2010). Guidelines for the control of pertussis outbreaks. Retrieved from http://www.cdc.gov/vaccines/pubs/pertussis-guide/guide.htm

Cincinnati Children's Hospital Medical Center. (2006a). Bronchiollitis in infants less than 1 year of age presenting with a first episode. Retrieved from http://www.cincinnatichildrens.org/svc/alpha/h/health-policy/bronchiolitis.htm

Cincinnati Children's Hospital Medical Center. (2006b). Evidence-based care guideline for community acquired pneumonia in children 60 days through 17 years of age. Retrieved from http://www.guideline.gov/content.aspx?id=9690

Crowcroft, N. S., & Pebody, R. G. (2006). Recent developments in pertussis. Lancet, 367(9526), 1926-1936.

Daneman, N., McGeer, A., Green, K., & Low, D. E. (2006). Macrolide resistance in bacteremic pneumococcal disease: Implications for patient management. Clinical Infectious Diseases, 43(4), 432-438.

Diagnosis and management of bronchiolitis. (2006). Pediatrics, 118(4), 1774-1793.

Eisner, M. D., Blanc, P. D., Yelin, E. H., Sidney, S., Katz, P. P., Ackerson, L., et al. (2008). COPD as a systemic disease: Impact on physical functional limitations. American Journal of Medicine, 121(9), 789-796.

Ernst, D., & Lee, A. (2010). Nurse practitioners prescribing reference. New York: Haymarket Media Publication.

Global Initative for Chronic Obstructive Lung Disease. (2009). Global strategy for the diagnosis, management, and prevention of chronic obstructive pulmonary disease. Retrieved from http://www.goldcopd.com/Guidelineitem.asp?l1=2&l2=1&intId=2003

Harper, S. A., Bradley, J. S., Englund, J. A., File, T. M., Gravenstein, S., Hayden, F. G., et al. (2009). Seasonal influenza in adults and children--diagnosis, treatment, chemoprophylaxis, and institutional outbreak management: Clinical practice guidelines of the infectious diseases society of america. Clinical Infectious Diseases, 48(8), 1003-1032.

Heron, M., Sutton, P. D., Xu, J., Ventura, S. J., Strobino, D. M., & Guyer, B. (2010). Annual summary of vital statistics: 2007. Pediatrics, 125(1), 4-15.

Hopewell, P. C., Pai, M., Maher, D., Uplekar, M., & Raviglione, M. C. (2006). International standards for tuberculosis care. Lancet Infectious Diseases, 6(11), 710-725.

Li, J. Z., Winston, L. G., Moore, D. H., & Bent, S. (2007). Efficacy of short-course antibiotic regimens for community-acquired pneumonia: A meta-analysis. American Journal of Medicine, 120(9), 783-790.

Mallia, P., & Johnston, S. L. (2006). How viral infections cause exacerbation of airway diseases. Chest, 130(4), 1203-1210.

Mandell, L. A., Wunderink, R. G., Anzueto, A., Bartlett, J. G., Campbell, G. D., Dean, N. C., et al. (2007). Infectious diseases society of america/american thoracic society consensus guidelines on the management of community-acquired pneumonia in adults. Clinical Infectious Diseases, 44 Suppl 2, S27-72.

Ostfeld, B. M., Esposito, L., Perl, H., & Hegyi, T. (2010). Concurrent risks in sudden infant death syndrome. Pediatrics, 125(3), 447-453.

Papi, A., Bellettato, C. M., Braccioni, F., Romagnoli, M., Casolari, P., Caramori, G., et al. (2006). Infections and airway inflammation in chronic obstructive pulmonary disease severe exacerbations. American Journal of Respiratory and Critical Care Medicine, 173(10), 1114-1121.

Qaseem, A., Snow, V., Shekelle, P., Sherif, K., Wilt, T. J., Weinberger, S., et al. (2007). Diagnosis and management of stable chronic obstructive pulmonary disease: A clinical practice guideline from the american college of physicians. Annals of Internal Medicine, 147(9), 633-638.

Rihkanen, H., Ronkko, E., Nieminen, T., Komsi, K. L., Raty, R., Saxen, H., et al. (2008). Respiratory viruses in laryngeal croup of young children. Journal of Pediatrics, 152(5), 661-665.

Sarkar, M., Hennessy, S., & Yang, Y. X. (2008). Proton-pump inhibitor use and the risk for community-acquired pneumonia. Annals of Internal Medicine, 149(6), 391-398.

Screening for chronic obstructive pulmonary disease using spirometry: U.S. Preventive services task force recommendation statement. (2008). Annals of Internal Medicine, 148(7), 529-534.

Shazberg, G., Revel-Vilk, S., Shoseyov, D., Ben-Ami, A., Klar, A., & Hurvitz, H. (2000). The clinical course of bronchiolitis associated with acute otitis media. Archives of Disease in Childhood, 83(4), 317-319.

Siva, R., Green, R. H., Brightling, C. E., Shelley, M., Hargadon, B., McKenna, S., et al. (2007). Eosinophilic airway inflammation and exacerbations of COPD: A randomised controlled trial. European Respiratory Journal, 29(5), 906-913.

Strausbaugh, S. D., & Davis, P. B. (2007). Cystic fibrosis: A review of epidemiology and pathobiology. Clinics in Chest Medicine, 28(2), 279-288.

Tiwari, T., Murphy, T. V., & Moran, J. (2005). Recommended antimicrobial agents for the treatment and postexposure prophylaxis of pertussis: 2005 CDC guidelines. MMWR Recomm Rep, 54(RR-14), 1-16.

16

SEXUALLY TRANSMITTED DISEASES

Sexually Transmitted Diseases

Human Immunodeficiency Virus (HIV) 625

Bacterial Vaginosis 628

Chlamydia 629

Gonorrhea 631

Syphilis 633

Genital Herpes 635

Human Papilloma Virus 637

Pelvic Inflammatory Disease 639

Trichomoniasis 641

References *643*

HUMAN IMMUNODEFICIENCY VIRUS (HIV) INFECTION

DESCRIPTION

Viral infection that causes CD4 cell death and gradual decline in immune function resulting in opportunistic infections, malignancies, and neurologic lesions.

CD4 cell count <200 cells/mm3 is classified as AIDS.

ETIOLOGY

- Retrovirus (human immunodeficiency virus) that infects cells, most notably the CD4 lymphocytes (T helper cells)
- Is transmitted through sexual intercourse, transfusion of blood or blood products, and perinatally from mother to infant

INCIDENCE

- HIV considered a chronic disease
- Occurs mostly among young adults ages 25-44 years
- Males > Females

RISK FACTORS

- Sexual activity (most common risk factor)
- Prostitution
- Multiple sexual partners or sexual partner has multiple partners
- Engaging in sex for money
- Sexual partner of injecting drug user
- Men who have sex with men
- Injecting drug use and sharing of contaminated needles
- Hemophiliacs who have received pooled plasma products
- Infants born to HIV-infected women
- Infants breast fed by HIV-infected mother
- Health care workers

Viral load in the HIV positive patient is the best predictor of viral transmission in heterosexuals.

ASSESSMENT FINDINGS

Initial infection:
- Fever
- Pharyngitis
- Nonpruritic maculopapular skin rash
- Myalgia/arthralgia
- Malaise
- Diarrhea
- Headache
- Lymphadenopathy
- Hepatosplenomegaly
- Self-limiting viral-type syndrome occurring about 6-8 weeks postinfection; often goes unnoticed by patient
- An asymptomatic period of variable length follows the initial infection
- The time between infection and development of AIDS ranges from a few months to 17 years with the median time being 10 years

Established HIV:
- Anemia
- Leukopenia
- Thrombocytopenia
- Involuntary weight loss
- Diarrhea
- Dementia
- Pneumocystis carinii pneumonia (PCP), which is characterized by nonproductive cough, dyspnea, and fever that persists for days or weeks.
- Candidal infections: esophageal, bronchial, pulmonary, oral, vaginal
- Other opportunistic infections
- Herpes zoster, may be disseminated
- Pulmonary tuberculosis
- Kaposi's sarcoma: nodule or papule that appears purple or dark brown, found on skin, mucous membranes, and/or viscera

TB is co-epidemic with HIV. All persons who test positive for TB should be screened for HIV.

DIAGNOSTIC STUDIES

- ELISA for screening (sensitivity and specificity > 98%)
- Western blot or immunofluorescence assay (IFA) for confirmation
- May be negative in first 6-12 weeks after initial infection
- Informed consent must be obtained before HIV testing is performed
- In infants born to HIV-infected mothers, maternally

acquired HIV IgG antibodies and infant-derived IgG antibodies cannot be differentiated. A positive ELISA or Western blot, therefore, does not confirm an infection in the child < 18 months of age

Consider early referral to an HIV care specialist to complete workup and deliver care.

PREVENTION

- Avoid unprotected sexual intercourse
- Use of condoms
- Avoid contact with intravenous products and fluids
- HIV screening for all persons at risk of infection
- Screening recommended for all pregnant women and newborn infants at risk for HIV infection

POSTEXPOSURE PROPHYLAXIS (PEP):

- HIV PEP warranted in exposure to known HIV exposure or exposure thought to be highly likely
- Initiate as soon as possible after exposure
- PEPline at http://www.nccc.ucsf.edu/Hotlines/PEPline.html, telephone 888-448-4911

NONPHARMACOLOGIC MANAGEMENT

- Counseling regarding behavioral, psychosocial, and medical implications of HIV infection
- Encourage regular exercise and good nutrition
- Avoid raw eggs, raw seafood, unpasteurized milk, and other potentially contaminated foods
- Review immunization status and bring up to date (pneumococcal, influenza, Td, hepatitis A & B)
- Education regarding methods of transmission
- Teach how to minimize risk to others
- Partner notification (sexual partners and those who share needles or other injected drug equipment)
- Notification of local health department
- Polymerase chain reaction (PCR) RNA assays detect presence of virus and are used to monitor progression and response to therapy
- Once HIV is confirmed:
    - ◊ CBC with differential and platelets
    - ◊ Chemistry profile
    - ◊ Syphilis serology
    - ◊ Baseline CD4 count
    - ◊ Viral load (HIV RNA) tests are increasingly being used to monitor progression of disease and determining when to initiate treatment
    - Hepatitis profile
    - Chest x-ray
    - PPD with controls (> 5mm considered positive)
    - Toxoplasmosis antibody test
    - Serology for cytomegalovirus and toxoplasmosis
    - Pap smear every 6 months
    - Cervical culture for gonorrhea and chlamydia
    - Wet prep

CD4 counts should be checked at least every 3-6 months.

PHARMACOLOGIC MANAGEMENT

- Antiretroviral therapy – current standard: requires multidrug therapy to prevent emergence of resistance (HARRT-highly active antiretroviral therapy)
- PCP prophylaxis (indicated if CD4 count < 200/mm3 and for infants born to HIV-infected mothers):
    - ◊ Trimethoprim-sulfamethoxazole (Bactrim DS®) 15 mg/kg/day based on trimethoprim component for 14-21 days
- Toxoplasmosis prophylaxis (indicated if CD4 count < 100/mm3):
    - ◊ Same as PCP prophylaxis
- Mycobacterium avium complex prophylaxis if CD4 count < 50/mm3 and no HARRT:
    - ◊ Clarithromycin (Biaxin®) 500 mg twice daily or azithromycin (Zithromax®) 1200 mg PO weekly
- Pneumococcal vaccine every 5 years
- Influenza vaccine in fall annually
- Td booster if > 5 years since last dose
- Hepatitis B vaccine if not immune

Commonly used drugs:

- Nucleoside reverse transcriptase inhibitors: abacavir (ABC®, Ziagen®), didanosine (ddI or Videx®), lamivudine (3TC or Epivir®), stavudine (Zerit®), zidovudine (AZT or Retrovir®)
- Protease inhibitors: atazanavir (Reyataz®), darunavir (Prezista®), fosamprenavir (Lexiva®) indinavir (Crixivan®), lopinavirritonavir (Kaletra®), ritonavir (Norvir®), nelfinavir (Viracept®)
- Nonnucleoside reverse transcriptase inhibitors: nevirapine (Viramune®), delavirdine (Rescriptor®), efavirenz (Sustiva®)

At least 3 different drugs from different classes are recommended to decrease viral load and delay onset of AIDS.

PREGNANCY/LACTATION CONSIDERATIONS

- Antiretroviral therapy during pregnancy and the first 6 weeks of an infant's life has been shown to decrease incidence of transmission to infant from 25% to 8%
- CDC recommends all women be offered HIV counseling and testing
- Breastfeeding is contraindicated in women who are HIV-infected due to the risk of transmission
- Trimethoprim-sulfamethoxazole DS (Bactrim DS®) is indicated for PCP prophylaxis in all HIV-infected women who are pregnant. Dapsone may be substituted in first trimester.
- Azithromycin (Zithromax®) is the drug of choice in pregnancy for Mycobacterium avium complex (MAC) prophylaxis

CONSULTATION/REFERRAL

- Refer to health care professional experienced in management of HIV infection

FOLLOW-UP

- Patients on antiretroviral therapy need close monitoring due to significant drug toxicities

Close follow up needed for evaluation of neurological symptoms which could indicate CNS infection.

EXPECTED COURSE

- Life expectancy after HIV progresses to AIDS is 2-3 years. With development of better treatment life expectancy is increasing
- Opportunistic infections usually begin to develop when CD4 count are < 200 mm3
- The majority of children who are infected have a gradual course and do not meet criteria for case definition until about age 3 years. A smaller number of children become symptomatic early and die before age 1 year

POSSIBLE COMPLICATIONS

- Immunodeficiency
    - ◊ Candidal infections
    - ◊ Staphylococcal infections
    - ◊ Salmonella bacteremia
    - ◊ Genital warts
    - ◊ Herpes simplex and zoster
- Depression
- Suicide

BACTERIAL VAGINOSIS (BV)

(Gardnerella Vaginosis, Nonspecific Vaginosis)

DESCRIPTION

Clinical syndrome resulting from replacement of the normal vaginal flora, Lactobacillus sp., with high concentrations of anaerobic bacteria (e.g., *Prevotella sp.* and *Mobiluncus sp., Gardnerella. vaginalis,* and *Mycoplasma hominis*).

BV is not an STD, however, it is more common in women who are sexually active.

ETIOLOGY

- Cause of the microbacterial overgrowth not completely understood

INCIDENCE

- 4-33% of women affected depending on setting
- Most prevalent vaginal infection in women of reproductive age in the U.S. (most common vaginal infection according to NHANES data)

RISK FACTORS

- African American race
- Multiple sexual partners
- New sexual partner
- Douching

ASSESSMENT FINDINGS

- Asymptomatic in about 50% of women
- Grayish-white malodorous vaginal discharge
- Unpleasant, fishy, or musty vaginal odor
- Profuse discharge
- Pruritus and burning of vulvovaginal area

Suspect BV in patients who complain of malodorous discharge after sexual intercourse.

DIFFERENTIAL DIAGNOSIS

- Candidiasis
- Chlamydia trachomatis infection
- Gonorrhea
- Trichomoniasis
- Atrophic vaginitis
- Atrophic vaginitis
- Staphylococci infection
- Foreign body

Atrophic vaginitis is associated with the following findings: negative amine and potassium hydroxide (KOH), greater numbers of white blood cells (WBCs), and immature epithelial cells.

DIAGNOSTIC STUDIES

- Amsel's clinical criteria for diagnosis requires three of the following symptoms or signs be present:
  - ◊ A homogeneous, white, noninflammatory discharge that smoothly coats the vaginal walls
  - ◊ The presence of clue cells on microscopic examination
  - ◊ A pH of vaginal fluid > 4.5
  - ◊ A fishy odor of vaginal discharge before or after addition of 10% KOH ("positive whiff test")
- Wet mount: vaginal discharge on slide with normal saline; look for WBCs (not numerous), clue cells present
- Gram stain: absence or decreased lactobacilli

Atrophic vaginitis is associated with the following findings: negative amine and potassium hydroxide (KOH), greater numbers of white blood cells (WBCs), and immature epithelial cells.

PREVENTION

- Good hygiene
- Avoid use of feminine pads, liners
- Use of condoms
- Avoid douching as this may reduce recurrences
- Screen for STIs

NONPHARMACOLOGIC MANAGEMENT

- Consider screening for sexually transmitted disease
- Avoid sexual intercourse until treatment completed
- No alcohol if on metronidazole due to a disulfiram-type reaction
- Stress good personal hygiene

- Avoid douching to prevent recurrences
- Treatment of the male sex partner has not been beneficial in reducing recurrence of BV

Treatment of sexual partners is not considered standard of care. However, it is observed in clinical practice.

PHARMACOLOGIC MANAGEMENT

- Consider
  - ◊ Tinidazole: 2 g stat, repeat in 24 hours (Alternative treatment: Tinidazole: 1 g by mouth daily for 5 days - may have advantage of fewer side effects compared to metronidazole)
    OR
  - ◊ Metronidazole (Flagyl®) 500 mg twice daily
    OR
  - ◊ Clindamycin 2% vaginal cream 5 g for 7 days
    OR
  - ◊ Metronidazole vaginal gel 0.75% 5 g intravaginally for 7 days
- Consider treating partner, especially if infection recurrent. However, treatment of the male does not reduce recurrence or symptoms

Patient must refrain from use of alcohol while taking metronidazole.

PREGNANCY/LACTATION CONSIDERATIONS

- BV during pregnancy is associated with adverse pregnancy outcomes (e.g., preterm labor, premature rupture of membranes, and premature birth)
- CDC recommends use of metronidazole or clindamycin orally in symptomatic women
- Clindamycin cream may be used until 22 weeks gestation
- Screen in second trimester if woman at high risk for preterm labor (e.g., has had previous preterm delivery or labor)

CONSULTATION/REFERRAL

- Not usually indicated

FOLLOW-UP

- Not usually indicated but may be associated with lower recurrence rate
- One month follow-up during pregnancy recommended

Follow up after treatment ensures that infection has cleared. Symptomatic relief is not an objective measure of cure since 50% of patients are asymptomatic.

EXPECTED COURSE

- Recurrences common

POSSIBLE COMPLICATIONS

- Acquisition and transmission of other sexually transmitted infections
- Urinary tract infections
- May be a factor in premature rupture of membranes and preterm delivery
- Associated with postpartal endometritis
- Pelvic inflammatory disease
- Postoperative infections after gynecologic surgery

CHLAMYDIA

DESCRIPTION

Sexually transmitted infection with an often asymptomatic clinical course with serious sequelae.

ETIOLOGY

- *Chlamydia trachomatis*

INCIDENCE

- Most prevalent STI in United States
- Over 4 million cases diagnosed annually
- Highest incidence among adolescents and young adults

RISK FACTORS

- Sexually active
- New sexual partner
- Multiple sexual partners or partner of person with multiple partners
- African American females
- Lower socioeconomic groups
- Women at greater risk for contraction of chlamydia than are men
- Age < 21 years

Incidence of chlamydia infection declines with age, especially after age 21 years.

ASSESSMENT FINDINGS

Females:
- Often asymptomatic
- Mucopurulent cervicitis
- Edematous, congested friable cervix
- Vaginal discharge
- Discharge from Bartholin's gland when milked
- Cervical motion tenderness
- Dysuria
- Urethritis
- Salpingitis

Males:
- Dysuria (urethritis)
- Proctitis (rectal pain)
- Epididymitis (scrotal pain)
- Prostatitis (prostate pain)

Infants:
- Afebrile
- Pneumonia
- Conjunctivitis

Test for Chlamydia in any patient with urethritis, cervical discharge, pelvic, rectal, or testicular pain.

DIFFERENTIAL DIAGNOSIS

- Gonorrhea
- Vaginitis
- Pelvic inflammatory disease
- Salpingitis
- Urinary tract infection

DIAGNOSTIC STUDIES

- Nucleic acid amplification test (NAAT)
- GenProbe (chlamydia and gonorrhea)
- Urinalysis: positive for WBCs
- Wet prep: > 20 WBC/high-powered field
- Culture: not usually used, however it is the gold standard for diagnosis

PREVENTION

- Use of condoms
- Screening should be done for target populations:
  - ◊ Sexually active females
  - ◊ Women 20-24 years old who meet either of two following criteria:
    - * Inconsistent use of barrier contraception
    - * New or more than one sex partner during the past three months
    - * In the third trimester of pregnancy
- Screen sexually active males < 25 years who are high risk populations (controversial)
- Screen for other STIs if positive for chlamydia

Pelvic inflammatory disease is a common sequelae of untreated chlamydia infections.

NONPHARMACOLOGIC MANAGEMENT

- Education regarding serious sequelae of chlamydia infection
- Abstinence until treatment completed
- Evaluate and treat sexual partners
- Sexual abuse should be considered for any child with confirmed chlamydia after the neonatal period
- Report to local health department

PHARMACOLOGIC MANAGEMENT

- Consider
  - ◊ Doxycycline (Vibramycin®) 100 mg twice daily for 7 days OR
  - ◊ Azithromycin (Zithromax®) 1 gm single dose OR
  - ◊ Doxycycline for 10-14 days if epididymis involved or for pelvic inflamatory disease
  - ◊ Erythromycin 500 mg four times a day for 7

days if patient unable to take doxycycline

- ◊ Second line: levofloxacin 500 mg PO daily for 7 days; or ofloxacin 300 mg twice daily for 7 days

Children:

- < 45 kg: erythromycin base
- > 45 kg and < 9 years old: azithromycin
- > 8 years old: azithromycin OR doxycycline

PREGNANCY/LACTATION CONSIDERATIONS

- Prevalence among pregnant women in U.S. is 5%
- Treat with azithromycin, erythromycin base or amoxicillin
- Teteracyclines, quinolones contraindicated during pregnancy
- Screen in third trimester in women at risk (e.g., < 25 years old, recent new sexual partner, more than one sexual partner)
- Test of cure recommended in pregnant patients

FOLLOW-UP

- Test of cure is not needed unless symptoms persist or reinfection suspected
- Screen for HIV, gonorrhea and syphilis in persons with chlamydia infection
- Re-infection rate is very high; recommendation is to rescreen in 3 months after treatment

EXPECTED COURSE

- Complete resolution with early and compliant therapy
- Due to asymptomatic nature of disease, many persons develop complications

POSSIBLE COMPLICATIONS

- Transient oligospermia
- Post epididymitis urethral stricture
- Pelvic inflamatory disease
- Infertility: most common cause of acquired infertility in US
- Ectopic pregnancy
- Chronic pelvic pain
- Acute or chronic salpingitis
- Fitz-Hugh-Curtis syndrome (perihepatitis)
- Conjunctivitis in infants born to infected mothers
- Pneumonia in infants born to infected mothers

GONORRHEA

DESCRIPTION

A sexually transmitted disease that produces a purulent inflammation of mucous membranes.

ETIOLOGY

- *Neisseria gonorrhoeae* infection transmitted by sexual contact or from infected mother to infant during childbirth

INCIDENCE

- Incidence highest among females aged 15-19 years

RISK FACTORS

- New sexual partners
- Sexual exposure to an infected individual without barrier protection
- Multiple sexual partners
- Men having sex with other men (MSM)
- Infant born to infected mother
- Sexually abused children
- Use of IUD increases risk of pelvic inflamatory disease

ASSESSMENT FINDINGS

Males:

- Purulent urethral discharge
- Dysuria
- Testicular pain
- Asymptomatic

Females:

- Often asymptomatic
- Endocervical discharge
- Vaginal discharge

- Dysuria
- Bartholin's gland abscess
- Abnormal vaginal bleeding
- Abdominal/pelvic pain
- Adnexal tenderness
- Cervical motion tenderness

Males & Females:
- Rectal discharge
- Tenesmus
- Rectal burning or itching
- Exudative pharyngitis
- Purulent discharge from eye

Infants:
- Most common:
  - ◊ Eye infection (ophthalmia neonatorum)
- Less common:
  - ◊ Sepsis
  - ◊ Serious systemic disease

Disseminated disease:
- Fever
- Chills
- Arthralgias of small joints
- Pustular, red, and tender skin lesions
- Septic arthritis, usually symmetric, polyarticular, especially seen in elbow, knee and distal joints

DIFFERENTIAL DIAGNOSIS

- Chlamydia
- Urinary tract infection
- Vaginitis/urethritis from another etiologic agent
- Pelvic inflammatory disease

DIAGNOSTIC STUDIES

- NAAT (nucleic acid amplification test is most sensitive and specific so is recommended)
- Gram stain of exudate for urethritis
- DNA probe
- Culture of exudate or joint aspirate on Thayer-Martin agar (also called chocolate agar)
- Cervical culture or DNA probe for *C. trachomatis*
- Syphilis serology
- HIV testing if appropriate

PREVENTION

- Use of condoms
- Neonatal ocular prophylaxis: silver nitrate, erythromycin, or tetracycline eye drops
- Screening during pregnancy if high-risk

NONPHARMACOLOGIC MANAGEMENT

- Avoid sexual intercourse until treatment completed
- Treatment of sexual contacts
- Sexual abuse should be considered for any child with confirmed gonorrhea after neonatal period
- Report all cases to local health department
- Screen for other STDs

PHARMACOLOGIC MANAGEMENT

- Consider
  - ◊ Ceftriaxone (Rocephin®) 125 mg IM OR
  - ◊ Cefixime (Suprax®) 400 mg oral as single dose (tablet or liquid)

  PLUS (treat chlamydia unless ruled out)
  - ◊ Doxycycline (Vibramycin®) 100 mg twice daily for 7 days or azithromycin (Zithromax®) 1 gm as single dose for treatment of chlamydia because of frequent coinfection
- If pharyngitis or conjunctivitis: 1g Ceftriaxone

Infants/Children:
- < 45 kg: 125 mg Ceftriaxone IM (full adult dose is given)

PREGNANCY/LACTATION CONSIDERATIONS

- Ceftriaxone is the treatment of choice
- Consider test of cure
- All pregnant women should be screened at first prenatal visit
- For high-risk women an additional screen should be done in third trimester
- Cephalosporin is treatment of choice
- Tetracycline contraindicated

CONSULTATION/REFERRAL

- Not usually needed unless dissemination occurs or resistance to treatment

FOLLOW-UP

- Test of cure not necessary unless symptoms persist or noncompliance is an issue

EXPECTED COURSE

- Complete resolution

POSSIBLE COMPLICATIONS

- Urethral stricture in men
- Infertility in women
- Pelvic inflamatory disease (PID)
- Destruction of joints and cardiac valves
- Meningitis
- Endocarditis
- Pneumonia
- Endometritis

Infants:
- Corneal scarring in infants
- Disseminated disease in infants
- Ophthalmia neonatorum

SYPHILIS

DESCRIPTION

Sexually transmitted disease characterized by sequential stages and involving multiple systems. Syphilis has the following stages:
- Primary
- Secondary
- Latent (infection present at least 12 months)
- Tertiary

ETIOLOGY

- *Treponema pallidum,* a spirochete, penetrates intact skin or mucous membrane during sexual intercourse, enters the bloodstream and is transported to other tissues
- Congenital syphilis is acquired transplacentally from an infected mother

INCIDENCE

- > 110,000 new cases annually
- More prevalent among persons 15-25 years of age
- Males > Females (6:1)

RISK FACTORS

- Multiple sexual partners
- Injecting drug use
- Men who have sex with men
- HIV infection
- Presence of another sexually transmitted disease

ASSESSMENT FINDINGS

Primary syphilis:
- Chancre at site of inoculation begins as papule then ulcerates with a hard edge and clean, yellow base; indurated and painless; usually located on genitalia; may be solitary or multiple; persists for 1-5 weeks and heals spontaneously
- Chancre may go unnoticed in females
- Regional lymphadenopathy

Secondary syphilis:
- Rash that is bilaterally symmetrical, polymorphic, nonpruritic, frequently on soles and palms, and usually persists for 2-6 weeks then spontaneously resolves
- Condyloma lata which are moist, pink, peripheral warty lesions. These may be present on glans, perianal, vulval areas, and intertriginous areas
- Mucous patches in mouth, throat, cervix
- Generalized lymphadenopathy
- Flu-like symptoms
- Mild hepatosplenomegaly

Latent syphilis:
- Asymptomatic

Tertiary syphilis:
- Cardiovascular manifestations: aortic valve disease, aneurysms
- Neurological manifestations: meningitis, encephalitis, tabes dorsalis, dementia
- Integumentary manifestations: gummas
- Orthopedic manifestations: Charcot joints, osteomyelitis

Congenital syphilis:
- Early
  - ◊ Failure to thrive
  - ◊ Stillbirths
  - ◊ Hydrops fetalis
  - ◊ Prematurity
  - ◊ Rhinitis
  - ◊ Lymphadenopathy
  - ◊ Jaundice
  - ◊ Anemia
  - ◊ Hepatosplenomegaly

- ◊ Nephrosis
- ◊ Hallmark rash similar to secondary syphilis in adult, may be bullous or vesicular
- Late (due to chronic inflammation or hypersensitivity)
  - ◊ CNS changes
  - ◊ Bony abnormalities
  - ◊ Dental deformities
  - ◊ Cataracts, blindness
  - ◊ Stage of congenital syphilis is dependent on the maternal stage of syphilis

DIFFERENTIAL DIAGNOSIS

Primary syphilis:

- Chancroid
- Lymphogranuloma venereum
- Granuloma inguinale
- Herpes simplex
- Behçet's syndrome
- Trauma

Secondary syphilis:

- Pityriasis rosea
- Guttate psoriasis
- Drug eruption

DIAGNOSTIC STUDIES

- Nontreponemal tests
  - ◊ Rapid plasma reagin (RPR)
  - ◊ Venereal Disease Research Laboratory (VDRL)
- Treponemal tests (usually positive for life after treatment):
  - ◊ Fluorescent treponemal antibody absorbed (FTA-ABS)
  - ◊ Microhemagglutination assay for antibody to *T. pallidum* (MHA-TP)
- Lumbar puncture for CSF serologies when neurologic symptoms are present and in all children diagnosed after the newborn period
- Darkfield microscopy or direct fluorescent antibody test of exudate or tissue

PREVENTION

- Use of condoms
- Screening for syphilis in asymptomatic persons
- Screening for HIV in persons with syphilis infection

NONPHARMACOLOGIC MANAGEMENT

- Avoid sexual intercourse until treatment complete
- Sexual abuse should be considered for any child with confirmed syphilis
- Treatment of all sexual partners
- Evaluate for other STIs

PHARMACOLOGIC MANAGEMENT

- Consider
  - ◊ Benzathine penicillin G (Bicillin® LA) intramuscular in adults and children
    2-4 million units IM for primary and secondary stage
- Late latent without evidence of neurosyphilis:
  - ◊ Benzathine penicillin G, 2.4 million units IM weekly for 3 doses
- Neurosyphilis:
  - ◊ Aqueous crystalline penicillin G intravenous (3-4 million units) every 4 hours for 10-14 days
- Congenital:
  Patients with penicillin allergy:
  - ◊ Doxycycline (Vibramycin®) 100 mg PO twice daily for 2 weeks OR
  - ◊ Tetracycline 500 mg PO 4 times daily for 2 weeks OR
  - ◊ Ceftriaxone, 1g IM or IV daily for 8-10 days
- Desensitization is recommended for penicillin-allergic persons in the following cases:
  - ◊ HIV-positive
  - ◊ Children
  - ◊ Pregnancy

Sexual contact is ill advised until 4 fold decrease in titer is observed.

PREGNANCY/LACTATION CONSIDERATIONS

- If penicillin allergic, desensitization is recommended
- All pregnant women should be screened for syphilis at the first prenatal visit
- Those at high risk should be screened again in the third trimester and at delivery

CONSULTATION/REFERRAL

- Consultation with or referral to obstetrician in pregnant women
- Report to local health department

FOLLOW-UP

- Repeat syphilis serology for 3, 6, 9, 12 months, then annually to confirm treatment (should observe

a 4-fold decrease in titer to determine adequate treatment)
- HIV-positive patients: repeat serology at 3 month intervals
- Infants: repeat syphilis serology at 3, 6, and 12 months or until nonreactive

EXPECTED COURSE

- Excellent prognosis except in late syphilis complications and in HIV-infected patients

POSSIBLE COMPLICATIONS

- Cardiovascular disease
- Central nervous system disease
- Membranous glomerulonephritis
- Paroxysmal cold hemoglobinemia
- Organ damage that cannot be reversed
- Multiple disorders
- Jarisch-Herxheimer reaction often occurs among people being treated for early syphilis. Antipyretics may be used, but there is no proven method to prevent this reaction. May induce early labor in pregnant women, but this concern should not prevent treatment in pregnancy

GENITAL HERPES
(Herpes Simplex II, Herpes Genitalis)

DESCRIPTION

Recurrent, incurable cutaneous or mucous membrane infection.

ETIOLOGY

- Herpes simplex virus type 1 or 2 (usually HSV-2)
- Transmitted by direct contact with active lesions or by virus-containing fluid
- An asymptomatic patient can be infectious while shedding virus
- Usual incubation period is 2-12 days

The incubation period after exposure is 1-45 days.

INCIDENCE

- 300,000-700,000 cases annually in the U.S.

Prevalence studies indicate 1 in 6 Americans is infected with genital herpes, 48% of African American females are infected, and 1 in 3 women over age 30 years is infected. The incidence increases with increasing age.

Source: NHANES data, 2010

RISK FACTORS

- Sexual activity

ASSESSMENT FINDINGS

Primary infection:
- Asymptomatic often
- Painful papules followed by vesicles on an erythematous base that ulcerate, crust, and resolve within 21 days
- Hyperesthesia
- Fever
- Headache
- Malaise
- Myalgia
- Dysuria
- Lymphadenopathy

Recurrent infections:
- Prodrome of pain, burning, and/or paresthesia over area of eruption
- Burning genital pain
- Lesions as above that resolve within 7-10 days

DIFFERENTIAL DIAGNOSIS

- Primary syphilis
- Atypical genital warts
- Candidiasis
- Herpes zoster

DIAGNOSTIC STUDIES

- Viral tissue culture (notify lab since this requires a

special culture tube)
- DNA prep has the highest sensitivity
- Serologic assays (usually positive 4-6 weeks after onset of symptoms); many point of care tests (POCT) available commercially
- Tzanck prep
- ELISA
- Syphilis serology

Varicella zoster will give same results as Tzanck prep.

PREVENTION

- Use of condoms
- Cesarean section indicated in women with lesions to prevent infection in newborn

Screen for other sexually transmitted infections.

NONPHARMACOLOGIC MANAGEMENT

- Counseling
  - Natural course of disease
  - Asymptomatic viral shedding
  - Potential for recurrent episodes
  - Sexual transmission
  - Implications for pregnancy
- Cool compresses with Burow's solution
- Ice packs to lesion area
- NSAIDs or acetaminophen for pain
- Good hygiene
- Avoid sexual contact during symptomatic periods, for 48 hours after symptoms resolve, and during prodromal symptoms
- Use of condoms during all sexual exposures to decrease risk of transmission when asymptomatic
- Avoidance of triggers to recurrent infection when possible (e.g., genital trauma, emotional stress, concurrent infection)
- Sexual abuse should be considered for any child with confirmed herpes infection

Patient education: During asymptomatic shedding, genital infections can be transmitted.

PHARMACOLOGIC MANAGEMENT

Primary infection:
- Treatment for 7-10 days or until clinical resolution attained
  - ◊ acyclovir (Zovirax®) 400 mg three times daily for 7-10 days OR
  - ◊ acyclovir 200 mg 5x/day for 7-10 days OR
  - ◊ famciclovir (Famvir®) 250 mg three times daily 7-10 days OR
  - ◊ valacyclovir (Valtrex®)1 gm PO twice daily for 7-10 days

Recurrent episodes:
- Should be started during prodrome or within one day of onset of lesion:
  - ◊ acyclovir (Zovirax®) 400 mg three times daily for 5 days OR
  - ◊ famciclovir (Famvir®) 125mg twice daily for 5 days OR
  - ◊ valacyclovir (Valtrex®) 500 mg twice daily for 5 days OR 1 gm daily for 5 days

Suppressive therapy:
- Use in persons with 6 or more recurrences annually:
  - ◊ acyclovir (Zovirax®) 400 mg twice daily OR
  - ◊ famciclovir (Famvir®) 250 mg twice daily up to one year OR
  - ◊ valacyclovir (Valtrex®) 1 g daily for 1 year (Cr Cl < 29 mL: 500 mg daily)

Reassess after one year of daily suppressant therapy.

PREGNANCY/LACTATION CONSIDERATIONS

- Acyclovir may be used during pregnancy for treatment of an initial episode
- Cesarean section is indicated if genital herpetic lesions are present during labor

CONSULTATION/REFERRAL

- If symptoms persist or frequent recurrences
- Immunocompromised persons

FOLLOW-UP

- Re-evaluate in one week if no improvement
- Screen for other STDs
- Annual Pap smear

EXPECTED COURSE

- Resolution of primary lesions in 14-21 days
- Resolution of recurrent lesions 7-10 days
- Recurrences occur in 50% of persons within 6 months of primary infection

POSSIBLE COMPLICATIONS

- Prolonged severe local disease
- Disseminated disease
- Secondary bacterial infection
- Increased risk for HIV infection

HUMAN PAPILLOMA VIRUS
(Condyloma Acuminata, Genital Warts)

DESCRIPTION

Viral infection transmitted sexually through an epidermal defect that produces warts on genital area. Generally benign and produce no symptoms except the cosmetic appearance.

High degree of cervical dysplasia associated with HVP 16, 18, 31, and 33.

ETIOLOGY

- Human papilloma virus Types 6 and 11 most commonly cause genital warts. These have very low oncogenic potential and usually do not cause cancer
- Types 16, 18, 31, 35, 45, 51, 52, 56, and 58 have the highest oncogenic potential and are usually associated with subclinical infections, but may be found in warts

HPV is present in nearly ALL cervical cancers.

INCIDENCE

- > 25% of women in the US are HPV positive
- 0.5-1 million new cases annually
- Approximately 50% of all sexually active college women may be infected

RISK FACTORS

- Sexual activity
- Multiple sexual partners
- Exposure without barrier protection

ASSESSMENT FINDINGS

- Soft, flesh-colored warts
- Warts are usually painless
- Surface smooth to very rough
- Multiple finger-like projections
- May be confluent
- Perianal warts usually rough and cauliflower-like
- Penile lesions often smooth and papular
- Pruritus
- Irritation
- Bleeding secondary to trauma
- Asymptomatic in subclinical infections
- Common sites of male infection: penile glans and shaft, anus, buttocks; scrotal involvement uncommon
- Common sites of female infection: labia, clitoris, periurethral area, perineum, vagina, cervix, anus, buttocks

DIFFERENTIAL DIAGNOSIS

- Condyloma lata (syphilitic wart)
- Molluscum contagiosum
- Herpes simplex
- If anal genital warts present, must consider biopsy to rule out high grade lesions

DIAGNOSTIC STUDIES

- Acetowhitening can make subclinical lesions visible
- Biopsy for persistent warts or if diagnosis uncertain
- Pap smear
- Colposcopy with biopsy when Pap smear positive (or ASC-H, or persistent HPV even if two

consecutive negative Pap in women 30 and over) or for visible lesions on the cervix

PREVENTION

- Use of condoms provides limited protection
- Immunizations for HPV (Gardasil®, Cervarix®)
- Screen for other STDs

Immunization against HPV is part of the routine schedule from CDC. Ideally, these are offered prior to the onset of sexual activity.

NONPHARMACOLOGIC MANAGEMENT

- Use of condoms
- Abstinence until therapy completed
- CO_2 laser for external genital warts

Sexual abuse should be considered for any child with confirmed papilloma infection.

PHARMACOLOGIC MANAGEMENT

- Consider
  - ◊ Podophyllin resin 10-25% topically every 1-2 weeks
  - ◊ Trichloroacetic acid (TCA) 80-90%
  - ◊ Topical 5-fluorouracil is not recommended by CDC

Self-treatment options for external warts:

- ◊ Imiquimod 5% cream (Aldara®) applied three times weekly until resolution or maximum 16 weeks whichever is less
- ◊ Podofilox 0.5% gel or solution (Condylox®) applied two times daily for 3 days, off 4 days; may repeat every week for 1-4 weeks

PREGNANCY/LACTATION CONSIDERATIONS

- Often grow larger during pregnancy and regress spontaneously after delivery
- May need cesarean section if large and obstruct vagina, otherwise not indicated
- Cryotherapy is treatment of choice
- Podofilox and podophyllin contraindicated during pregnancy
- Imiquimod safety not established in pregnancy

CONSULTATION/REFERRAL

- Refer patients with extensive or refractory disease and intraurethral warts, to gynecologist or dermatologist

FOLLOW-UP

- Every 1-2 weeks for treatment until resolved
- Screen for syphilis
- Pap smear annually
- Monitor sexual partners

EXPECTED COURSE

- Warts clear with treatment or spontaneously regress
- Recurrence is common with all forms of therapy
- Growth may be stimulated by oral contraceptives, immunosuppression, and local trauma

POSSIBLE COMPLICATIONS

- Male urethral obstruction
- Secondary infection
- Aspiration of secretions from infected mothers at delivery may result in laryngeal papillomas in 2-5% of infants

PELVIC INFLAMMATORY DISEASE (PID)

(Salpingitis, Salpingo-oophoritis)

DESCRIPTION

Sexually transmitted infection caused by ascent of microorganisms from vagina and endocervix to uterus, fallopian tubes, ovaries, and contiguous structures.

ETIOLOGY

- Can be caused by *N. gonorrhea, C. trachomatis, Bacteroides, Peptostreptococcus, Peptococcus, E. coli, Diphtheroids, Gardnerella vaginalis*, and other microorganisms

Most infections are polymicrobial, but chlamydia and/or gonorrhea are common pathogens.

INCIDENCE

- 1 million women annually are treated for PID

PID is very rare before puberty and after menopause. Pregnant women and adolescents are very susceptible to PID.

RISK FACTORS

- Intrauterine device
- Sexual activity
- Age < 25 years
- Adolescence
- Multiple sexual partners
- Previous history of PID

ASSESSMENT FINDINGS

- Asymptomatic
- Symptoms often begin during or within one week of menses
- Unusual or new onset menorrhagia, dysmenorrhea
- Lower abdominal pain
- Fever, malaise
- Vaginal discharge or lesion
- Urinary discomfort
- Nausea and vomiting
- Abdominal tenderness
- Cervical motion tenderness
- Adnexal tenderness

PID is often a diagnostic challenge since women may present in a variety of manners.

DIFFERENTIAL DIAGNOSIS

- Appendicitis
- Ectopic pregnancy
- Ruptured ovarian cyst
- Endometriosis

DIAGNOSTIC STUDIES

- Pregnancy test
- CBC (WBC: > 10,500)
- Wet prep
- Pelvic ultrasound
- Complete screen for STDs
- Hepatitis serology
- Syphilis serology
- HIV screen

Start the laboratory assessment with a pregnancy test since this may alter the treatment plan.

DIAGNOSTIC CRITERIA

- Suggested criteria for diagnosis (sufficient for empiric therapy)
    - ◊ Lower abdominal tenderness
    - ◊ Cervical motion tenderness
    - ◊ Adnexal tenderness
- Additional criteria
    - ◊ Temperature > 101°F (38.3°C)
    - ◊ WBC > 10,500
    - ◊ Purulent material obtained with culdocentesis
    - ◊ Abnormal cervical or vaginal discharge
    - ◊ Elevated C-reactive protein/ESR
    - ◊ Adnexal mass
    - ◊ Laboratory evidence of gonorrhea or chlamydia
    - ◊ Cervical specimen on saline slide: increased WBCs
- Elaborate criteria
    - ◊ Histopathologic endometritis on biopsy

◊ Transvaginal sonography or other imaging techniques showing thickened fluid-filled tubes with or without free pelvic fluid or tubo-ovarian complex
◊ Laparoscopic evidence of PID

Minimum criteria for diagnosis by CDC: cervical motion tenderness in an at risk patient.

PREVENTION

- Use of condoms and spermicide provide some degree of protection
- Use of oral contraceptives has been shown to decrease incidence of pelvid inflamatory disease

NONPHARMACOLOGIC MANAGEMENT

- Abstinence until treatment completed
- Evaluation and treatment of sexual partners
- Screen regularly for STDs in at risk patients

PHARMACOLOGIC MANAGEMENT

Outpatient management: CDC recommends any of several different regimens

No specific regimen is considered superior because treatment is empiric until cultures confirm organisms present. However, antibiotic coverage for chlamydia, gonorrhea, anaerobes, gram negative rods, and streptococcus should be included

Outpatient Regimen:

- Consider
  ◊ Cefoxitin (Mefoxin®) 250 mg intramuscular in a single dose PLUS
  ◊ Doxycycline (Vibramycin®) 100 mg orally twice a day for 14 days WITH OR WITHOUT
  ◊ Metronidazole 500 mg orally twice a day for 14 days
- Optional Regimen A
  ◊ Cefoxitin 2 g intramuscular in a single dose and Probenecid 1 g orally administered concurrently in a single dose PLUS
  ◊ Doxycycline 100 mg orally twice a day for 14 days WITH OR WITHOUT
  ◊ Metronidazole 500 mg orally twice a day for 14 days
- Optional Regimen B
  ◊ Other parenteral third-generation cephalosporin (e.g., ceftizoxime or cefotaxime) PLUS
  ◊ Doxycycline 100 mg orally twice a day for 14 days WITH OR WITHOUT
  ◊ Metronidazole 500 mg orally twice a day for 14 days

  (See CDC.gov for alternate treatments)

PID is always associated with anaerobic organisms. As such, many PID experts recommend always giving metronidazole with PID. Doxycycline is not particularly effective in eradicating anaerobic organisms.

PREGNANCY/LACTATION CONSIDERATIONS

- Hospitalization required during pregnancy

CONSULTATION/REFERRAL

- Hospitalization for the following:
  ◊ Can not exclude surgical emergency
  ◊ Pregnancy
  ◊ No clinical response (at 72 hours)
  ◊ Unable to follow-up
  ◊ Tubo-ovarian abscess
  ◊ Severe nausea, vomiting or high fever

FOLLOW-UP

- Close observation of clinical course with re-evaluation in 72 hours; sooner if symptoms worsen
- Test of cure in 7-10 days and at 4-6 weeks posttreatment
- Use of intrauterine device is contraindicated in women with a previous episode of PID

Patient should feel better within 72 hours if empiric selection of antibiotics was appropriate.

EXPECTED COURSE

- Good prognosis if treated early with effective treatment
- Poor prognosis related to poor compliance and repeated infections

POSSIBLE COMPLICATIONS

- Recurrent infection
- Increased risk of ectopic pregnancy
- Infertility
- Sepsis

TRICHOMONIASIS

DESCRIPTION

Sexually transmitted disease which can infect vagina, Skene's ducts, and lower genitourinary tract in women and lower genitourinary tract in men.

ETIOLOGY

- Trichomonas vaginalis, a single-celled, flagellated protozoan parasite

INCIDENCE

- Accounts for 10-25% of all vaginal infections
- Most common in African Amercian women compared to all other races/genders

RISK FACTORS

- Multiple sexual partners
- History of previous STDs

ASSESSMENT FINDINGS

Female:
- Asymptomatic (up to 75%)
- Vaginal discharge that is frothy, copious, and pale yellow to gray-green in color
- Vulvovaginal irritation
- Dysuria
- Foul, fishy odor
- Intense erythema of the vaginal mucosa
- Dyspareunia
- Symptoms may worsen during menstruation

Cervical petechiae ("strawberry cervix") can be visible secondary to tiny hemorrhages.

Male:
- Asymptomatic (almost 80%)
- Urethral discharge
- Dysuria
- Epididymitis
- Prostatitis

DIFFERENTIAL DIAGNOSIS

- Vaginal candidiasis
- Bacterial vaginosis
- Atrophic vaginitis
- Gonococcal or chlamydial infections in women
- Chlamydia urethritis in men

Incubation period is 3-28 days.

DIAGNOSTIC STUDIES

- Wet prep:
  - ◊ Visualization of trichomonads as flagellated, motile cells slightly larger than WBCs
  - ◊ Polymorphonuclear cells
- Vaginal secretion pH: > 4.5 (usually 5.5-6.0)
- Culture usually not needed but may be needed if motile trichomonads not identified and/or symptoms persist/recur
- Pap smear

PREVENTION

- Use of condoms
- Screen for other STDs

NONPHARMACOLOGIC MANAGEMENT

- Abstinence until treatment completed
- Abstain from alcohol if taking metronidazole

PHARMACOLOGIC MANAGEMENT

- Consider
  - ◊ Metronidazole (Flagyl®) 2 g orally in single dose
  - ◊ Tinidazole 2 g orally in a single dose
  - ◊ If still symptomatic: Metronidazole 500 mg twice daily for 7 days
- Treat sexual partner(s)

PREGNANCY/LACTATION CONSIDERATIONS

- Metronidazole 2 g orally in single dose if patient is symptomatic

CONSULTATION/REFERRAL

- None usually needed
- Consider consult regarding treatment of pregnant women

FOLLOW-UP

- No follow-up needed if symptoms resolve

EXPECTED COURSE

- Complete resolution
- Recurrent infection raises possibility of noncompliance, reinfection, or infection with resistant organism

Test of cure is not necessary if both partners have been treated AND patient symptoms resolve.

POSSIBLE COMPLICATIONS

- Recurrent infections

References

Allsworth, J. E., & Peipert, J. F. (2007). Prevalence of bacterial vaginosis: 2001-2004 national health and nutrition examination survey data. Obstetrics and Gynecology, 109(1), 114-120.

Bernstein, K. T., Zenilman, J., Olthoff, G., Marsiglia, V. C., & Erbelding, E. J. (2006). Gonorrhea reinfection among sexually transmitted disease clinic attendees in baltimore, maryland. Sexually Transmitted Diseases, 33(2), 80-86.

Branson, B. M., Handsfield, H. H., Lampe, M. A., Janssen, R. S., Taylor, A. W., Lyss, S. B., et al. (2006). Revised recommendations for HIV testing of adults, adolescents, and pregnant women in health-care settings. MMWR Recomm Rep, 55(RR-14), 1-17; quiz CE11-14.

Centers for Disease Control and Prevention. (2009). 2008 sexually transmitted diseases surveillance. Retrieved from http://www.cdc.gov/std/stats08/main.htm

Dunne, E. F., & Markowitz, L. E. (2006). Genital human papillomavirus infection. Clinical Infectious Diseases, 43(5), 624-629.

Ernst, D., & Lee, A. (2010). Nurse practitioners prescribing reference. New York: Haymarket Media Publication.

Geisler, W. M., Wang, C., Morrison, S. G., Black, C. M., Bandea, C. I., & Hook, E. W., 3rd. (2008). The natural history of untreated chlamydia trachomatis infection in the interval between screening and returning for treatment. Sexually Transmitted Diseases, 35(2), 119-123.

Greer, L., & Wendel, G. D., Jr. (2008). Rapid diagnostic methods in sexually transmitted infections. Infectious Disease Clinics of North America, 22(4), 601-617, v.

Hall, C. S., & Marrazzo, J. D. (2007). Emerging issues in management of sexually transmitted diseases in HIV infection. Curr Infect Dis Rep, 9(6), 518-530.

Hobbs, M. M., van der Pol, B., Totten, P., Gaydos, C. A., Wald, A., Warren, T., et al. (2008). From the nih: Proceedings of a workshop on the importance of self-obtained vaginal specimens for detection of sexually transmitted infections. Sexually Transmitted Diseases, 35(1), 8-13.

Johnston, C., Magaret, A., Selke, S., Remington, M., Corey, L., & Wald, A. (2008). Herpes simplex virus viremia during primary genital infection. Journal of Infectious Diseases, 198(1), 31-34.

Kaplan, J. E., Benson, C., Holmes, K. H., Brooks, J. T., Pau, A., & Masur, H. (2009). Guidelines for prevention and treatment of opportunistic infections in HIV-infected adults and adolescents: Recommendations from CDC, the national institutes of health, and the HIV medicine association of the infectious diseases society of america. MMWR Recomm Rep, 58(RR-4), 1-207; quiz CE201-204.

Mahilum-Tapay, L., Laitila, V., Wawrzyniak, J. J., Lee, H. H., Alexander, S., Ison, C., et al. (2007). New point of care chlamydia rapid test--bridging the gap between diagnosis and treatment: Performance evaluation study. BMJ, 335(7631), 1190-1194.

Majeroni, B. A., & Ukkadam, S. (2007). Screening and treatment for sexually transmitted infections in pregnancy. American Family Physician, 76(2), 265-270.

Markowitz, L. E., Dunne, E. F., Saraiya, M., Lawson, H. W., Chesson, H., & Unger, E. R. (2007). Quadrivalent human papillomavirus vaccine: Recommendations of the advisory committee on immunization practices (acip). MMWR Recomm Rep, 56(RR-2), 1-24.

McClelland, R. S., Sangare, L., Hassan, W. M., Lavreys, L., Mandaliya, K., Kiarie, J., et al. (2007). Infection with trichomonas vaginalis increases the risk of HIV-1 acquisition. Journal of Infectious Diseases, 195(5), 698-702.

Ness, R. B., Smith, K. J., Chang, C. C., Schisterman, E. F., & Bass, D. C. (2006). Prediction of pelvic inflammatory disease among young, single, sexually active women. Sexually Transmitted Diseases, 33(3), 137-142.

Nsuami, M., Taylor, S. N., Sanders, L. S., & Martin, D. H. (2006). Missed opportunities for early detection of chlamydia and gonorrhea in school-based health centers. Sexually Transmitted Diseases, 33(12), 703-705.

Rieg, G., Lewis, R. J., Miller, L. G., Witt, M. D., Guerrero, M., & Daar, E. S. (2008). Asymptomatic sexually transmitted infections in HIV-infected men who have sex with men: Prevalence, incidence, predictors, and screening strategies. Aids Patient Care and STDS, 22(12), 947-954.

Sena, A. C., Miller, W. C., Hobbs, M. M., Schwebke, J. R., Leone, P. A., Swygard, H., et al. (2007). Trichomonas vaginalis infection in male sexual partners: Implications for diagnosis, treatment, and prevention. Clinical Infectious Diseases, 44(1), 13-22.

Seroprevalence of herpes simplex virus type 2 among persons aged 14--49 years --- United States, 2005--2008. (2010). MMWR CDC Surveillance Summaries, 59(15), 456-459.

Syphilis testing algorithms using treponemal tests for initial screening --- four laboratories, New York City, 2005--2006. (2008). MMWR Weekly, 57(32), 872-875.

Update to CDC's sexually transmitted diseases treatment guidelines, 2006: Fluoroquinolones no longer recommended for treatment of gonococcal infections. (2007). MMWR, 56(14), 332-336.

Walker, C. K., & Wiesenfeld, H. C. (2007). Antibiotic therapy for acute pelvic inflammatory disease: The 2006 centers for disease control and prevention sexually transmitted diseases treatment guidelines. Clinical Infectious Diseases, 44 Suppl 3, S111-122.

Workowski, K., Berman, S., & Centers for Disease Control and Prevention. (2006). Sexually transmitted diseases treatment guidelines, 2006. MMWR Recomm Rep, 55(RR-11), 1-94.

Zetola, N. M., Engelman, J., Jensen, T. P., & Klausner, J. D. (2007). Syphilis in the United States: An update for clinicians with an emphasis on HIV coinfection. Mayo Clinic Proceedings, 82(9), 1091-1102.

17

SOCIAL AND PSYCHIATRIC DISORDERS

Psychiatric and Social Disorders

Anxiety 649

Depression and Suicide 653

Alcohol Use Disorder 660

Substance Use Disorder 662

Smoking Cessation 665

Domestic Violence 667

Sexual Assault 669

Anorexia Nervosa 671

Bulimia Nervosa 673

Insomnia 676

References *681*

ANXIETY

DESCRIPTION

A psychic and physical experience of dread, foreboding, apprehension, or panic in response to emotional or physiologic stimuli; may be acute or chronic

Common types of anxiety: acute situational anxiety, generalized anxiety disorder, and panic disorder

Acute situational anxiety: triggered by a specific and identifiable event
Generalized anxiety disorder: anxiety and worry occur most days for > 6 months
Panic disorder: Intense fear that occurs with somatic symptoms (chest pain, palpitations, shortness of breath, dizziness, etc.)

ETIOLOGY

- Behavioral theory: anxiety is the conditioned response to specific environmental stimuli
- Biologic theories
  - ◊ Norepinephrine, serotonin, and γ-aminobutyric acid (GABA) are poorly regulated
  - ◊ The autonomic nervous system responds inappropriately to stimuli
  - ◊ Functional cerebral pathology causes anxiety disorder symptoms

INCIDENCE

- 6-25% lifetime prevalence in general population of U.S.
- Females > Males
- Most prevalent in 20-45 year olds
- Separation anxiety is the most common reason given for school refusal (mean age 9 years)

Anxiety is the most common psychiatric disorder in the U.S.

RISK FACTORS

Organic causes:
- Organic syndromes: endocrinopathies, cardiorespiratory disorders, anemia
- Use of or withdrawal from medications and substances
  - ◊ Alcohol
  - ◊ Antihypertensives
  - ◊ Caffeine, including analgesics containing caffeine
  - ◊ Cocaine, marijuana, hallucinogens
  - ◊ Corticosteroids
  - ◊ Lidocaine
  - ◊ Oral contraceptives
  - ◊ Nonsteroidal anti-inflammatories (NSAIDs)
  - ◊ Withdrawal from selective serotonin reuptake inhibitors (SSRIs)
- Family history

Psychosocial stress:
- Marital discord
- Medical illness
- Job-related stress
- Financial problems

Psychiatric disorders:
- Major depression
- Panic disorders
- Personality disorders
- Schizophrenia

ASSESSMENT FINDINGS

Children:
- Excessive anxiety about separation after preschool age
- Unrealistic worry about harm to self or family
- Somatic complaints in absence of physical illness
- Persistent worry about past behavior, competence, or future events

Adults:
- Complaints of apprehension, restlessness, edginess, distractibility
- Insomnia
- Somatic complaints
  - ◊ Fatigue
  - ◊ Paresthesias, near syncope, derealization, dizziness
  - ◊ Palpitations, tachycardia, chest pain/tightness
  - ◊ Dyspnea, hyperventilation
  - ◊ Nausea, vomiting, diarrhea
- Excessive rumination

DIFFERENTIAL DIAGNOSIS

- Any medical condition that involves stimulation of the sympathetic nervous system
  - ◊ Arrhythmias, MI, valvular disease
  - ◊ Endocrinopathies: hyperthyroidism, Cushing's syndrome, hypoglycemia, electrolyte imbalances, menopause
  - ◊ Medication and substance reactions
  - ◊ Medication and substance withdrawal
  - ◊ Anemia
  - ◊ Asthma, COPD, pulmonary embolism, pneumothorax

DIAGNOSTIC STUDIES

- TSH
- CBC, urinalysis
- Urine drug screen
- Focus on medical conditions for which patient is already being treated
- Direct attention toward arrhythmias, hyperthyroidism, drugs
- Evaluate prominent constellation of symptoms
- Psychologic testing
  - ◊ Interview based on DSM-IV criteria
  - ◊ Hamilton Anxiety Scale
  - ◊ Zung Anxiety Self-Assessment

NONPHARMACOLOGIC MANAGEMENT

- Psychotherapy
  - ◊ Education regarding diagnosis, treatment plan, and prognosis
  - ◊ Support and empathic listening
- Behavioral therapy
  - ◊ Relaxation techniques
  - ◊ Reconditioning: exposure to feared stimuli in controlled setting to develop tolerance and eventually eradicate the anxiety response
- General measures
  - ◊ Regular exercise
  - ◊ Serial office visits

Limiting caffeine intake may help reduce symptoms of anxiety. Avoid alcohol consumption because this increases the risk of drug interactions and is associated with high rates of abuse.

PHARMACOLOGIC MANAGEMENT

- Should be of limited duration, with intent of allowing patient to benefit from behavioral treatments
  - ◊ Drugs should play an adjunctive role, except in panic disorder
  - ◊ Drugs reduce, but do not eradicate symptoms

Tricyclic antidepressants (TCAs) and Selective Serotonin Re-uptake Inhibitors (SSRIs) may take 2-4 weeks before therapeutic response is realized by patient.
Use of benzodiazepines (BNZ) until TCA or SSRI become effective is a commonly employed strategy.

- Situational anxiety
  - ◊ Benzodiazepines (BNZ) (short-term, up to one month)
- Generalized anxiety disorder
  - ◊ BuSpar®
    Adult: 7.5 mg twice daily, usual range 20-30 mg/day
    Child: < 6 yr: not recommended
    6-17 yr: 7.5 mg-30 mg twice daily
    Tabs: 5 mg, 10 mg, 15 mg, 30 mg
  - ◊ Selective Serotonin Re-uptake Inhibitors (SSRIs)
- Panic disorder
  - ◊ Selective Serotonin Re-uptake Inhibitors (SSRIs)
  - ◊ Tricyclic antidepressants (TCAs)
  - ◊ Benzodiazepines (BNZ)
- Obsessive-compulsive disorder
  - ◊ Tricyclic antidepressants (TCAs)
  - ◊ Selective Serotonin Re-uptake Inhibitors (SSRIs)

ANXIETY PHARMACOLOGIC MANAGEMENT

Class	Drug Generic name (Trade name®)	Dosage How supplied	Comments
Benzodiazepines *binds at stereo specific receptors at several sites in the CNS* **General comments** Depressant activity is produced from mild impairment to hypnosis. Do not engage in activities that require mental alertness while taking All benzodiazepines have abuse potential Do not mix with other CNS depressants, like alcohol, sedative effect is enhanced Tolerance develops with daily use Use for short periods of time (2-4 weeks)	**alprazolam**	**Immediate Release** **Adults > 18 years:** *Initial*: 0.25 mg to 0.5 mg three times daily *Max*: 4 mg daily in divided doses **Elderly or debilitated:** 0.25 mg 2-3 times daily **Extended Release** **Adult:** 0.5-1 mg daily in the AM; increase at intervals of at least 3-4 days *Usual*: 3-6 mg per day *Max*: 10 mg/day	• Pregnancy Category D; Class IV • May increase dose at intervals of 3-4 days. Do not increase by more than 1 mg daily • Lowest effective dose should be used • Reassess need to discontinue treatment frequently • Elderly are especially sensitive to the effects of benzodiazepines • DO NOT MIX WITH ketoconazole, itraconazole • Monitor for seizures during withdrawal • Withdrawal can occur with abrupt withdrawal, especially after 12 weeks • Caution in using in patients with renal, hepatic, or pulmonary dysfunction
	Xanax	*Tabs: 0.25 mg, 0.5 mg, 1 mg, 2 mg*	
	Xanax XR	*Ext release tabs: 0.5 mg, 1 mg, 2 mg, 3 mg*	
	diazepam	**Adults:** *Initial*: 2-10 mg two to four times daily depending on severity of symptoms **Elderly or debilitated**: 2-2.5 mg 1 or 2 times initially; increase gradually as tolerated	• Pregnancy Category D; Class IV • Lowest effective dose should be used • Reassess need to discontinue treatment frequently • Elderly are especially sensitive to the effects of benzodiazepines • Contraindicated in acute narrow angle glaucoma • Monitor for seizures during withdrawal • Caution in using in patients with renal, hepatic, or pulmonary dysfunction
	Valium	*Tabs: 2 mg, 5 mg, 10 mg*	
	lorazepam	**Adults:** *Initial*: 2-3 mg/d given two or three times daily **Elderly or debilitated**: 1-2 mg/day in divided doses	• Pregnancy Category D; Class IV • Increase gradually to avoid adverse effects • Contraindicated in narrow angle glaucoma • Lowest effective dose should be used • Reassess need to discontinue treatment frequently • Elderly are especially sensitive to the effects of benzodiazepines • Caution in using in patients with renal, hepatic, or pulmonary dysfunction
	Ativan	*Tabs: 0.5 mg, 1 mg, 2 mg scored*	

continued

Social/Psych Disorders

Social/Psych Disorders

ANXIETY PHARMACOLOGIC MANAGEMENT

Class	Drug Generic name (Trade name®)	Dosage How supplied	Comments
Non-Benzodiazepine Anti-anxiety Agents	**buspirone** Buspar	**Adults**: *Initial*: 7.5 mg twice daily; *Max initial dose:* 15 mg daily Increase dose 5 mg/day at intervals of 2-3 days *Usual*: 20-30 mg/day *Max*: 60 mg/day *Tabs: 5 mg, 7.5 mg, 10 mg, 15 mg, 30 mg*	• Pregnancy Category B • Do not administer to patients taking MAO inhibitors • May produce functional impairment; but not usually as much as benzodiazepines • Drug interactions with 3A4 medications including calcium channel blockers, grapefruit juice, others • Dose adjustment needed for patients with renal, hepatic function
	duloxetine Cymbalta	**Adults**: 60 mg once daily *Alternative*: 30 mg once daily for one week, then increase to 60 mg once daily *Max*: 120 mg but no evidence that doses > 60 mg confer greater benefit *Caps: 20 mg, 30 mg, 60 mg caps*	• Pregnancy Category C • May increase the risk of suicidal thinking and behavior in patients with major depressive disorder • Do not administer to patients taking MAO inhibitors • Avoid in patients with uncontrolled narrow angle glaucoma • May be given without regard to meals • Increased risk of bleeding with NSAIDs, aspirin, warfarin • Do not prescribe for patients with substantial alcohol use • Monitor for orthostatic hypotension and syncope within first week of therapy
	escitalopram Lexapro	**Adults:** 10 mg once daily *Max*: 20 mg daily *Tabs: 5 mg, 10 mg, 20 mg* *Susp: 5 mg/5 mL*	• Pregnancy Category C • May increase the risk of suicidal thinking and behavior in patients with major depressive disorder • Increased dose should occur after a minimum of one week • Separate MAO inhibitors by at least 14 days • Dosage adjustment needed for severe renal impairment, hepatic impairment and elderly • Gradual dose reduction is recommended

PREGNANCY/LACTATION CONSIDERATIONS

- Benzodiazepines contraindicated in pregnancy and lactation
- TCAs contraindicated in pregnancy
- SSRIs contraindicated in first trimester but may be continued by midwife/obstetrician

CONSULTATION/REFERRAL

- Parent/child or family intervention
- Evidence of substance abuse
- Disabling symptoms
- Symptoms that worsen despite treatment

FOLLOW-UP

- Regular follow-up visits are important to reinforce education regarding nonpharmacologic management and proper use of medications
- Avoid prescribing anxiolytics by telephone
- Remain alert to signs of medication misuse
- Tricyclic antidepressants require periodic serum levels

EXPECTED COURSE

- Anxiety in children can be a precursor to agoraphobia or panic disorder in adulthood
- Treatment of medical cause usually, but not always, initiates improvement
- Short-term anxiety disorders usually respond well to treatment
- Obsessive compulsive disorder requires long-term pharmacologic therapy along with psychotherapy

Generalized anxiety disorder is a chronic disease with many exacerbations and relapses. Exacerbations are more common during times of stress; relapses more common in the first year of if medication is discontinued.

POSSIBLE COMPLICATIONS

- Work and school related difficulties
- Self medication leading to alcohol abuse, benzodiazepine dependence
- Social impairment
- Cardiac arrhythmias related to TCA use
- Falls due to sedating effects of medications, especially in the elderly

DEPRESSION AND SUICIDE

DESCRIPTION

- Depression is a constellation of signs and symptoms that is an abnormal reaction to life's difficulties. Disturbances in cognitive, emotional, behavioral, and somatic regulations are involved. Depressed mood, and loss of interest or pleasure are the major symptoms.
- Suicide is self-inflicted death. Attempted suicide is a potentially lethal act that does not result in death.

Anhedonia is a loss of pleasure or interest in things which had always given joy or pleasure. Depressed patients exhibit anhedonia.

ETIOLOGY

- Impaired synthesis and/or metabolism of the neurotransmitters norepinephrine, serotonin, and/or dopamine
- Evidence indicates genetic basis

Serotonin produces calmness and relaxed states of being.
Norepinephrine and dopamine enhance productivity, ambition, and ability to concentrate.

INCIDENCE

Depression:

- Will affect 5-20% of the U.S. population at some time
- 1.5-3 times more common among those with an affected first-degree relative
- Affects 2% of preadolescents and 5% of adolescents in the U.S.

Suicide:

- Successful suicide: Males > Females
- Suicide attempts: Females > Males
- Threefold increase in adolescent suicide reports over the last 40 years
- 9-18% of preadolescents with nonpsychiatric diagnoses entertain suicidal ideations

RISK FACTORS

- Female gender
- Psychosocial stressors
- Postpartum period
- Physical or chronic illness, especially migraines and back pain
- Prior episodes of depression
- Family history
- Alcohol or substance abuse
- Children with behavioral disorders, especially hyperactivity
- Retirement, aging, significant losses (death of a spouse, loss of a job, etc.)

ASSESSMENT FINDINGS

Children:

- Anorexia
- Sleep disturbance
- Apathy
- Developmental delay
- Anxiety, irritability, cries easily
- Aggression, hyperactivity
- School problems
- GI or other somatic complaints

Adolescents:

- Similar to adults
- Impulsivity
- Fatigue
- Hopelessness
- Substance abuse

Adults:

- Depressed mood
- Anhedonia
- Decreased or increased appetite
- Sleep disorder
- Psychomotor agitation or retardation
- Fatigue, loss of energy
- Feelings of worthlessness, inappropriate guilt
- Recurrent thoughts of death

In adults, depression is likely if the patient experiences anhedonia or depression and (any 4 or more of the following): change in appetite, sleep pattern, fatigue, psychomotor retardation or agitation, poor self-image, difficulty concentrating, or suicidal ideation.

DIFFERENTIAL DIAGNOSIS

Children:

- Bipolar disorder
- Attention deficit disorder
- Separation anxiety
- Chronic physical illness
- Conduct disorder
- Physical or sexual abuse

Adults:

- Bipolar disorder
- Substance abuse
- Physical illness: organic brain diseases, diabetes, liver, or renal failure
- Grief reaction
- Other psychiatric disorders
- Medication abuse/use
- Medication withdrawal
- Hypothyroidism, B12 deficiency
- Dementia

DIAGNOSTIC STUDIES

Structured interviews/questionnaires:

- The Children's Depression Inventory
- Children's Depression Scale
- Depression Self-Rating Scale
- Center for Epidemiological Studies Depression Scale for Children
- Beck's Depression Inventory
- Child Behavior Checklist for Ages 4-18 Years
- Pediatric Symptom Checklist
- Zung Self-rating Depression Scale
- Halstead-Reitan battery: helps distinguish dementia from depression
- Yesavage's Geriatric Depression scale

Laboratory studies do not diagnose depression, but, are used to rule out other conditions.

Laboratory studies:

- TSH; indicated for women >age 50 years to rule out hypothyroidism
- Laboratory tests specific to depression are under clinical investigation (serotonin, dopamine,

norepinephrine levels)
- Urine screen for substance use disorders
- ECG as baseline to rule out arrhythmias or heart block before instituting tricyclic antidepressants (TCAs)

TCA may provoke arrhythmias in patients with subclinical sinus node dysfunction.

PREVENTION

- Maintain a high index of suspicion in adolescents and adults with family or personal history of depression, or with chronic illness or recent loss
- Question persons suspected of suicide intent regarding plan and availability of method
- Routine questioning regarding use of alcohol and drugs starting during adolescence

NONPHARMACOLOGIC MANAGEMENT

- Identify suicidal risk, plan, and intent
- Establish safe environment: ensure patient safety in least restrictive environment
  - ◊ Negotiate suicide contract
- Provide community resources, suicide hotline
- Suicide threats should be interpreted as a communication of desperation and are to be taken seriously
- Psychoeducation
  - ◊ Ongoing information regarding illness, symptoms, prognosis, and therapy
  - ◊ Include interpersonal relationships, work, other health related needs
  - ◊ Discourage major life changes while in a depressive state
  - ◊ Help set realistic, attainable, concrete goals
  - ◊ Educate regarding importance of avoiding alcohol
- Psychotherapy
  - ◊ Establish and maintain a supportive therapeutic relationship
  - ◊ Remain available during times of crisis
  - ◊ Maintain vigilance for signs of destructive impulses
  - ◊ Strengthen expectations of help and hope for the future
  - ◊ Enlist support of others in patient's social network
- Electroconvulsive therapy (ECT)
  - ◊ Indicated for depression in which a rapid antidepressant response is imperative: depression coupled with psychotic features, catatonic stupor, severe suicidality, or severe nutritional compromise
  - ◊ Indicated for patients who prefer this method of treatment, or who have responded unsatisfactorily to antidepressant medication in the past
  - ◊ High rate of therapeutic success
  - ◊ Chief side effect is transient postictal confusional state, and memory impairment which resolves in a few weeks
- Light therapy
  - ◊ Particularly effective for seasonal affective disorder
  - ◊ Exposure to bright white artificial light for 30 minutes or more in morning and/or evening
  - ◊ May be used along with pharmacotherapy

Psychotherapeutic interventions in conjunction with pharmacologic therapy are superior to either when used alone.

PHARMACOLOGIC MANAGEMENT

- Determine coexisting substance use disorders and general medical conditions
- Cyclic antidepressants (tri and tetracyclics)
- Selective serotonin-reuptake inhibitors
- Monoamine oxidase inhibitors are not used first or second line because of numerous food and drug interactions
- Others
  - ◊ Effexor®
  - ◊ Wellbutrin®

TCAs and SSRIs are equally efficacious but the SSRIs have a better side effect profile and would not be fatal if a month's supply were taken at once.

ANTI-DEPRESSANT PHARMACOLOGIC MANAGEMENT

Class	Drug Generic name (Trade name®)	Dosage How supplied	Comments
Selective Serotonin Reuptake Inhibitors (SSRIs) General comments May increase the risk of suicidal thinking and behavior in patients with major depressive disorder Monitor patient closely for clinical worsening, suicidality, unusual changes in behavior especially during the intial months of therapy	**fluoxetine**	**Adults:** 20 mg once daily Increase dose after several weeks if insufficient clinical response. Doses greater than 20 mg may be administered as single or twice daily dosing *Max*: 80 mg daily **Children 8-17 years:** *Initial*: 10-20 mg daily. If started on 10 mg/day, increase after 1 week to 20 mg/day. Lower weight children: start at 10 mg/day; may increase after several weeks to 20 mg/day	• Pregnancy Category C • Do not administer to patients within 5 weeks of taking MAO inhibitors • Avoid in patients with uncontrolled narrow angle glaucoma • No dosage adjustment recommended for renal dysfunction or elderly. However, elderly may have greater sensitivity • Monitor for weight change during treatment • May alter glycemic control (hypoglycemia during use, hyperglycemia after discontinuing) • Discontinuation should take place gradually rather than abruptly
Write Rx for smallest practical amount Full effect may be delayed for 4 weeks or longer	Prozac	*Tabs: 10 mg, 20 mg, 40 mg* *Solution: 20 mg/5 mL*	
May increase risk of bleeding especially in combination with aspirin, NSAIDs, warfarin Do not abruptly stop usage	Prozac weekly	*Caps: 90 mg e-c delayed release pellets*	• Pregnancy Category C • Used in maintenance phase • Start 7 days after last dose of fluoxetine 20 mg when switching from daily dose • See fluoxetine for precautions
Monitor for hyponatremia Drug interactions may occur with many medications given in combination with SSRIs. Check compatibility Treatment should be sustained for several months Avoid alcohol when taking SSRIs	**citalopram**	**Adults**: 20 mg once daily. May increase to 40 mg daily after at least one week in between dose increases **Elderly and hepatic impairment:** 20 mg daily; 40 mg/day only for nonresponding patients *Max*: 60 mg daily	• Pregnancy Category C • At least 14 days should elapse between MAO inhibitor and administration of citalopram • Avoid in patients with uncontrolled narrow angle glaucoma • No dosage adjustment necessary for renal impairment • Discontinuation should take place gradually rather than abruptly
May cause decrease in libido	Celexa	*Tabs: 10 mg, 20 mg, 40 mg*	

continued

Class	Drug Generic name (Trade name®)	Dosage How supplied	Comments
	paroxetine	**Adults**: *Initial*: 20 mg in morning; may increase dose in 10 mg increments at 1 week intervals *Max*: 50 mg daily **Elderly, debilitated:** *Initial*: 10 mg *Max*: 40 mg daily	• Pregnancy Category D • At least 14 days should elapse between MAO inhibitor and administration of paroxetine • Avoid in patients with uncontrolled narrow angle glaucoma • Cautious use in history of seizures
	Paxil	*Tabs: 10 mg, 20 mg, 30 mg, 40 mg* *Susp: 10 mg/5 mL*	• Discontinuation should take place gradually rather than abruptly; consider a 10 mg/day at weekly intervals before discontinuing
	Paxil CR	**Adults**: *Initial*: 25 mg daily; adjust by 12.5 mg/day at weekly intervals *Max*: 62.5 mg/day **Elderly, debilitated:** *Initial*: 12.5 mg/day *Max*: 50 mg/day	• See paroxetine
	sertraline	**Adults**: 50 mg daily in AM or PM; may increase at 1 week intervals *Max*: 200 mg/day	• Pregnancy Category C • At least 14 days should elapse between MAO inhibitor and administration of citalopram • Avoid in patients with uncontrolled narrow angle glaucoma
	Zoloft	*Tabs: 25 mg, 50 mg, 100 mg* *Oral concentrate: 20 mg/mL*	• No dosage adjustment necessary for renal impairment • Need dosage adjustment for hepatic dysfunction • Dilute oral concentrate before administering in 4 oz. water, ginger ale, lemon/lime soda, orange juice

continued

ANTI-DEPRESSANT PHARMACOLOGIC MANAGEMENT

Class	Drug Generic name (Trade name®)	Dosage How supplied	Comments
Serotonin and Norepinephrine Reuptake Inhibitors (SNRIs) **General comments** Antidepressants increase the risk of suicide in adolescents and young adults < 24 years. Close monitoring by family members and caregivers is advised especially during the first few months of treatment	**duloxetine** Cymbalta	**Adults**: 60 mg once daily *Alternative*: 30 mg once daily for one week, then increase to 60 mg once daily *Max*: 120 mg but no evidence doses > 60 mg confer greater benefit *Caps: 20 mg, 30 mg, 60 mg caps*	• Pregnancy Category C • May increase the risk of suicidal thinking and behavior in patients with major depressive disorder • Do not administer to patients taking MAO inhibitors • Avoid in patients with uncontrolled narrow angle glaucoma • May be given without regard to meals • Increased risk of bleeding with NSAIDs, aspirin, warfarin • Do not prescribe for patients with substantial alcohol use • Monitor for orthostatic hypotension and syncope within first week of therapy
Tricyclic Antidepressants **General comments** Antidepressants increase the risk of suicide in adolescents and young adults < 24 years. Close monitoring by family members and caregivers is advised especially during the first few months of treatment	**amitriptyline** Elavil	**Adults**: 75 mg in divided doses in late afternoon or at bedtime *Alternate*: 50 to 100 mg at bedtime. May increase by 25-50 mg *Max*: 150 mg/day **Elderly and adolescents**: 10 mg three times daily *Alternate*: 20 mg at bedtime *Tabs: 10 mg, 25 mg, 50 mg, 75 mg, 100 mg, 150 mg*	• Pregnancy Category C • Prescribe smallest amount feasible. Deaths may occur from overdosage with this class of medications • May cause sedation. Administer at bedtime if feasible • Do not administer to patients taking MAO inhibitors • Cautious use in patients with cardiovascular disorders. May cause sinus tachycardia, prolonged QT interval, or arrhythmias • Close supervision if given to patients with hyperthyroidism or being treated for hyperthyroidism • When possible, should be discontinued prior to elective surgery • Fluctuations in blood sugar are possible • Cautious use in patients with hepatic dysfunction

continued

ANTI-DEPRESSANT PHARMACOLOGIC MANAGEMENT

Class	Drug Generic name (Trade name®)	Dosage How supplied	Comments
Norepinephrine and Dopamine Reuptake Inhibitors General comments Antidepressants increase the risk of suicide in adolescents and young adults < 24 years. Close monitoring by family members and caregivers is advised especially during the first few months of treatment	**bupropion** Wellbutrin XL Wellbutrin SR	**Adults**: 150 mg initially with target of 300 mg daily given in the AM. If tolerated, can increase to 300 mg as soon as 4 days after starting 150 mg dose Tabs: 150 mg, 300 mg **Adults**: 150 mg given in AM initially. Target of 300 mg daily given in divided doses Must separate twice daily doses by 8 or more hours. If tolerated, can increase to 300 mg in divided doses as soon as 4 days after starting 150 mg dose. *Max*: 200 mg given twice daily	• Pregnancy Category C • Full antidepressant effect may not be seen for 4 weeks • Dosage adjustment in patients with renal or hepatic dysfunction • Contraindicated in seizure disorder, current or prior diagnosis of bulimia • Contraindicated in patients undergoing abrupt cessation of alcohol or benzodiazepines • At least 14 days should elapse between MAO inhibitors and bupropion • When switching patients from wellbutrin tablets or from Wellbutrin SR tablets, give the same total daily dose as a single dose of wellbutrin XR

CONSULTATION/REFERRAL

- Psychiatrist if patient has suicide plan, or for ECT if severe major depression is coupled with psychosis, nutritional compromise, or suicidality. Make appointment and referral at time of visit
- Indications for inpatient psychiatric treatment
  - ◊ Unable to adequately care for self or cooperate with outpatient treatment
  - ◊ Have suicidal or homicidal ideation and plan, particularly if method is violent
  - ◊ Lack of psychosocial support
  - ◊ Complicating psychiatric or medical conditions that make outpatient treatment unsafe

In the elderly, depression often coexists with dementia.

FOLLOW-UP

- Follow-up within 2 weeks after initiating medication or sooner if patient's condition dictates
- Antidepressant medications should be continued for at least 4-6 months after complete remission of symptoms
- Antidepressant medications should be tapered rather than abruptly discontinued
- Patients with multiple prior episodes of depression may require long-term pharmacologic management
- After recovery from a suicide attempt, explore frame of mind to determine whether suicidal thoughts persist
- Educate regarding constructive methods of seeking help for future problems

EXPECTED COURSE

- 60-70% response rates to antidepressants of all classes
- Patients take 4-6 weeks to fully respond to medication management
- High relapse rate during the first 8 weeks after resolution of symptoms

POSSIBLE COMPLICATIONS

- Suicide: overdose of tricyclics is potentially lethal
- Bizarre behavior may endanger social relationships and reputation
- Complicating psychiatric or medical conditions
- Substance abuse resulting from attempts to self medicate

ALCOHOL USE DISORDER

Social/Psych Disorders

DESCRIPTION

Alcohol *abuse* is a pattern of inappropriate alcohol consumption for one month or more, without the development of physical tolerance. This may include drinking in the presence of a medical condition, or when driving. It may or may not precede alcohol *dependence*. In alcohol dependence, tolerance develops, causing cellular changes, altered metabolism, and the withdrawal symptoms that result when blood alcohol levels drop.

ETIOLOGY

- Combination of social, cultural, biological and emotional factors
- Probable genetic influence

INCIDENCE

- Males > Females (3:1)
- Predominant age is 18-25 years
- Heavy drinking (> 5 drinks/day) is reported by 10% of adult men and 2% of women
- 40% of unintentional injuries involving adolescents are alcohol-related
- Alcohol abuse implicated in 50% of traffic fatalities, 67% of drowning and murders, 70-80% of deaths in fires, and 35% of suicides

RISK FACTORS

- Genetic vulnerability: family history
- Use of other psychoactive substances
- Alcohol use in peer group or by parents, cultural acceptance of alcohol abuse
- Recent stressful life events
- Low socioeconomic status
- Unemployment

ASSESSMENT FINDINGS

- Reliability of patient reporting is highly variable
- Medical problems associated with alcohol dependence
  - ◊ Psychosis, dementia, memory impairment, blackouts, insomnia
  - ◊ Nausea, vomiting, peptic ulcer disease, abdominal pain
  - ◊ Hepatitis, cirrhosis, pancreatitis
  - ◊ Thiamine deficiency: anorexia, weight loss, peripheral neuropathy, irritability, tremors
  - ◊ Cardiomyopathy, hypertension, arrhythmias
  - ◊ Aspiration pneumonia, bronchitis
  - ◊ Cancer of oropharynx, larynx, esophagus, and liver
  - ◊ Impotence
  - ◊ Cushingoid appearance, gynecomastia
  - ◊ Signs of accidents (e.g., fractures, bruises, burns)
  - ◊ Poor hygiene, plethoric facies
- Social consequences of alcohol abuse
  - ◊ Divorce
  - ◊ Depression
  - ◊ Suicide
  - ◊ Domestic violence
  - ◊ Arrests, legal problems
  - ◊ Unemployment, employment problems
  - ◊ Poverty
  - ◊ Unsafe sexual behavior, sexually transmitted diseases
  - ◊ Children may experience abnormal psychosocial development related to parental alcohol abuse

Delays in maturation and sexual development are common in adolescents who abuse alcohol.

DIFFERENTIAL DIAGNOSIS

- Depression, anxiety, bipolar disorder
- Essential hypertension, ischemic heart disease
- Peptic ulcer disease, viral gastroenteritis, cholelithiasis, viral hepatitis, pancreatitis
- Primary endocrine disorder
- Solar skin damage
- Primary seizure disorder

DIAGNOSTIC STUDIES

- Blood alcohol levels may be detected; breath alcohol commonly used
- Liver function tests (γ-glutamyltransferase, ALT, AST) abnormal in 50% of cases
- AST : ALT > 2.0
- Mean corpuscular volume (MCV): elevated
- Uric acid, PT, triglycerides elevated
- Brief screening questionnaires: all have limitations, may be less sensitive and specific in adolescents

◊ CAGE questionnaire: most popular; less sensitive for early or heavy drinking
◊ Michigan Alcoholism Screening Test (MAST): highly sensitive and specific, but too long for routine screening
◊ Alcohol Use Disorders Identification Test (AUDIT): sensitive and specific for hazardous or harmful drinking
- Biopsy of liver diagnostic of alcoholic hepatitis or cirrhosis

PREVENTION

- Screen all adolescents and adults concerning alcohol utilizing patient inquiry or standardized instruments
- Offer counseling to problem drinkers
- Careful discussion with all adolescents regarding alcohol use, including regular advice to abstain from alcohol
- Counsel parents regarding their use of alcohol in the home

NONPHARMACOLOGIC MANAGEMENT

- Substance abuse counseling
  ◊ Establish a therapeutic relationship
  ◊ Make medical office off-limits for substance abuse
  ◊ Present information about negative health consequences
  ◊ Involve family and other support
  ◊ Set goals
  ◊ Involve community treatment services
- Balanced diet: common deficiencies are folate, thiamine, magnesium, phosphate, and zinc
- Provide education about Alcoholics Anonymous
- Treatment for adolescents should be developmentally appropriate, peer oriented, and involve the family

PHARMACOLOGIC MANAGEMENT

- Detoxification: symptoms of withdrawal (e.g., seizures, hallucinations, and delirium) typically begin within 12 hours of cessation of alcohol use and resolve within 5 days
  ◊ Lorazepam (Ativan®) Initially 2-3 mg daily in 2-3 divided doses, elderly: 1-2 mg daily, divided
  ◊ Chlordiazepoxide (Librium®) Initially 5-10 mg 3-4 times daily Elderly: 5 mg 2-4 times daily
  ◊ Oxazepam (Serax®) Taper according to patient response. Elderly may require higher benzodiazepine doses and a longer detoxification period. Dosing: 10-15 mg 3-4 times daily Tabs: 10 mg, 15 mg, 30 mg
- Naltrexone (ReVia®) reduces craving for alcohol Dosage: 50 mg daily Mon-Fri and 100 mg on Saturdays. Tabs: 50 mg
- Disulfiram (Antabuse®)
  ◊ Produces sensitivity to alcohol which results in a highly unpleasant reaction when alcohol is ingested
  ◊ Patient must want to remain in a state of enforced sobriety
  ◊ Should never be administered to a patient who is in a state of denial, or who is intoxicated, or without his full knowledge
  ◊ Dosage: abstain for at least 12 hours prior, initial dose 500 mg daily for 1-2 weeks, then 250 mg daily. Tabs: 250 mg
- Thiamine (B1) supplementation due to poor thiamine absorption associated with alcohol ingestion (intramuscular or intravenous initially, then oral)
- Folic acid, B6, B12, multivitamin, magnesium sulfate

First dose of benzodiazepine should make patient sleepy. Dose is tapered to control withdrawal symptoms.

PREGNANCY/LACTATION CONSIDERATIONS

- Pregnant women at high risk for sexually transmitted diseases, hepatitis, anemia, tuberculosis, hypertension, and failure to obtain prenatal care
- Alcohol passes through the placenta, resulting in higher risk of birth defects, fetal alcohol syndrome, cardiovascular problems, impaired growth and development, prematurity, low birth weight, and stillbirth
- Neonate may suffer from withdrawal
- Abstinence recommended when planning conception, and throughout pregnancy
- Mothers with alcohol abuse problems often need education in parenting and nutrition

CONSULTATION/REFERRAL

- Indications for inpatient detoxification treatment:
  ◊ Patients in severe withdrawal or with a prior history of delirium tremens
  ◊ History of very heavy alcohol use and high tolerance
  ◊ Severe comorbid medical or psychiatric disorder
  ◊ History of repeatedly failing to benefit from outpatient detoxification
- Alcoholics Anonymous for support and education

- Family support groups (e.g., Al-Anon, Alateen)
- Addiction specialist

FOLLOW-UP

- Daily visits during detoxification, reduce to weekly, then less frequently
- Involvement in some form of aftercare is a strong predictor of a successful outcome
- Aftercare should include coping skills training to prevent relapse

The first 3 months after withdrawal are the most important in predicting long term success.

EXPECTED COURSE

- Relapses are common and should be expected
- Patients may learn from relapse, resulting in ability to pursue complete recovery
- Long-term sobriety is attainable

POSSIBLE COMPLICATIONS

- Accidents, trauma
- Social problems: financial, marital, occupational, legal, parental
- Psychiatric problems: suicide, depression
- Cirrhosis, GI malignancies
- Cardiovascular disorders
- Respiratory problems
- Neurologic problems
- Hematologic disorders
- Metabolic disorders
- Obstetric problems
- Oropharyngeal and esophageal cancers
- Fetal alcohol syndrome

SUBSTANCE USE DISORDERS

DESCRIPTION

A maladaptive pattern of substance use leading to impairment or distress; substances commonly abused are alcohol, amphetamines, cocaine, hallucinogens, inhalants, marijuana, sedatives, and steroids. Manifestations of impairment or distress involve school, work, family, legal, physical, or social difficulties.

ETIOLOGY

- Biological factors: the intrinsic addictiveness of a drug coupled with inherited familial biologic markers
- Psychological factors: increased prevalence of certain psychiatric problems (e.g., affective disorders, borderline personality, antisocial personality)
- Social factors: increased prevalence among economically and culturally impoverished

The brain's dopamine system is stimulated when mood altering substances are consumed.

INCIDENCE

- Predominant age is young adult (age 16-25 years)
- Males > Females

RISK FACTORS

- Personal history of substance abuse
- Family history of substance abuse
- Substance abuse among peers
- Psychiatric illness (e.g., depression, anxiety, bipolar disorder)
- Chronic pain
- Health professionals

ASSESSMENT FINDINGS

Results of intoxication or withdrawal:

- Accidents, trauma
- Legal difficulties
- Physical signs
  - ◊ Opioid intoxication: somnolence, bradycardia, hypotension, hypoventilation, pupillary constriction
  - ◊ *Opioid withdrawal*: tearing, anxiety, disturbed sleep, nausea, vomiting, diarrhea, pain,

restlessness, rhinorrhea

- ◊ *Inhalant intoxication*: sedation, slurred speech, unsteady gait, irritation of the nasal and ocular tissues, foul odor to breath, paint on the body or clothing, excitation, depression, impulsiveness, exhilaration
- ◊ *Sedative intoxication*: sedation, somnolence, disinhibition, staggering gait, slurred speech, depressed respirations, slowed pulse, diminished reflexes
- ◊ *Sedative withdrawal*: insomnia, restlessness, tremor, anxiety, poor sleep, poor appetite, limb twitching, agitation, seizures, fever
- ◊ *Cannabis reactions* (marijuana or hashish): distortion of time, space, sound, and color, paranoia, disorientation
- ◊ *Stimulant intoxication* (cocaine or amphetamine): confusion, paranoia, restlessness, irritability, delusions, tremor, anxiety, tachycardia, hypertension, high fever, convulsion, coma
- ◊ *Stimulant withdrawal*: somnolence, depressed mood, fatigue, strong desire to obtain more stimulants
- ◊ *Hallucinogen intoxication*: panic reaction, hallucinations, loss of contact with reality, disturbed behavior, increased pulse, elevated blood pressure, perspiration, blurred vision

Results of chronic use:

- Frequent infections: hepatitis B and C, tuberculosis, sexually transmitted diseases, endocarditis
- Regression or retardation of all aspects of personal and psychologic functioning (e.g., family, peers, marital, occupation, school)
- Needle tracks on skin
- Perforated nasal septum with cocaine use

Patients are often malnourished.

DIFFERENTIAL DIAGNOSIS

- Thyroid disorders
- Delirium, depression, anxiety
- Dementia secondary to HIV, syphilis, neurologic disease, alcohol abuse
- Hypo/hyperglycemia
- Hypo/hyperthyroidism
- Bipolar disorder, depression
- Schizophrenia, psychosis
- Stroke
- Head trauma

DIAGNOSTIC STUDIES

- Urine drug screen
  - ◊ Direct supervision of patient voiding helps ensure validity
  - ◊ Sensitive, but not specific; therefore, all positive results should be confirmed by radioimmunoassay
- CBC, glucose, metabolic panel, RPR
- TSH to rule out thyroid dysfunction
- Serum chemistries to rule out physiologic causes for bizarre behavior
- B_{12} and folate levels to rule out deficiencies as cause of memory impairment
- CT scan may be indicated in some cases especially if tumor or head injury is suspected
- Consider lumbar puncture

PREVENTION

- New innovative approaches and research regarding effective methods of prevention are needed
- Effective methods of drug use prevention are still unknown
- Education of patient and parents about risk factors and effects of substance abuse
- Early identification of substance abuse; clinicians should discuss drug use with all children and adolescents during routine visits

NONPHARMACOLOGIC MANAGEMENT

- Consider that denial is often an integral problem and anticipate defenses
- Behavioral therapies
  - ◊ Counseling
  - ◊ Cognitive therapy
  - ◊ Relaxation techniques (e.g., biofeedback and self-hypnosis) to help alleviate detoxification symptoms
- Self-help groups for patient: twelve-step programs (e.g., Narcotics Anonymous, Cocaine Anonymous)
- Self-help groups for families
- Nutritional education
- Detoxification if needed, must be done in appropriate environment
  - ◊ Most basic consideration is acceptance of treatment plan by patient
  - ◊ Consider financial resources
  - ◊ Consider risk of suicide or homicide
  - ◊ Consider patient's general and mental health status and comorbid conditions
  - ◊ Consider support resources
- Fundamental requirement is abstinence from use of

mood altering substances
- A caring, nonjudgmental attitude is essential to patient's acceptance of treatment

PHARMACOLOGIC MANAGEMENT

- Opiate withdrawal
  - ◊ Decreasing doses of methadone, a synthetic narcotic analgesic with actions similar to morphine; dispensed only to FDA-approved pharmacies, hospitals, and maintenance programs
  - ◊ Clonidine ameliorates abstinence-related withdrawal symptoms
  - ◊ Naltrexone blocks the subjective and physiologic effects of subsequently administered opioids
- Use of sedatives is discouraged. Short-term use of benzodiazepines may be necessary for physical withdrawal from amphetamines, cocaine, and other stimulant drugs if patient is severely agitated
- Intravenous diazepam (Valium®) is the drug of choice for treatment of cocaine toxicity characterized by agitation, seizures, and dysrhythmias. β-adrenergic blockers are **not** recommended
- Sedative withdrawal is accomplished by gradually decreasing the amount of drug available in order to avoid precipitating CNS rebound, hyperactivity
- Medications to treat comorbid psychiatric conditions

Thiamine is often added to the diet of substance abusing patients.

PREGNANCY/LACTATION CONSIDERATIONS

- Women who substantially reduce cocaine use during pregnancy have outcomes similar to nonusers
- Methadone maintenance is the usual treatment for opiate addiction in pregnancy. Withdrawal during pregnancy is dangerous. Methadone prolongs withdrawal in the infant, but can be done safely
- The most seriously affected drug users often present late in pregnancy, making treatment very difficult
- American College of Obstetrics and Gynecology recommends that clinicians take a thorough history of substance abuse in all pregnant women
- Substance abuse in pregnancy increases the risk of spontaneous abortion, pre-eclampsia, abruptio placentae, early labor, and prolonged labor

Opiates and cocaine are most likely to affect the fetus in the third trimester due to increased maternal blood flow rate and increased placental transport.

- Parenting behavior is likely to be affected by substance abuse

FOLLOW-UP

- Treatment for substance abuse needs to continue on a long-term basis and should include group and individual therapy

Medication intervention in conjunction with counseling yields higher success rates than either alone.

EXPECTED COURSE

- Relapse is common
- Absolute abstinence occurs in a minority of patients, but there is an excellent chance for improvement
- Ongoing encouragement and support is crucial to successful treatment
- When relapse occurs, it is important to identify triggers and modify life to prevent future relapse

POSSIBLE COMPLICATIONS

- Amotivational syndrome
- Depression, suicide
- Spouse battering
- Child abuse
- Hepatitis
- HIV
- Tuberculosis
- Unintentional overdose
- Cocaine poisoning: hyperpyrexia, vasoconstriction, vasospasm, seizures, MI, ischemic stroke, arrhythmias

SMOKING CESSATION

DESCRIPTION

Cigarette smoking is a behavior that involves the continuous use of tobacco and becomes addictive. As physiologic tolerance develops, the smoker increases the number of cigarettes smoked per day. Withdrawal from nicotine produces anxiety, craving, hunger, irritability, drowsiness, tremors, diaphoresis, insomnia, dizziness, and headaches. Successful smoking cessation is defined as abstaining from cigarette smoking for at least one year.

ETIOLOGY

- The two primary reasons people smoke are psychosocial stress and nicotine dependence. A patient's reasons for smoking, as well as motivation to quit, are age-related:
  - ◊ Teenagers smoke to appear older, due to peer pressure, and are influenced by media and marketing

Teenagers are motivated to quit by recognizing the immediate undesirable effects of cigarette smoking (e.g., bad odor, expense, decreased exercise capacity, relationship between smoking and acute respiratory illness).

  - ◊ Adults smoke due to physical dependence

Adults quit smoking if there is provision of healthy alternatives, if psychosocial issues are addressed, and if recognition of the relationship between smoking and acute illness occurs.

  - ◊ Older adults continue to smoke because they feel it is too late to undo damage that is already done

Older adults quit smoking because of immediate benefits (e.g., fewer upper respiratory infections, improved taste sensation, less coughing, and to save money) and the belief that if they quit they can prevent further damage.

INCIDENCE

- Smoking has generally declined in incidence, particularly in higher-educated groups, but children continue to start smoking at the same rate
- 3000 teenagers start smoking every day in the U.S. 60% of current smokers start by age 14 years
- There are 3 million users of smokeless tobacco under age 21 years in the U.S.
- 46 million adults smoke cigarettes
- 1/5 of annual deaths in the U.S. are attributable to smoking-related problems

RISK FACTORS

- Adolescent boys participating in team sports are at increased risk of using smokeless tobacco
- Low education level, low socioeconomic status
- Friends and household members who smoke
- Other substance abuse

ASSESSMENT FINDINGS

- Chronic cough
- Inflammation of oropharynx, sinuses, nose
- Cigarette odor to breath, hair, clothing
- Stained teeth and fingers
- Prematurely aged skin
- Frequent upper respiratory infections
- Chronic obstructive pulmonary disease
- Past attempts at quitting

Smokeless tobacco:

- Erythema of isolated areas of intraoral soft tissue
- Leukoplakia (white patches) on gums

DIAGNOSTIC STUDIES

- Fagerstrom Tolerance Questionnaire: an 8-item tool used to assess level of nicotine addiction
- Spirometry: abnormal indicates damage
- Lipid panel to determine risk factor for heart disease

Chest x-rays are not recommended as screening tools for patients who smoke.

PREVENTION

- Ask all patients and adolescents at each visit whether they use tobacco
- Educate regarding tobacco use and its consequences
- Target prevention programs to the less educated,

economically disadvantaged population, and toward adolescents and children

- Provide information about smoking cessation programs
- Link education regarding smoking cessation to the individual's age and to presenting complaints

NONPHARMACOLOGIC MANAGEMENT

- Advise all smokers to quit at each visit
- Suggest replacing smoking with some other activity (e.g., hobbies, exercise, sports)
- Address the patient's personal concerns:
  - ◊ Weight gain: average is an 8 pound weight gain
- Stop-smoking contracts may be helpful
- Identify triggers to smoking by journaling
- Involve friends and family as support system
- Recommend and instruct on relaxation techniques (e.g., deep breathing, guided imagery)
- Educate patients that chewing tobacco or snuff results in nicotine levels equal to that of smokers
- Meticulous oral hygiene and twice a year dental exams for all users of smokeless tobacco

PHARMACOLOGIC MANAGEMENT

- Nicotine replacement therapies
  - ◊ Help relieve the withdrawal symptoms while quitting
  - ◊ Should be used in conjunction with counseling
  - ◊ Patient should quit smoking before using nicotine replacement (do not use concurrently)
  - ◊ Transdermal patch releases a constant dose of nicotine through the skin
  - ◊ Not recommended for those less than 18 years of age, but recent studies indicate can be used safely in adolescents
  - ◊ Nicotine gum helps reduce the urge to smoke
  - ◊ Nicotine nasal spray is highly effective but carries the risk of dependence due to the rapid absorption of nicotine
- Non-nicotine based therapy
  - ◊ Bupropion (Zyban®): theorized to block noradrenergic and dopaminergic pathways, addiction receptors in the brain, resulting in a reduction in the urge to smoke and reduction in withdrawal symptoms
  - ◊ Patients should start taking bupropion before they stop smoking and stop smoking during the second week of therapy. It is continued for 7 to 12 weeks. If used in conjunction with nicotine replacement therapy, the nicotine replacement should be started only after the patient has stopped smoking
  - ◊ Verenicline (Chantix®)
    Adult: begin therapy one week before stop date
    Initial 0.5 mg daily for 3 days, then 0.5 mg twice daily for 4 days; then 1.0 mg daily. Treat 12 weeks
    Children < 18 years not recommended
    Tabs: 0.5 mg, 1.0 mg

The brain's dopamine system is stimulated when nicotine is consumed.

PREGNANCY/LACTATION CONSIDERATIONS

- Smoking during lactation exposes infant to secondhand smoke and nicotine in breast milk
- Nicotine decreases volume and fat content of breast milk and interferes with production of prolactin and oxytocin
- Premature birth and low birth weight are associated with smoking during pregnancy
- Increased incidence of upper respiratory infections is seen in children exposed to secondhand smoke
- Nicotine replacement therapy products are Pregnancy Category D drugs and should not be used
- Bupropion is a pregnancy category B drug, but not recommended

CONSULTATION/REFERRAL

- Smoking cessation programs report a cessation rate of 20-30% compared to a 2.5% success rate without participation in a program
- Dentist or ENT physician for any changes in the oral mucosa

Leukoplakia (white patches) on gums may be indicative of pre-malignant or malignant changes. They cannot be diagnosed clinically, but, must be biopsied.

FOLLOW-UP

- If patient is unwilling to quit, provide literature and broach subject again at subsequent visits
- Every 2 weeks is recommended (while quitting) to reinforce education and provide encouragement and support
- Weekly supportive phone calls may be helpful

EXPECTED COURSE

- Relapse usually occurs during the first 2 weeks due to withdrawal symptoms
- The use of a nicotine patch doubles the likelihood of abstinence from smoking at 6 months
- Abstinence rates 3 months after use of nicotine nasal spray is 45%
- 12-month abstinence rates with the use of nicotine gum is 18%

POSSIBLE COMPLICATIONS

- Side effects of nicotine replacement therapies and bupropion therapy
- Lung, pancreatic, bladder, esophageal, and head and neck carcinomas
- Chronic obstructive pulmonary disease
- Cardiovascular disease
- Peripheral vascular disease
- Stroke
- Premature aging of the skin
- Otitis media with effusion

Smokeless tobacco:

- Dental caries, gingivitis, discolored teeth, gum recession
- Soft tissue changes, dysplasia, carcinoma
- Elevated cholesterol
- Elevated blood pressure

DOMESTIC VIOLENCE

DESCRIPTION

Use of physical, emotional, economic, or sexual manipulation to control a family member or partner in an intimate relationship. Examples: withholding of money, barring means of transportation, making it difficult to hold a job, routine disparagement and humiliation, forced sexual intercourse, threats of violence, and preventing access to medical treatment.

ETIOLOGY

- Perpetrators generally share low self-esteem and a need for power and control. They presume injustice and the tension culminates in an act of violence.
- In elder abuse, immense responsibilities are often an overwhelming stressor, resulting in neglect
- Children who witness violence learn to use it as adults

INCIDENCE

- 1000 children annually die in the U.S. as a result of abuse or neglect
- 1-4 million women are battered annually by their husband or partner
- 150,000 men are victims each year of assault, robbery, or rape committed by their partner or ex-partner, over half of these result in minor injuries
- 7-18% of pregnant women are abused
- 4% of the elderly in the U.S. are abused by relatives or caretakers
- 90-95% of adult victims of domestic violence are female; 59% of spouse- murder victims are female

RISK FACTORS

- Female gender
- Dependence (physical, financial, or emotional)
- Alcohol or other substance abuse by perpetrator or victim
- Isolation, on part of perpetrator or victim
- Families with poor social support
- Single-parent families
- Unplanned or unwanted pregnancies
- Low socioeconomic status
- Victims of abuse
- Mental retardation or mental illness
- Children with congenital anomalies

ASSESSMENT FINDINGS

- Signs of neglect: poor hygiene, nutritional deficits, lack of dental or medical attention
- Chemical dependency
- Mental illness or mental retardation

- Fear, unwillingness to disclose causes of injuries
- Injuries to abdomen, breasts, genitals, and/or torso
- Burns to back, buttocks, genitals, soles, or palms
- Injuries inconsistent with explanation offered
- Gap between time of injury and presentation for treatment
- Multiple injuries in various stages of healing
- History of multiple pregnancies, spontaneous abortions, preterm labor, or low-birthweight infants
- Unexplained hearing loss
- Children with aggressive behavior, enuresis, excessive masturbation, poor school performance

DIFFERENTIAL DIAGNOSIS

- Burnout as distinguished from bullying, in reference to care of a dependent
- Accidental injuries
- Hypochondriasis

PREVENTION

- Routine patient histories should include questions concerning violence in the home
  - ◊ Has anyone at home ever threatened or hurt you?
  - ◊ Have your children ever been threatened or abused?
  - ◊ Has anyone ever forced you to have sex?
  - ◊ Are you afraid of anyone at home?
  - ◊ Do you feel safe at home?
  - ◊ Have you ever been denied access to medical care?
  - ◊ Have you ever been coerced to sign papers you didn't understand?
  - ◊ How do members of your household get along?
  - ◊ What type of punishment is used at home?
  - ◊ Repeat these questions during patient history updates periodically, but, especially in high risk patients (though, it may be difficult to identify those at high risk)
- Interview patients alone
- Family violence should be part of the differential diagnosis when treating any injury
- Direct questioning may substantially increase reports of episodes of domestic violence

NONPHARMACOLOGIC MANAGEMENT

- Direct victims toward resources to assist in developing survival skills
- Do not recommend joint counseling; abuser may punish victim for exposure
  - ◊ Two independent adults who resolve disagreements with physical fights might benefit from family counseling regarding alternative methods of arbitration
- Maintain a supportive, nonjudgmental attitude
- Assist in development of a safety plan including availability of clothes, keys, documents, and cash
- Reinforce to patients that abuse and violence is never justified. Confirm alliance with the patient
- Reporting of abuse is mandatory if the victim is a child or an elderly adult
- Some states mandate reporting of suspected domestic violence
- Refrain from attempting to make decisions for competent adults
- Recommend emergency shelter if there seems to be a life-threatening situation
- Assure patient's safety before releasing from care
- Meticulous documentation is crucial in case of future legal action
  - ◊ Include photographs if patient consents
  - ◊ Describe events using patient's own words

PHARMACOLOGIC MANAGEMENT

- Dependent on extent of injuries
- Treat underlying psychiatric illness if appropriate

PREGNANCY/LACTATION CONSIDERATIONS

- Pregnant victims are more likely to defer prenatal care until the third trimester, perhaps in part due to forced isolation by abusers

CONSULTATION/REFERRAL

- National Resource Center on Domestic Violence
  - ◊ Provides information
  - ◊ 1-800-537-2238
- National Domestic Violence Hotline
  - ◊ Immediate crisis intervention
  - ◊ 1-800-799-SAFE (7233)
- Local shelters
- Family therapists, if appropriate
- Nursing home placement

FOLLOW-UP

- Dependent on extent of injuries and needs of patient
- Report of abuse against children and elderly adults is mandatory

EXPECTED COURSE

- Most cases of domestic violence begin early in a relationship and escalate with time
- Battered individuals may eventually resort to violence themselves, against children, or possibly against the batterer

POSSIBLE COMPLICATIONS

- Women with a history of domestic abuse are more likely to abuse alcohol
- Women with a history of domestic abuse are more likely to attempt suicide
- Victims are more likely to be killed when there is escalating violence, substance abuse, death threats, or a weapon in the home
- Adolescents and adults who were abused as children are more likely to abuse tobacco and alcohol, attempt suicide, and exhibit violent or criminal behavior
- Psychological trauma related to child sexual abuse often persists into adulthood
- Sexually transmitted diseases

SEXUAL ASSAULT
(Rape Crisis Syndrome)

DESCRIPTION

Any penetration of a person's intimate parts using force or coercion which occurs against his/her will; forcible carnal knowledge. Includes a range of sexual acts, including rape, incest, sodomy, oral copulation, or penetration of genital or anal opening by a foreign object.

Definitions vary from state to state.

ETIOLOGY

- Pedophiles seem to develop propensity for children during their own adolescence
- Father's need for sexual gratification and a daughter's need for nurturance may lead to incest

INCIDENCE

- 100,000 cases reported annually in U.S.
- Females > Males in both adults and children
- Prevalent age is teens and twenties

Reported sexual assault in children is 1 in 15-20 occurrences. Reported sexual assault in adults is 1 in 5-10 occurrences.

RISK FACTORS

- Child sexual abuse is often multigenerational
- Alcohol or drug use
- Closely knit, socially isolated family

PHYSICAL ASSESSMENT

Children:

- Sexually transmitted diseases are often the first indication of sexual abuse in children
- Dysuria
- Genital or perianal rash or pain
- Vaginal, penile, or rectal discharge or bleeding
- Presence of sperm and/or semen
- Enuresis, encopresis
- Regressive behaviors (e.g., thumb-sucking, bedwetting, reluctance to sleep alone)
- Compulsive behaviors, unusual fears
- Change in school performance, peer relationships, or behavior
- Inappropriate sexually oriented behavior
- Depression, anger, suicide attempts
- Substance abuse
- Running away
- Recurrent gastrointestinal or gynecological complaints
- Hymenal lacerations
- Gaping anal opening
- Genital or rectal injuries inconsistent with explanation
- Pregnancy

Adults:

- Report of sexual contact without consent
- Evidence of use of forceful sexual contact
- Presence of semen and/or sperm

DIFFERENTIAL DIAGNOSIS

- Consenting sex among adults
- Straddle injury to genital or rectal area
- Perinatally acquired STD
- Lichen sclerosis
- Poor hygiene
- Pinworm infestation

DIAGNOSTIC STUDIES

- Collection of forensic specimens:
  - ◊ Specimens are of limited value if > 72 hours since event
  - ◊ All specimens must be handled carefully, maintaining chain of custody
  - ◊ Clothing
  - ◊ Hair specimens obtained by combing pubic hair of victims
  - ◊ Vaginal fluid to test for sperm (motile or nonmotile)
- Rectal, throat, urethral, and/or endocervical cultures for *N. gonorrhoeae* and *C. trachomatis*
- Syphilis serology
- In selected cases as appropriate:
  - ◊ Herpes simplex
  - ◊ Hepatitis B, C
  - ◊ Bacterial vaginosis
  - ◊ Human papillomavirus
  - ◊ *Trichomonas vaginalis*
- Colposcopic examination of genital and rectal area by an expert may be requested by law enforcement agencies
- Pregnancy test, if appropriate
- Initial HIV test, if indicated, should be completed within 7 days

PREVENTION

- Instruct parents and caregivers to educate child about self-defense regarding inappropriate sexual advances
- Early referral of known victims for counseling to prevent future psychological problems
- Educate that children are at risk and unsafe around a pedophile
- Prompt reporting of suspected abuse to child protection authorities
- Assertiveness training, self-defense training

NONPHARMACOLOGIC MANAGEMENT

- Consider SANE (Sexual Assault Nurse Examiner) for exam (shown to be more beneficial for victim)
- Careful documentation of history and physical examination findings for medicolegal purposes
- Supportive and understanding communication, respecting privacy and allowing patient to ventilate feelings
- If emergency contraception is objectionable to patient, inform that fertilization may occur
- All those involved in patient care must be prepared to testify in court
- Inform of need to return at appropriate times for follow-up assessment and/or treatment

A complete genital and rectal exam should be performed with careful attention to documentation.

PHARMACOLOGIC MANAGEMENT

Emergency contraception:

- Failure rate of < 2%
- Levonorgestrel 0.75 mg (Plan B)
  Rule out pregnancy first
  >18yr: 1 tab as soon as possible, no later than 72 hours after unprotected intercourse, then repeat one tab in 12 hours after first dose

Prophylactic antibiotics:

- Ceftriaxone (Rocephin®) or cefixime (Suprax®) for prevention of gonorrhea
- Azithromycin (Zithromax®), doxycycline (Vibramycin®) for prevention of chlamydia
  - ◊ Substitute azithromycin for tetracycline in children < 9 years of age
  - ◊ May be given along with pharmacologic treatment for gonorrhea
- Tetanus prophylaxis

PREGNANCY/LACTATION CONSIDERATIONS

- Antibiotic prophylaxis for pregnant women:
  - ◊ Amoxicillin/probenecid, or ceftriaxone (Rocephin®) for prevention of gonorrhea and syphilis
  - ◊ Azithromycin for prevention of chlamydia
- Sedation may be indicated
- Tetanus prophylaxis
- Hepatitis B immune globulin within 14 days, followed by hepatitis B vaccine series

CONSULTATION/REFERRAL

- If possible, victims of sexual assault should be referred to providers who specialize in performing

the examination
- Refer to expert in field of sexual abuse for psychosocial interview and crisis counseling

FOLLOW-UP

- Report cases of sexual assault or abuse to law enforcement agency and to social services
- Periodic observation and involvement of patient in social support
- 7-10 days: pregnancy testing and counseling
- Repeat cervical culture, VDRL, and pregnancy test in 2 weeks
- 5-6 weeks: tests for syphilis and gonorrhea
- Repeat HIV and hepatitis B in 6 months

EXPECTED COURSE

- Acute phase usually lasts 3 weeks, involves anxiety, fear, pain, mood swings, guilt, shame, grief
- Chronic phase may develop, involving flashbacks, nightmares, fear of intercourse, fear of men, depression, anxiety, and post-traumatic stress syndrome
- Patients who are provided with counseling and are able to express themselves after the event usually recover more quickly

POSSIBLE COMPLICATIONS

- Sexually transmitted disease
- Pregnancy
- Post- traumatic stress disorder
- Emotional trauma
- Physical trauma

ANOREXIA NERVOSA
(AN)

DESCRIPTION

Disorder characterized by morbid fear of obesity and nutritionally significant weight loss.

ETIOLOGY

- Unknown, but serotonergic dysregulation is thought to play a major role
- May be related to underlying metabolic, psychological, and/or genetic predisposition

INCIDENCE

- Females > Males
- Most common in adolescents and young adults (1-4%)
- Predominantly a disease of white, middle and upper class, but increasing in males, minorities, and women of all ages
- May coexist with depression (50-75%) or obsessive-compulsive disorder (10-13%)

RISK FACTORS

- Meticulous, compulsive personality
- Low self-esteem
- High self-expectations
- Multiple responsibilities
- Early puberty
- Family history

ASSESSMENT FINDINGS

- Insidious initially
- Significant and noticeable weight loss (generally 15% below body weight)
- Preoccupation about weight loss and being fat is primary symptom
- Denial that there is a problem (prominent feature of the disease)
- Disturbance in body image (i.e., complaints of feeling bloated and being fat despite emaciation)
- Strenuous exercise to lose weight
- Resistance to medical treatment
- Possible depression
- Elaborate food rituals
- Amenorrhea (absence of 3 consecutive menstrual cycles) may appear before significant weight loss

The following findings are related to starvation:
- Sparse scalp hair, dry skin
- Growth arrest, arrested sexual maturation

- Lanugo on extremities, face, and trunk
- Cognitive decline
- Bradycardia, hypotension, cardiovascular compromise
- Hypothermia
- Weight loss of 30% in 6 months requires hospitalization

DIFFERENTIAL DIAGNOSIS

- Bulimia
- Severe depression
- Food phobia
- Schizophrenia
- Physical disorder (e.g., malignancy, diabetes mellitus)

Anorexia is commonly accompanied by other psychiatric illnesses like depression, social phobias, or obsessive compulsive disorder.

DIAGNOSTIC STUDIES

- No lab or imaging can diagnose anorexia nervosa
- Tests done to determine level of malnutrition
  - ◊ CBC: anemia
  - ◊ LFTs
  - ◊ LH, FSH, T_3: all are diminished
  - ◊ BUN, total protein: decreased
  - ◊ Fasting blood glucose: low
  - ◊ Potassium level: low

PREVENTION

- Enhance self-esteem
- Encourage healthy attitude about weight and self
- Encourage reasonable self-expectations

NONPHARMACOLOGIC MANAGEMENT

- Usually treated on outpatient basis
- Restoration of weight is primary goal and may result in cessation of obsessive focus on food
- Monitor physical, psychological and nutritional status
- Supportive therapy in an eating disorders clinic or group
- Build trust with patient
- Consider bedrest if physical and nutritional status is severe (inpatient treatment is preferable for patients who are 70% of weight for height)
- Involve patient and family in treatment plan and establishing target weight
- Supervised meals
- Increase calories gradually by about 300 kcal/day as tolerated
- Weigh 3 times in first 1-2 weeks, then weekly
- Goal is 1-2 pound weight gain per week until target is reached
- Discuss fear of weight gain as part of program
- Slowly increase patient's activity level as weight is gained
- Goal is weight stabilization and resumption of normal eating pattern

PHARMACOLOGIC MANAGEMENT

- May treat anxiety before meals to lessen anxiety about weight gain
- Careful dosing of medications required because patients may have compromised hepatic and/or renal function
- Consider treatment with antidepressants if depression is persistent

Underweight patients are more sensitive to usual dosages of medications. Dose carefully!

CONSULTATION/REFERRAL

- Refer to psychiatrist for initial treatment plan
- Consult support group or eating disorders clinic
- Refer to psychiatrist for weight less than 75% expected for age and height; compromised physical status (hypothermia, hypotension, bradycardia, etc.)
- Registered dietitian for meal planning

FOLLOW-UP

- Monitor weight weekly until stable, then monthly
- Monitor for depression, possible suicide
- Monitor abnormal lab values
- Participation in long-term maintenance program is recommended to help prevent relapse

EXPECTED COURSES

- Relapses are common
- Fewer than 50% completely recover
- Poor prognosis for failed inpatient hospitalization and for patients with a history of disturbed family relationships
- Possible depression during or after recovery
- Food rituals, low self-esteem, and distorted body image may persist even after treatment and recovery

POSSIBLE COMPLICATIONS

- 5% mortality (often due to suicide)
- Cardiac arrhythmias from electrolyte imbalances
- Osteoporosis
- Congestive heart failure
- Necrotizing colitis
- Seizures

BULIMIA NERVOSA

DESCRIPTION

Disorder characterized by distorted body image, recurrent episodes of overeating and either self-induced vomiting, use of laxatives, diuretics, rigorous exercise, dieting, or any combination of these. Diagnostic criteria according to DSM-IV: 2 binge episodes per week for at least 3 months.

ETIOLOGY

- Unknown

INCIDENCE

- Females > Males (5:1)
- Young adults and adolescents are at highest risk
- College females thought to have the highest incidence, however, <2% prevalence rate in this group
- Actual incidence is unknown because of the secretive nature of the disease

RISK FACTORS

- Meticulous, compulsive personality
- Low self-esteem
- High self-expectations
- Multiple responsibilities
- Increased stress levels
- Individuals considered at high risk to develop: ballet dancers, cheerleaders, gymnasts, weightlifters, jockeys, runners
- Obesity
- History of sexual abuse
- Chemical dependency
- Anxiety

ASSESSMENT FINDINGS

- May exist concurrently with anorexia
- Belief that they are fat despite weight that is average or higher
- Frequent weight fluctuations
- Express extreme concern about weight gain; preoccupation with weight
- Expression of feelings of "lack of control" during binge episodes
- May hoard food
- Secret abuse of diet pills, laxatives, diuretics, syrup of ipecac
- Erosion of dental enamel from acid in vomitus
- Abdominal pain, esophagitis, enlargement of the parotid glands, gastric dilation
- Scarring on knuckles from inducing vomiting
- Denial that eating habits are a problem
- Depression may follow recovery initiation
- May feel guilty about behavior when asked about it
- More prone to impulsive behavior than anorexics

DIFFERENTIAL DIAGNOSIS

- Anorexia
- Depression
- Gastrointestinal disorder
- Schizophrenia
- Psychogenic vomiting

DIAGNOSTIC STUDIES

- Electrolyte levels: all may be low, especially potassium, chloride (alkalosis from vomiting), and magnesium from laxative abuse; or may be normal values
- BUN: elevated
- Other chemistries as patient condition dictates
- Consider ECG if electrolytes are severely decreased
- Consider a urine drug screen

PREVENTION

- Encourage healthy attitudes about weight and self
- Encourage reasonable self-expectations
- Appropriate stress management

NONPHARMACOLOGIC MANAGEMENT

- Cognitive behavioral therapy (CBT) should be considered first line treatment
- Most treated on outpatient basis
- Consider inpatient if suicidal, severe concurrent chemical dependency, or if entirely out of control and unresponsive to outpatient treatment
- Monitor physical, psychological and nutritional status
- Supportive therapy in an eating disorders clinic or group
- Build trust with patient. Development of trust is good prognostic indicator
- Involve patient and family in treatment plan and in establishing goals
- Monitor exercise and eating patterns
- Supervised meals, supervised bathroom privileges for at least 2 hours after meals
- Discuss fear of weight gain and use this challenge as part of recovery
- Slowly increase patient's activity level
- Goal is weight stabilization and resumption of normal eating pattern

Non-compliance with treatment regimen and lack of honesty with counselor, health care provider is common.

BULIMIA PHARMACOLOGIC MANAGEMENT

Class	Drug Generic name (Trade name®)	Dosage How supplied	Comments
Selective Serotonin Reuptake Inhibitors (SSRIs) General comments May increase the risk of suicidal thinking and behavior in patients with major depressive disorder Monitor patient closely for clinical worsening, suicidality, unusual changes in behavior especially during the initial months of therapy Write Rx for smallest practical amount Full effect may be delayed for 4 weeks or longer May increase risk of bleeding especially in combination with aspirin, NSAIDs, warfarin Do not abruptly stop usage Monitor for hyponatremia	**fluoxetine**	**Adults**: 20 mg initially with target dose of 60 mg. Titrate over several days. Administer in the AM. Consider treatment for 1 year	• Pregnancy Category C • Periodically re-assess to determine continued need for maintenance therapy. • Do not administer to patients within 5 weeks of taking MAO inhibitors • Avoid in patients with uncontrolled narrow angle glaucoma • No dosage adjustment recommended for renal dysfunction or elderly. However, elderly may have greater sensitivity • Monitor for weight change during treatment • May alter glycemic control (hypoglycemia during use, hyperglycemia after discontinuing) • Discontinuation should take place gradually rather than abruptly

continued

BULIMIA PHARMACOLOGIC MANAGEMENT

Class	Drug Generic name (Trade name®)	Dosage How supplied	Comments
Drug interactions may occur with many medications given in combination with SSRIs. Check compatibility Treatment should be sustained for several months Avoid alcohol when taking SSRIs May cause decrease in libido	Prozac	*Tabs: 10 mg, 20 mg, 40 mg* *Solution: 20 mg/5 mL*	

Avoid bupropion because it is associated with seizures in patients who purge.

PREGNANCY/LACTATION CONSIDERATIONS

- Pregnancy may worsen or improve disorder
- Danger to fetus due to poor nutritional status

CONSULTATION/REFERRAL

- Consult physician for all new diagnoses and for development of treatment plan
- Psychologist for behavioral therapy
- Dietitian for meal planning

FOLLOW-UP

- Dictated by severity of patient disorder
- Attendance at eating disorders clinic should be coordinated with routine follow-up
- Monitor potassium as long as patient is purging

EXPECTED COURSES

- Expect noncompliance and frequent relapses
- Expect improvement, but some symptoms often persist over a period of years

POSSIBLE COMPLICATIONS

- Erosion of dental enamel
- Gastric dilation
- Esophagitis
- Life threatening arrhythmias from electrolyte imbalances, cardiomyopathy, and sudden death related to vomiting
- Suicide
- Abuse of drugs or alcohol

INSOMNIA

DESCRIPTION

Insomnia is defined as difficulty initiating or maintaining sleep, or non-restorative sleep. This is a diagnosis of subjective clinical report, which may be purely subjective without daytime impairment or may be objectively measured with daytime consequences such as drowsiness or functional impairments.

Insomnia may be acute or chronic.

ETIOLOGY

Acute Insomnia

- Occurrence: 1 night occasionally, lasting up to one month
- Can be attributed to emotional or physical complaints including
  - ◊ Life stressors
  - ◊ Acute illness
  - ◊ Environmental issues: noise, light, temperature
  - ◊ Jet lag

Chronic Insomnia

- 3 or more nights per week for greater than one month
- Can be attributed to multiple factors
  - ◊ Psychological
  - ◊ Mood and anxiety disorders
  - ◊ Dementia
  - ◊ Pain
  - ◊ Stimulants
  - ◊ Illicit drugs: heroin, cocaine, other stimulants
    Drugs such as stimulating antidepressants, steroids, decongestants, beta blockers
    Caffeine, alcohol, tobacco
  - ◊ Medical conditions
    Asthma
    Gastroesophageal reflux disease
    Hormone changes in pregnancy, perimenopause and menopause
  - ◊ Sleep disorders
  - ◊ Restless leg syndrome
  - ◊ Sleep apnea
  - ◊ Circadian rhythm disorders

INCIDENCE

- 30-40% adults report acute insomnia
- 10% adults have chronic insomnia
- More common in women
- Chronic insomnia more common after age 60

RISK FACTORS

- Alcohol Abuse
- Psychiatric disorder

ASSESSMENT FINDINGS

- Difficulty falling asleep
- Difficulty staying asleep
- Early morning awakenings
- Non-restorative sleep
- Daytime sleepiness or fatigue
- Irritability

DIFFERENTIAL DIAGNOSES

- Mood and anxiety disorders
- Post traumatic stress disorder
- Sleep related breathing problems
- Restless leg syndrome
- Medical (pain, gastroesophageal reflux disease, nocturia, orthopnea, medications)

DIAGNOSTIC STUDIES

- Sleep history
- Sleep laboratory studies
- Evaluate for anemia, uremia, and thyroid disorders
- Brain CT or MRI for severe daytime sleepiness or acute onset

PREVENTION

- Sleep hygiene measures
  - ◊ Awaken at same time each day
  - ◊ No caffeine within 4-6 hours of bedtime
  - ◊ Avoid alcohol, nicotine, and heavy meals prior to bedtime
  - ◊ Minimize noise, light and temperature extremes
  - ◊ Move alarm clock from side of bed

◊ Warm bath prior to bed
◊ Restrict in bed time for sleep and sex
◊ Increase daytime activity patterns

NONPHARMACOLOGIC MANAGEMENT

- Behavioral therapy
- Relaxation therapy
- Sleep restriction therapy
  - ◊ Stay in bed only to sleep, if not sleeping, get up
  - ◊ Biofeedback to learn how to fall asleep
  - ◊ Cognitive therapy to address underlying stress issues

INSOMNIA PHARMACOLOGIC MANAGEMENT

Class	Drug Generic name (Trade name®)	Dosage How supplied	Comments
Benzodiazepines *Helpful for patients with difficulty initiating sleep* **General comments** Side effects and falls are substantially increased in elderly patients	**flurazepam** Dalmane	**Adult and > 15 years**: 15-30 mg at bedtime **< 15 yr**: not recommended **Elderly**: *Initial*: 15 mg at bedtime *Tabs: 15 mg, 30 mg*	• Pregnancy Category X; controlled substance • Used for patients with difficulty falling asleep, frequent nocturnal or early morning awakenings • Re-evaluate insomnia that does not remit after 7-10 days of treatment • Avoid use with alcohol or other CNS hypnotics • Extreme caution advised in patients with hepatic or renal dysfunction; or pulmonary insufficiency • Elderly: limit dose to 15 mg if alternative therapy not helpful • Be alert for drug abuse and dependence

continued

INSOMNIA PHARMACOLOGIC MANAGEMENT

Class	Drug Generic name (Trade name®)	Dosage How supplied	Comments
	temazepam Restoril	**Adults > 18 years**: *Initial*: 7.5 mg *Usual*: 15 mg at bedtime *Max*: 30 mg **Children < 18 years**: not recommended *Tabs: 7.5 mg, 15 mg, 22.5 mg, 30 mg*	• Pregnancy Category X; controlled substance • Used short term for treatment of insomnia (7-10 days) • Re-evaluate insomnia that does not remit after 7-10 days of treatment • Avoid use with alcohol or other CNS hypnotics • Extreme caution advised in patients with hepatic or renal dysfunction; or pulmonary insufficiency • Be alert for drug abuse and dependence
	triazolam Halcion	**Adults > 18 yearr:** *Initial*: 0.125 mg - 0.25 mg at bedtime *Max*: 0.5 mg **Elderly or debilitated:** *Initial*: 0.0625 mg *Max*: 0.25 mg *Tabs: 0.125 mg, 0.25 mg, scored*	• Pregnancy Category X; controlled substance • Used short term for treatment of insomnia (7-10 days) • Do not prescribe in quantities exceeding 1 month supply • Avoid use with alcohol or other CNS hypnotics • Be alert for drug abuse and dependence
Hypnotics *Helpful for patients with difficulty initiating sleep* <u>General comments</u> Monitor for abnormal thinking and behavior changes Side effects and falls are substantially increased in elderly patients Effect delayed if taken with high fat heavy meal	**eszopiclone** Lunesta	**Adults and > 18 years:** 2-3 mg immediately at bedtime. Take only if able to get 8 hours sleep before becoming active again **Elderly:** 1 mg; may give 2 mg if difficulty remaining asleep *Tabs: 1 mg, 2 mg, 3 mg*	• Pregnancy Category C; controlled substance • Cautious use in patients with depression, compromised respiratory function • Dosage adjustment needed for hepatic dysfunction • Avoid alcohol or drugs when taking eszopiclone • Write Rx for smallest practical amount • May cause unpleasant taste in mouth

continued

INSOMNIA PHARMACOLOGIC MANAGEMENT

Class	Drug Generic name (Trade name®)	Dosage How supplied	Comments
	ramelteon	**Adult:** 8 mg taken within 30 minutes of bedtime	• Pregnancy Category C • Cautious use in patients with depression • Not recommended in patients with hepatic dysfunction • Watch for drug interactions, especially fluvoxamine • Monitor for cognitive and behavioral changes
	Rozerem	*Tabs: 8 mg*	
	zolpidem	Ambien **Adults**: 10 mg at bedtime (take only if able to get 7-8 hours of sleep before becoming active again) **Elderly, debilitated, or hepatic insufficiency:** *Initial*: 5 mg at bedtime *Max*: 10 mg	• Pregnancy Category B; controlled substance • May potentiate other CNS depressants • Rapid onset of action: take only immediately before going to bed • NO dosage adjustment needed for renal impairment, but monitor closely
		Ambien CR **Adults**: 12.5 mg at bedtime (take only if able to get 7-8 hours of sleep before becoming active again) **Elderly, debilitated, or hepatic insufficiency**: *Initial*: 6.25 mg	• Pregnancy Category C; controlled substance • May potentiate other CNS depressants • Rapid onset of action: take only immediately before going to bed • NO dosage adjustment needed for renal impairment, but monitor closely
	Ambien	*Tabs: 5 mg, 10 mg*	
	Ambien CR	*Ext Rel tabs: 6.25 mg, 12.5 mg*	

Sleep Management Pharmacology				
Drug	Indications	Half life Adults	Half life Elderly	Tablet Form
Eszopiclone (Lunesta®)	Insomnia, decreases sleep latency and improves sleep maintenance	6 hr	9 hr	1 mg, 2 mg, 3 mg
Zaleplon (Sonata®)	Short term insomnia, decreases time to sleep	1 hr	1 hr	5 mg, 10 mg
Zolpidem (Ambien®)	Short term insomnia, decreases sleep latency and increases duration of sleep	2.5 hr	2.9 hr	5 mg, 10 mg
Ramelteon (Rozerem®)	Insomnia related to difficulty with sleep onset	1-2.6 hr	2.6 hr	8 mg

CONSULTATION/REFERRAL

- For excessive daytime sleepiness (narcolepsy, sleep related breathing disorders)
- Night time behavior suggestive of parasomnia
- Severe insomnia not improved with basic treatment

FOLLOW UP

- Re-evaluate in two weeks for effectiveness of management plan

References

Ait-Daoud, N., Malcolm, R. J., Jr., & Johnson, B. A. (2006). An overview of medications for the treatment of alcohol withdrawal and alcohol dependence with an emphasis on the use of older and newer anticonvulsants. Addictive Behaviors, 31(9), 1628-1649.

Allen, N. E., Beral, V., Casabonne, D., Kan, S. W., Reeves, G. K., Brown, A., et al. (2009). Moderate alcohol intake and cancer incidence in women. Journal of the National Cancer Institute, 101(5), 296-305.

Appelbaum, P. S. (2007). Clinical practice. Assessment of patients' competence to consent to treatment. New England Journal of Medicine, 357(18), 1834-1840.

Bolton, J. M., Cox, B. J., Afifi, T. O., Enns, M. W., Bienvenu, O. J., & Sareen, J. (2008). Anxiety disorders and risk for suicide attempts: Findings from the baltimore epidemiologic catchment area follow-up study. Depression and Anxiety, 25(6), 477-481.

Cigarette smoking among adults - - - United States, 2007. (2008). MMWR, 57(45), 1221-1226.

Cipriani, A., Furukawa, T. A., Salanti, G., Geddes, J. R., Higgins, J. P., Churchill, R., et al. (2009). Comparative efficacy and acceptability of 12 new-generation antidepressants: A multiple-treatments meta-analysis. Lancet, 373(9665), 746-758.

Dejesus, R. S., Vickers, K. S., Melin, G. J., & Williams, M. D. (2007). A system-based approach to depression management in primary care using the patient health questionnaire-9. Mayo Clinic Proceedings, 82(11), 1395-1402.

Eaton, D. K., Kann, L., Kinchen, S., Shanklin, S., Ross, J., Hawkins, J., et al. (2008). Youth risk behavior surveillance--United States, 2007. MMWR. Surveillance Summaries, 57(4), 1-131.

Ebmeier, K. P., Donaghey, C., & Steele, J. D. (2006). Recent developments and current controversies in depression. Lancet, 367(9505), 153-167.

Eckert, L. O., & Sugar, N. F. (2008). Older victims of sexual assault: An underrecognized population. American Journal of Obstetrics and Gynecology, 198(6), 688 e681-687; discussion 688 e687.

Ellsberg, M., Jansen, H. A., Heise, L., Watts, C. H., & Garcia-Moreno, C. (2008). Intimate partner violence and women's physical and mental health in the WHO multi-country study on women's health and domestic violence: An observational study. Lancet, 371(9619), 1165-1172.

Ernst, D., & Lee, A. (2010). Nurse practitioners prescribing reference. New York: Haymarket Media Publication.

Ernst, D. B., Pettinati, H. M., Weiss, R. D., Donovan, D. M., & Longabaugh, R. (2008). An intervention for treating alcohol dependence: Relating elements of medical management to patient outcomes with implications for primary care. Ann Fam Med, 6(5), 435-440.

Fancher, T., & Kravitz, R. (2007). In the clinic. Depression. Annals of Internal Medicine, 146(9), ITC5-1-ITC5-16.

Fiore, M. C., Jaen, C. R., Baker, T. B., Bailey, W. C., Curry, S. J., Dorfman, S. F., et al. (2008). Treating tobacco use and dependence: 2008 update. Clinical practice guideline. Rockville, MD.

Fournier, J. C., DeRubeis, R. J., Hollon, S. D., Dimidjian, S., Amsterdam, J. D., Shelton, R. C., et al. (2010). Antidepressant drug effects and depression severity: A patient-level meta-analysis. JAMA, 303(1), 47-53.

Gale, C., & Davidson, O. (2007). Generalised anxiety disorder. BMJ, 334(7593), 579-581.

Grant, B. F., Hasin, D. S., Stinson, F. S., Dawson, D. A., June Ruan, W., Goldstein, R. B., et al. (2005). Prevalence, correlates, co-morbidity, and comparative disability of dsm-iv generalized anxiety disorder in the USA: Results from the national epidemiologic survey on alcohol and related conditions. Psychological Medicine, 35(12), 1747-1759.

Hasin, D. S., Stinson, F. S., Ogburn, E., & Grant, B. F. (2007). Prevalence, correlates, disability, and comorbidity of dsm-iv alcohol abuse and dependence in the United States: Results from the national epidemiologic survey on alcohol and related conditions. Archives of General Psychiatry, 64(7), 830-842.

Hawton, K., & van Heeringen, K. (2009). Suicide. Lancet, 373(9672), 1372-1381.

Hudson, J. I., Hiripi, E., Pope, H. G., Jr., & Kessler, R. C. (2007). The prevalence and correlates of eating disorders in the national comorbidity survey replication. Biological Psychiatry, 61(3), 348-358.

Keski-Rahkonen, A., Hoek, H. W., Susser, E. S., Linna, M. S., Sihvola, E., Raevuori, A., et al. (2007). Epidemiology and course of anorexia nervosa in the community. American Journal of Psychiatry, 164(8), 1259-1265.

Kroenke, K., Spitzer, R. L., Williams, J. B., Monahan, P. O., & Lowe, B. (2007). Anxiety disorders in primary care: Prevalence, impairment, comorbidity, and detection. Annals of Internal Medicine, 146(5), 317-325.

MacMillan, H. L., Wathen, C. N., Jamieson, E., Boyle, M. H., Shannon, H. S., Ford-Gilboe, M., et al. (2009). Screening for intimate partner violence in health care settings: A randomized trial. JAMA, 302(5), 493-501.

Miller, K. K., Grinspoon, S. K., Ciampa, J., Hier, J., Herzog, D., & Klibanski, A. (2005). Medical findings in outpatients with anorexia nervosa. Archives of Internal Medicine, 165(5), 561-566.

Moeller, K. E., Lee, K. C., & Kissack, J. C. (2008). Urine drug screening: Practical guide for clinicians. Mayo Clinic Proceedings, 83(1), 66-76.

Pope, H. G., Jr., Lalonde, J. K., Pindyck, L. J., Walsh, T., Bulik, C. M., Crow, S. J., et al. (2006). Binge eating disorder: A stable syndrome. American Journal of Psychiatry, 163(12), 2181-2183.

Qaseem, A., Snow, V., Denberg, T. D., Forciea, M. A., & Owens, D. K. (2008). Using second-generation antidepressants to treat depressive disorders: A clinical practice guideline from the american college of physicians. Annals of Internal Medicine, 149(10), 725-733.

Schuckit, M. A. (2009). Alcohol-use disorders. Lancet, 373(9662), 492-501.

Solberg, L. I., Maciosek, M. V., & Edwards, N. M. (2008). Primary care intervention to reduce alcohol misuse ranking its health impact and cost effectiveness. American Journal of Preventive Medicine, 34(2), 143-152.

World Health Organization. (2008). WHO report on the global tobacco epidemic, 2008: The MPOWER package. Geneva: World Health Organization.

18

UROLOGIC DISORDERS

Urologic Disorders

Asymptomatic Bacteriuria 687

Urinary Tract Infection 688

Acute Pyelonephritis 694

Urethritis 695

Urinary Incontinence 697

* Enuresis 702

Hematuria 704

Urolithiasis 705

Poststreptococcal Glomerulonephritis 707

Renal Insufficiency 708

* Wilm's Tumor 710

References *711*

*Denotes pediatric diagnosis

Urologic Disorders

ASYMPTOMATIC BACTERIURIA

DESCRIPTION

Significant bacterial count present in the urine of a person without symptoms of a urinary tract infection.

ETIOLOGY

- Bacteria (e.g., *E. coli, Proteus mirabilis, Klebsiella pneumoniae*, or *Staphylococcus saprophyticus*)
- More commonly caused by gram negative bacteria

INCIDENCE

- 20% of elderly women living in the community
- 30-50% of institutionalized elderly women
- 4-7% of pregnancies

RISK FACTORS

- Female
- Perimenopausal
- Increasing age
- Structural abnormalities that impede the flow of urine
- Indwelling urinary catheter

ASSESSMENT FINDINGS

- By definition, none

DIFFERENTIAL DIAGNOSIS

- Contaminated specimen
- Symptomatic bacteriuria

DIAGNOSTIC STUDIES

- Urinalysis: WBCs
- Urine culture may be positive

PHARMACOLOGIC MANAGEMENT

- Pharmacological treatment is controversial. It is generally recommended in persons with diabetes, polycystic renal disease, AIDS, and before urological procedures

Treatment is recommended in patients undergoing a procedure in which mucosal bleeding might be anticipated.

PREGNANCY/LACTATION CONSIDERATIONS

- Associated with acute pyelonephritis, preterm labor, and low birthweight infants
- Screening of all pregnant women should be done at the initial prenatal visit
- Treatment recommended in pregnancy
- Recommended medications for treatment during pregnancy are nitrofurantoin (Macrodantin®), ampicillin, an extended spectrum penicillin, OR a cephalosporin
- Trimethoprim-sulfamethoxazole (Bactrim®) and quinolones should not be used in pregnancy

CONSULTATION/REFERRAL

- None usually needed

FOLLOW-UP

- None unless patient becomes symptomatic

POSSIBLE COMPLICATIONS

- Development of symptomatic bacteriuria
- Disseminated infection
- Acute pyelonephritis in pregnancy
- Delivery of low birth weight infant

URINARY TRACT INFECTION
(Cystitis, UTI)

DESCRIPTION

Infection and inflammation of the bladder mucosa; presence of bacteria in the urine. Upper urinary tract infections (acute pyelonephritis) can result in renal scarring, hypertension or end-stage renal disease.

ETIOLOGY

- Bacteria [e.g., *E. coli* (most common pathogen in children and adults), *Proteus mirabilis, Klebsiella pneumoniae, Enterobacter*, or *Staphylococcus saprophyticus*)]
- More commonly caused by gram negative bacteria of colonic origin
- Most UTI in adult women are due to ascending infections from the urethra
- Hematogenous spread is rarely the cause

INCIDENCE

- 43% of women aged 14-61 years have had at least one UTI
- Females > Males
- Uncommon in men < 50 years old
- 4-7% prevalence in pregnant women
- Most common of all bacterial infections in women
- In girls is most common in ages 7-11 years
- In children, UTI is highest in boys < 1 year and girls < 4 years

Females are more likely than males to have urinary tract infections because females have short urethras compared to males.

RISK FACTORS

- Previous urinary tract infection
- Diabetes mellitus in women
- Pregnancy
- Increase in frequency of sexual activity
- Use of spermicides and/or diaphragm, oral contraceptive use
- Urinary tract abnormalities (e.g., tumors, calculi, strictures, anomalies, neuropathic bladder, vesicoureteral reflux or polycystic kidneys)
- Benign prostatic hyperplasia
- Fecal/urinary incontinence
- Cognitive impairment
- Immunocompromised host
- Infrequent voiding
- Indwelling urinary catheter

Always assess risk factors for UTI in pediatric patients with suspected UTI.

ASSESSMENT FINDINGS

- Burning, frequency, and/or urgency during urination
- Pain during or after urination
- Sensation of incomplete bladder emptying
- Fever, chills
- Hematuria: gross or microscopic
- Lower abdominal and/or back pain
- Dribbling of urine in men
- Small volume voiding
- Foul-smelling urine

The most common symptom of upper urinary tract infection in young children is fever.

DIFFERENTIAL DIAGNOSIS

- Vaginitis
- Sexually transmitted disease
- Hematuria from another cause
- Pregnancy
- Pelvic inflammatory disease
- Prostatitis, epididymitis
- Enuresis

DIAGNOSTIC STUDIES

- Urinalysis: WBCs present, positive leukocyte esterase, positive nitrites
- Bacterial count > 100,000 CFU/mL of urine if midstream catch
- Urine culture with sensitivity for recurrent infections, infection refractory to treatment, and in children
- Blood pressure and temperature
- Routine imaging recommended for girls < 3 years with first UTI, boys with a first UTI (any age), children with febrile UTI or recurrent UTI,

or child with a UTI and family history of renal disease, abnormal pattern of voiding, poor growth, hypertension
- Imaging in children: renal ultrasound to detect obstruction; voiding cystourethrogram to establish vesicoureteral reflux

The preferred method of collection of a urine specimen in children who are not toilet-trained is catheterization.

Urine culture results will be altered if patient has taken an antibiotic prior to collection of urine for culture.

PREVENTION

- Good hydration
- Emptying bladder immediately after sexual intercourse
- Estrogen therapy in postmenopausal women
- Good perineal hygiene
- Frequent voiding
- Prophylactic antibiotics

NONPHARMACOLOGIC MANAGEMENT

- Good hydration
- Voiding after intercourse if infection associated with sexual intercourse
- Good perineal hygiene

URINARY TRACT INFECTION PHARMACOLOGIC MANAGEMENT

Class	Drug Generic name (Trade name®)	Dosage How supplied	Comments
Sulfa Agents *Block synthesis of folic acid by bacteria and thus inhibit bacterial replication*	**sulfamethoxazole (SMZ) - trimethoprim (TMP)**	**Adult:** one DS or 2 regular strength tabs twice daily for 10-14 days **Children > 2 months:** give 8 mg/kg/day of trimethoprim and 40 mg/kg/day of sulfamethoxazole in 2 divided doses daily	• Pregnancy Category C • Avoid use during pregnancy • Hypersensitivity reactions like Stevens-Johnson syndrome, toxic epidermal necrolysis and blood dyscrasias have been associated with sulfa use • Photosensitivity may occur with these drugs
	Bactrim Septra	*Tabs: 400 mg SMZ- 80 mg TMP* *Susp: 200 mg SMZ- 40 mg TMP/5 mL*	
	Bactrim DS	*Tabs: 800 mg SMZ-160 mg TMP*	
Fluoroquinolones *Inhibit the action of DNA gyrase which is essential for the organism to be able to replicate* <u>**General comments**</u> Fluoroquinolones, are associated with an increased risk of tendinitis and tendon rupture in all ages. This risk is further increased in older patients usually over 60 years of age, in patients taking corticosteroid drugs, and in patients with kidney, heart or lung transplants	**ciprofloxacin**	**Adult**: <u>Acute uncomplicated</u> 250 mg twice daily for 3 days <u>Mild/moderate</u> 250 mg twice daily for 7-14 days <u>Severe/complicated</u> 500 mg twice daily for 7-14 days **Children**: not recommended	• Pregnancy Category C • Avoid with theophylline, antacids, iron, zinc or NSAIDs at higher doses • Use with caution with drugs that lower the seizure threshold • Hypersensitivity reactions like Stevens-Johnson syndrome may occur • CNS disturbances such as seizure, dizziness, insomnia, nervousness may occur

continued

URINARY TRACT INFECTION PHARMACOLOGIC MANAGEMENT

Class	Drug Generic name (Trade name®)	Dosage How supplied	Comments
May exacerbate myasthenia gravis, therefore use in caution with this population Patients may experience moderate to severe photosensitivity while on medication Monitor for prolongation of QT interval May alter blood glucose levels in patients on antidiabetic agents	Cipro	*Tabs: 250 mg, 500 mg*	
	levofoxacin	**Adult**: Acute uncomplicated 250 mg daily for 3 days Complicated 250 mg daily for 10 days OR 750 mg daily for 5 days **Children:** not recommended	• Pregnancy Category C • Concomitant use with NSAIDs may increase risk of CNS stimulation and seizures
	Levaquin	*Tabs: 250 mg, 500 mg, 750 mg*	
	ofloxacin	**Adult**: Acute uncomplicated 200 mg twice daily for 3 days Complicated 200 mg twice daily for 10 days **Children**: not recommended	• Pregnancy Category C • Concomitant use with NSAIDs may increase risk of CNS stimulation and seizures • Maintain adequate hydration
	Floxin	*Tabs: 200 mg*	
	norfloxacin	**Adult**: Acute uncomplicated 400 mg twice daily for 3 days Complicated 400 mg twice daily for 10-21 days **Children**: not recommended	• Pregnancy Category C • Reduce dose if renal insufficiency present • Concomitant use with NSAIDs may increase risk of CNS stimulation and seizures
	Noroxin	*Tabs: 400 mg*	
Penicillins *Inhibit cell wall synthesis* In species that produce beta-lactamase, amoxicillin, and ampicillin are ineffective Amoxicillin/potassium clavulanate is effective against organisms that produce beta-lactamase	**amoxicillin**	**Adult**: Mild/Moderate 500 mg twice daily OR 250 mg three times daily for 10 days Severe 875 mg twice daily OR 500 mg three times daily for 10 days	• Pregnancy Category B • Adjust dose if renal insufficiency • Avoid if history of hypersensitivity to penicillin

continued

Urologic Disorders

URINARY TRACT INFECTION PHARMACOLOGIC MANAGEMENT

Class	Drug Generic name (Trade name®)	Dosage How supplied	Comments
		Children: Mild/Moderate 20 mg/kg/day in divided doses every 8 hours OR 40 mg/kg/day in divided doses every 12 hours *Max:* 500 mg/dose Severe 20 mg/kg/day in divided doses every 8 hours *Max:* 875 mg/dose	
	Amoxil Trimox	*Caps: 250 mg, 500 mg* *Tabs: 500 mg, 875 mg* *Susp: 125 mg/5 mL, 250 mg/5mL, 400 mg/5 mL*	
	amoxicillin and potassium clavulanate	**Adult**: Mild/Moderate 500 mg twice daily OR 250 mg three times daily for 10 days Severe 875 mg twice daily OR 500 mg three times daily for 10 days **Children**: Mild/Moderate 20 mg/kg/day in divided doses every 8 hours OR 40 mg/kg/day in divided doses every 12 hours *Max:* 500 mg/dose Severe 20 mg/kg/day in divided doses every 8 hours *Max:* 875 mg/dose	• Pregnancy Category B • Adjust dose if renal insufficiency • Avoid if history of hypersensitivity to penicillin • **TWO 250 mg tablets SHOULD NOT be substituted for a 500 mg dose due to the clavulanic acid dose**
	Augmentin	*Tabs: 250 mg, 500 mg, 875 mg* *Susp: 125 mg/5 mL, 250 mg/5 mL, 400 mg/5 mL*	

continued

URINARY TRACT INFECTION PHARMACOLOGIC MANAGEMENT

Class	Drug Generic name (Trade name®)	Dosage How supplied	Comments
	ampicillin	**Adult**: 500 mg four times/day for 10 days **Children < 20 kg:** 100 mg/kg/day every six hours for 10 days *Max:* 2-3 g/day **> 20 kg:** See adult	• Pregnancy Category B • Take on empty stomach • Avoid use if suspect *N. gonorrhoeae*
	Principen	*Caps: 250 mg, 500 mg*	
Cephalosporins - Second Generation *Inhibits cell wall synthesis of bacteria* General comments ~ 2-10% cross sensitivity with penicillin; contraindicated if patient has history of penicillins anaphylactic response or hives	**cefaclor**	**Adults**: 250-500 mg three times daily **Children**: 20-40 mg/kg/day in three divided doses *Max:* 500 mg/dose	• Pregnancy Category B
	Ceclor	*Tabs: 250 mg, 500 mg* *Susp: 125 mg/5 mL, 187 mg/5 mL, 250 mg/5 mL, 375 mg/5mL*	
	cefuroxime	**Adults**: Uncomplicated 250 mg twice daily for 7-10 days **Children**: not recommended	• Pregnancy Category B • May be taken without regard to meals • Ceftin tablets and Ceftin suspension are NOT bioequivalent • Renal dysfunction prolongs half-life of product
	Ceftin	*Tabs: 250 mg* *Susp: 125 mg/5 mL, 250 mg/5 mL*	
Cephalosporins - Third Generation *Inhibits cell wall synthesis of bacteria* General comments ~ 2-10% cross sensitivity with penicillin; contraindicated if patient has history of penicillins anaphylactic response or hives	**cefixime**	**Adults:** 400 mg once daily for 3-7 days **Children**: not approved	• Pregnancy Category B • Reduce dose by 25% if renal dysfunction
	Suprax	*Tabs: 400 mg* *Susp: 100 mg/5 mL, 200 mg/5 mL*	
	cefpodoxime	**Adults:** 100 mg twice daily for 7 days	• Pregnancy Category B • Avoid antacids 2 hours before and after dose
	Vantin	*Tabs: 100 mg* *Susp: 50 mg/5 mL, 100 mg/5 mL*	

continued

URINARY TRACT INFECTION PHARMACOLOGIC MANAGEMENT

Class	Drug Generic name (Trade name®)	Dosage How supplied	Comments
Miscellaneous	**nitrofurantoin**	**Adult**: 100 mg twice daily for 7 days (with food) **Children < 12 years:** not recommended **> 12 years:** see adult	• Pregnancy Category B • Contraindicated if patient has anuria, oliguria, or impaired renal function • Should be taken with food • Avoid concurrent use of antacids
	Macrobid	*Caps: 100 mg*	
Anti-spasmodic *Inhibits smooth muscle spasm of the bladder and urinary tract*	**flavoxate**	**Adult**: 100 mg-200 mg three or four times a day **Children**: not recommended	• Pregnancy Category B • Must be used in conjunction with an antibiotic for treatment of UTI • Do not use in patients with glaucoma, intestinal obstruction
	Urispas	*Tabs: 100 mg*	
	phenazopyridine	**Adult:** 200 mg three times daily after meals; maximum 2 days of therapy **Children:** not recommended	• Pregnancy Category B • The dye exerts an analgesic effect on the bladder and urinary tract mucosa via unknown means • Must be used in conjunction with an antibiotic to treat UTI • Discolors urine orange and can stain undergarments • Use with caution in patients with hepatic or renal dysfunction • Maximum of 6 doses per UTI because accumulation of drug can occur and toxicity can result • May discolor soft contact lens
	Pyridium	*Tabs: 100 mg, 200 mg*	

- Women: three day treatment usually adequate for uncomplicated UTI; consider 7-14 days if complicated
- Men: treat for 7-10 days
- Children: 7-10 days
- Preferred antibiotic for children is a second or third generation cephalosporin because of Gram negative coverage and palatability

PREGNANCY/LACTATION CONSIDERATIONS

- Urine culture recommended
- Penicillin, cephalosporin, or nitrofurantoin are good first choices but consider regional resistance rates to *E. coli*
- Treat for 10-14 days
- May need prophylactic antibiotics for duration of pregnancy
- Avoid quinolones and sulfa drugs

CONSULTATION/REFERRAL

- Consultation with urologist for recurring infections, infection in child under 4 months, pyelonephritis in children, and in presence of acute illness
- Referral to urologist is indicated if anatomic abnormality is suspected or diagnosed
- Hospitalization may be required in patients with severe symptoms

FOLLOW-UP

- Post treatment culture if patient having frequent or recurrent UTI
- Evaluate children one week after therapy started

EXPECTED COURSE

- Complete resolution without complications within 2-3 days after starting treatment

POSSIBLE COMPLICATIONS

- Pyelonephritis
- Renal abscess

ACUTE PYELONEPHRITIS

DESCRIPTION

Infection of the upper urinary tract and renal parenchyma; is usually uncomplicated but if not managed appropriately can lead to bacteremia and death.

ETIOLOGY

- 75% caused by *E. coli*
- Other gram negative bacteria (e.g., *Proteus mirabilis, Klebsiella pneumoniae*, or *Enterobacter* sp.) are responsible for 10-15%
- Gram positive bacteria (e.g., *Staphylococcus aureus* and *saprophyticus*) account for another 10-15%
- In older children and adults the most common route of infection is movement of bacteria from bladder to upper urinary tract
- In neonates, the most common route is hematogenous spread to the kidneys

INCIDENCE

- 15.7/100,000 persons develop pyelonephritis annually

RISK FACTORS

Adults:
- Urinary tract abnormalities
- Recent untreated or undertreated UTI
- Indwelling urinary catheter
- Urinary tract instrumentation
- Renal calculi
- Diabetes mellitus
- Immunocompromised host
- Elderly
- Institutionalization, especially women
- Recent pyelonephritis
- Obstruction of normal urine flow (e.g., urethral stricture, benign prostatic hyperplasia)
- Fecal, stress incontinence
- Pregnancy

Children:
- Vesicoureteral reflux
- Anatomical abnormalities in the renal system
- Behavioral factors (e.g., deferral of voiding, poor hygiene)
- Lack of circumcision in male infants

ASSESSMENT FINDINGS

Adolescents and adults:
- Fever, chills
- Costovertebral angle tenderness
- Flank pain
- Abdominal tenderness
- Malaise, myalgia
- Hematuria
- Nausea and vomiting
- Headache
- Dysuria, frequency, urgency

Infants and children:
- Fever which can progress to sepsis
- Failure to thrive
- Irritability
- Enuresis
- Nausea and vomiting

DIFFERENTIAL DIAGNOSIS

- Renal calculi
- Prostatitis, epididymitis

- Low back pain secondary to disc disease, aortic aneurysm, strain
- Urinary tract tumors
- Herpes zoster
- Ectopic pregnancy

DIAGNOSTIC STUDIES

- Urinalysis: pyuria, positive leukocyte esterase test, possibly hematuria, proteinuria, alkaline pH, WBC casts
- Urine culture with sensitivity
- CBC: leukocytosis

For patients with acute pyelonephritis who do not improve within 48-72 hours and who are on an appropriate antibiotic, renal ultrasound or CT scan should be considered.

NONPHARMACOLOGIC MANAGEMENT

- Requires inpatient treatment if patient appears toxic, pregnant, intolerant of oral medications, fluids, and food, or in young children
- Encourage fluids

PHARMACOLOGIC MANAGEMENT

- Initial treatment is broad spectrum antibiotic until culture and sensitivity available (consider quinolone or third generation cephalosporin, broad spectrum penicillin until culture available): See Urinary Tract Infection, page 689
- Do not use nitrofurantoin since poor tissue levels are achieved in the renal parenchyma

PREGNANCY/LACTATION CONSIDERATIONS

- Requires hospitalization during pregnancy
- Common reason for hospitalization during pregnancy

CONSULTATION/REFERRAL

- Consult urologist if patient has been febrile > 72 hours (probable invasive/extensive workup: IVP, cysto, spiral CT)
- Refer if patient is pregnant
- Refer if no improvement after 48 hours of outpatient treatment
- Refer for inpatient treatment if acutely ill
- Refer to urologist for urologic workup if recurring infections occur

FOLLOW-UP

- Follow up urine culture not needed if patient resolution of symptoms and an unremarkable course; otherwise, consider a follow up urine culture

EXPECTED COURSE

- Good prognosis with adequate treatment
- Should see improvement in 48 hours in outpatient setting

POSSIBLE COMPLICATIONS

- Sepsis
- Preterm labor/delivery
- Chronic renal insufficiency
- Chronic pyelonephritis

URETHRITIS

DESCRIPTION

Inflammation of the urethra; generally due to infection with gonorrhea, but maybe non-gonococcal.

ETIOLOGY

- Usually a sexually transmitted disease
- Most common organisms: *N. gonorrhoeae, C. trachomatis, Ureaplasma urealyticum, Trichomonas vaginalis*, and viruses
- May be due to foreign bodies, irritating soaps, indwelling urinary catheter

INCIDENCE

- Gonococcal urethritis usually found in males
- Non-gonococcal usually found in females

RISK FACTORS

- Sexual activity
- Multiple sexual partners
- Previous sexually transmitted disease

ASSESSMENT FINDINGS

- Asymptomatic (especially females)
- Fever
- Dysuria
- Frequency
- Urethral discharge
- Suprapubic discomfort
- Urethral tenderness
- Pruritus of urethra
- Dyspareunia

- Tenderness, edema, and inflammation of the urethra, especially in women
- Vaginitis, cystitis, and cervicitis may also be present in women
- Proctitis, pharyngitis, and conjunctivitis may also be present

Males usually report symptoms 3-5 days after exposure to an STD. Females are usually asymptomatic initially.

DIFFERENTIAL DIAGNOSIS

- Cystitis
- Epididymitis, prostatitis
- Trauma
- Atrophic vaginitis
- Intraurethral foreign bodies or growths
- Allergic or sensitivity reaction

DIAGNOSTIC STUDIES

- All patients with suspected or confirmed urethritis should be tested for gonorrhea and chlamydia
- Diagnosis made if > 5 WBC per high power field (HPF)
- Gram stain and culture of discharge
- Urinalysis not as sensitive as direct culture
- Wet prep of discharge: WBCs, trichomonads may be visible

Encourage screening for other STDs, hepatitis B & C, and HIV.

PREVENTION

- Use of condoms
- Urinating immediately after sexual intercourse
- Screen for STDs

NONPHARMACOLOGIC MANAGEMENT

- Evaluation and treatment of sexual partners
- Abstinence until treatment completed
- Sexual abuse should be investigated in children with any STD

Treat all known sexual partners in the last 60 days.

PHARMACOLOGIC MANAGEMENT

- Treat initially for gonorrhea and chlamydia
- Consider:
  - ◊ ceftriaxone 125 mg IM in a single dose OR cefixime 400 mg in a single dose *plus*
  - ◊ azithromycin 1 gram orally in a single dose OR doxycycline 100 mg orally twice daily for 7 days

Do not wait until cultures are available to treat.

PREGNANCY/LACTATION CONSIDERATIONS

- Avoid use of tetracycline
- Do not use metronidazole (Flagyl®) in first trimester
- Test of cure recommended after treatment complete

FOLLOW-UP

- Test of cure not necessary if course of treatment completed

EXPECTED COURSE

- Improvement of symptoms in 48-72 hours
- Complete resolution with effective treatment

POSSIBLE COMPLICATIONS

- Stricture formation
- Pelvic inflammatory disease in women

URINARY INCONTINENCE

(Stress Incontinence, Urge Incontinence, Overflow Incontinence)

DESCRIPTION

Involuntary loss of urine (in an adult patient) from the urethra which is usually recognized by the patient as a problem or inconvenience.

Involuntary loss of urine in children usually termed enuresis.

ETIOLOGY

Urge Incontinence (detrusor instability):
- Urinary tract infection
- Chronic cystitis
- Dementia
- Parkinson's disease
- Aging
- Stroke
- Irradiation of bladder

Conditions that mimic urge incontinence
- ◊ **Dementia**
- ◊ **Infection**
- ◊ **Atrophic vaginitis**
- ◊ **Pharmaceuticals (retention)**
- ◊ **Excess urinary output**
- ◊ **Restricted mobility**
- ◊ **Stool impaction**

Stress Incontinence (sphincter incompetence):
- Aging
- Pelvic floor muscle weakness
- Estrogen deficiency
- Perineal trauma
- Prostatic/pelvic surgery

Reflex Incontinence:
- Disc herniation
- Diabetes mellitus
- Neurologic tumors
- Spinal cord disease
- Multiple sclerosis

Overflow Incontinence:
- Prostatic enlargement
- Medications (e.g., antidepressants, anticholinergics)
- Outflow tract obstruction
- Diabetic neuropathy

Functional Incontinence:
- Severe mental illness
- Sedating medications
- Physical or mental disability

Mixed incontinence is stress incontinence coupled with urge incontinence.

INCIDENCE

- 5-15% of elderly in the community
- Approximately 12 million in the United States
- Up to 50% of nursing home residents
- Females > Males

RISK FACTORS

- Increasing age in men and women
- Declining estrogen levels
- Multiparity
- Dementia
- Diabetes mellitus
- Spinal cord injury/lesion, other neurological conditions
- Prostatic hypertrophy
- Stroke
- Certain medications (e.g., diuretics)
- Immobility

ASSESSMENT FINDINGS

- Involuntary loss of urine
- Urinary urgency
- Burning with urination
- Perineal irritation
- Pelvic exam: may detect GU pathology
- Rectal exam: may demonstrate prostatic pathology, fecal impaction
- Abdomen: may palpate distended bladder

DIFFERENTIAL DIAGNOSIS

- Urinary tract infection

- Effect of medications
- Undiagnosed diabetes, benign prostatic hyperplasia, STD
- Psychiatric illness

DIAGNOSTIC STUDIES

- Voiding diary for 2-3 days indicating when incontinent episodes occur
- Urinalysis: normal unless some underlying condition is present
- BUN, creatinine
- Post-voiding residual volume measurement
- Voiding cystourethrogram or uroflowmetry when obstruction is suspected

PREVENTION

- Kegel exercises, especially following childbirth
- Regular
- Treatment of prostatic hyperplasia

NONPHARMACOLOGIC MANAGEMENT

- Treat underlying problem if present
- Use of a voiding diary for 3 days to provide information about the patient's voiding habits
- Good perineal hygiene
- Regular emptying of bladder even if no urge is sensed
- Kegel exercises
- Intermittent self-catheterization for urinary retention
- Use of incontinence pads, vaginal cones in women
- Condom catheters in male patients
- Dietary/medication modifications (e.g., caffeine restriction, avoidance of alcohol, etc.)
- Biofeedback
- Surgery in selected patients (e.g., TURP, bladder suspension)
- Treat constipation

Urologic Disorders

URGE INCONTINENCE PHARMACOLOGIC MANAGEMENT

Class	Drug Generic name (Trade name®)	Dosage How supplied	Comments
Anticholinergics *Antispasmodic effect on smooth muscle and inhibits the muscarinic action of acetylcholine on smooth muscle* General comments Use in caution in myasthenia gravis patients (who have decreased cholinergic activity at the neuromuscular junction) May cause dry mouth, blurred vision May produce constipation	**oxybutynin**	**Immediate Release** **Adult:** *Initial*: 5 mg 2-3 times daily *Max*: 5 mg four times daily **Frail elderly**: *Initial*: 2.5 mg 2-3 times daily **Children > 5 yr:** 5 mg twice daily **Extended Release** **Adult:** *Initial*: 5-10 mg once daily (Same time each day) *Max*: 30 mg once daily **Children:** *Initial*: 5 mg/day *Max*: 20 mg/day	• Pregnancy Category B • NOTE DOSAGE FORMS • Do not crush XL formulation • May aggravate symptoms of hyperthyroidism, congestive heart failure, arrhythmias, tachycardia, prostatic hypertrophy, myasthenia gravis • Use in caution in patients with bladder outflow obstruction
	Ditropan	*Tabs: 5 mg*	
	Ditropan XL	*Tabs: 5 mg, 10 mg, 15 mg*	

continued

URGE INCONTINENCE PHARMACOLOGIC MANAGEMENT

Class	Drug Generic name (Trade name®)	Dosage How supplied	Comments
	tolterodine	<u>**Immediate Release**</u> **Adult:** 2 mg twice daily **Renal or hepatic patients:** 2 mg daily **Children:** not recommended <u>**Extended Release**</u> **Adult:** *Initial*: 2-4 mg once daily *Usual*: 4 mg once daily *Max*: 4 mg once daily	• Pregnancy Category C • NOTE DOSAGE FORMS • Do not crush LA formulation • May prolong QT interval • Contraindicated in patients with urinary retention, gastric retention, uncontrolled narrow-angle glaucoma • May cause dizziness or drowsiness • Not recommended in patients with severe renal impairment
	Detrol	*Tabs: 1 mg, 2 mg*	
	Detrol LA	*Ext. Rel. Tabs: 2 mg, 4 mg*	
	trospium	<u>**Immediate Release**</u> **Adult:** 20 mg twice daily **Adult > 75 years:** 20 mg once daily **Renal or hepatic patients:** 20 mg once nightly **Children:** not recommended <u>**Extended Release**</u> **Adult:** 60 mg daily on an empty stomach	• Pregnancy Category C • NOTE DOSAGE FORMS • Should be taken on empty stomach • Has effect on QT interval • Avoid XL formulation in patients with renal or hepatic impairment • Contraindicated in patients with narrow angle glaucoma
	Sanctura	*Tabs: 20 mg*	
	Sanctura XL	*Caps: 60 mg*	
	solifenacin	**Adult:** *Initial*: 5 mg daily *Max*: 10 mg daily **Renal Impairment:** *Max*: 5 mg daily **Children:** not recommended	• Pregnancy Category C • Has effect on QT interval • Contraindicated in patients with urinary retention, gastric retention, uncontrolled narrow-angle glaucoma • May cause dizziness or drowsiness • Not recommended in patients with severe renal impairment
	Vesicare	*Tabs: 5 mg, 10 mg*	• Use in caution in patients with reduced hepatic function

OVERFLOW INCONTINENCE PHARMACOLOGIC MANAGEMENT

Prior to initiating therapy with these products must include appropriate evaluation to identify other conditions such as BPH, infection, prostate cancer, stricture disease, hypotonic bladder or other neurogenic disorders

Class	Drug Generic name (Trade name®)	Dosage How supplied	Comments
Alpha adrenergic antagonists *blockade of the alpha adrenergic receptors causes relaxation of smooth muscle in the prostate and neck of the bladder* **General comments** May cause orthostatic hypotension Must be used with caution in patients taking erectile dysfunction medications Seek medical attention for priapism	**doxazosin**	**Adult:** *Initial*: 1 mg/day *Usual*: Titrate for effect *Max*: 8 mg/day **Extended Release** **Adult:** *Initial*: 4 mg/day *Usual*: Titrate for effect *Max*: 8 mg/day	• Pregnancy Category C • Drug therapy must be individualized • Increase immediate release dose at 7-14 day intervals; increase extended dose at 3-4 week interval • Extended release form contraindicated in patients with hepatic dysfunction • Extended release form should be taken daily with breakfast • Do not crush or chew extended release form
	Cardura	*Tabs: 1 mg, 2 mg, 4 mg, 8 mg scored*	
	Cardura XL	*Ext. Rel. Tabs: 4 mg, 8 mg*	
	tamsulosin	**Adult:** *Initial*: 0.4 mg/day *Max*: 0.8 mg/day	• Pregnancy Category B • Doses should be taken at a consistent time each day • May increase dose after 2-4 weeks • If higher doses are held for extended periods, resume at lower dose and titrate back
	Flomax	*Caps: 0.4 mg*	
	terazosin	**Adult:** *Initial*: 1 mg/day at HS *Usual*: titrate for effect *Max*: 20 mg/day	• Pregnancy Category C • Syncope most likely timed with dosage administration • If higher doses are held for extended periods, resume at lower dose and titrate back
	Hytrin	*Tabs: 1 mg, 2 mg, 5 mg, 10 mg* *Caps: 1 mg, 2 mg, 5 mg, 10 mg*	
Antiandrogenic agents *inhibit conversion of testosterone to the androgen, DHT. Enlargement of the prostate gland is caused by DHT*	**dutasteride**	As Monotherapy **Adult:** *Initial*: 0.5 mg/day *Max*: 0.5 mg/day As Combination Therapy *Initial*: 0.5 mg/day *Max*: 0.5 mg/day in combination with tamsulosin (0.4 mg) daily	• Pregnancy Category C • Do not crush or chew • If higher doses are held for extended periods, resume at monotherapy dose and titrate back
	Avodart	*Caps: 0.5 mg*	

continued

OVERFLOW INCONTINENCE PHARMACOLOGIC MANAGEMENT

Prior to initiating therapy with these products must include appropriate evaluation to identify other conditions such as BPH, infection, prostate cancer, stricture disease, hypotonic bladder or other neurogenic disorders

Class	Drug Generic name (Trade name®)	Dosage How supplied	Comments
General comments Pregnant women should not handle product May take 6-12 months to assess benefit of therapy PSA levels will decrease while on this therapy	**finasteride** Proscar	As Monotherapy **Adult:** *Initial*: 5 mg/day *Max*: 5 mg/day As Combination Therapy **Adult:** *Initial*: 5 mg/day *Max*: 5 mg/day in combination with doxazosin daily *Tabs: 5 mg*	• Pregnancy Category X • Do not crush or chew • May be taken without regard to meals • May decrease amount of ejaculate

PREGNANCY/LACTATION CONSIDERATIONS

- Stress incontinence may occur in pregnancy
- Should be treated non-pharmacologically with Kegel exercises, good hygiene, frequent voiding, and use of incontinence pads

CONSULTATION/REFERRAL

- Refer to urologist or gynecologist (depending on etiology) when refractory to initial medication measures or lifestyle modification
- Refer if neurologic abnormalities present

FOLLOW-UP

- Frequent visits for assessment of therapy and support
- Assess BP in men on alpha blockers
- Ophthalmologist for measurement of intraocular pressure in patients with family history of glaucoma

EXPECTED COURSE

- Variable prognosis depending on underlying cause, but good improvement seen with medication management for urge and overflow incontinence
- Stress incontinence best managed (eradicated) with surgical intervention

POSSIBLE COMPLICATIONS

- Intolerable side effects from medication
- Urinary tract infection
- Hydronephrosis
- Renal failure
- Skin excoriation and breakdown
- Social isolation
- Depression and/or anxiety

ENURESIS
(Bed-wetting)

DESCRIPTION

Involuntary urination beyond the age of 5 years in children; nocturnal enuresis is defined as 2 episodes weekly of bedwetting having occurred for 3 months or more.

TERMS

Nocturnal enuresis	Most common form, occurs during sleep
Diurnal enuresis	Incontinence during waking hours
Primary enuresis	Child who has never achieved continence
Secondary enuresis	Child who has return of involuntary urination after achieving continence

ETIOLOGY

- Multifactorial
- Inheritance plays a role (75% of patients with enuresis have/had a first degree relative with enuresis)
- Other contributing factors may be:
  - ◊ Lack of normal increase in nocturnal ADH secretion
  - ◊ Reduced bladder capacity
  - ◊ Food allergies
  - ◊ Disorders of the genitourinary or nervous system (3-4 %)
  - ◊ Psychological factors may play a role
- Causes of secondary enuresis may be:
  - ◊ Bacteriuria
  - ◊ Inability to concentrate urine due to insufficient ADH or renal tubular defect
  - ◊ Glucosuria
  - ◊ Pelvic mass
  - ◊ Spinal cord malformation

INCIDENCE

- Approximately 10% of children
- Occurs in 40% of 3 year olds, 13% of 6 year olds, 3% of 12 year olds, and 1% of > 15 year olds
- Males > Females (2:1)

RISK FACTORS

- History of at least one parent having been enuretic
- First born child
- Dysfunctional family, stressful life events for children
- Children with sleep disorders

ASSESSMENT FINDINGS

- Inability to keep from urinating while asleep at least once/month
- Wetting may occur during daytime
- Stress factors may be present

Assess for constipation. This is an often missed cause of secondary enuresis.

DIFFERENTIAL DIAGNOSIS

- Diabetes insipidus
- Diabetes mellitus
- Renal tubular defects
- Spinal cord malformations or tumors, especially seen with secondary and diurnal enuresis
- Urinary tract infection
- Genitourinary or neurologic anomalies

DIAGNOSTIC STUDIES

- Urinalysis
- Urine culture if infection present
- Pregnancy test if indicated
- If enuresis complicated by severe voiding dysfunction, encopresis, or abnormal neurologic exam consider:
  - ◊ Renal ultrasound
  - ◊ Intravenous pyelogram
  - ◊ Voiding cystourethrogram

Urinalysis screens for diabetes insipidis, can indicate the presence of glucose, ketones, white cells and bacteria. A urinalysis should include a urine specific gravity.

NONPHARMACOLOGIC MANAGEMENT

- Counseling and behavior modification if enuresis due to apparent stressor or family dysfunction
- Positive reinforcement, rewards and praise for dry nights
- No fluids within 2 hours of bedtime
- Avoidance of stimulants before bedtime (caffeinated drinks, chocolate, spicy foods, etc.)
- Voiding immediately before bedtime
- No punishment of child for enuresis
- Child should not be made to feel guilty
- Bed-wetting alarms (70% rate of success)
- Bladder capacity and stretching exercises (most children with nocturnal enuresis have small bladder capacity)

Bed wetting alarms have a higher success rate than medications for eradication of enuresis.

Most cases resolve spontaneously.

ENURESIS PHARMACOLOGIC MANAGEMENT

Class	Drug Generic name (Trade name®)	Dosage How supplied	Comments
Tricyclic antidepressants	**imipramine**	**Children 6-12 years:** *Initial*: 25 mg given 1 hour before bedtime; may increase to 50 mg night after one week **Children > 12 years:** 75 mg one hour before bedtime (if not using split dose therapy) *Max*: 2.5 mg/kg/day	• Pregnancy Category C • Effectiveness may decrease with continued drug administration • For older children, consider split dose therapy; 25 mg in afternoon and 50 mg 1 hour before bedtime • Avoid MAO Inhibitors
	Tofranil	*Tabs: 10 mg, 25 mg, 50 mg*	
Vasopressin	**desmopressin**	**Children 6-17 years:** *Initial*: 0.2 mg at bedtime *Max*: 0.6 mg at bedtime	• Pregnancy Category B • Must address possible hyponatremia and water intoxication with caregiver • Contraindicated in patients with several renal impairment
	DDAVP	*Tabs: 0.1 mg, 0.2 mg*	

CONSULTATION/REFERRAL

- Presence of emotional problem may require referral
- Neurological or genitourinary dysfunction requires referral to specialist

FOLLOW-UP

- Frequent visits for support and encouragement

EXPECTED COURSE

- Self-limiting problem
- Eventual resolution as child ages

HEMATURIA

DESCRIPTION

The presence of blood in an uncontaminated specimen of urine detected by dipstick, microscopic examination, or the naked eye.

Microscopic hematuria occurs when 3000-4000 RBCs/minute are excreted in the urine. Macroscopic hematuria occurs when the rate exceeds 1 million/minute.

ETIOLOGY

Adults:
- Malignant neoplasms in the GU tract
- Infection
- Renal calculi
- Coagulopathy
- Glomerular disease
- Hydronephrosis
- Polycystic kidneys
- Trauma
- Medications (e.g., heparin, warfarin, aspirin)
- Benign prostatic hyperplasia
- Exercise-induced

Children:
- Urinary tract infection
- Perineal or urethral irritation
- Sickle cell disease
- Trauma

ASSESSMENT FINDINGS

- May be associated with pain
- May be intermittent or persistent
- Assessment findings consistent with underlying problem

DIFFERENTIAL DIAGNOSIS

- Urinary tract infection
- Polycystic kidney disease
- Neoplasm
- Lupus erythematosus
- Renal calculi
- Benign prostatic hyperplasia
- Wilm's tumor
- Sickle cell disease
- Drugs (e.g., heparin, warfarin, aspirin)
- Hemophilia
- Thrombocytopenia purpura
- Glomerulonephritis
- Epididymitis
- Vaginal bleeding
- Presence of pigment from various sources (e.g., porphyria, foods, medications)
- Strenuous exercise and long-distance running
- Fever
- Trauma
- False positive urine dipstick from some confounding substance
- Cigarette smoking

DIAGNOSTIC STUDIES

- Urinalysis: RBCs, RBC casts
- BUN, creatinine
- CBC to assess for anemia
- 24-hour urine specimen (to quantify RBC loss)
- IVP (good initial test)
- Renal ultrasound (differentiates cysts from solid masses), cystoscopy
- Renal biopsy
- CT scan (best to assess/identify renal masses or stone)
- MRI (evaluates renal masses, expensive)
- Sickle cell assessment
- Other specific tests as indicated

A cast is a mucoprotein formed in the renal tubules. An RBC cast is one which contains trapped RBCs. The presence of an RBC cast indicates glomerular injury and may be seen in freshly voided specimens.

MANAGEMENT

- Dependent on underlying etiology

CONSULTATION/REFERRAL

- Need consultation with referral to urologist/ nephrologist depending on diagnostic work-up
- Patients with persistent hematuria should be referred to a nehprologist

FOLLOW-UP

- Repeat urinalysis within 4-6 weeks if uncomplicated urinary tract infection

EXPECTED COURSE

- Dependent on underlying etiology

POSSIBLE COMPLICATIONS

- Dependent on underlying etiology

UROLITHIASIS
(Urinary Tract Stones)

DESCRIPTION

Stones in the urinary tract generally composed of calcium (most common), uric acid, cystine, magnesium, aluminum, phosphate, etc.

ETIOLOGY

- Supersaturation of urine with stone-forming salts
- Cause of this phenomenon is multifactorial and dependent on type of stone

Calcium oxalate/calcium phosphate stones are most common (65-85% incidence). However, in warm, dry climates, uric acid stones account for up to 40% of stones.

INCIDENCE

- Males > Females (4:1)
- 2-5% of the population may have urolithiasis during their lifetime

RISK FACTORS

- Renal tubular acidosis
- Alkaline pH of urine
- Cystinuria
- Genetic defects
- Low water intake or high Vitamin C or D consumption
- Calcium supplementation
- Thiazide diuretic use, gout
- High animal protein diet
- Sedentary lifestyle

ASSESSMENT FINDINGS

- Sudden onset of back and flank pain (usually severe) that waxes and wanes
- Pain may radiate to groin, testicles, suprapubic area, and labia
- Costovertebral angle tenderness
- Flank pain
- Hematuria
- Dysuria
- Urinary frequency
- Diaphoresis
- Restlessness
- Tachycardia
- Tachypnea
- Chills and fever if infection secondary to obstruction
- Nausea and/or vomiting

If stone is very large or unable to move outside the kidney, patient may be asymptomatic. Eventually, the stone will move or the patient will develop an infection.

DIFFERENTIAL DIAGNOSIS

- Acute peritonitis
- Pyelonephritis
- Acute appendicitis
- Abdominal aortic aneurysm
- Colitis, diverticulitis
- Salpingitis, other GYN disorder
- Cholecystitis
- Peptic ulder disease
- Pancreatitis

DIAGNOSTIC STUDIES

- Urinalysis: hematuria, pyuria may or may not be present
- CBC: within normal limits
- BUN, creatinine, metabolic panel
- Urine culture: may be positive if obstruction to urinary flow has occurred
- 24-hour urine collection for calcium, uric acid, magnesium, oxalate, citrate, and creatinine if recurrent problem
- Stone analysis
- Spiral CT considered gold standard (most sensitive test and helpful in evaluating cause of pain if not due to a stone)
- KUB x-ray (will not identify uric acid stones, small stones or stones overlying a bony prominence)
- Intravenous pyelogram (IVP)
- Ultrasonography, if cannot use CT because of radiation exposure (example: pregnant patient)

If urine pH is < 5.5, stone is likely uric acid in composition.
If urine pH is > 7.5, stone is likely a "staghorn calculus". "Staghorn calculus" refers to the shape of the stone in the renal pelvis which forms as a result of high urinary pH. The stone is usually composed of magnesium ammonium nitrate (struvite).

Urologic Disorders

PREVENTION

- Adequate fluids

NONPHARMACOLOGIC MANAGEMENT

- Low animal fat diet
- Increased fiber in diet
- Fluid intake to maintain urinary output at 2-3 L/day
- Strain urine for presence of stones for 72 hours after symptoms resolve
- Observation with periodic evaluation is recommended for initial treatment
- For larger stones > 6 mm:
  - ◊ Extracorporeal shock wave lithotripsy
  - ◊ Ureteroscopy
  - ◊ Percutaneous nephrolithotomy
  - ◊ Open surgery for removal of the stone

Calcium stones:

- Restriction of:
  - ◊ Protein
  - ◊ Sodium
  - ◊ Dairy products
  - ◊ Calcium-rich foods
- Moderate calcium restriction (1000-1500 mg/day)

Uric acid stones:

- Alkalinization of urine for uric acid stones

There is a > 60% chance of passing a stone < 6 mm. If stone > 6 mm, chance of passing stone is < 20%.

PHARMACOLOGIC MANAGEMENT

- Medication for pain usually includes: narcotic analgesics or NSAIDs (ketorolac 60 mg IM) until referral to urologist or emergency department
- Antiemetic if nausea is present

CONSULTATION/REFERRAL

- Refer for hospitalization if:
  - ◊ Infection present
  - ◊ Stone > 6 mm in diameter
  - ◊ Excessive nausea and vomiting present
  - ◊ Intractable pain
  - ◊ Gross hematuria
- Urological consult, if obstruction suspected or if symptoms persist > 3-4 days
- Dietary consultation, if dietary modifications are planned

FOLLOW-UP

- Creatinine level weekly
- Parathormone level if stones are calcium
- Abdominal x-ray at 1-2 week intervals
- Monitor potassium levels and blood pressure in persons on hydrochlorothiazide (HCTZ®)

EXPECTED COURSE

- Up to 90% pass spontaneously
- Usually resolves within 4 weeks
- Recurrences common in up to 50% of patients within 5 years

POSSIBLE COMPLICATIONS

- Complete urinary obstruction
- Hydronephrosis
- Renal failure
- Infection

POSTSTREPTOCOCCAL GLOMERULONEPHRITIS

DESCRIPTION

Immune response to an infection which causes damage to the glomeruli; characterized by diffuse inflammatory changes in the glomeruli and clinically by gross hematuria.

ETIOLOGY

- Follows infection of throat or skin with bacteria, usually *Streptococcus* sp. (Group A **β**-hemolytic)
- The patient typically develops an acute glomerulonephritis 1-3 weeks after a streptococcal infection

INCIDENCE

- 20/100,000 cases annually in U.S.
- Most common in children between 2-12 years of age

RISK FACTORS

- More common in children
- Recent streptococcal infection (e.g., pharyngitis or impetigo)

ASSESSMENT FINDINGS

- Skin or pharyngeal streptococcal infection within the past 2-3 weeks
- Hematuria, abrupt onset (100% exhibit)
- Oliguria/anuria
- Proteinuria
- Edema, particularly of face, hands, and feet
- Hypertension (82%)
- Malaise
- Fever
- Abdominal or flank pain

DIFFERENTIAL DIAGNOSIS

- Glomerulonephritis secondary to something other than *Streptococcus*
- Systemic lupus erythematosus
- Anaphylactoid purpura
- Subacute bacterial endocarditis

DIAGNOSTIC STUDIES

- Antistreptolysin O (ASO): increased in 60-80% of cases
- Urinalysis: proteinuria, hematuria
- Throat and skin cultures: positive for streptococcal organism
- Total serum complement: decreased
- BUN/Creatinine

PREVENTION

- Early and aggressive treatment of streptococcal infections

It is unusual to have acute glomerulonephritis secondary to *Streptococcus* more than once because immunity usually develops after the first episode.

NONPHARMACOLOGIC MANAGEMENT

- Treatment inpatient until edema and hypertension under control; followed as outpatient
- No-added salt diet
- Fluid restriction
- Dialysis may be needed

PHARMACOLOGIC MANAGEMENT

- Management is focused on treating symptoms
- Volume overload if present (loop diuretics)
- Hypertension if present (antihypertensive agents specific to patient's age and severity)
- Treatment of Group A streptococcal infection if evidence supports its presence

CONSULTATION/REFERRAL

- Refer for inpatient management in the acute stage

FOLLOW-UP

- Depends on severity of illness
- Generally done by nephrologist

EXPECTED COURSE

- Usually self-limited
- Complete recovery in 95% of patients
- Resolution within 2-3 weeks
- Prognosis excellent in children; may have more morbidity in adults or in those with preexisting renal disease
- Proteinuria usually persists for up to 3 months, but may be present for up to 2 years

POSSIBLE COMPLICATIONS

- Glomerulonephritis which progresses to acute renal failure
- Persistence of abnormal urinalysis: hematuria, proteinuria
- Chronic renal failure is rare
- Nephrotic syndrome
- Congestive heart failure

RENAL INSUFFICIENCY

DESCRIPTION

Decrease in glomerular filtration rate (GFR) of the kidneys. Due to the difficulty of measuring GFR, another marker such as serum creatinine concentration or 24-hour urinary creatinine clearance may be used to define renal failure.

ETIOLOGY

- Numerous etiologies: tubular, glomerular, and/or vascular in origin
- Uncontrolled hypertension, diabetes
- Infection
- Metabolic disease
- Collagen vascular disease
- Exposure to nephrotoxic substances or medications

INCIDENCE

- 100 million annually develop end-stage renal failure
- Incidence is greater in nonwhites
- Males > Females

ASSESSMENT FINDINGS

- May be asymptomatic until end-stage renal disease
- Normochromic, normocytic anemia
- Fatigue and weakness
- Pruritus
- Nausea and vomiting
- Hematuria and proteinuria
- Lethargy
- Increased skin pigmentation
- Impaired urine concentrating ability in early stages resulting in polydipsia, polyuria, and nocturia
- Oliguria in later stages of failure
- Hypertension
- Edema including pulmonary edema

DIAGNOSTIC STUDIES

- Urinalysis: hematuria, proteinuria, casts
- BUN: elevated
- Creatinine: elevated
- 24-hour urine creatinine: elevated
- Potassium: elevated
- Serum calcium: decreased
- Sodium level: increases as insufficiency worsens
- Phosphate level: increased
- Uric acid levels: increased
- CBC: anemia
- Impaired platelet function
- Bleeding studies: prolonged

Cockroft and Gault Equation
Creatinine clearance (which closely correlates with GFR in most patients) can be estimated by using the following formula: **Creatinine clearance =({140-age in years} x ideal body weight in kg) / serum creatinine (mg/dL) x 72 (x 0.85 for females)**

GFR and Serum Creatinine Concentration Correlation with Renal Failure				
	Males		Females	
	GFR	Creat Conc	GFR	Creat Conc
Normal renal function	130 +15 mL/min	< 1.3 mg/dL	120 +15 mL/min	< 1 mg/dL
Early renal failure	56-100 mL/min	1.3-1.9 mg/dL	56-100 mL/min	1-1.9 mg/dL
Mod renal failure	25-55 mL/min	2-4 mg/dL	25-55 mL/min	2-4 mg/dL
Severe renal failure	< 24 mL/min	> 4 mg/dL	< 24 mL/min	> 4 mg/dL

NONPHARMACOLOGIC MANAGEMENT

- Treatment of underlying renal disease
- Discontinue nephrotoxic medications, especially NSAIDs
- Increase fluid intake (when tolerated) to 3000 mL daily
- Reduction of dietary protein intake to 0.5 g/kg/day of high quality protein
- Smoking cessation
- Fluid restriction when oliguria develops
- Sodium restriction of 4 grams/day when hypertension, oliguria, or congestive heart failure present
- Potassium restriction when patient becomes oliguric
- Restriction of uric acid if gout develops
- Peritoneal dialysis
- Hemodialysis
- Renal transplantation

Goal in treating contributing causes is to slow progression.

PHARMACOLOGIC MANAGEMENT

- Angiotensin converting-enzyme inhibitors are the drugs of choice for blood pressure control in renal insufficiency. Monitor potassium, BUN, creatinine levels CAREFULLY!
- Allopurinol (Zyloprim®) for prevention of gout
  Adult: 200-300 mg daily
  Children: not usually recommended
  Tabs: 100 mg, 300 mg scored tabs
- Recombinant erythropoietin when patient becomes symptomatic from anemia
- Loop diuretic therapy for treatment of fluid overload
  - ◊ furosemide
    Adult: initial 20-80 mg daily
    Children: initially 2 mg/kg, max 80 mg daily
    Tabs: 20 mg, 40 mg, 80 mg, scored

Thiazide diuretics are ineffective if GFR < 30 mL/min.

- Calcium citrate for correction of hyperphosphatemia
- Oral ferrous sulfate for iron deficiency anemia
- Multivitamin with folate
- Antiemetics
- Antihistamines for treatment of pruritus
- Dosages of medication which are excreted renally must be adjusted
- Avoid nephrotoxic drugs

ACE inhibitors are used to decrease proteinuria.

CONSULTATION/REFERRAL

- Early referral to nephrologist

FOLLOW-UP

- Must be followed closely with frequent visits and diagnostic testing

Many medications will require renal dose adjustment.

EXPECTED COURSE

- Largely determined by underlying renal disease
- Most patients develop end-stage renal failure within 1-5 years after initial diagnosis

POSSIBLE COMPLICATIONS

- Impotence and infertility
- Seizures
- Metabolic acidosis
- Coma
- Hypertension
- Hemorrhagic diathesis

WILM'S TUMOR
(Nephroblastoma)

DESCRIPTION

Embryonal renal neoplasm that is the major cause of renal malignancy in children.

ETIOLOGY

- Familial form is autosomal dominant trait

INCIDENCE

- 1 in 10,000 children < 16 years of age
- Most commonly occurs in children from infancy to age 15 years
- 2/3 of cases are in children <4 years old

RISK FACTORS

- Family member with Wilm's tumor

ASSESSMENT FINDINGS

- Usually asymptomatic
- Hematuria
- Abdominal mass
- Low grade fever
- Anemia
- Fatigue
- Anorexia
- Weight loss
- Associated anomalies: aniridia (absence of the iris of the eye), cryptorchidism, hypospadias, duplicated renal collecting systems, hemihypertrophy

DIFFERENTIAL DIAGNOSIS

- Neuroblastoma
- Hepatic tumors
- Sarcoma
- Abdominal mass

DIAGNOSTIC STUDIES

- Urinalysis: hematuria
- CBC: normocytic, normochromic anemia
- LDH: may be elevated
- KUB
- Abdominal ultrasound
- Chest x-ray
- CT scan of chest and abdomen
- MRI of abdomen

The chest is the usual site of recurrence of tumors or for metastasis. Therefore, it is prudent to order a chest x-ray and consider a chest CT.

PREVENTION

- Diagnostic work-up of children with associated anomalies

NONPHARMACOLOGIC MANAGEMENT

- Radiation therapy
- Radical nephrectomy

PHARMACOLOGIC MANAGEMENT

- Chemotherapy

CONSULTATION/REFERRAL

- Refer to pediatric oncologist and/or urologist upon diagnosis

EXPECTED COURSE

- Good prognosis with favorable histology and staging

POSSIBLE COMPLICATIONS

- Second malignancy

References

Bogart, L. M., Berry, S. H., & Clemens, J. Q. (2007). Symptoms of interstitial cystitis, painful bladder syndrome and similar diseases in women: A systematic review. *Journal of Urology, 177*(2), 450-456.

Brown, J. S., Bradley, C. S., Subak, L. L., Richter, H. E., Kraus, S. R., Brubaker, L., et al. (2006). The sensitivity and specificity of a simple test to distinguish between urge and stress urinary incontinence. *Annals of Internal Medicine, 144*(10), 715-723.

Burns, C. E., Dunn, A. M., Brady, M. A., Starr, N. B., & Blosser, C. (2008). *Pediatric primary care: A handbook for nurse practitioners*. Philadelphia: W. B. Saunders.

Chang, S. L., & Shortliffe, L. D. (2006). Pediatric urinary tract infections. *Pediatric Clinics of North America, 53*(3), 379-400, vi.

Colgan, R., Johnson, J. R., Kuskowski, M., & Gupta, K. (2008). Risk factors for trimethoprim-sulfamethoxazole resistance in patients with acute uncomplicated cystitis. *Antimicrobial Agents and Chemotherapy, 52*(3), 846-851.

Conway, P. H., Cnaan, A., Zaoutis, T., Henry, B. V., Grundmeier, R. W., & Keren, R. (2007). Recurrent urinary tract infections in children: Risk factors and association with prophylactic antimicrobials. *JAMA, 298*(2), 179-186.

Cook, R. L., Hutchison, S. L., Ostergaard, L., Braithwaite, R. S., & Ness, R. B. (2005). Systematic review: Noninvasive testing for chlamydia trachomatis and neisseria gonorrhoeae. *Annals of Internal Medicine, 142*(11), 914-925.

Curhan, G. C. (2007). Epidemiology of stone disease. *Urologic Clinics of North America, 34*(3), 287-293.

Czaja, C. A., Scholes, D., Hooton, T. M., & Stamm, W. E. (2007). Population-based epidemiologic analysis of acute pyelonephritis. *Clinical Infectious Diseases, 45*(3), 273-280.

Czaja, C. A., Stamm, W. E., Stapleton, A. E., Roberts, P. L., Hawn, T. R., Scholes, D., et al. (2009). Prospective cohort study of microbial and inflammatory events immediately preceding escherichia coli recurrent urinary tract infection in women. *Journal of Infectious Diseases, 200*(4), 528-536.

Demertzis, J., & Menias, C. O. (2007). State of the art: Imaging of renal infections. *Emerg Radiol, 14*(1), 13-22.

Domino, F., Baldor, R., Golding, J., Grimes, J., & Taylor, J. (2011). *The 5-minute clinical consult 2011*. Philadelphia: Lippincott Williams & Wilkins.

Drugs facts and comparisons 2010. (2010). St. Louis: Wolters Kluwer Health.

German, D. (2010). *Nurse practitioners prescribing reference*. New York: Haymarket Media Publication.

Goode, P. S., Burgio, K. L., Richter, H. E., & Markland, A. D. (2010). Incontinence in older women. *JAMA, 303*(21), 2172-2181.

Gross, P. A., & Patel, B. (2007). Reducing antibiotic overuse: A call for a national performance measure for not treating asymptomatic bacteriuria. *Clinical Infectious Diseases, 45*(10), 1335-1337.

Harris, S. S., Link, C. L., Tennstedt, S. L., Kusek, J. W., & McKinlay, J. B. (2007). Care seeking and treatment for urinary incontinence in a diverse population. *Journal of Urology, 177*(2), 680-684.

Hewitt, I. K., Zucchetta, P., Rigon, L., Maschio, F., Molinari, P. P., Tomasi, L., et al. (2008). Early treatment of acute pyelonephritis in children fails to reduce renal scarring: Data from the italian renal infection study trials. *Pediatrics, 122*(3), 486-490.

Holroyd-Leduc, J. M., Tannenbaum, C., Thorpe, K. E., & Straus, S. E. (2008). What type of urinary incontinence does this woman have? *JAMA, 299*(12), 1446-1456.

Ishani, A., Grandits, G. A., Grimm, R. H., Svendsen, K. H., Collins, A. J., Prineas, R. J., et al. (2006). Association of single measurements of dipstick proteinuria, estimated glomerular filtration rate, and hematocrit with 25-year incidence of end-stage renal disease in the multiple risk factor intervention trial. *Journal of the American Society of Nephrology, 17*(5), 1444-1452.

Johnson, L., Sabel, A., Burman, W. J., Everhart, R. M., Rome, M., MacKenzie, T. D., et al. (2008). Emergence of fluoroquinolone resistance in outpatient urinary escherichia coli isolates. *American Journal of Medicine, 121*(10), 876-884.

Koeijers, J. J., Kessels, A. G., Nys, S., Bartelds, A., Donker, G., Stobberingh, E. E., et al. (2007). Evaluation of the nitrite and leukocyte esterase activity tests for the diagnosis of acute symptomatic urinary tract infection in men. *Clinical Infectious Diseases, 45*(7), 894-896.

Lin, K., & Fajardo, K. (2008). Screening for asymptomatic bacteriuria in adults: Evidence for the U.S. Preventive services task force reaffirmation recommendation statement. *Annals of Internal Medicine, 149*(1), W20-24.

Mardon, R. E., Halim, S., Pawlson, L. G., & Haffer, S. C. (2006). Management of urinary incontinence in medicare managed care beneficiaries: Results from the 2004 medicare health outcomes survey. *Archives of Internal Medicine, 166*(10), 1128-1133.

Metzger, M. L., & Dome, J. S. (2005). Current therapy for wilms' tumor. *The Oncologist, 10*(10), 815-826.

Montini, G., Zucchetta, P., Tomasi, L., Talenti, E., Rigamonti, W., Picco, G., et al. (2009). Value of imaging studies after a first febrile urinary tract infection in young children: Data from italian renal infection study 1. *Pediatrics, 123*(2), e239-246.

Neveus, T., von Gontard, A., Hoebeke, P., Hjalmas, K., Bauer, S., Bower, W., et al. (2006). The standardization of terminology of lower urinary tract function in children and adolescents: Report from the standardisation committee of the international children's continence society. *Journal of Urology, 176*(1), 314-324.

Nicolle, L. E., Bradley, S., Colgan, R., Rice, J. C., Schaeffer, A., & Hooton, T. M. (2005). Infectious diseases society of america guidelines for the diagnosis and treatment of asymptomatic bacteriuria in adults. *Clinical Infectious Diseases, 40*(5), 643-654.

O'Connor, O. J., McSweeney, S. E., & Maher, M. M. (2008). Imaging of hematuria. *Radiologic Clinics of North America, 46*(1), 113-132, vii.

Oreskovic, N. M., & Sembrano, E. U. (2007). Repeat urine cultures in children who are admitted with urinary tract infections. *Pediatrics, 119*(2), e325-329.

Pearle, M. S., Calhoun, E. A., & Curhan, G. C. (2005). Urologic diseases in america project: Urolithiasis. *Journal of Urology, 173*(3), 848-857.

Prevalence of chronic kidney disease and associated risk factors--United States, 1999-2004. (2007). *MMWR. Morbidity and Mortality Weekly Report, 56*(8), 161-165.

Radvanska, E., Kovacs, L., & Rittig, S. (2006). The role of bladder capacity in antidiuretic and anticholinergic treatment for nocturnal enuresis. *Journal of Urology, 176*(2), 764-768; discussion 768-769.

Rodriguez-Iturbe, B., & Musser, J. M. (2008). The current state of poststreptococcal glomerulonephritis. *Journal of the American Society of Nephrology, 19*(10), 1855-1864.

Routh, J. C., Alt, A. L., Ashley, R. A., Kramer, S. A., & Boyce, T. G. (2009). Increasing prevalence and associated risk factors for methicillin resistant staphylococcus aureus bacteriuria. *Journal of Urology, 181*(4), 1694-1698.

Scales, C. D., Jr., Curtis, L. H., Norris, R. D., Springhart, W. P., Sur, R. L., Schulman, K. A., et al. (2007). Changing gender prevalence of stone disease. *Journal of Urology, 177*(3), 979-982.

Schneider, V., Levesque, L. E., Zhang, B., Hutchinson, T., & Brophy, J. M. (2006). Association of selective and conventional nonsteroidal antiinflammatory drugs with acute renal failure: A population-based, nested case-control analysis. *American Journal of Epidemiology, 164*(9), 881-889.

Scholes, D., Hooton, T. M., Roberts, P. L., Gupta, K., Stapleton, A. E., & Stamm, W. E. (2005). Risk factors associated with acute pyelonephritis in healthy women. *Annals of Internal Medicine, 142*(1), 20-27.

Screening for asymptomatic bacteriuria in adults: U.S. Preventive services task force reaffirmation recommendation statement. (2008). *Annals of Internal Medicine, 149*(1), 43-47.

Shaikh, N., Morone, N. E., Lopez, J., Chianese, J., Sangvai, S., D'Amico, F., et al. (2007). Does this child have a urinary tract infection? *JAMA, 298*(24), 2895-2904.

Sureshkumar, P., Jones, M., Cumming, R., & Craig, J. (2009). A population based study of 2,856 school-age children with urinary incontinence. *Journal of Urology, 181*(2), 808-815; discussion 815-806.

U S Food and Drug Administration. (2007). Safety information. Desmopressin acetate (marketed as ddavp nasal spray, ddavp rhinal tube, ddavp, ddvp, minirin, and stimate nasal spray). Retrieved from http://www.fda.gov/Safety/MedWatch/SafetyInformation/SafetyAlertsforHumanMedicalProducts/ucm079928.htm

Van Hoeck, K., Bael, A., Lax, H., Hirche, H., Van Dessel, E., Van Renthergem, D., et al. (2007). Urine output rate and maximum volume voided in school-age children with and without nocturnal enuresis. *Journal of Pediatrics, 151*(6), 575-580.

Workowski, K., Berman, S., & Centers for Disease Control and Prevention. (2006). Sexually transmitted diseases treatment guidelines, 2006. *MMWR Recomm Rep, 55*(RR-11), 1-94.

19

WOMEN'S HEALTH DISORDERS

Women's Health Disorders

Menstrual Cycle 719

Abnormal Vaginal Bleeding 720

Amenorrhea 722

Dysmenorrhea 723

Premenstrual Syndrome/Premenstrual Dysphoric Disorder 725

Abnormal Pap Smear 726

Cervical Cancer 729

Atrophic Vaginitis 730

Vulvovaginal Candidiasis 732

Bartholin's gland Cyst/Abscess 733

Polycystic Ovarian Disease 734

Benign Ovarian Tumors 736

Ovarian Cancer 737

Contraception 738

Menopause 747

Breast Cancer 749

Fibrocystic Breast Disease 750

Fibroadenoma 752

Intraductal Papilloma 753

References... *754*

MENSTRUAL CYCLE

NORMS

Age of menarche (1st menstrual cycle)	Average: 12-13 years Normal range: 10-16 years
Length of menstrual cycle	Average: 28 days
Length of menses	Normal range: 4-6 days
Blood loss with menses	25-60 mL/cycle

The menstrual cycle includes two cycles occurring simultaneously: *ovarian* and *endometrial*. View the summary of the two cycles.

Ovarian Cycle			
Timing in cycle	**Phase**	**Prominent Hormones**	**Description**
Day 1-14	Follicular	Follicular-stimulating hormone (FSH) Estrogen	Maturation of ovarian follicle
Day 14	Ovulation	Luteinizing hormone (LH)	Ovulation occurs 36 hours after LH surge. Basal body temperature elevation occurs
Day 15-28	Luteal	Progesterone Estrogen	Follicle becomes corpus luteum

Endometrial/Ovarian Cycle			
Timing in cycle	**Phase**	**Prominent Hormones**	**Description**
Day 1-5 (variable)	Menses (part of proliferative phase)	Prostaglandin	Endometrium sloughs if fertilization of ovum does not occur
Day 1-14	Proliferative	Estrogen	Endometrium proliferates
Day 14-28	Secretory	Progresterone	Endometrium thickens in preparation for implantation

Women's Health Disorders

ABNORMAL VAGINAL BLEEDING

DESCRIPTION

Vaginal bleeding that is not related to normal menses.

TERMS

Menorrhagia (hypermenorrhagia)	Heavy or prolonged bleeding at normal intervals
Metrorrhagia	Intermenstrual bleeding, spotting or breakthrough
Polymenorrhea	Normal bleeding with menstrual interval < 21 days
Oligomenorrhea	Menstrual interval > 35 days
Hypomenorrhea	Decreased menstrual flow
Amenorrhea	Absence of menstrual bleeding

ETIOLOGY

- Anovulation is most frequent cause
- Multiple causes

Trauma:
- Tampon use
- Foreign body, especially in 4-8 year olds
- Intrauterine device
- Sexual abuse

Pregnancy-related:
- Ectopic pregnancy
- Spontaneous abortion
- Placenta previa
- Abruptio placenta

Medications:
- Aspirin, NSAIDs, anticoagulants
- Oral contraceptives
- Tranquilizers
- Neuroleptics
- Corticosteroids
- Tamoxifen (Nolvadex®)
- Hormone replacement therapy

Reproductive tract origin:
- Dysfunctional uterine bleeding
- Endometriosis
- Uterine fibroids
- Carcinoma
- Ovarian cysts
- Inflammation and/or infection of the vagina, cervix, uterus, or adnexa

Systemic disease:
- Bleeding disorder
- Thyroid disease
- Adrenal disease
- Renal or hepatic disease

Other:
- Influence of maternal hormones on newborn
- Precocious puberty

INCIDENCE

- Common
- Approximately 40,000 new cases annually
- 50% occur after age 40 years

RISK FACTORS

- Anovulation
- Hormone replacement

ASSESSMENT FINDINGS

- Anemia
- Heavy bleeding during menstrual cycle
- Bleeding lasting > 7 days
- Frequent passage of clots during menses

DIFFERENTIAL DIAGNOSIS

- See *Etiology*

DIAGNOSTIC STUDIES

- Pregnancy test
- Cervical screening with cytology
- Wet prep of vaginal secretions
- CBC with platelet count to determine severity of blood loss

- STD testing
- Depending on history and physical:
  - ◊ TSH
  - ◊ Chemistry profile
  - ◊ Liver function tests
  - ◊ BUN and creatinine
  - ◊ Bleeding/clotting studies
  - ◊ Endometrial biopsy in perimenopausal and postmenopausal women
  - ◊ Ultrasonography if mass palpated or suspected

Serum hCG should always precede evaluation of a female of menstruating age who presents with vaginal bleeding.

NONPHARMACOLOGIC MANAGEMENT

- Rule out pregnancy
- Removal of foreign bodies if present
- Hospitalization may be required if bleeding severe
- Surgical intervention may be required if bleeding severe: dilatation and curettage or hysterectomy in extreme cases

PHARMACOLOGIC MANAGEMENT

- Antibiotics as indicated for infection (sexually transmitted infections)
- Consider topical estrogen cream if vaginal atrophy present
  - ◊ Premarin Vaginal Cream®
    0.5-2.0 g intravaginally cyclically (3 weeks on, one week off)
    Cream: 0.625 mg/g conjugated estrogens
- Iron replacement therapy for anemia
- For less severe bleeding:
  - ◊ Oral contraceptives
  - ◊ Medroxyprogesterone acetate (Provera®)
    Initially 5-10 mg daily for 5-10 days beginning on day 16 or 21 of menstrual cycle
    Tabs: 2.5 mg, 5 mg, 10 mg scored
- Prostaglandin inhibitors (e.g., NSAIDs)
- Danazol (Danocrine®) may be indicated in some cases caused by dysfunctional uterine bleeding
  Mild cases 200-400 mg in 2 divided doses daily
  Severe cases 800 mg in 2 divided doses daily
  Tabs: 50 mg, 100 mg, 200 mg

CONSULTATION/REFERRAL

- Hospitalization may be required for severe bleeding
- Consult gynecologist if bleeding is moderate and cause is not evident or if bleeding is severe
- Consult hematologist if apparent cause is hematological

FOLLOW-UP

- Re-evaluate in 1-2 weeks, review diagnostic studies with patient, and determine response to intervention
- Monitor hemoglobin and hematocrit if bleeding moderate to severe

EXPECTED COURSE

- Dependent on cause and severity of bleeding

POSSIBLE COMPLICATIONS

- Anemia

AMENORRHEA

DESCRIPTION

Primary	Absence of menses by age 14 years in the absence of secondary sexual characteristics By age 16 years regardless of appearance of secondary sexual characteristics
Secondary	Absence of menses for 6 months or three cycles after having at least one spontaneous menstrual period

ETIOLOGY

Primary:
- Gonadal dysgenesis
- Uterovaginal anomalies (e.g., imperforate hymen, uterine agenesis, Turner's syndrome)
- Hypothalamic/pituitary disorders
- Immature hypothalamic-pituitary axis
- Thyroid disease

Secondary:
- Pregnancy, breast feeding, menopause
- Prolactin-secreting adenoma
- Hypothalamic/pituitary disorders (stress, excessive weight loss, low BMI)
- Excessive exercise
- Polycystic ovarian disease (Stein-Leventhal syndrome)
- Anorexia nervosa
- Systemic lupus erythematosus
- Crohn's disease
- Sheehan's syndrome
- Diabetes mellitus, uncontrolled
- Systemic corticosteroids
- Use of danazol (Danocrine®)
- Oral contraceptive pill
- Thyroid disease

The most common cause of amenorrhea is pregnancy.

INCIDENCE

- Primary: 0.3% of women
- Primary and secondary combined: 3.3% of women of childbearing age in the U.S.

RISK FACTORS

- Strenuous physical exercise (long distance runners, cyclists, gymnasts, dancers, etc.)
- Eating disorders
- Emotional crisis
- Extreme levels of stress

ASSESSMENT FINDINGS

- Absence of menses
- Temperature intolerance
- Signs and symptoms of pregnancy
- Signs of androgen excess (e.g., hirsutism)

DIAGNOSTIC STUDIES

- hCG
- TSH
- FSH
- Prolactin
- Blood glucose
- Chromosomal analysis if suspect abnormality (e.g., Turner's syndrome)

PREVENTION

- Maintenance of appropriate body mass index (BMI)
- Avoid overtraining

NONPHARMACOLOGIC MANAGEMENT

- Depends on etiology
- Correction of over- or underweight state

PHARMACOLOGIC MANAGEMENT

- Depends on etiology
- Progesterone challenge will result in withdrawal bleeding if pituitary-ovarian axis is intact and patient is NOT pregnant
- Oral contraceptives

CONSULTATION/REFERRAL

- Refer any patient with primary amenorrhea to gynecologist

FOLLOW-UP

- Discontinue hormone (oral contraceptives) therapy after 6 months to assess for menses

EXPECTED COURSE

- Dependent on underlying cause
- If due to pituitary-ovarian suppression, 99% will resume normal menses in 6 months

POSSIBLE COMPLICATIONS

- Infertility
- Vaginal dryness
- Vasomotor instability
- Osteoporosis
- Cardiovascular disease

DYSMENORRHEA

DESCRIPTION

Painful cramping associated with menstruation.

ETIOLOGY

Primary:
- Increased prostaglandins cause platelet aggregation, vasoconstriction, and uterine contractions which increases the likelihood of uterine ischemia
- No underlying pathology

Secondary:
- Congenital anomaly of the uterus or vagina
- Pelvic infection, STDs
- Adenomyosis
- Endometriosis
- Pelvic tumors (e.g., leiomyomata)

INCIDENCE

- 40% of women of childbearing age in the U.S. have dysmenorrhea
- Primary: predominant age is teens to early twenties
- Secondary: predominant age is twenties and thirties

RISK FACTORS

Primary:
- Nulliparity
- Positive family history
- Cigarette smoking

Secondary:
- Pelvic infection or STDs
- Endometriosis

ASSESSMENT FINDINGS

- Pelvic cramping
- Sensation of heaviness in pelvis
- Malaise
- Headache
- Nausea, vomiting, diarrhea
- Back, thigh pain
- Urinary frequency

Primary:
- Occurs usually in first 2 days of menstruation
- Located in suprapubic area and radiates to back and thighs
- May be associated with diarrhea, nausea, and vomiting

Secondary:
- Pain may refer to area of underlying pathology

DIFFERENTIAL DIAGNOSIS

- Intrauterine polyps
- Presence of intrauterine device
- Pelvic/genital infection

- Endometriosis
- Uterine/ovarian tumors
- Adhesions
- Incomplete abortion
- Ectopic pregnancy
- Complication of pregnancy
- Intrauterine device in use
- Ovarian cysts
- Polyps

Non-gynecologic causes:
- Urinary tract infection
- Adhesions

In a diagnosis of primary dysmenorrhea, the physical and pelvic exams should always be normal.

DIAGNOSTIC STUDIES

Primary:
- None usually indicated

Secondary:
- WBC: elevated in infections
- Cervical cultures
- As history and physical indicate

NONPHARMACOLOGIC MANAGEMENT

Primary:
- Heating pad to abdomen
- Hot bath
- Exercise (raises endorphins)
- Pelvic exercises
- Relaxation therapy
- Low fat diet may help

PHARMACOLOGIC MANAGEMENT

Primary:
- NSAIDs at onset of menses or cramping and continued for duration of pain
  - ◊ Ibuprofen 400-600 mg po every 4-6 hr prn OR
  - ◊ Naproxen sodium 550 mg, one every 12 hr prn
- Oral contraceptives
- Vitamin B6 and Vitamin E may be helpful

Secondary:
- As diagnosis indicates

Primary dysmenorrhea typically abates as patient ages or has children.

CONSULTATION/REFERRAL

- For primary dysmenorrhea, if no improvement after 6 months of therapy
- For secondary dysmenorrhea if unable to achieve improvement in symptoms after 3-6 months

FOLLOW-UP

- 2 months after initial diagnosis to evaluate treatment

EXPECTED COURSE

Primary:
- Improves with age and parity

Secondary:
- Likely to require therapy based on underlying cause

POSSIBLE COMPLICATIONS

Primary:
- Anxiety
- Depression

Secondary:
- Infertility from underlying pathology

PREMENSTRUAL SYNDROME (PMS) / PREMENSTRUAL DYSPHORIC DISORDER (PMDD)

DESCRIPTION

Group of symptoms that occurs most commonly during the luteal phase of the menstrual cycle (5-11 days before menses) and abates within 1-2 days of onset of menses. When primary symptoms are emotional, PMDD.

DSM IV criteria are used to diagnose PMDD.

ETIOLOGY

- Unknown
- Presumed multifactorial and hormonally influenced; worsened by stress
- Fluid imbalance and increased prostaglandins thought to play a role

INCIDENCE

- 20-90% of women experience some symptoms of PMS, but PMS occurs in only about 5% of women
- Most common in women 25-40 years of age

RISK FACTORS

- Caffeine intake
- Pre-existing depression
- High fluid and/or sodium intake
- Stress
- Increasing age
- History of postpartal depression or affective disorder
- Obesity

ASSESSMENT FINDINGS

- Irritability, fatigue
- Depression
- Insomnia
- Crying spells
- Mood swings/depressed mood
- Difficulty concentrating
- Edema
- Sleep disturbances
- Appetite changes (carbohydrate craving)
- Libido changes
- Breast tenderness
- Nervousness
- Headache
- Lethargy
- Food cravings

Symptoms disappear at menopause.

DIFFERENTIAL DIAGNOSIS

Diagnosis of exclusion:
- Depression
- Anxiety disorder
- Marital discord
- Alcohol/drug abuse
- Eating disorder
- Dysmenorrhea
- Thyroid disorder

DIAGNOSTIC STUDIES

- None indicated except to rule out other disorders

NONPHARMACOLOGIC MANAGEMENT

- Menstrual diary for 2 menstrual cycles to establish pattern of symptoms
- Decrease sodium intake
- Limit/avoid alcohol, caffeine, highly processed foods, foods high in fat
- Diet high in complex carbohydrates and lower in protein may be beneficial
- Regular, daily exercise
- Smoking cessation
- Adequate sleep and rest
- Stress reduction techniques
- Support groups

PHARMACOLOGIC MANAGEMENT

- Vitamin and mineral supplementation, especially B6, E, calcium, magnesium
- NSAIDs

- Oral contraceptives
- Diuretics can be used cautiously if edema is present
  ◊ spironolactone (Aldactone®)
  Adult: initially 25-200 mg daily, usually starting dose 100 mg/day, maintain for 5 days then re-titrate dosage
  Tabs: 25 mg, 50 mg, 100 mg scored
- Antidepressants: SSRIs (fluoxetine, others)
- Anxiolytics
  ◊ buspirone (BuSpar®)
  Adult: initially 7.5 mg BID, max 60 mg/day
  Tabs; 5 mg, 10 mg, 15 mg, 30 mg scored (bi-trisected tabs at 15 mg and 30 mg)

Avoid using spironolactone concomitantly with ACE inhibitors and ARBs because of risk of hyperkalemia.

CONSULTATION/REFERRAL

- Refer if refractory to above treatments

FOLLOW-UP

- Re-evaluate in 2 months and review diary, then every 3-6 months.

PMS symptoms can continue after hysterectomy.

EXPECTED COURSE

- Usually symptoms can be adequately controlled

POSSIBLE COMPLICATIONS

- Severe depression
- Social isolation

ABNORMAL PAP SMEAR
(Abnormal Cervical Cytology)

DESCRIPTION

Papanicolaou smears are used for the early detection of abnormal cervical cells. An abnormal Pap smear is defined as any classification of cervical cytology other than within normal limits.

ETIOLOGY

Infection:
- Human papilloma virus (HPV)
- Herpes simplex virus
- Bacterial vaginosis
- Trichomoniasis
- Gonorrhea
- Chlamydia

Inflammation:
- Chemotherapy
- Radiation
- Use of intrauterine device
- DES exposure

Neoplasia:
- Vaginal
- Endometrial
- Cervical

The most common reason females have abnormal cervical cytology is from HPV infections.

INCIDENCE

- 13,000-14,000 new cases of cervical cancer in U.S. annually
- Sixth most common malignancy in women
- Average age of diagnosis of cervical cancer is 45 years

RISK FACTORS

- Early age of first sexual intercourse
- Multiple sexual partners
- Sexual partner with multiple sexual partners
- Cigarette smoking
- Previous abnormal Pap smear
- History of sexually transmitted disease
- Sexual partner with cancer of the penis
- Early age of first pregnancy (before age 18 years)
- Exposure to certain viruses: (herpes simplex, human papilloma virus)
- Immunocompromised state
- African-American ancestry
- Low socioeconomic status
- DES exposure in utero

ASSESSMENT FINDINGS

- Asymptomatic
- Vaginal discharge, especially if infectious etiology
- Vaginal bleeding
- External lesions related to HPV

PREVENTION

- Delaying onset of sexual activity
- Mutual monogamy
- Use of condom if non-monogamous relationship
- Routine screening with PAP smear every 1-3 years depending on risk factors

SCREENING RECOMMENDATIONS

- American College of Obstetrics & Gynecology Pap Smear Guidelines 2010

Time Frame	ACOG Recommended Screening Guidelines
Initial Pap Smear	All women first pap at age 21 years
Routine Pap Smear	Age 21-29 years may be screened every 2 years with either traditional Pap or liquid-based cytology
3 consecutive normal pap smears	Women aged 30 and older who have had 3 consecutive negative Paps may be screened once every 3 years with either traditional Pap or liquid-based cytology
	Women aged 65-70 years may discontinue paps after 3 consecutive normal pap smears and no abnormal pap history in previous 10 years
Hysterectomy patients	Total hysterectomy: No pap smear recommended after total hysterectomy unless surgery due to cancer or precancerous conditions in GYN tract
	Partial hysterectomy (with intact cervix): follow same guidelines as other women

- U.S. Preventive Task Force recommends that screening stop at age 65 years, if all previous Pap smears have been negative

BETHESDA SYSTEM OF REPORTING PAP SMEARS

Common causes of unsatisfactory specimens are scant number or no cervical cells present, poor fixation, the presence of foreign material, obscuring inflammation, obscuring blood, or excess cytolysis.

Thin Prep® is a method used to improve sensitivity of the sampling process by dispersing cervical cells in a fluid medium. It is more expensive than traditional methods.

PREGNANCY CONSIDERATIONS

- If conization is indicated, delay until after delivery.

EXPECTED COURSE

- Depends on categorization of lesion

Bethesda System for Reporting PAP Smear Results			
Section		**Categories**	**Management**
Specimen adequacy		Unsatisfactory can be due to: 1. Scant or no squamous cellularity 2. Air drying artifacts or foreign materials 3. Obscured by RBC or WBC 4. Excess cytolysis 5. Poor fixation	If unsatisfactory, repeat pap smear
Categorization	Negative for intraepithelial lesion or malignancy		Repeat pap at next regularly scheduled interval
	Epithelial cell abnormalities	Atypical squamous cells of undetermined origin (ASCUS)	Colposcopy & biopsy on 2 paps within 4-6 months apart
		Atypical cells cannot exclude high grade SIL (ASC-H)	Colposcopy & biopsy
		Low grade squamous intraepithelial lesion (LSIL) *Mild dysplasia (CIN 1); often secondary to HPV, 16% progress to cervical cancer without treatment*	Colposcopy & biopsy, with LEEP for abnormal findings
		High grade squamous intraepithelial lesion (HSIL) *Moderate to severe intraepithelial, 20% progress to cervical cancer without treatment (CIN 2 or 3)*	Colposcopy & biopsy on initial pap result LEEP
	Glandular cells	*Atypical glandular cells (AGS)*	Colposcopy & biopsy
		Endocervical adenocarcinoma in situ	

CERVICAL CANCER

DESCRIPTION

Malignancy of the cervix usually originating at the squamocolumnar junction.

ETIOLOGY

- Probable relation to viral infections
- Human papilloma virus (HPV) type 16, 18, 31, 33, and 35 implicated in many cases

INCIDENCE

- 4,800 deaths annually

RISK FACTORS

- Infection with HPV (current or previous)
- HIV infection
- Cigarette smoking
- Multiple sexual partners
- Early age of first sexual intercourse
- DES exposure in utero
- Immunocompromised state

ASSESSMENT FINDINGS

- Often asymptomatic
- Irregular vaginal bleeding
- Postcoital vaginal bleeding
- Dyspareunia
- Pelvic pain
- Enlarged cervix

DIFFERENTIAL DIAGNOSIS

- Severe cervicitis
- Cervical polyp
- Endometrial carcinoma
- Metastatic cancer

DIAGNOSTIC STUDIES

- Pap smear
- LEEP (loop electrosurgical excision procedure)
- Colposcopy with endocervical biopsy

A common finding is invasive squamous cell carcinoma or invasive adenocarcinoma.

PREVENTION

- Screening for cervical cytology starting at age 21 years. Women at high risk should continue to be screened annually
- Smoking cessation
- Barrier contraceptive method and spermicides during intercourse

NONPHARMACOLOGIC MANAGEMENT

- Surgical intervention:
  - ◊ Hysterectomy
  - ◊ Cone biopsy
  - ◊ Lymph node dissection
  - ◊ Pelvic exenteration
- Radiation therapy

PHARMACOLOGIC MANAGEMENT

- Fluorouracil, cisplatin, hydroxyurea, others as supplemental therapy to radiation

PREGNANCY/LACTATION CONSIDERATIONS

- Can occur in pregnancy
- Choice of therapy dependent on stage of malignancy and gestational age of fetus

CONSULTATION/REFERRAL

- Surgical/oncology physician referral

FOLLOW-UP

- Physical exam and Pap smear after initial diagnosis and treatment:
  - ◊ Every three months for 1-2 years
  - ◊ Every six months until 5 years
  - ◊ Annually after 5 years

EXPECTED COURSE

Five-year survival:

- Stage 0 (carcinoma in situ): > 99%
- Stage I (confined to uterus): 90%
- Stage II (invasion beyond uterus, but not to pelvic wall or lower third of vagina): 50-70%
- Stage III (invasion to pelvic wall, lower third of vagina, or causes hydronephrosis): 40%-60%
- Stage IV (invasion of bladder, rectum, or beyond true pelvis): 20%

POSSIBLE COMPLICATIONS

- Recurrence
- Ureteral fistula
- Rectovaginal fistula
- Hydronephrosis
- Uremia

Common signs of recurrence of cervical cancer are weight loss, pelvic or thigh pain, and edema in the lower extremities.

ATROPHIC VAGINITIS
(Estrogen Deficient Vulvovaginitis)

DESCRIPTION

Thinning and atrophy of vaginal tissue resulting in friability and associated with urinary incontinence.

ETIOLOGY

- Estrogen deficiency secondary to:
  - ◊ Menopause (natural or surgically induced)
  - ◊ Oophorectomy
  - ◊ Pelvic radiation

INCIDENCE

- Common in postmenopausal women especially if not on hormone replacement therapy

ASSESSMENT FINDINGS

- Vaginal dryness, atrophy, absence or decreased vaginal rugae
- Pruritus
- Blood-tinged vaginal discharge
- Bleeding after intercourse
- Erythematous and petechial patches on vaginal mucosa
- Dyspareunia

Another name used to describe atrophic vaginitis is urogenital atrophy. Urinary incontinence is commonly seen accompanying decreased estrogenic states.

DIFFERENTIAL DIAGNOSIS

- Candida vaginitis
- Bacterial vaginosis
- Trichomoniasis or another STD

DIAGNOSTIC STUDIES

- Wet prep: normal vaginal flora
- FSH level to confirm menopause: increased in menopause
- Estradiol level to measure circulating estrogen level: decreased in menopause
- Pap smear and mammogram before initiation of estrogen therapy

PREVENTION

- Hormone replacement therapy in estrogen deficient states is a personal decision which should be made after consultation with a health care provider

Average age of menopause in the U.S. is 52.5 years.

NONPHARMACOLOGIC MANAGEMENT

- Water-soluble lubricants before intercourse
- Cool baths and compresses for discomfort
- Cotton underwear

PHARMACOLOGIC MANAGEMENT

- Consider low dose oral estrogen daily
- Progesterone should be added in women who have not had a hysterectomy
- Conjugated estrogen vaginal cream may be used for vaginal symptoms
  - ◊ Premarin Vaginal Cream®
    Initially 0.5-2 g intravaginally 3 weeks on and 1 week off
    Conjugated estrogens 0.625 mcg/g cream
  - ◊ Vagifem®
    Adult: 1 tab intravaginally daily for 2 weeks then 1 tab twice weekly
    Tabs: 10 mcg estradiol vaginal tabs

Estrogen replacement is absolutely contraindicated in patients with history of breast cancer, undiagnosed vaginal bleeding, carcinoma, and/or active liver disease.

Lactation can produce a hypoestrogenic state and thus, dyspareunia or other symptoms of vaginal dryness may prevail. Use of vaginal lubricants may provide symptomatic relief. Symptoms usually resolve once breastfeeding is stopped.

CONSULTATION/REFERRAL

- Not usually required

FOLLOW-UP

- Re-evaluate 1-2 months after beginning drug therapy
- Annual physical examination

EXPECTED COURSE

- Symptoms should resolve in 1-2 months after treatment instituted
- Most will be relieved by estrogen replacement therapy

POSSIBLE COMPLICATIONS

- Secondary infections
- Vaginal fissures or ulcerations

VULVOVAGINAL CANDIDIASIS
(Monilial Vulvovaginitis)

DESCRIPTION

Vulvovaginal infection, not considered a sexually transmitted disease.

ETIOLOGY

- Candida albicans most common, but may be caused by other organisms (e.g., *C. glabrata, C. tropicalis*)
- Occurs when a change in the balance of microorganisms of the vagina allows proliferation of yeast

INCIDENCE

- Very common in women from menarche to menopause
- Accounts for 33% of all vaginal infections
- 13 million cases reported annually in the U.S.
- Rare in children

RISK FACTORS

- Recent antibiotic therapy
- Immunocompromised states, recent corticosteroid use
- Pregnancy
- Hypothyroidism, diabetes
- Anemia, especially iron deficiency
- Oral contraceptives
- Wearing tight-fitting, synthetic (non-cotton) clothing
- Previous candidal vulvovaginitis
- Obesity

ASSESSMENT FINDINGS

- Thick, white, curd-like vaginal discharge
- Thick, white patches on vaginal mucosa
- Vulvar itching, erythema, edema
- Dyspareunia
- Usually no malodor
- Dysuria

DIFFERENTIAL DIAGNOSIS

- Bacterial vaginosis
- Gonorrhea
- Chlamydial infection
- Atrophic vaginitis
- Allergic reaction
- Trichomoniasis
- Pinworm vaginitis, especially in children
- Vaginal foreign body

DIAGNOSTIC STUDIES

- 10% KOH prep: budding yeast and pseudohyphae
- Vaginal secretions pH: < 4.5
- Blood glucose if diabetes suspected
- HIV if suspect immunocompromise is underlying problem

PREVENTION

- Good perineal hygiene
- Cotton underwear
- Sleeping without underwear
- Avoid tight fitting clothing, especially jeans
- Weight loss if indicated
- Management of elevated glucose
- Frequent change of tampons and use of pad at night
- Use of unscented, mild soap
- Avoid frequent douching
- Consider screening and treating sexual partner if female has recurrent infection
- With recurrent vaginal candidiasis, consider screening for Type 2 diabetes in at-risk patients

Growth of yeast is facilitated in a warm, dark, moist environment.

NONPHARMACOLOGIC MANAGEMENT

- Refrain from sexual intercourse until symptoms resolved
- Creams and/or suppositories used for treatment may weaken latex condoms and diaphragms
- Good perineal hygiene
- Treatment of male sexual partner is not indicated unless balanitis present

PHARMACOLOGIC MANAGEMENT

- Many medications available
  - ◊ Fluconazole (Diflucan®) orally
    Adult: 50-200 mg daily, may be given as single dose or daily for 3 days for uncomplicated cases; longer with complicated situations
    Tabs: 100 mg, 200 mg OR
  - ◊ Miconazole nitrate (Monistat®) vaginal suppository or cream
    Suppository: vaginally once at HS
    Cream: apply BID up to 7 days
    Suppository: 100 mg
    Cream 2%, tube 9 gm cream OR
  - ◊ Butoconazole nitrate (Femstat®) vaginal cream
    Cream: apply 1 applicator intravaginally at HS for 3 nights OR
  - ◊ Terconazole (Terazol®) vaginal suppository or cream
    Apply one applicator or one suppository at HS for 3 nights
    Cream: 0.8%, suppository: 80 mg

Terconazole is a good choice for atypical yeast.

PREGNANCY/LACTATION CONSIDERATIONS

- Increased risk during pregnancy due to elevated levels of glycogen and reproductive hormones
- Only topical azole therapies should be used during pregnancy
- Treat for 7-14 days during pregnancy
- The triazole, fluconazole (Diflucan®) and ketoconazole (Nizoral®) are excreted in breast milk and should be avoided during lactation

CONSULTATION/REFERRAL

- None usually needed

FOLLOW-UP

- None usually needed
- Treat sexual partner if infections are frequent or recalcitrant to therapy
- Culture if infection recurs 3 or more times annually

EXPECTED COURSE

- Complete resolution
- Recurrences common

POSSIBLE COMPLICATIONS

- Secondary bacterial infection

BARTHOLIN'S GLAND CYST/ABSCESS

DESCRIPTION

Obstruction of the major duct of Bartholin's gland resulting in cyst formation. Infection and obstruction of the duct will lead to an abscess.

ETIOLOGY

- Mechanical irritation from tight fitting undergarments resulting in chronic inflammation
- STDs

RISK FACTORS

- Vulvovaginal infection
- Poor perineal hygiene

ASSESSMENT FINDINGS

- Firm labia mass or cyst
- Pain, erythema, induration
- Edema of labia minora
- Low grade fever

DIFFERENTIAL DIAGNOSIS

- Sebaceous cyst
- Malignancy

DIAGNOSTIC STUDIES

- None usually indicated unless other infection suspected

- Culture and sensitivity of cyst contents
- Culture for STDs especially, *Neisseria gonorrhoeae*

PREVENTION

- Good perineal hygiene
- Early treatment

NONPHARMACOLOGIC MANAGEMENT

- Application of local moist heat
- Warm sitz baths
- Incision and drainage of fluctuant abscess
- No treatment needed if only 1-2 mm and patient is asymptomatic

Goal is to facilitate drainage of cyst contents. Warm baths provide comfort and may help to facilitate drainage.

PHARMACOLOGIC MANAGEMENT

- Base on culture and sensitivity, but consider trimethoprim-sulfamethoxazole, quinolone
- Analgesics

CONSULTATION/REFERRAL

- Consider referral to surgeon or gynecologist if cyst is large and initial treatment ineffective

FOLLOW-UP

- Re-evaluate in 7-10 days

EXPECTED COURSE

- Complete resolution with conservative treatment is usual

POSSIBLE COMPLICATIONS

- Cellulitis of surrounding tissue

POLYCYSTIC OVARIAN DISEASE
(Stein-Leventhal Syndrome)
POLYCYSTIC OVARIAN SYNDROME
(PCOS)

DESCRIPTION

Chronic, complex endocrine disorder associated with oligo-ovulation and/or anovulation; characterized by formation of cysts in the ovaries.

ETIOLOGY

- Hypothalamic suppression
- Pituitary suppression
- Disharmonious gonadotropin and estrogen production
- Inability of the ovary to respond to gonadotrophic stimulation
- Increased androgen production from the adrenals or ovaries

INCIDENCE

- Leading cause of oligomenorrhea and/or amenorrhea in premenopausal women
- 6% of premenopausal women

RISK FACTORS

- Endometrial hyperplasia
- Obesity, diabetes mellitus
- Infertility

ASSESSMENT FINDINGS

- Onset occurs at onset of menses or months to years after the onset of menses
- Hyperinsulinemia
- Hyperandrogenism
  - ◊ Hirsutism
  - ◊ Acne
  - ◊ Seborrhea
  - ◊ Alopecia
  - ◊ Voice changes
  - ◊ Hypertrophy of the clitoris
- Irregular menstrual cycles
- Amenorrhea
- Infertility
- Asymptomatic in majority of patients
- Enlarged ovaries

Polycystic Ovarian syndrome (PCOS) should be suspected in females who are overweight, have infrequent menses, hirsutism, and infertility.

DIFFERENTIAL DIAGNOSIS

- Cushing's syndrome
- Endocrine tumor: androgen-producing ovarian or adrenal tumor
- Prolactin-producing pituitary adenoma
- Adult-onset adrenal hyperplasia
- HAIR-An syndrome (includes hyperandrogenism, insulin resistance, acanthosis nigricans)
- Endometrial carcinoma

DIAGNOSTIC STUDIES

- Pregnancy test
- LH/FSH ratio: > 2.5:1
- Testosterone: increased
- Prolactin level: elevated
- Doppler ultrasound of ovaries: multiple cysts on the ovaries ("string of pearls")
- Fasting insulin level: increased
- Lipid panel, TSH, and glucose tolerance tests

NONPHARMACOLOGIC MANAGEMENT

- Weight loss if overweight
- Stress management
- Hair removal therapy

PHARMACOLOGIC MANAGEMENT

If pregnancy not desired:

- Low dose oral contraceptives OR
  - ◊ Medroxyprogesterone acetate (Depo-Provera®)
    Adult: 150 mg IM every 3 months
    If pregnancy desired:
  - ◊ Metformin (Glucophage®) daily
    Adult: initially 500 mg daily, may increase after 2 weeks
    Tabs: 500 mg
  - ◊ Clomiphene citrate (Clomid®)
    Dosage: 50 mg daily for 5 days OR
  - ◊ Menotropins (Pergonal®)
    Dosage: 225 mg FSH and 225 mg LH injected subcutaneously OR
  - ◊ Bromocriptine (Parlodel®)
    Adult: initially 1.25-2.5 mg daily
    Tabs: 2.5 mg scored

Consider referring patients who desire pregnancy and to fertility specialist.

FOLLOW-UP

- Frequent monitoring

POSSIBLE COMPLICATIONS

- Endometrial, breast, ovarian cancer
- Hyperlipidemia, hyperinsulinemia, hyperglycemia
- Insulin resistance
- Diabetes mellitus
- Cardiovascular disease
- Infertility

BENIGN OVARIAN TUMORS

DESCRIPTION

Nonmalignant tumor of the ovary; may be solid or cystic.

ETIOLOGY

- Unknown
- Endometriosis
- Physiologic cysts

Many different types of cells in the ovaries and so they are susceptible to benign and malignant tumors.

INCIDENCE

- Unknown

RISK FACTORS

- Age: post-menopausal

ASSESSMENT FINDINGS

- Asymptomatic in most cases
- Pain, abdominal or lower back
- Abdominal distention
- Bowel and/or bladder pressure

DIFFERENTIAL DIAGNOSIS

- Malignant tumor of the ovary
- Polycystic ovary
- Ectopic pregnancy
- Uterine tumors
- Urinary tract infection
- PID with tubo-ovarian abscess

DIAGNOSTIC STUDIES

- Pregnancy test
- Urinalysis
- CA-125: <35 μg /mL
- Pelvic ultrasound

PREVENTION

- Risk may be decreased by use of oral contraceptives

Physical and pelvic exam, along with history play important role in diagnosis.

NONPHARMACOLOGIC MANAGEMENT

- Surgical removal of tumor

PHARMACOLOGIC MANAGEMENT

- Oral contraceptives in premenopausal women for physiologic cysts may help resolve more rapidly

CONSULTATION/REFERRAL

- Gynecologic/surgical consultation to assist with diagnosis if needed

FOLLOW-UP

- Annual examination

EXPECTED COURSE

- Complete cure

POSSIBLE COMPLICATIONS

- Torsion
- Rupture
- Hemorrhage

OVARIAN CANCER

DESCRIPTION

A malignancy of the ovaries with origins in the epithelium, stroma, or germ cells.

Ovarian cancer is the leading cause of gynecological death in women.

ETIOLOGY

- Unknown

INCIDENCE

- 26,500 new cases annually
- Causes 14,500 deaths annually in U.S.
- 4th leading cause of cancer death in women
- Usual age: 40-75 years of age

The incidence of ovarian cancer has not decreased in the last 6 decades.

RISK FACTORS

- History of breast cancer especially before age 40
- Nulliparity or low parity
- Pregnancy after age 30 years
- Family history in first-degree or second-degree relatives
- Increasing age
- Presence of BRCA-1, BRCA-2 genes

ASSESSMENT FINDINGS

- Bloating
- Dyspepsia
- Abdominal pressure, fullness, or pain
- Irregular vaginal bleeding
- Ascites
- Pelvic mass
- Dyspareunia
- Weight loss
- Vaginal discharge

DIFFERENTIAL DIAGNOSIS

- GI malignancy
- Uterine fibroid
- Other gynecologic malignancy
- Irritable bowel syndrome
- Inflammatory bowel syndrome

DIAGNOSTIC STUDIES

- Ultrasound of pelvis
- Surgical exploration
- CA-125 (normal < 35 μ/mL) possibly helpful but not a good screening tool

CA-125 may be elevated in benign ovarian conditions, endometriosis, liver disease, CHF. Therefore, this test lacks specificity.

PREVENTION

- Oral contraceptives have role in prevention
- Multiparity
- Women who have breastfed their infants have lower rates of ovarian cancer

Women with a history of breast cancer before age 40 should be screened at least annually for ovarian cancer because the risk of ovarian cancer is 17-fold more than in women without history of breast cancer.

NONPHARMACOLOGIC MANAGEMENT

- Surgery
    - ◊ Total abdominal hysterectomy for epithelial malignancies
    - ◊ Salpingo-oophorectomy for germ cell cancers
- Radiation therapy

PHARMACOLOGIC MANAGEMENT

- Chemotherapy

CONSULTATION/REFERRAL

- Refer for surgical/oncological evaluation and treatment

FOLLOW-UP

- Follow with CA-125 for response to therapy (a 7-fold decrease in CA-125 suggests good response to therapy)

EXPECTED COURSE

Five-year survival rates:
- Stage I (limited to ovaries): 80%
- Stage II (confined to pelvis): 60%
- Stage III (involvement of regional lymph nodes or upper abdomen): 15-30%
- Stage IV (distant or visceral metastasis): 10%

POSSIBLE COMPLICATIONS

- Adverse effects of treatment
- Ascites

CONTRACEPTION

COMBINED ORAL CONTRACEPTIVES

DESCRIPTION

Oral contraceptive containing both estrogen and progestin.

MECHANISM OF ACTION

- Suppresses pituitary gonadotropins (FSH and LH) which inhibits ovulation

3 Types of Combination Oral Contraceptives	
Monophasic	Fixed dosage of estrogen to progestin throughout the cycle
Biphasic	Amount of estrogen remains the same for the first 21 days of the cycle. Decreased progestin:estrogen ratio in first half of cycle; increased ratio in second half
Triphasic	Estrogen amount remains the same or varies throughout cycle. Progestin amount varies

- Phasic pills developed to mimic hormonal fluctuations in the menstrual cycle

Most women should receive an oral contraceptive with no more than 35 mcg of ethinyl estradiol.

Dose Related Side Effects of Oral Contraceptives	
Too Much Estrogen	Nausea, bloating, hypertension, breast tenderness, edema
Too Little Estrogen	Early or midcycle breakthrough bleeding, increased spotting
Too Much Progestin	Increased appetite, weight gain, fatigue, changes in mood
Too Little Progestin	Late breakthrough bleeding, amenorrhea

EFFECTIVENESS

- Theoretical effectiveness rate of 99.7%
- Actual effectiveness is 90-96%

ADVANTAGES

- Very reliable temporary method of contraception when used properly
- No interference with sexual activity
- Health-related benefits
  - ◊ Decreased menstrual flow and diminished reports of dysmenorrhea

◊ Improvement of acne
◊ Regularity of menses
◊ Protection against anemia

DISADVANTAGES

May cause life-threatening or serious complications
◊ Thrombophlebitis/thromboembolism
◊ Hepatocellular adenomas
◊ Stroke
◊ Gallbladder disease
◊ Hypertension
Must remember to take pill every day
Provide no protection against STIs
May decrease milk production in lactating women

SIDE EFFECTS

- Nausea
- Breast fullness and/or tenderness
- Cyclic weight gain and fluid retention
- Breakthrough bleeding, especially in first three months of use
- Decreased menstrual flow and/or amenorrhea
- Fatigue
- Acne
- Mild headaches
- Increased appetite

Cigarette smoking increases the risk of cardiovascular side effects. The risk increases with age (35 years) and heavy smoking (15 or more cigarettes per day). Women who use hormonal contraceptives should not smoke.

ABSOLUTE CONTRAINDICATIONS

- History of, or current thrombophlebitis, or thromboembolic disorder
- Stroke
- Age > 35 years and hypertensive or diabetic
- Migraine with aura
- LDL > 160 or Triglycerides > 250
- Ischemic heart disease or coronary artery disease
- Known or suspected breast cancer
- Diabetes with vascular complications
- Known or suspected estrogen-dependent neoplasia
- Pregnancy, known or suspected
- Hepatic adenomas
- Undiagnosed gynecologic bleeding
- Uncontrolled hypertension
- Active liver disease

RELATIVE CONTRAINDICATIONS

- Over 35 years old and a heavy smoker
- Migraine headaches that start after initiation of oral contraceptives
- Hypertension with resting diastolic blood pressure > 90 mm Hg; or resting systolic > 140 mm Hg on three separate visits; or a diastolic > 110 mm Hg on a single visit
- Diabetes mellitus
- Elective major surgery requiring immobilization within next 4 weeks
- Sickle cell anemia
- Lactation
- Active gall bladder disease
- Congenital hyperbilirubinemia (Gilbert's disease)
- Age > 50 years
- Conditions that make it difficult for a woman to take pills consistently and correctly (e.g., mental retardation, psychiatric illness, substance abuse)
- Family history of hyperlipidemia
- Family history of death of a parent or sibling from myocardial infarction before age 50 years

DIAGNOSTIC STUDIES

Before prescribing:
- Pap smear
- Pregnancy test
- STD screening as indicated
- Lipid profile

PATIENT EDUCATION

Danger signs of oral contraceptives (OCS): ACHES
A: severe abdominal pain (may be indicative of hepatic tumors)
C: severe chest pain or shortness of breath
H: severe headache
E: eye problems (blurred vision, flashing lights, or blindness)
S: severe leg pain

- Oral contraceptives do not provide STD prevention
- Smoking cessation
- Maintenance of ideal body weight
- Exercise program
- Must use back-up method if on any of these medications:
  ◊ Rifampin
  ◊ Barbiturates
  ◊ Phenytoin (Dilantin®)
  ◊ Phenylbutazone

◊ Griseofulvin (Fulvicin®)
◊ Ampicillin
◊ Tetracycline
◊ Carbamazepine (Tegretol®)

- Pill should be taken each day at same time
- If one pill is missed, take missed pill as soon as remembered. If not remembered until time for next pill, take two pills
- If two consecutive pills are missed, take two pills per day for the next two days, and then resume one pill per day. Use vaginal spermicide and condoms for remainder of cycle
- 50% of patients have breakthrough bleeding during the first 3 months on oral contraceptives, but then usually abates. Breakthrough bleeding does not indicate decrease in effectiveness of pills

FOLLOW-UP

- Evaluate 3 months after beginning pills then annually
- Check weight and blood pressure after 3 months on pills
- Breast examination and Pap smear annually

PROGESTIN-ONLY ORAL CONTRACEPTIVE (MINI-PILL)

DESCRIPTION

Oral contraceptive that contains no estrogen, only progestin

MECHANISM OF ACTION

- Suppression of ovulation
- Creation of a thin, atrophic endometrium
- Thickening of cervical mucous making sperm penetration difficult

EFFECTIVENESS

- 97-99% rate of effectiveness
- Failure rate highest in women younger than 40 years
- Rate nearly 100% in lactating women

ADVANTAGES

- May be used in lactating women, does not alter quality or quantity of breast milk
- May be used in women with cardiovascular risk factors
- Health benefits similar to combined oral contraceptives: protection against developing endometrial cancer and decreased risk of pelvic inflammatory disease
- Decreased menstrual cramps
- Less heavy bleeding and shorter menses
- Decreased premenstrual syndrome symptoms
- Decreased breast tenderness

DISADVANTAGES

- Increased chance of ectopic pregnancy
- Must be taken each day at same time
- Missing only one pill will substantially increase risk of pregnancy
- Menstrual cycle changes

SIDE EFFECTS

Serious:

- Same as combined oral contraceptives

Other:

- Functional ovarian cysts
- Menstrual cycle changes including spotting, breakthrough bleeding, prolonged cycles, and amenorrhea

INDICATIONS

- Women who experience unacceptable estrogen-related side effects (e.g., GI upset, breast tenderness, or decreased libido)
- Women who have developed severe headaches or hypertension while on combined oral contraceptives
- Women who have an absolute or relative contraindication to estrogen and combined oral contraceptives
  ◊ Age > 40 years
  ◊ History of severe headaches
  ◊ Stable hypertension
  ◊ Well-controlled diabetes
  ◊ Chloasma
  ◊ Mental depression
  ◊ Lactation

CONTRAINDICATIONS

- Active thrombophlebitis or thromboembolic disorder
- History of myocardial infarction, ischemic heart disease, or coronary artery disease
- Known or suspected breast cancer
- Pregnancy, known or suspected

- Liver disease
- Undiagnosed gynecologic bleeding
- Medical condition which is worsened by fluid retention (e.g., CHF, mitral stenosis, pulmonary hypertension)
- Use of rifampin, barbiturates, phenytoin, carbamazepine, and/or phenylbutazone

DIAGNOSTIC STUDIES

Before prescribing:
- Pap smear
- STD screening as indicated
- Pregnancy test

PATIENT EDUCATION

- If changing from combined to mini pills, start pill on first day of menses or anytime during combined oral contraceptive cycle
- If no history of unprotected postpartal intercourse and not currently taking oral contraceptives, start mini-pills immediately
- Use backup method for one month following initiation of pills
- If pill is taken more than 3 hours late, use back-up method for remainder of pill pack
- If one pill is missed, take it as soon as possible
- If more than one pill is missed, the chance of pregnancy is great. A back-up method should be used for remainder of pill pack
- Most women will experience irregular menstrual bleeding with spotting, breakthrough bleeding, prolonged cycles, and/or amenorrhea

FOLLOW-UP

- Evaluate 3 months after beginning pills then annually
- Notify health care provider when discontinuing breastfeeding

DIAPHRAGM

DESCRIPTION

Dome-shaped latex cup with a flexible spring rim which is filled with spermicide and placed in the upper vagina to cover the cervix completely.

MECHANISM OF ACTION

- The latex dome forms a barrier between the cervix and semen, preventing sperm from entering the uterus. The spermicidal cream or jelly is used with the diaphragm for additional protection, killing any sperm that accidentally slip past the rim of the diaphragm

EFFECTIVENESS

- About 82%
- 94% with consistent, perfect use

ADVANTAGES

- Helpful in prevention of STDs
- No serious side effects
- Insertion may be incorporated into foreplay
- Decreased incidence of cervical neoplasia

DISADVANTAGES

- Must be used each time intercourse occurs
- May be embarrassing for women who dislike touching their genitals
- May be considered “messy” by some women
- Decreased effectiveness with increased frequency of intercourse
- Must be refitted if change in weight and after delivery or cervical surgery

SIDE EFFECTS

- May be uncomfortable once inserted
- Recurrent bladder infections
- Possible allergic reaction to latex and/or spermicide
- Foul smelling, profuse vaginal discharge if diaphragm forgotten or left in place too long
- Toxic shock syndrome
- Vaginal trauma or ulceration caused by excessive rim pressure or prolonged wear

CONTRAINDICATIONS

- Latex allergy
- Allergy to spermicide
- History of toxic shock syndrome
- History of frequent UTI
- Abnormalities of uterine anatomy that prevent a satisfactory fit:
  - ◊ Uterine prolapse
  - ◊ Extreme uterine retroversion

- ◊ Vaginal septum
- ◊ Severe cystocele or rectocele

- Inability of patient or partner to learn correct insertion technique
- Full-term pregnancy delivered within the past 6 weeks

DIAGNOSTIC STUDIES

- Pap smear
- STD screening

PATIENT EDUCATION

- Proper insertion and removal
- May insert diaphragm up to six hours prior to intercourse
- Remove diaphragm 6-8 hours after intercourse
- Always use diaphragm with spermicidal cream/jelly
- Return for refitting if weight gain of 10-20 lbs, after pregnancy, and after pelvic surgery
- Periodic inspection of integrity of diaphragm
- Signs and symptoms of toxic shock syndrome
- To decrease risk of toxic shock syndrome:
  - ◊ Do not use diaphragm during menses
  - ◊ Do not wear diaphragm longer than 24 hours
  - ◊ Wash hands carefully before inserting or removing diaphragm

FOLLOW-UP

- 1-3 weeks return with diaphragm in place for evaluation of proper position and size
- Annual examination

MALE CONDOMS

DESCRIPTION

Latex or rubber sheath used to cover the penis during intercourse; may be used with or without spermicide.

MECHANISM OF ACTION

- Mechanical barrier which prevents sperm from entering cervix

EFFECTIVENESS

- 88-98% in prevention of pregnancy

ADVANTAGES

- Most effective method for preventing the spread of STDs including HIV
- Relatively inexpensive
- Easily attainable, do not require prescription

DISADVANTAGES

- May decrease sexual pleasure for either partner
- Putting on condom may interrupt foreplay
- Possibility of breakage

CONTRAINDICATIONS

- Latex allergy
- Allergy to spermicide

PATIENT EDUCATION

- Use spermicide to increase effectiveness of condom
- Proper usage: place on erect penis before penis comes into contact with vulvar area; leave about 1/2 inch space at end of condom; after intercourse, hold onto condom as the penis is withdrawn
- Condoms should be used only once
- Condoms should not be kept in a wallet, glove compartment of a car, or other warm area that may cause deterioration
- Avoid use of oil-based vaginal creams or lubricants that may weaken condoms (e.g., petroleum jelly, antifungals)

NATURAL FAMILY PLANNING

DESCRIPTION

Method of determining days of each month when it is most likely for a woman to be fertile and then, abstaining from intercourse during that time. Use of basal body temperature tracking and assessment of cervical mucous greatly increases effectiveness of this method over the old rhythm-type calendar method.

EFFECTIVENESS

- Theoretical effectiveness is 87%
- Actual effectiveness is 79%

ADVANTAGES

- Involves no chemicals or devices
- Few religious objections to its use
- Low cost

DISADVANTAGES

- May require long periods of abstinence
- No protection against STDs

CONTRAINDICATIONS

- Irregular intervals between menses
- History of anovulatory cycles
- During the perimenopausal period

INTRAUTERINE DEVICE (IUD)

DESCRIPTION

Device made of copper or other material that is placed and retained within the uterine cavity

- Three types available in the U.S.:
  - ◊ Progestasert®: contains progesterone
  - ◊ ParaGard Copper T380A®: contains copper
  - ◊ Mirena: contains levonorgestrel

MECHANISM OF ACTION

- Not exactly known. Hypotheses are:
  - ◊ Increased motility of ovum in fallopian tubes
  - ◊ Inflammatory effects on the endometrium
  - ◊ Local foreign body inflammatory response that interferes with sperm survival, motility, and/or capacitation
  - ◊ The copper in the ParaGard® interferes with estrogen uptake and its effect on the endometrium
  - ◊ The progesterone in Progestasert® thickens cervical mucus, blocking entry to uterine cavity

EFFECTIVENESS

- Progestasert®: 98%
- ParaGard®: 99.2%

ADVANTAGES

- No action required for contraception
- Intrauterine device not detectable during intercourse
- No systemic effect on hormones
- Long-term contraception
- Cost-effective if used long-term
- Good choice for lactating women: no effect on milk production and if using ParaGard®, no hormone secreted in milk

DISADVANTAGES

- 2-5% of patients spontaneously expel intrauterine device
- Limited population of women are candidates
- Do not protect against STDs

SIDE EFFECTS

- Abdominal infection or adhesions
- Sepsis
- Cervical infection or erosion
- Ovarian cysts
- Ectopic pregnancy
- Embedment of intrauterine device in uterine tissue
- Infertility
- Spotting between periods
- Dysmenorrhea
- Pregnancy
- Prolonged or heavy menstrual flow

INDICATIONS

- Contraception in women who have had at least one full-term pregnancy
- Women who are in a stable, mutually monogamous sexual relationship
- Women aged 21 years or older
- No history of PID
- Desire for long-term contraception

CONTRAINDICATIONS:

- < 6 weeks postpartum
- < 2 weeks postabortion
- History of pelvic inflammatory disease
- Multiple sexual partners or sexual partner of person with multiple sexual partners
- Acute or subacute infection of cervix, uterus, fallopian tubes, postpartal endometritis or infected abortion
- Cancer of the uterus, cervix, or fallopian tubes
- Untreated dysplasia on recent Pap smear
- Undiagnosed gynecologic bleeding
- Current abnormal vaginal discharge or infection
- Current or suspected pregnancy

- Immunocompromised state
- Abnormal uterine cavity
- Current genital actinomycosis
- Active herpes simplex virus
- Valvular heart disease

ParaGard®:
- Wilson's disease
- Allergy to copper, if copper device is used

Progestasert®:
- Presence of, or history of STDs (e.g., chlamydia or gonorrhea)
- History of pelvic surgery that may be associated with increased risk of ectopic pregnancy (e.g., surgery on fallopian tubes, endometriosis)
- History of ectopic pregnancy or condition that predisposes to ectopic pregnancy
- Incomplete involution after abortion or birth
- Factors predisposing patient to PID

DIAGNOSTIC STUDIES

Before insertion:
- Pap smear
- Hematocrit
- STD screening (HIV, gonorrhea, chlamydia)
- Pregnancy test
- Vaginal wet prep

PATIENT EDUCATION

- Complications of intrauterine device use
- Barrier method of contraception until re-evaluation after next menses
- Monthly string checks after menses and notify health care provider if cannot locate
- Progestasert® needs to be changed every year, ParaGard® every 10 years
- Educate about signs and symptoms of infection
- Warning signs associated with intrauterine device use:
  - ◊ Late or missed period
  - ◊ Abdominal pain
  - ◊ Fever or chills
  - ◊ Delayed period, followed by scanty or irregular bleeding
  - ◊ Exposure to STD
  - ◊ Foul smelling vaginal discharge
  - ◊ Genital lesion
  - ◊ Fever with vaginal discharge
  - ◊ Severe or prolonged menstrual bleeding
  - ◊ String disappearance
  - ◊ Dyspareunia

FOLLOW-UP

- Evaluate after next menses, then annually
- Pregnancy test if amenorrheic

MEDROXYPROGESTERONE ACETATE
(Depo-Provera®)

DESCRIPTION

Injectable progestin which is administered intramuscularly is slowly released and provides contraception for thirteen weeks.

MECHANISM OF ACTION

- Suppression of ovulation
- Creation of a thin, atrophic endometrium
- Thickening of cervical mucous making sperm penetration difficult

EFFECTIVENESS

- 99.7% effective in pregnancy prevention

ADVANTAGES

- No increased risk of thromboembolism, hypertension, and other estrogenic side effects
- Decreased or no menstrual flow or cramping
- 13 week period of effectiveness
- No effect on milk production in lactating women

DISADVANTAGES

- Fertility may not return for up to two years following last injection, but most women will be fertile within 12 months
- Requires injection for administration

Significant loss of bone mineral density can occur with use. Bone loss increased by duration of use and may not be reversible. Treat with Vitamin D and calcium to reduce risk of bone loss.

SIDE EFFECTS

- Side effects of menstrual changes: amenorrhea, irregular spotting or bleeding, or heavy vaginal bleeding

- Headaches
- Weight changes, especially gain
- Libido changes
- Depression
- Dizziness

CONTRAINDICATIONS

- Undiagnosed gynecologic bleeding
- Suspected or confirmed pregnancy
- Breast cancer
- Active thrombophlebitis
- Active liver disease
- Active gallbladder disease
- Coronary artery disease
- History of stroke
- Known sensitivity to medroxyprogesterone

DIAGNOSTIC STUDIES

Before administering:
- Pap smear
- Pregnancy test
- STD screening as indicated

PATIENT EDUCATION

- Side effect profile of drug
- Menses may not return for three to 12 months following last Depo-Provera® injection
- Change of contraceptive method 6-18 months before attempting pregnancy
- Use of barrier method for prevention of STDs

FOLLOW-UP

- Repeat injections every 13 weeks
- Annual examination
- Hematocrit or hemoglobin if history of heavy or persistent menstrual bleeding
- Pregnancy test if no regular menses and/or symptoms of pregnancy are present

SPERMICIDES

DESCRIPTION

Spermicidal product (usually nonoxynol-9) placed in the vagina for contraceptive purposes; can be used alone or with condom or diaphragm

MECHANISM OF ACTION

Composed of chemicals which are toxic to sperm

EFFECTIVENESS

- 80-85% when used alone
- 99% when used with condom

ADVANTAGES

- Helps prevent STDs, especially gonorrhea and chlamydia
- Available over-the-counter
- Provides lubrication
- Relatively inexpensive
- Can serve as back up method of other contraceptives
- Does not affect milk production in lactating women

DISADVANTAGES

- Some women consider the use of foam "messy"
- Must be consistently used with each act of intercourse
- High user-failure rate

SIDE EFFECTS

- Irritation or burning
- Temporary skin irritation on vulva or penis

CONTRAINDICATIONS

- Allergy to product

DIAGNOSTIC STUDIES

- Pap smear
- STD screening

PATIENT EDUCATION

- Proper usage: place a full applicator of spermicide deep into the vagina while in supine position
- Spermicide should remain in vagina for 8 hours following intercourse
- Do not douche within 8 hours after intercourse
- Increased efficacy with barrier method (e.g., diaphragm or condom)
- Wash applicator with soap and water at each use

- Additional spermicide and fresh condom for subsequent acts of intercourse

FOLLOW-UP

- Annual examination

EMERGENCY CONTRACEPTION

DESCRIPTION

Use of a birth control method after sexual intercourse has occurred

EFFECTIVENESS

- 75% effective in preventing pregnancy if taken within 72 hours of intercourse

MECHANISM OF ACTION

- Inhibit or delay ovulation
- May inhibit fertilization or implantation of a fertilized egg

ADVANTAGES

- Back up method for barrier method failure (e.g., torn diaphragm, condom) and missed oral contraceptives
- May use this method more than once in a cycle
- No reports of teratogenic effects when emergency contraception failed

DISADVANTAGES

- Health care providers not familiar with use
- 72-hour window for use

SIDE EFFECTS

- Nausea
- Vomiting

INDICATIONS

- Women who have had unprotected intercourse within the past 72 hours and do not desire pregnancy

CONTRAINDICATIONS

- Same as combined oral contraceptives

DIAGNOSTIC STUDIES

- Pregnancy test before administering

PATIENT EDUCATION

- The first dose of pills must be taken within 72 hours of intercourse and the second dose must be taken 12 hours after the first
- Danger signs (as above in combined oral contraceptives)
- Take antiemetic one hour before ingestion of emergency oral contraceptive
- Need for routine contraceptive and health care

FOLLOW-UP

- If no menstrual bleeding within 3 weeks of emergency oral contraception
- If menstrual bleeding less than 2 days duration
- If development of early pregnancy signs: breast tenderness, fatigue, loss of appetite

MENOPAUSE

DESCRIPTION

Cessation of menstrual cycle for 12 months; premature menopause is defined as occurring before age 40 years.

ETIOLOGY

- Physiologic due to depletion of follicles in ovaries and decreased estrogen synthesis and resultant cessation of menses
- Surgical
- Medical due to administration of medications for treatment of breast cancer and endometriosis

INCIDENCE

- 30-40 million women in the U.S. with the number growing
- 10% by age 38 years
- 20% by age 43 years
- 50% by age 48 years
- 90% by age 54 years
- 99% by age 58 years
- Surgical menopause is present in 25-33% of women by age 55 years

ASSESSMENT FINDINGS

- Cycles become farther and farther apart and irregular with eventual cessation of menses
- Vasomotor instability (hot flashes, night sweats): 85% of women experience
- Depression
- Nervousness
- Headache
- Fatigue
- Palpitations
- Paresthesias
- Insomnia
- Vaginal atrophy (mucosa appears thin, pale, friable)
- Decrease in vaginal lubrication resulting in itching, discharge, bleeding, dyspareunia, increased risk of urethritis
- May have decreased libido

DIFFERENTIAL DIAGNOSIS

- Pregnancy
- Diabetes mellitus
- Thyroid disease
- Hyperparathyroidism
- Polycystic ovarian disease
- Pituitary adenoma
- Hypothalamic dysfunction

DIAGNOSTIC STUDIES

- Usually none required to diagnose
- FSH: elevated > 40 mIU/mL
- LH: > 30 mIU/mL FSH:LH ratio: >1
- Progesterone challenge: absence of withdrawal bleeding suggests menopause
- Pap smear
- Mammogram
- Bone density measurement in high-risk patients

NONPHARMACOLOGIC MANAGEMENT

- Avoid factors which precipitate vasomotor instability (e.g., hot drinks, alcohol, caffeine, stress, warm environment, and overdressing)
- Wear layered clothing
- Smoking cessation
- Regular exercise program to promote feeling of well-being and prevention of osteoporosis
- Weight bearing exercise to prevent osteoporosis
- Kegel exercises
- Self-breast examination monthly
- Use of contraceptive during perimenopausal period unless pregnancy desired
- Low fat, high calcium diet

PHARMACOLOGIC MANAGEMENT

- Hormone therapy should be carefully considered
  - ◊ oral
  - ◊ transdermal
- Estrogen alone if uterus removed
  Examples of oral estrogens:
  - ◊ Conjugated estrogens, initially 0.3 mg to 1.25 mg daily depending on symptoms
  - ◊ Estradiol; initial 0.5 mg to 2.0 mg daily

    - ◊ Esterified estrogens: start at 0.5 mg, may increase up to 1.25 mg daily
    - ◊ Estropipate 0.625-2.5 mg daily
- Estrogen with progestin if uterus intact
- Calcium supplement

Estrogen therapy should not be used in patients with history of breast cancer, undiagnosed vaginal bleeding, known or suspected pregnancy, active thrombosis or thrombophlebitis, endometrial adenocarcinoma, and/or active liver disease.

CONSULTATION/REFERRAL

- Cardiologist referral for signs/symptoms of cardiovascular disease

FOLLOW-UP

- Re-evaluate 1-2 months after beginning drug therapy for effectiveness of therapy
- Mammogram every 1-2 years between ages 40-49 years then annually after age 50 years

EXPECTED COURSE

Without hormone therapy:
- Gradual disappearance of vasomotor symptoms over years
- Development of osteoporosis and cardiovascular disease

With hormone therapy:
- Minimal effects of estrogen depletion

Women who experience early menopause are at increased risk of osteoporosis and so should be screened and treated if necessary.

POSSIBLE COMPLICATIONS

- Stress incontinence
- Osteoporosis
- Cardiovascular disease

BREAST CANCER

DESCRIPTION

Malignant tumor of the breast occurring primarily in women but may occur in men.

ETIOLOGY

- 20% of patients have a family history
- Etiology is otherwise unknown

The presence of BRCA 1 and BRCA 2 genes are strongly associated with the development of breast cancer.

INCIDENCE

- 1 in 8 women in the US will develop breast cancer at some time
- >150,000 new cases annually
- Account for 50,000 deaths annually
- Females > Males

77% of women with breast cancer are over age 50 years.

RISK FACTORS

- Age, median age at time of diagnosis is 54 years
- History of previous breast cancer
- Family history of breast cancer in first-degree relative
- Early menarche (< 11 years)
- Onset of menopause after age 55 years
- Nulliparity
- First term pregnancy after age 30 years
- Obesity in postmenopausal women
- Ashkenazi Jewish descent
- Presence of BRCA1 or BRCA2 gene
- Possible risk factors:
  - ◊ Estrogen use
  - ◊ High dietary fat
  - ◊ High alcohol use
  - ◊ Obesity

ASSESSMENT FINDINGS

- Painless, firm, fixed mass
- No changes in mass with menstruation
- Spontaneous nipple discharge that is usually clear
- Dimpling of skin (peau d'orange appearance)
- Nipple retraction
- Increased vascular pattern of breast
- Significant asymmetry of breasts
- Axillary, supraclavicular, and/or infraclavicular lymph node enlargement
- Skin ulcerations
- Scaly lesions of nipple (Paget's disease)

DIFFERENTIAL DIAGNOSIS

- Fibrocystic breast disease
- Intraductal papilloma
- Fibroadenoma
- Mastitis

DIAGNOSTIC STUDIES

- Mammography
- Ultrasound of breast to differentiate fluid-filled cyst from solid mass
- Fine needle aspiration biopsy
- Open biopsy
- MRI

PREVENTION

- Baseline mammography by age 35 years; every 1-2 years between ages 40-49 years; then annually starting at age 50 years. Women who have higher than average risk for breast cancer may need more frequent mammography
- Monthly self-breast examinations

NONPHARMACOLOGIC MANAGEMENT

- Lumpectomy
- Mastectomy
- Radiation therapy
- Assessment of estrogen receptors in tumor
- Baseline bone scan, chest x-ray, liver scan

A breast mass in conjunction with a normal mammogram is NOT normal. An ultrasound must be performed.

PHARMACOLOGIC MANAGEMENT

- Hormone therapy
  - ◊ tamoxifen (Nolvadex®)
    Adult: 20-40 mg daily, if more than 20 mg given, divide doses to bid
    Tab: 10 mg, 20 mg
- Chemotherapy, radiation

CONSULTATION/REFERRAL

- Refer all palpable masses to surgeon for evaluation and biopsy if indicated

FOLLOW-UP

- Mammogram at least annually
- Bone scan with development of bone pain or elevated alkaline phosphate

EXPECTED COURSE

10-year survival rates:
- Noninvasive (tumors < 1 cm with no axillary node involvement): 95%
- Stage I (tumors > 1 cm with no axillary node involvement): 90%
- Stage II (tumors < 5 cm or axillary node involvement): 40%
- Stage III (tumors > 5 cm or with chest wall or skin extension, inflammatory changes, or supraclavicular involvement): 15%
- Stage IV (metastatic): 0%

POSSIBLE COMPLICATIONS

- Postoperative lymphedema
- Limited shoulder movement after surgery
- Side effect of chemotherapy: nausea, vomiting, alopecia, leukopenia, stomatitis, fatigue
- Radiation side effects: skin reactions

FIBROCYSTIC BREAST DISEASE

(Benign Breast Disease)

DESCRIPTION

Benign breast disorder

ETIOLOGY

- Unknown
- Possible causes:
  - ◊ Luteal phase defect
  - ◊ Increased estrogen
  - ◊ Hyperprolactinemia
  - ◊ Hypersensitivity to estrogen
  - ◊ Sensitivity to methylxanthines
  - ◊ Dietary fat intake

INCIDENCE

- 50% of women in the U.S. have fibrocystic breast disease to some extent

RISK FACTORS

- None definitively known
- Possible ingestion of methylxanthines (e.g., caffeine-containing beverages, chocolate)

ASSESSMENT FINDINGS

- Asymptomatic
- Palpation of smooth, movable masses
- Breast pain or tenderness which diminishes after menses
- Breast engorgement
- Breast thickening
- Worsening of symptoms premenstrually
- Nipple discharge of varying color and consistency

Mastoplasia is thickening of the breast tissue in a rope-like manner that predominates during the menstrual cycle.

DIFFERENTIAL DIAGNOSIS

- Breast cancer
- Chest wall syndrome
- Neuralgia
- Intraductal papilloma
- Fibroadenoma
- Mastitis

DIAGNOSTIC STUDIES

- Prolactin level
- TSH
- Mammogram
- Ultrasound of breast differentiates cysts from solid masses
- Needle or open biopsy

NONPHARMACOLOGIC MANAGEMENT

- Evaluate to rule out malignancy
- Reassurance
- Cold compresses
- Supportive brassiere
- Wearing brassiere 24 hours may help
- Sodium restriction 10 days before onset of menstruation
- Decrease or eliminate caffeine
- Biopsy often needed to differentiate from malignant mass

PHARMACOLOGIC MANAGEMENT

- Consider
  - ◊ Spironolactone (Aldactone®) for swelling and pain premenstrually
    Adult: Initially 25-200 mg daily, usual starting dose is 100 mg daily, maintain for 5 days, then re-titrate
    Tabs: 25 mg, 50 mg, 100 mg scored
  - ◊ Vitamin B6, E
  - ◊ Oral contraceptives
  - ◊ Danazol (Danocrine®)
    Adult: 200-400 mg in divided doses
    Tabs: 50mg, 100 mg, 200 mg
  - ◊ Bromocriptine (Parlodel®) may be used for more severe disease
    Adult: 1.25-2.5 mg daily
    Tabs: 2.5 mg scored

PREGNANCY/LACTATION CONSIDERATIONS

- No known effect on lactation

CONSULTATION/REFERRAL

- Refer to surgeon for evaluation of especially painful masses or any abnormalities on mammogram or ultrasound

FOLLOW-UP

- Mammogram by age 35, every 1-2 years between ages 40-49 years, and annually after age 50 years

EXPECTED COURSE

- Benign but chronic condition

POSSIBLE COMPLICATIONS

- May have an increased risk of malignancy if atypical hyperplasia is present on biopsy.

FIBROADENOMA

DESCRIPTION

A benign tumor containing fibrous tissue which occurs in the breast.

ETIOLOGY

- Unknown, thought to be hormonally induced

INCIDENCE

- Most common benign tumor in the female breast
- Occurs most in ages 20-30 years

ASSESSMENT FINDINGS

- Single, nontender, and firm mass
- Multiple lesions in 10-15% of cases
- Freely movable
- No change in mass with menstrual cycle
- No nipple discharge

DIFFERENTIAL DIAGNOSIS

- Fibrocystic breast disease
- Intraductal papilloma
- Breast cancer
- Other benign breast disease

DIAGNOSTIC STUDIES

- Mammography
- Ultrasound to differentiate fluid-filled cyst from solid mass
- Fine needle aspiration biopsy
- Open biopsy

NONPHARMACOLOGIC MANAGEMENT

- Surgical excision

PREGNANCY/LACTATION CONSIDERATIONS

- Pregnancy stimulates growth
- No known effect on lactation

CONSULTATION/REFERRAL

- Surgical referral for excision

FOLLOW-UP

- None needed

EXPECTED COURSE

- Complete resolution after surgical removal without recurrence

POSSIBLE COMPLICATIONS

- Postoperative infection

INTRADUCTAL PAPILLOMA

DESCRIPTION

Benign tumor within the ductal system of the breast

ETIOLOGY

- Unknown
- Thought to be due to overgrowth of ductal epithelium

INCIDENCE

- Usually occurs perimenopausally during ages 40-50 years

ASSESSMENT FINDINGS

- Bloody or serous nipple discharge
- Usually unilateral unless multiple ducts involved

DIFFERENTIAL DIAGNOSIS

- Breast cancer
- Galactorrhea

DIAGNOSTIC STUDIES

- Mammography
- Ultrasound to differentiate fluid-filled cyst from solid mass

NONPHARMACOLOGIC MANAGEMENT

- Surgical excision

PREGNANCY/LACTATION CONSIDERATIONS

- Removal does not affect ability to breastfeed

CONSULTATION/REFERRAL

- Surgical consult for excision

FOLLOW-UP

- None indicated

EXPECTED COURSE

- Complete resolution after surgical removal without recurrence

2006 consensus guidelines for the management of women with abnormal cervical cancer screening tests. 2009 addendum. (2009). Retrieved from http://www.guideline.gov/content.aspx?id=14698

Adams Hillard, P., & Deitch, H. (2005). Menstrual disorders in the college age female. Pediatric Clinics of North America, 52(1), 179-197, ix-x.

Alsharif, M., Kjeldahl, K., Curran, C., Miller, S., Gulbahce, H., & Pambuccian, S. (2009). Clinical significance of the diagnosis of low-grade squamous intraepithelial lesion, cannot exclude high-grade squamous intraepithelial lesion. Cancer Cytopathology, 117(2), 92-100.

Barnhart, K., & Schreiber, C. (2009). Return to fertility following discontinuation of oral contraceptives. Fertility and Sterility, 91(3), 659-663.

BÈlisle, S., Blake, J., Basson, R., Desindes, S., Graves, G., Grigoriadis, S., et al. (2006). Canadian consensus conference on menopause, 2006 update. Journal of Obstetrics and Gynaecology Canada, 28(2 Suppl 1), S7-S94.

Benedetti Panici, P., Manci, N., Bellati, F., Di Donato, V., Marchetti, C., Calcagno, M., et al. (2007). Co2 laser therapy of the bartholin's gland cyst: Surgical data and functional short- and long-term results. Journal of Minimally Invasive Gynecology, 14(3), 348-351.

Berry, D., Cronin, K., Plevritis, S., Fryback, D., Clarke, L., Zelen, M., et al. (2005). Effect of screening and adjuvant therapy on mortality from breast cancer. New England Journal of Medicine, 353(17), 1784-1792.

Bilimoria, K., Cambic, A., Hansen, N., & Bethke, K. (2007). Evaluating the impact of preoperative breast magnetic resonance imaging on the surgical management of newly diagnosed breast cancers. Archives of Surgery, 142(5), 441-445; discussion 445-447.

Blithe, D. (2008). Male contraception: What is on the horizon? Contraception, 78(4 Suppl), S23-27.

Buggs, C., & Rosenfield, R. (2005). Polycystic ovary syndrome in adolescence. Endocrinology and Metabolism Clinics of North America, 34(3), 677-705, x.

Bulletins-Gynecology, A. C. o. P. (2006). ACOG practice bulletin. No. 73: Use of hormonal contraception in women with coexisting medical conditions. Obstetrics and Gynecology, 107(6), 1453-1472.

Burkman, R. (2007). Transdermal hormonal contraception: Benefits and risks. American Journal of Obstetrics and Gynecology, 197(2), 134.e131-136.

Burns, C. E., Brady, M. A., Blosser, C., Starr, N. B., & Dunn, A. M. (2009). Pediatric primary care: A handbook for nurse practitioners (4th ed.). Philadelphia: W.B. Saunders.

Canfell, K., Kang, Y., Clements, M., Moa, A., & Beral, V. (2008). Normal endometrial cells in cervical cytology: Systematic review of prevalence and relation to significant endometrial pathology. Journal of Medical Screening, 15(4), 188-198.

Care, A. C. o. A. H. (2006). ACOG committee opinion no. 350, november 2006: Breast concerns in the adolescent. Obstetrics and Gynecology, 108(5), 1329-1336.

Costantino, D., & Guaraldi, C. (2008). Effectiveness and safety of vaginal suppositories for the treatment of the vaginal atrophy in postmenopausal women: An open, non-controlled clinical trial. European Review for Medical and Pharmacological Sciences, 12(6), 411-416.

Davey, D., Cox, J., Austin, R., Birdsong, G., Colgan, T., Howell, L., et al. (2008). Cervical cytology specimen adequacy: Patient management guidelines and optimizing specimen collection. Journal of Lower Genital Tract Disease, 12(2), 71-81.

Davis, A., Westhoff, C., O'Connell, K., & Gallagher, N. (2005). Oral contraceptives for dysmenorrhea in adolescent girls: A randomized trial. Obstetrics and Gynecology, 106(1), 97-104.

Dawood, M. (2006). Primary dysmenorrhea: Advances in pathogenesis and management. Obstetrics and Gynecology, 108(2), 428-441.

Diaz, A., Laufer, M., Breech, L., Adolescence, A. A. o. P. C. o., Care, A. C. o. O., & Health, G. C. o. A. (2006). Menstruation in girls and adolescents: Using the menstrual cycle as a vital sign. Pediatrics, 118(5), 2245-2250.

Domino, F., Baldor, R., Golding, J., Grimes, J., & Taylor, J. (2011). The 5-minute clinical consult 2011. Philadelphia: Lippincott Williams & Wilkins.

Drugs facts and comparisons. (2010). St. Louis: Wolters Kluwer Health.

Ernst, D., & Lee, A. (2010). Nurse practitioners prescribing reference. New York: Haymarket Media Publication.

Greydanus, D., Matytsina, L., & Gains, M. (2006). Breast disorders in children and adolescents. Primary Care; Clinics in Office Practice, 33(2), 455-502.

Guray, M., & Sahin, A. (2006). Benign breast diseases: Classification, diagnosis, and management. The Oncologist, 11(5), 435-449.

Gynecologists, A. C. o. O. a. (2007). ACOG practice bulletin. Management of adnexal masses. Obstetrics and Gynecology, 110(1), 201-214.

Haider, Z., Condous, G., Kirk, E., Mukri, F., & Bourne, T. (2007). The simple outpatient management of bartholin's abscess using the word catheter: A preliminary study. Australian and New Zealand Journal of Obstetrics and Gynaecology, 47(2), 137-140.

Holt, V., Scholes, D., Wicklund, K., Cushing-Haugen, K., & Daling, J. (2005). Body mass index, weight, and oral contraceptive failure risk. Obstetrics and Gynecology, 105(1), 46-52.

James, A. (2005). More than menorrhagia: A review of the obstetric and gynaecological manifestations of bleeding disorders. Haemophilia, 11(4), 295-307.

Jayasinghe, Y., Moore, P., Donath, S., Campbell, J., Monagle, P., & Grover, S. (2005). Bleeding disorders in teenagers presenting with menorrhagia. Australian and New Zealand Journal of Obstetrics and Gynaecology, 45(5), 439-443.

Jemal, A., Siegel, R., Ward, E., Hao, Y., Xu, J., & Thun, M. (2009). Cancer statistics, 2009. CA: A Cancer Journal for Clinicians, 59(4), 225-249.

Joste, N. (2008). Overview of the cytology laboratory: Specimen processing through diagnosis. Obstetrics and Gynecology Clinics of North America, 35(4), 549-563; viii.

Kost, K., Singh, S., Vaughan, B., Trussell, J., & Bankole, A. (2008). Estimates of contraceptive failure from the 2002 national survey of family growth. Contraception, 77(1), 10-21.

LandÈn, M., Erlandsson, H., Bengtsson, F., Andersch, B., & Eriksson, E. (2009). Short onset of action of a serotonin reuptake inhibitor when used to reduce premenstrual irritability. Neuropsychopharmacology, 34(3), 585-592.

Martin, K., Chang, R., Ehrmann, D., Ibanez, L., Lobo, R., Rosenfield, R., et al. (2008). Evaluation and treatment of hirsutism in premenopausal women: An endocrine society clinical practice guideline. Journal of Clinical Endocrinology and Metabolism, 93(4), 1105-1120.

McDonald, J., Doran, S., DeSimone, C., Ueland, F., DePriest, P., Ware, R., et al. (2010). Predicting risk of malignancy in adnexal masses. Obstetrics and Gynecology, 115(4), 687-694.

Medicine, P. C. o. t. A. S. f. R. (2006). Current evaluation of amenorrhea. Fertility and Sterility, 86(5 Suppl 1), S148-155.

Nam, E., Yun, M., Oh, Y., Kim, J., Kim, J., Kim, S., et al. (2010). Diagnosis and staging of primary ovarian cancer: Correlation between pet/ct, doppler us, and ct or mri. Gynecologic Oncology, 116(3), 389-394.

North American Menopause Society. (2007). The role of local vaginal estrogen for treatment of vaginal atrophy in postmenopausal women: 2007 position statement of the North American Menopause Society. Menopause, 14(3 Pt 1), 355-369; quiz 370-351.

North American Menopause Society. (2010). Estrogen and progestogen use in postmenopausal women: 2010 position statement of the North American Menopause Society. Menopause, 17(2), 242-255.

Pappas, P., Kauffman, C., Andes, D., Benjamin, D. J., Calandra, T., Edwards, J. J., et al. (2009). Clinical practice guidelines for the management of candidiasis: 2009 update by the infectious diseases society of america. Clinical Infectious Diseases, 48(5), 503-535.

Peters, N., Borel Rinkes, I., Zuithoff, N., Mali, W., Moons, K., & Peeters, P. (2008). Meta-analysis of mr imaging in the diagnosis of breast lesions. Radiology, 246(1), 116-124.

Salley, K., Wickham, E., Cheang, K., Essah, P., Karjane, N., & Nestler, J. (2007). Glucose intolerance in polycystic ovary syndrome--a position statement of the androgen excess society. Journal of Clinical Endocrinology and Metabolism, 92(12), 4546-4556.

Schiffman, M., Castle, P., Jeronimo, J., Rodriguez, A., & Wacholder, S. (2007). Human papillomavirus and cervical cancer. Lancet, 370(9590), 890-907.

Shah, N., Jones, J., Aperi, J., Shemtov, R., Karne, A., & Borenstein, J. (2008). Selective serotonin reuptake inhibitors for premenstrual syndrome and premenstrual dysphoric disorder: A meta-analysis. Obstetrics and Gynecology, 111(5), 1175-1182.

Siebers, A., Klinkhamer, P., Grefte, J., Massuger, L., Vedder, J., Beijers-Broos, A., et al. (2009). Comparison of liquid-based cytology with conventional cytology for detection of cervical cancer precursors: A randomized controlled trial. JAMA, 302(16), 1757-1764.

Singh, H., Sethi, S., Raber, M., & Petersen, L. (2007). Errors in cancer diagnosis: Current understanding and future directions. Journal of Clinical Oncology, 25(31), 5009-5018.

Sobel, J. (2007). Vulvovaginal candidosis. Lancet, 369(9577), 1961-1971.

Turnbull, L., Brown, S., Harvey, I., Olivier, C., Drew, P., Napp, V., et al. (2010). Comparative effectiveness of mri in breast cancer (comice) trial: A randomised controlled trial. Lancet, 375(9714), 563-571.

Westhoff, C., Heartwell, S., Edwards, S., Zieman, M., Cushman, L., Robilotto, C., et al. (2007). Initiation of oral contraceptives using a quick start compared with a conventional start: A randomized controlled trial. Obstetrics and Gynecology, 109(6), 1270-1276.

Workowski, K., Berman, S., & Centers for Disease Control and Prevention. (2006). Sexually transmitted diseases treatment guidelines, 2006. MMWR Recomm Rep, 55(RR-11), 1-94.

Yonkers, K., Holthausen, G., Poschman, K., & Howell, H. (2006). Symptom-onset treatment for women with premenstrual dysphoric disorder. Journal of Clinical Psychopharmacology, 26(2), 198-202.

Zakhireh, J., Gomez, R., & Esserman, L. (2008). Converting evidence to practice: A guide for the clinical application of mri for the screening and management of breast cancer. European Journal of Cancer, 44(18), 2742-2752.

Zhao, C., Austin, R., Pan, J., Barr, N., Martin, S., Raza, A., et al. (2009). Clinical significance of atypical glandular cells in conventional pap smears in a large, high-risk U.S. West coast minority population. Acta Cytologica, 53(2), 153-159.

INDEX

Abnormal Pap Smear 726
Abnormal Vaginal Bleeding 720
Abruptio Placentae 552
Acne Vulgaris 87
Actinic Keratosis 92
Acute Bacterial Prostatitis 402
Acute Bronchitis 573
Acute Coronary Syndrome 52
Acute Gastroenteritis 267
Acute Pyelonephritis 694
ADD/ADHD 452
Addison's Disease 246
Adolescent Pregnancy 566
Adult Health Promotion and Disease Prevention 311
Alcohol 389
Alcohol Use Disorder 660
Allergic Rhinitis 190
Alzheimer's Disease 449
Amenorrhea 722
Amniocentesis 549
Anemia of Chronic Disease 361
Ankle Edema 545
Anorexia Nervosa 671
Anxiety 649
Appendicitis 280
Assessment of Fetal Well-Being 549
Asthma 588
Asymptomatic Bacteriuria 687
Atopic Dermatitis 95
Atrophic Vaginitis 730
Backache 546
Bacterial Infections of the Skin 100
Bacterial Vaginosis 628
Bartholin's gland Cyst/Abscess 733
Bell's palsy 454
Benefits of Breastfeeding 387
Benign Ovarian Tumors 736
Benign Prostatic Hyperplasia 399
Biophysical Profile 549
Blepharitis 481
Breast Cancer 749
Breast Care 389
Breastfeeding Technique 388
Bronchiolitis 608
Bulimia Nervosa 673
Burns 104
Bursitis 505
Cafe' au lait Spots 107
Candidal Infection of Nipples 392
Carpal Tunnel Syndrome 455
Cat Scratch Fever 108
Cataract 476
Cellulitis 109
Cervical Cancer 729
Chalazion 480
Chemoprophylaxis 316
Chlamydia 629
Cholecystitis 270
Chronic Bronchitis 576
Chronic Heart Failure 22
Chronic Prostatitis 403
Clavicular Fracture 515
Colic 297
Common Benign Pediatric Skin Lesions 113
Common Cold 194
Common Discomforts of Pregnancy 545
Common Problems of Lactation 390
Complications Associated with Pregnancy 552
Congenital Heart Disease 70
Conjunctivitis 469
Constipation 546
Contact Dermatitis 114
Contraception 738
Contraception 738
Contraction Stress Test 550
Contraindications to Breastfeeding 387
Corneal Abrasion 466
Crohn's Disease 285
Croup (Laryngotracheobronchitis) 610
Cryptorchidism 406
Cushing's Syndrome 245
Cystic Fibrosis 613
Dacryostenosis 483
Deep Vein Thrombosis 66
Depression and Suicide 653
Determination of Adequate Intake 388
Developmental Dysplasia of the Hip 523
Diabetes Mellitus Type 1 229
Diabetes Mellitus Type 2 231
Diaper Dermatitis 119
Disadvantages of Breastfeeding 387
Disease Prevention for the International Traveler 318
Diverticulitis 277
Domestic Violence 667

Down Syndrome 555
Drugs/Medications 389
Dysmenorrhea 723
Early Adolescence (11, 12, 13, and 14 Years) 346
Ectopic Pregnancy 553
Education and Counseling 313
Eight Years (School Age) 344
Eighteen Months (Toddler) 338
Emphysema 582
Encopresis 300
Engorgement 391
Enuresis 702
Epididymitis 407
Epiglottitis 211
Epistaxis 197
Erectile Dysfunction 417
Febrile Seizures 440
Fibroadenoma 752
Fibrocystic Breast Disease 750
Fifteen Months (Toddler) 337
Fifth Disease 121
Five Years (Preschool) 342
Flat or Inverted Nipples 390
Folic Acid Deficiency 372
Foreign Body Aspiration 612
Four Months (Infant) 332
Four Years (Preschool) 341
Fractures 512
Gastroesophageal Reflux Disease (GERD) 259
Genetic Disorders 554
Genital Herpes 635
Gestational Trophoblastic Disease 555
Glaucoma 477
Glucose-6-Phosphate Dehydrogenase Deficiency 362
Gonorrhea 631
Gout 497
Gynecomastia 248
Hand Foot and Mouth Disease 122
Headaches 425
Hearing Loss 175
Heart Murmurs 73
Heartburn 546
Hematuria 704
Hemorrhoids 293, 547
Herpangina 123
Herpes Zoster 124
Hidradenitis Suppurativa 127
Hirschsprung's Disease 295
Human Immunodeficiency Virus (HIV) 625
Human Papilloma Virus 637
Hydrocele 410
Hyperemesis Gravidarum 556
Hyperlipidemia 29
Hypertension 5
Hyperthyroidism 240
Hyphema 468
Hypoglycemia 239
Hypospadias 415
Hypothyroidism 242
Idiopathic Thrombocytopenia Purpura 376
Immunizations 349
Impetigo 128
Inadequate Let-Down Reflex 392
Incompetent Cervix 557
Infectious Mononucleosis 212
Inflammatory Bowel Disease 285
Influenza 198
Inguinal Hernia 414
Insomnia 676
Intraductal Papilloma 753
Intussusception 296
Iron Deficiency Anemia 357
Irritable Bowel Syndrome 281
Jaundice 392
Kawasaki Syndrome 78
Late Adolescence (18, 19, 20, and 21 Years) 348
Lead Toxicity 364
Leaking 391
Leg Cramps 547
Legg-Calve-Perthes Disease 524
Leukemia 373
Leukorrhea 547
Low Back Pain 502
Lyme Disease 130
Lymphoma 375
Mastitis 391
Mastoiditis 177
Maternal Assessment of Fetal Activity 550
Maternal Nutrition 388
Meningitis 441
Menopause 747
Menstrual Cycle 719
Metatarsus Adductus 530
Middle Adolescence (15, 16, and 17 Years) 347
Multiple Gestation 558
Multiple Sclerosis 443
Nasal Congestion and Epistaxis 547
Nausea and Vomiting 545
Neonatal Conjunctivitis 473

Neonatal Hyperbilirubinemia 378
Newborn (Birth to One Month) 328
Nine Months (Infant) 334
Nonstress Testing 550
Obesity 319
Ocular Chemical Burn 467
Ocular Foreign Body 465
Oral Candidiasis 132
Osgood-Schlatter Disease 522
Osteoarthritis 491
Osteoporosis 517
Otitis Externa 178
Otitis Media 180
Ovarian Cancer 737
Parkinson's Disease 445
Paronychia 134
Pediculosis 137
Pelvic Inflammatory Disease 639
Peptic Ulcer Disease (PUD) 263
Peripheral Vascular Disease 68
Peritonsillar Abscess (Quinsy) 214
Pertussis 606
Pharyngitis/Tonsillitis 215
Phimosis 416
Physiologic and Psychologic Changes of Pregnancy 541
Physiology of Lactation 387
Pinworms 298
Pityriasis Rosea 139
Placenta Previa 559
Plantar Fasciitis 531
Plugged Milk Duct 390
Pneumonia 596
Polycystic Ovarian Disease 734
Poststreptococcal Glomerulonephritis 707
Post-term Labor 562
Precocious Puberty 249
Preconceptual Care 539
Pre-eclampsia, Eclampsia 559
Premenstrual Syndrome/Premenstrual Dysphoric Disorder 725
Prenatal Care 542
Pre-term Labor 561
Primary Lung Malignancies 616
Primary Prevention 327
Primary, Secondary, Tertiary Prevention 311
Prolapsed Umbilical Cord 563
Prostate Cancer 404
Psoriasis 142
Pyloric Stenosis 294
Recurrent Abdominal Pain 301
Refractive Errors/Color Blindness 475
Renal Insufficiency 708
Rh Incompatibility 379
Rheumatic Fever 76
Rheumatoid Arthritis 494
Roseola, Exanthem Subitum 143
Rotator Cuff Syndrome 516
Round Ligament Pain 548
Rubella 144
Rubeola 146
Scabies 147
Scarlet Fever 149
Scoliosis 527
Seborrheic Dermatitis 150
Secondary Prevention 327
Seizure Disorders 437
Sexual Assault 669
Sickle Cell Anemia 366
Sinusitis 202
Six Months (Infant) 333
Six Years (School Age) 343
Skin Cancer 152
Slipped Capital Femoral Epiphysis 525
Smoking 390
Smoking Cessation 665
Sore Nipples 390
Special Considerations: Elderly Adults 317
Spermatocele 411
Spider/Insect Bites and Stings 154
Spontaneous Abortion 563
Sprain 511
Stable Angina 39
Storage of Breast Milk 389
Strabismus 474
Stress Fracture 514
Subluxation of the Radial Head 510
Substance Abuse in Pregnancy 564
Substance Use Disorder 662
Sudden Infant Death Syndrome (SIDS) 615
Syncope 433
Syphilis 633
Talipes Equinovarus 529
Tanner Stages of Physical Development 327
Ten Years (School Age) 345
Tertiary Prevention 327
Testicular Cancer 412
Testicular Torsion 408
Thalassemia 368
Three Years (Toddler) 340

Thyroid Nodule 244
Tinea Infections 158
Transient Ischemic Attack 435
Transient Synovitis of the Hip 526
Trichomoniasis 641
Trigeminal Neuralgia 431
Tuberculosis (TB) 602
Twelve Months (Toddler) 335
Two Months (Infant) 331
Two Years (Toddler) 339
Ulcerative Colitis 287
Ultrasound 551
Upper Extremity Joint Derangement 509
Urethritis 695
Urinary Frequency 548
Urinary Incontinence 697
Urinary Tract Infection 688
Urolithiasis 705
Vaccine Schedule for Adults 314
Varicella 162
Varicocele 411
Varicose Veins 65, 548
Vertigo 187
Viral Hepatitis 274
Vitamin B12 Deficiency Anemia 370
Vitamin Supplementation of the Breastfed Infant 388
Vulvovaginal Candidiasis 732
Warts 163
Weaning 389
Wilm's Tumor 710